Keri Johnson   2002

P9-ELX-463

Keri Johnson   2002

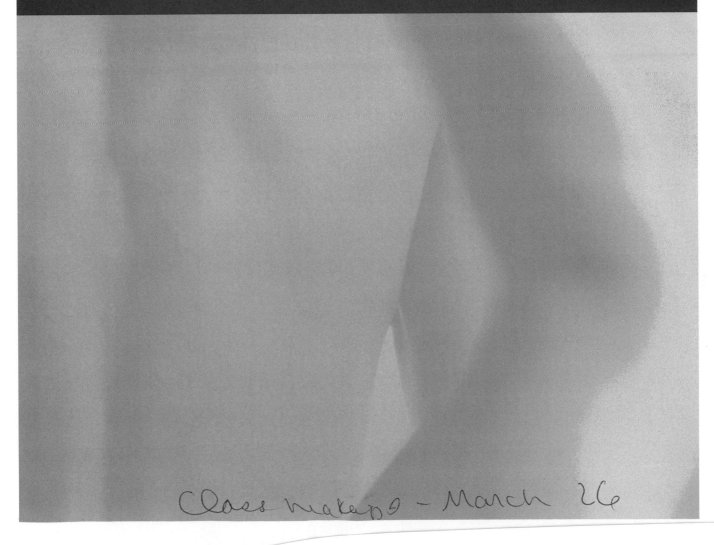

a
massage therapist's
guide to

PATHOLOGY

Class makeup - March 26

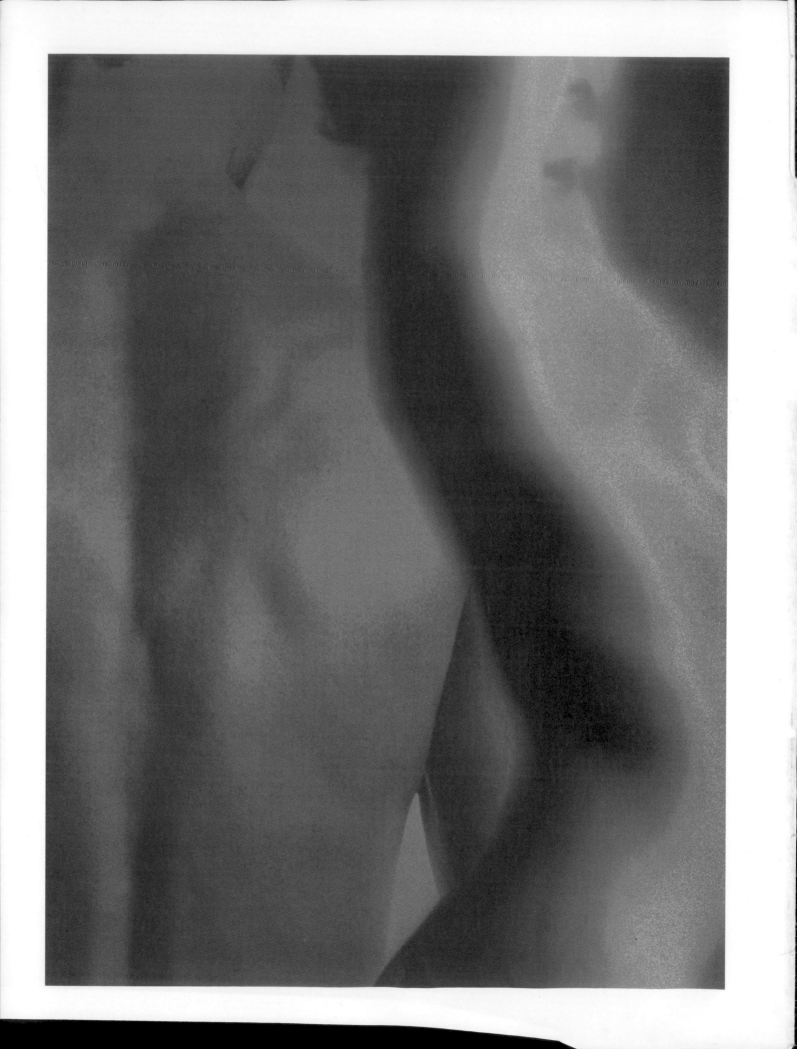

a

massage therapist's

guide to

PATHOLOGY

RUTH WERNER, LMP,
MEMBER NCTMB, AMTA

BEN E. BENJAMIN, PhD
Associate Editor

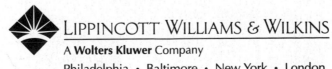

LIPPINCOTT WILLIAMS & WILKINS
A **Wolters Kluwer** Company
Philadelphia • Baltimore • New York • London
Buenos Aires • Hong Kong • Sydney • Tokyo

Editor: Rina Steinhauer
Managing Editors: Sue Kimner, Cecilia Reilly
Marketing Manager: Chris Kushner
Project Editor: Lisa J. Franko
Original Illustrations: Sandra M. Dean Illustration

Copyright © 1998 Lippincott Williams & Wilkins
351 West Camden Street
Baltimore, Maryland 21201-2436 USA

All rights reserved. This book is protected by copyright. No part of this book may be reproduced in any form or by any means, including photocopying, or utilized by any information storage and retrieval system without written permission from the copyright owner.

The publisher is not responsible (as a matter of product liability, negligence or otherwise) for any injury resulting from any material contained herein. This publication contains information relating to general principles of medical care which should not be construed as specific instructions for individual patients. Manufacturers' product information and package inserts should be reviewed for current information, including contraindications, dosages, and precautions.

For many of the conditions in this book, massage is described as "indicated," at least at some stage of the healing process. The authors want to make very clear that to call massage "indicated" does not imply that massage will fix something that is wrong. There are times when massage can definitely influence the healing process for the better: the subacute stage of a sprained ankle, for instance. There are other times when massage may have no affect on the severity of a condition whatsoever, for instance, with fibroid tumors. Massage is called "indicated" for both of these situations which, in this case, simply means that massage won't make the situation any worse.

Printed in the United States of America

Library of Congress Cataloging-in-Publication Data

A massage therapist's guide to pathology / [by] Ruth Werner, — 1st ed.
   p.   cm.
    Includes bibliographical references and index.
    ISBN 0-683-30210-8
    1. Massage therapy.   2. Diagnosis, Differential.   I. Werner, Ruth
(Ruth A.) 1994-   .
    [DNLM: 1. Massage. 2. Diagnosis, Differential.   WB 537 M4147
1998]
RM721.M366   1998
615.8'22—DC21
DNLM/DLC
for Library of Congress   98-4257
                                        CIP

The publishers have made every effort to trace the copyright holders for borrowed material. If they have inadvertently overlooked any, they will be pleased to make the necessary arrangements at the first opportunity.

To purchase additional copies of this book, call our customer service department at **(800) 638-3030** or fax orders to **(301) 824-7390.** For other book services, including chapter reprints and large quantity sales, ask for the Special Sales Department. International customers should call **(301) 714-2324.**

Visit Lippincott Williams & Wilkins on the Internet: **http://www.lww.com.** Lippincott Williams & Wilkins customer service representatives are available from 8:30 am to 6:00 pm, EST.

01 02 03
7 8 9 10

This book is dedicated to the
memory of my grandmother,
Dora C. Beckhard, who probably
never got a massage in her
life—but she sure could have
used one.

—RW

Preface

Dear Students and Practitioners,

This book is a compilation of years of massage teaching and experience, collaboration with dozens of professionals in the field, a variety of printed resources, and hundreds of articles about ongoing research. In the old days, when we all had to walk 10 miles to school through raging blizzards, carrying our massage tables with us (and we *liked* it!), students were responsible for owning several different medical texts to have information concerning a variety of diseases. Such texts are important resources, but this book contains the pertinent information that has been extracted from hundreds of resources and reexamined in light of how massage may effect each condition.

Why do massage therapists need this book?

Massage therapy is one of the fastest-growing fields in the health care industry. Public interest in massage is at an all-time high. As massage therapy continues to enter the mainstream, massage students and practicing therapists can expect to be confronted with numerous conditions that they've never seen and probably only vaguely heard about. It is the responsibility of every massage therapist to know when our work can be helpful and when we need to send certain clients elsewhere for relief. This book is for students and practitioners who need to make decisions quickly and accurately about whether or not massage is appropriate for their clients.

What types of bodywork are covered here?

Judgments about the appropriateness of massage expressed in this book are based on mechanical (rather than reflexive or energetic) types of bodywork. Most conditions that are contraindicated for massage are contraindicated because of the effect massage has on the lymphatic and circulatory systems: massage can spread microorganisms or cancer cells through the bloodstream, or it can contribute to the accumulation of lymphatic congestion. In many cases massage can make a bad situation worse. However, although circulatory massage may be locally or systemically contraindicated for some conditions, reflexive or energetic work may not only be safe, but may contribute substantially to the healing process.

There are some conditions, though, for which any kind of hands-on work—mechanical, reflexive, or energetic—is strictly contraindicated. These are mainly acute and contagious conditions, which bodyworkers can not only catch but can spread to other people as well. *This is why any practitioner of any kind of bodywork needs to have a reference of this sort.*

A nod to political correctness:

In this book the terms "therapist" and "practitioner" are synonymous, and refer to the person performing bodywork. The people who have conditions are called "patients" in the context of medical care, and "clients" in the context of receiving massage. Patients or clients are referred to as "he" or "she" depending on what statistics indicate is the more likely gender to experience the condition. Thus, although it is possible for a woman to have hemophilia, for instance, the large majority of hemophiliacs are male and patients are therefore referred to as males. When there is no particular gender-related risk factor, patients or clients have been referred to as males or females more or less randomly.

Is this the definitive text?

Please don't fall into the trap of believing that this book is a permanent, definitive massage pathophysiology text. Our understanding of how the body works in the disease process is elementary at best, and our understanding of how massage can influence the disease process is positively primitive. The basic pathophysiology is presented here, and the effects of massage have been extrapolated from those points. We all anticipate that future research will reveal much more about massage and disease, perhaps even research that some of you will conduct.

And finally . . .

On a final note, one of the items on my personal agenda in writing this book is to share with you the wonder of the human body. It's amazing that we function as well as we do. It's even more miraculous that we can recover from injury and disease. As massage practitioners, we work to create an internal environment in our clients that fosters healing and recovery. Having conscious intention in our work makes us even better at achieving this goal. My purpose in writing this book is to help each practitioner develop that specific sense of intention: you should know *why* you're doing what you're doing every minute that you're working with a client.

So, happy reading. Do more research if it interests you, and remember that some of the questions dealt with here will probably never be completely answered. And what we think we know now may someday be revised or proved wrong. Isn't that terrific?!

Ruth Werner
Spring 1998

Acknowledgments

No book is written in a vacuum although it may sometimes seem that way. Many people contributed to the development of this work, and it is important—for me, anyway—to recognize them publicly, and with gratitude.

To Susanne Carlson, MA, LMT, who first made it clear to all of us how important it was to know this material—years before we were required to;

and to Brian Utting, LMP, teacher, boss, Big Kahuna, commissioner of the original work, source of inspiration to constantly strive to do something that might be too hard:

The two of you formed the germinal material from which this work grew. My thanks and admiration are with you always.

To the students of the Brian Utting School of Massage:

All of you convinced me that there was something important to write about in this topic. Through my years at the school, I learned far more *from* you than I could ever hope to teach *to* you.

To Ben Benjamin, PhD, teacher, helper, guide;

To Cecilia Reilly (have a pink squirrel on me);

To my reviewers—I didn't always agree with you, but I always appreciated everything you did to make this book better:

I am humbled by your efforts on my behalf. I am grateful for your time and energy. I am hopeful that we have created something that will be useful to many people for a long time. Thank you.

And finally, to my family: Curt, Nate-the-Great, and Lilybug:

This book wouldn't have been the same without you. You have put up with a lot of crankiness. Know that I love you, all the time, every minute, no matter what.

—RW

Reviewer Acknowledgments

The publisher and authors gratefully acknowledge the dedication, hard work, and perspective of the reviewers of this text.

Andre F. Fountain, RN, Director
Linda Young, RN, Faculty
in consultation with selected faculty and staff members
Praxis College of Health Arts and Sciences
Oklahoma City, OK

Kathleen M. Paholsky, PhD
Owner
Optimum Health Center,
Troy, MI
Director of Education
Health Enrichment Center
Lapeer, MI

Tracy Walton, MS, LMT, NCTMB
Head of Science Department
Muscular Therapy Institute
Cambridge, MA

A special thanks goes to:
William J. Ryan, PhD, RN
Assistant Professor
Allied Health Department
Slippery Rock University
Slippery Rock, PA
Dr. Ryan accepted the monumental task of closely reviewing the pathology information for this text. His guidance was invaluable.

How To Use This Book

One of the best definitions of health I've ever heard is, "Health is the ability to adapt to changes in the environment." In other words, health is not a noun; it's a verb. Health means being able to cope with changes in external conditions, but even more, being healthy means being able to adapt to changes in the *internal* environment of the body. Health is not simply the absence of infection or injury; it is an active state of adjustment and counteradjustment that allows the body to function under a broad variety of circumstances. When that ability to adapt is compromised, when a person's homeostatic processes are threatened, then the whole organism becomes weak and vulnerable to sickness, to disease.

The term *pathology* (from the Greek *pathos*, disease, and *logos*, science), is the study of the nature and causes of disease as related to structure and function of the body. This discipline can be divided into two specialties: *anatomic pathology* (the examination of tissues removed from cadavers or living people for the diagnosis of disease), and *clinical pathology* (also known as laboratory medicine: a broad field involving chemistry, histology, microbiology, hematopathology, immunopathology and other specialties). So pathology can be viewed as the laboratory study of cell and tissue changes associated with disease and/or injury.

Patho*physiology*, on the other hand, involves the study of functional or physiologic changes in the body that result from various disease processes. It explains the processes within the body that create the signs and symptoms of a disorder and examines how normal functions are altered by disease.

Massage therapy is intimately involved with anatomic and histological changes associated with disease and injury. More importantly, we work with how these diseases or conditions change the way our clients function. Therefore, massage therapists need to be familiar with the principles of pathophysiology to be able to judge whether our work is appropriate for each client. This book is designed to assist in the formation of that judgment.

Massage therapists challenge homeostasis. We create changes in the internal environment of our clients' bodies. We influence the diameter of blood vessels and the direction of fluid flow. Massage changes the chemical balance of the body, reducing some types of hormones while increasing others, shifting neurotransmitter secretion, altering the protein levels in interstitial tissues. Our first job, before we ever touch a client, is to determine whether that person is capable of adjusting to the changes massage precipitates.

This book has been written for two audiences: massage students who are learning about the body in health and disease for the first time, and practicing therapists working with a wide variety of people who may present a broad spectrum of disorders. It is written to present a wealth of complicated, interrelated, and convoluted material in an orderly fashion, but it can also provide easy reference and quick answers to the practitioner who needs to make a fast, well-informed decision.

The conditions that have been chosen to appear in this book are here for one of two reasons: either they occur frequently enough that practicing massage therapists will probably encounter them at some point, or because massage may have such a profound affect on certain conditions that practitioners are obligated to be well-informed about them.

Some controversy exists concerning what constitutes a disease rather than just a symptom; the dividing line between the two sometimes seems completely arbitrary. Although "jaundice" is considered a disease, it is really a description of the yellow skin and mucous membranes that occur when the liver is malfunctioning: it is, in fact, just a symptom. At a very basic level, most "diseases" could be considered to be symptoms of other underlying problems. These are usually simple but insidious situations like inadequate sleep, too much stress, poor nutrition, or genetic predisposition. These issues, after all, determine the body's susceptibility to a variety of infectious agents and disorders. So an argument could be made that the common cold is not really a disease at all; it is a symptom of a compromised immune system that is vulnerable to infection because of lack of sleep, stress, or poor nutrition. In this book, no particular division is drawn between conditions that could be labeled symptoms and those that could be labeled diseases; medical convention has been followed and traditional terminology used, and, when necessary, convention clarified how those terms were to be used within each article.

The material is presented by body system, following the order most anatomy and physiology texts use. Each chapter begins with a brief overview of how the system works, in order to provide the context for a discussion of what happens when things break down. Then the disorders are arranged by category, so that related conditions will appear together in the text. Each article is accompanied by an "in brief" box that presents the basic information in abbreviated form. Within each article is information about the condition, including, where applicable, the demographics of the disorder, the etiology and progression of the disease, signs and symptoms, the standard medical approach to diagnosis and treatment, and the applicability of massage.

The applicability of massage is described in terms of being "indicated" or "contraindicated" for each condition. Where massage is contraindicated, there are guidelines to explain whether this is a local caution, in other words, only the affected area must be avoided, or whether this is a systemic situation, in which case the client needs to be referred to a primary care physician or needs to reschedule his or her appointment for massage. Further explanations describe specific phases or stages of healing when massage is most appropriate.

For many of the conditions in this book massage is described as "indicated," at least at some stage of the healing process. I want to make very clear that to call massage "indicated" does *not* imply that massage will *fix* something that is wrong. There are times when massage can definitely influence the healing process for the better: the subacute stage of a sprained ankle, for instance. There are other times when massage may have no affect on the severity of a condition whatsoever, for instance, with fibroid tumors. Massage is called "indicated" for both of these situations which, in this case, simply means that massage won't make the situation any worse.

Diseases, like everything else in the body, are interconnected. References are therefore made within each article to other related conditions, even though they may not be listed under the same body system. It will be worthwhile to review those references to obtain the most thorough understanding of the relationships between different kinds of disorders.

Sidebars, boxes, and appendices contain information that doesn't necessarily fit within discussions of individual conditions. Nonetheless, this material is important for massage therapists to understand in the context of how massage affects the disease process. The quick reference chart in the appendices is by no means a "Cliff's Notes" version of the text, but may serve as a reminder of the key points each condition entails to the practitioner who needs to know in a hurry. A thorough index is provided to facilitate the reader's ability to find information quickly.

Study aides have been included in the form of chapter objectives and review questions. A reader may claim mastery of this material when he or she can answer these questions, as well as independently recreate the material included in the "in brief" boxes.

—RW

Table of Contents

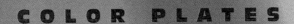

COLOR PLATES

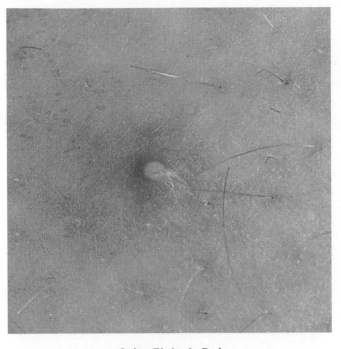

Color Plate 1. Boil

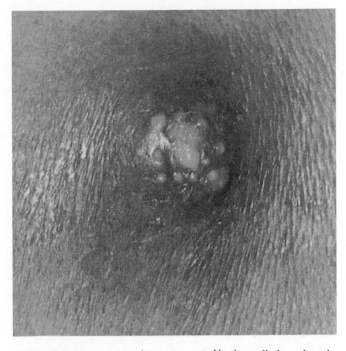

Color Plate 2. A group of interconnected boils is called a carbuncle

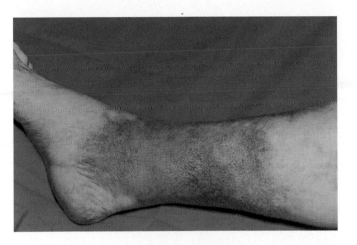

Color Plate 3. Erysipelas

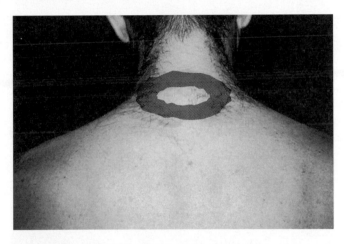

Color Plate 4. Tinea corporis: body ringworm

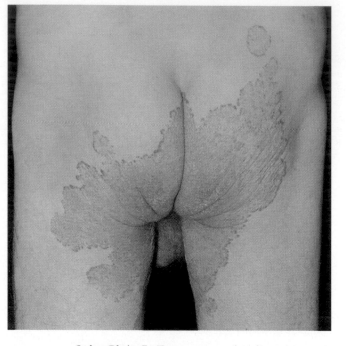

Color Plate 5. Tinea cruris: jock itch

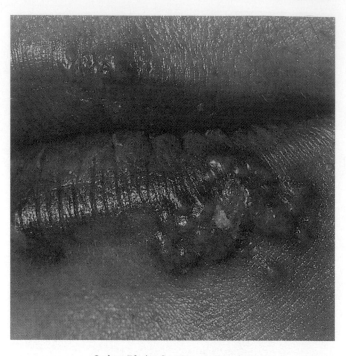

Color Plate 6. Herpes Simplex

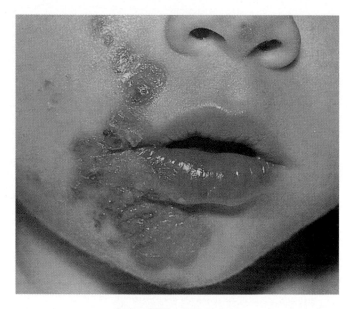

Color Plate 7. Impetigo

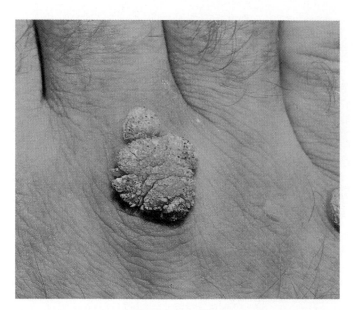

Color Plate 8. Wart

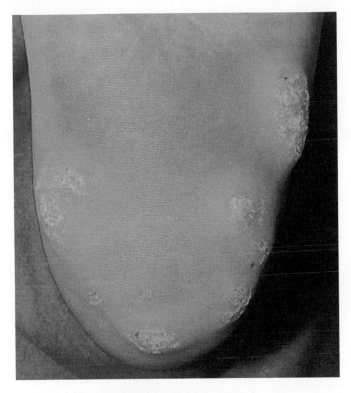

Color Plate 9. Plantar warts

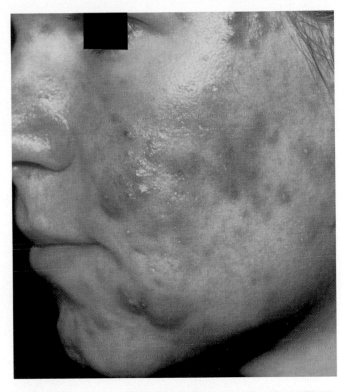

Color Plate 10. Acne

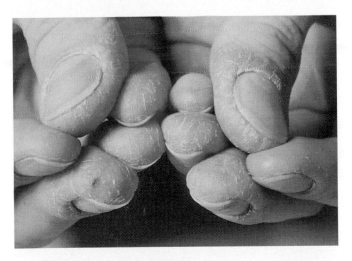

Color Plate 11. Eczema

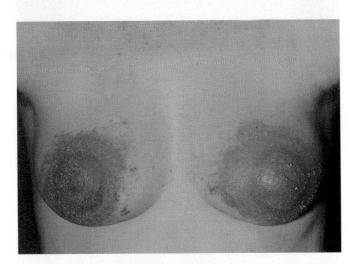

Color Plate 12. Dermatitis

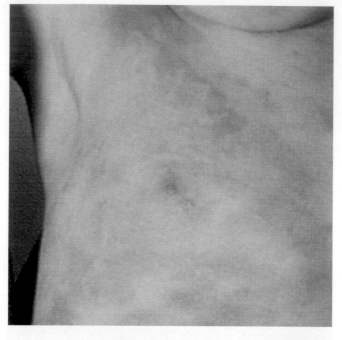

Color Plate 13. Hives

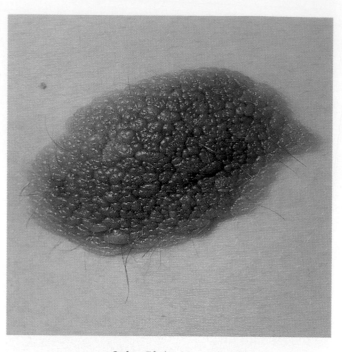

Color Plate 14. Mole

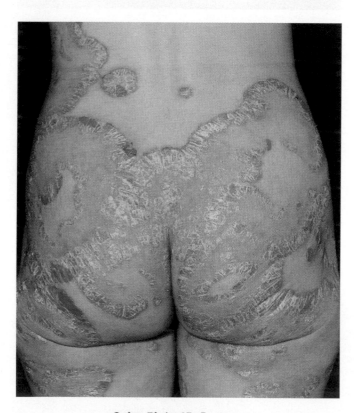

Color Plate 15. Psoriasis

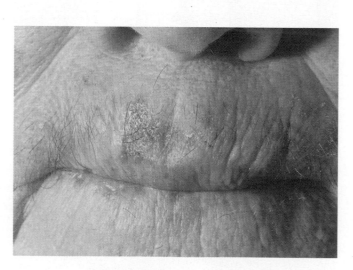

Color Plate 16. Actinic keratosis

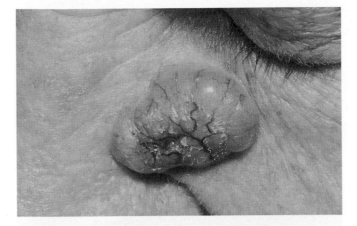

Color Plate 17. Basal cell carcinoma

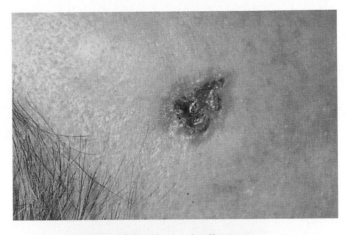

Color Plate 18. Basal cell carcinoma

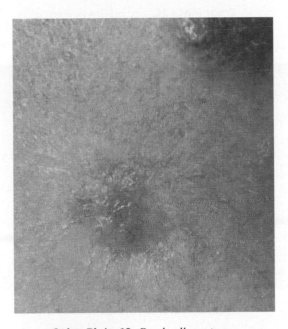

Color Plate 19. Basal cell carcinoma

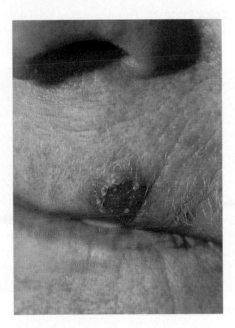

Color Plate 20. Squamous cell carcinoma

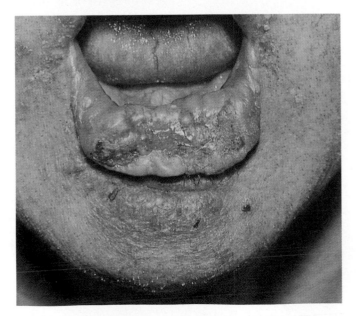

Color Plate 21. Squamous cell carcinoma

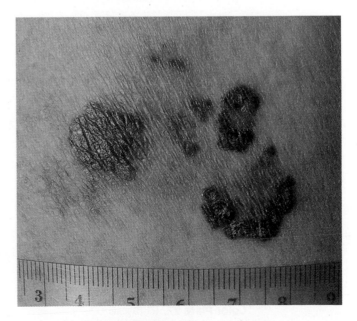

Color Plate 22. Malignant melanoma

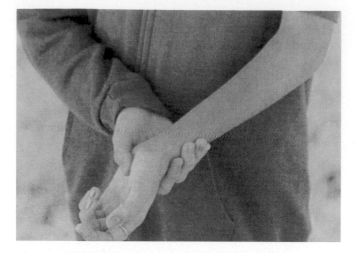

Color Plate 23. First-degree burn (sunburn)

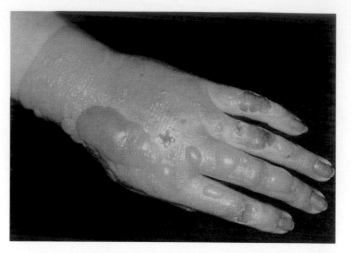

Color Plate 24. Second-degree burn

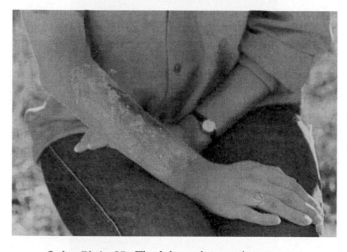

Color Plate 25. Third-degree burn with scar tissue

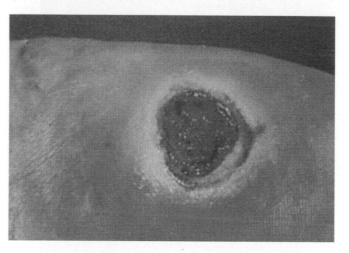

Color Plate 26. Decubitus ulcer

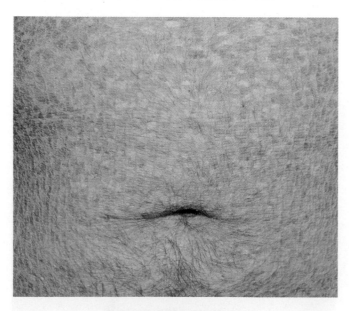

Color Plate 27. Ichthyosis

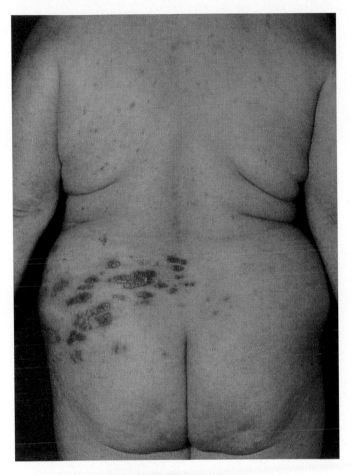

Color Plate 28. Herpes zoster

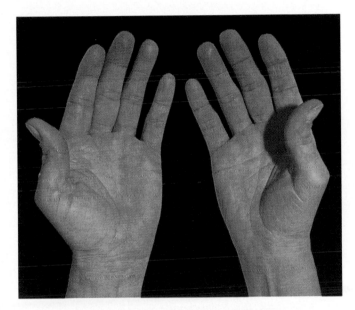

Color Plate 29. Raynaud's syndrome

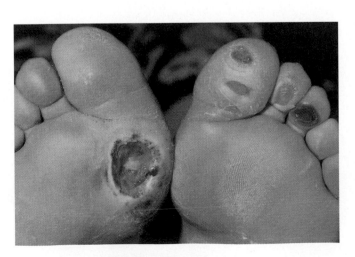

Color Plate 30. Diabetic ulcers

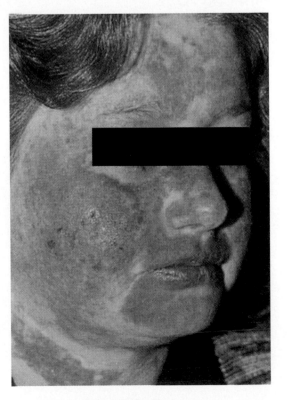

Color Plate 31. Lupus

Integumentary System Conditions

OBJECTIVES

After reading this chapter, you should be able to tell . . .

- What the disorder is.
- How to recognize it.
- Whether massage is indicated or contraindicated for that condition.
- Whether a contraindication is local or systemic, or refers to a specific stage of development or healing.
- Why those choices for massage are correct.

In addition to this basic information, you should be able to . . .

- Tell why massage is contraindicated in the presence of broken skin.
- Name three differences between a boil and acne.
- Name three variations on fungal infections of the skin.
- Name what kind of bacteria are usually associated with boils and acne.
- Name what kind of bacteria are usually associated with erysipelas.
- Name two dangers associated with widespread burns.
- Name three dangers associated with long-term use of corticosteroid creams.
- Name the ABCDEs of melanoma.
- Name the cardinal sign of non-melanoma skin cancer.
- Name a feature that distinguishes plantar warts from calluses.

INTRODUCTION

Massage practitioners speak in a language of touch. The messages practitioners give are invitations to a number of different possibilities: to enjoy a state of well-being; to heal and repair what is broken; to reacquaint a client with his or her own body. All this happens through the skin, a medium equipped like no other tissue in the body to take in information and respond to it, mostly on a subconscious level. The goal of massage practitioners is to anticipate these reactions and set the stage for them in a way that is most beneficial for their clients.

FUNCTIONS OF THE SKIN

A student once said that the purpose of skin is to keep our insides from falling out. That's true, but that's not all skin does; its functions are manifold. Among them are several devices to keep the body healthy and safe, all wrapped up in one tidy eighteen-to-thirty pound package.

Protection

The skin keeps pathogens *out* of the body, just by being intact, and it discourages their growth on its surface by secreting the acidic lubricants otherwise needed for keeping hair shafts oiled. Furthermore, by constantly sloughing off dead cells, it sloughs off potential invaders as well.

The skin is the first line of defense against invasion, and the superficial fascia is especially well supplied with immune system cells that are constantly on the lookout for potential sources of infection. These mast cells and other nonspecific white blood cells can create an extreme inflammatory response very quickly. When these defense mechanisms become hyperactive, they can cause certain types of rashes and other skin problems. For more details on hypersensitivity reactions, see the introduction to Lymph and Immune System Conditions, chapter 5, page 219.

Homeostasis

The skin protects us from fluid loss, a top homeostatic priority, and one of the most dangerous functions to lose when the skin is damaged. The skin is the membrane that connects inner bodies to the outside world. It helps to maintain a constant internal temperature in spite of what's happening outside because blood supply to the skin far exceeds the need for local nutrition: capillaries will dilate or constrict according to what is needed at the time. The fat in the subcutaneous layer also acts as insulation.

Sensory Envelope

With as many as 19,000 sensory receptors in every square inch of skin, it's obvious that this is the organ (or tissue, or membrane, or system—depending on the source of information) that tells us the most about our environment. Eyes and ears appear to be indispensable, but look how far Helen Keller got with just her skin to take in information. Massage therapists must develop the skill of becoming *conscious* of the subtle information their hands give them when they touch their clients, and must understand that every sensation created on a client's skin is also causing ripples of reactions all through the body.

Absorption, Excretion

To a small extent, the skin *does* absorb and excrete. Fat-soluble materials can be absorbed through the capillaries in hair shafts. Some massage oil is also absorbed this way. Compounds like DMSO are completely absorbed, a phenomenon called *transcutaneous absorption*.

The skin can help to excrete metabolic wastes, but it does so only as a last ditch option. When the liver, colon, or especially kidneys are so congested that they can't handle any more waste products, sweat can carry noxious chemicals out of the body.

CONSTRUCTION OF THE SKIN

Skin varies from being very thin (on the lips) to remarkably thick (on the heels). It remodels according to stresses put upon it. *Callus* is an example of this phenomenon: extra thick, extra hard epidermis develops on places that really take a beating.

The construction of the skin is important to understand, because it has relevance for how disease occurs, and how easily it might spread. There are three basic layers of skin, and within those layers there are more layers. (See Figure 1.1.)

- The **_subcutaneous tissue_** is probably familiar; it is also called superficial fascia.
- The **_dermis_**, or "true skin," is the location of hair shafts, oil and sweat glands, and some nerve endings. The outermost layer of dermis, the basal layer, lies just below the epidermis and has the best capillary supply. This is where new skin cells are born. Pigment cells (called *melanocytes*) are here, helping to protect people from harmful UV rays. Some of the worst diseases are born here, too, for reasons described later in this chapter. New cells are cloned near the border of the epidermis and migrate toward the surface, dying of starvation and becoming *keratinized*, or scaly, in the process, which takes about a month. By the time they get to the surface they are long dead, and will soon be sloughed off to become the major ingredient of household dust.
- The **_epidermis_** is made of epithelium. Epithelium heals faster than any other type of tissue, which is good because no other tissue type is as vulnerable to damage as skin. It would be nice if the central nervous system healed as readily as the skin does, but consider the priorities: compare the number of neurological traumas a person is likely to experience to the number of cuts, scrapes, scratches, tears, and punctures he will endure. Nevertheless, healing quickly has its disadvantages. Cells that have instructions to replicate at the drop of a hat sometimes replicate *without* the hat dropping, and that causes trouble.

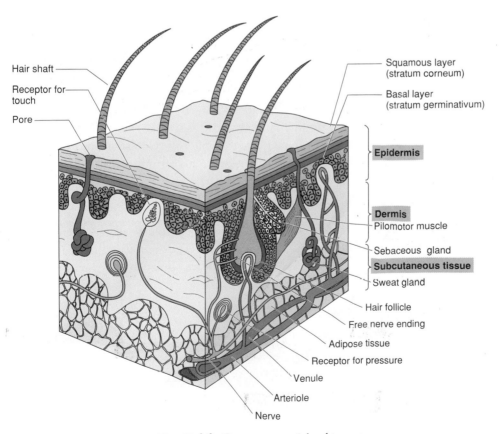

Figure 1.1. Cross section of the skin

INTEGUMENTARY SYSTEM CONDITIONS

Contagious Skin Disorders
- Boils
- Erysipelas
- Fungal Infections
- Herpes Simplex
- Impetigo
- Lice and Mites
- Warts

Noncontagious Inflammatory Skin Disorders
- Acne
- Dermatitis/Eczema
- Hives

Neoplastic Skin Disorders
- Moles
- Psoriasis
- Skin Cancer

Skin Injuries
- Burns
- Decubitus Ulcers
- Open Wounds and Sores
- Scar Tissue

Other Conditions
- Ichthyosis

RULES FOR MASSAGE

Skin conditions have a special relevance for massage therapists, because we are in a position to notice lesions and blemishes that clients often don't know are there. That's why it is especially important to be able to recognize most common skin conditions, at least as far as being able to recommend that clients investigate further with their own doctors. Many kinds of skin conditions contraindicate massage because they might be contagious. Beyond that danger, there is one cardinal rule for skin conditions and massage: if the intactness of the skin has been compromised in any way, the client is a walking invitation for infection. Open skin, broken skin, scabbed skin, any skin that allows access to the blood vessels inside is a red flag for massage practitioners. No matter how much a person scrubs, pathogens will always be present on the skin. By considering any compromised area of skin at least a local contraindication, practitioners take the responsibility to ensure that their microorganisms don't jump into their clients' vulnerable spots. At the same time, practitioners must prevent *clients'* pathogens jumping into the tiny cracks in the practitioner's skin.

Contagious Skin Disorders

Boils

BOILS
Furuncle comes from the Latin *furunculus*, which means "petty thief." The association between petty thievery and boils is obscure, unless it refers to the extreme irritation caused by both.

DEFINITION: WHAT IS IT?

Boils, also called *furuncles*, and acne are closely related, with one main difference: boils do *not* require excess testosterone and sebum production to develop.

ETIOLOGY: WHAT HAPPENS?

Like acne, boils are staphylococcus infections of sebaceous glands that are clogged by dirt, dead skin cells, or other debris. But in this case, the staph is not simply taking advantage of a stagnant pool of oil, but is actively attacking living tissue.

SIGNS AND SYMPTOMS

Boils tend to be bigger and more painful than acne, but they usually occur only one at a time, instead of being spread over general areas. (See Figure 1.2, Color Plate 1.) A cluster of boils connected by channels under the skin is called a *carbuncle*. (See Figure 1.3, Color Plate 2.)

TREATMENT

As long as the infection stays localized, boils are not dangerous, although they are *extremely* painful. Conservative treatment begins with hot compresses, which will sometimes help them to burst and then drain, relieving the pressure and therefore the pain. If compresses don't do the trick, doctors may lance the boil for the draining effects. Antibiotics are sometimes prescribed, but they tend to be slow-acting, and have the best effect for people who are plagued with a recurring problem.

It is important never to try to squeeze or pop a boil. This could force the infection deeper into tissues. Boils also carry a risk of complications brought about by the possibility of the staph bacteria spreading to other parts of the body, or even to different bodies altogether.

Chronically repeating boils may indicate a compromised immune system. They are also a warning sign for *diabetes* (chapter 4, page 210) or kidney problems.

MASSAGE?

The cautions for dealing with boils are exactly the same as for dealing with acne, only stronger. This is a local infection with extremely virulent, hardy bacteria that can spread

BOILS IN BRIEF

What are they?
Boils are local staphylococcus infections similar to acne, but they are not related to adolescence or liver dysfunction.

How are they recognized?
Boils look like acne, too, except that the lesions are bigger and they usually occur singly rather than being spread over a large area. They are also more painful than typical acne lesions.

Is massage indicated or contraindicated?
Boils at least locally contraindicate massage, and care should be taken to make sure the infection is not systemic (screen the client for other symptoms such as swelling, fever, or discomfort other than at the site of the lesion). The bacteria that cause boils are extremely virulent and communicable. The sheets of a client with boils should be treated with extra care.

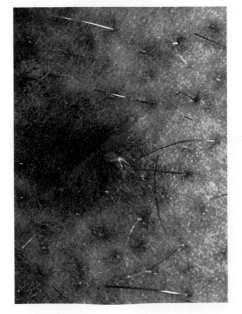

Figure 1.2. Boil

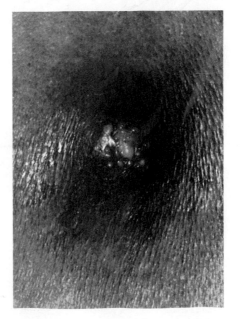

Figure 1.3. A group of interconnected boils is called a carbuncle

ERYSIPELAS IN BRIEF

What is it?
Erysipelas is a streptococcus infection that kills skin cells, leading to painful inflammation of the skin. It usually occurs on the face or lower leg.

How is it recognized?
A distinct margin between the reddened, affected area and the surrounding unaffected areas marks this condition. When it occurs on the face, it often creates a red "butterfly" shape over the cheeks and bridge of the nose. Fever and signs of systemic infection can accompany it.

Is massage indicated or contraindicated?
This is a bacterial infection that can invade both the lymph and circulatory systems. Massage is systemically contraindicated until the infection has completely passed.

ERYSIPELAS
This term comes from the Greek roots *eryth*, for "redness" (think of *erythema* or *erythrocyte*) and *pello*, for "skin." Red skin with a sharply demarcated border is a hallmark of erysipelas.

to anyone who touches it. Staphylococcus is often drug resistant, and it can be extremely difficult to kill. A client who has a boil with no signs of systemic infection may receive massage, but not on or near the lesion. If indications of a systemic infection *do* exist (fever, swelling at nearby lymph nodes, discomfort anywhere other than the site of the boil), it will be necessary to reschedule the massage.

The sheets of a client who has a boil will require special treatment. Isolate them and wash them with extra bleach to ensure that any staph bacteria will be eradicated.

Erysipelas

DEFINITION: WHAT IS IT?

Erysipelas is a streptococcal infection of the cells in the skin. "Erys" means *red*, referring to the characteristic red patches an infection of this kind can cause.

ETIOLOGY: WHAT HAPPENS?

Colonies of bacteria are always growing on the skin: under the fingernails, between the toes, everywhere. It is virtually impossible to remove all the bacteria from a living person's skin. These colonies include both staphylococcus and streptococcus bacteria. Staph is usually responsible for small, localized infections such as boils and pimples; it seems to have an affinity for sebum. But once *strep* gets under the skin—usually through a cut or a sore—the local infection may become systemic, involving first the lymphatic, then the circulatory system. The enzymes produced by strep bacteria, which break down and kill skin cells, cause erysipelas.

SIGNS AND SYMPTOMS

Erysipelas begins with a tender, red swelling at the portal of entry. (See Figure 1.4, Color Plate 3.) It's unclear why, exactly, but erysipelas usually begins on the face or the lower leg. The wound soon shows signs of infection, which can include red streaks running toward the nearest set of lymph nodes. If the infection starts on the face, a raised, red, hot, tender area will develop, which spreads laterally across the bridge of the nose. It looks like

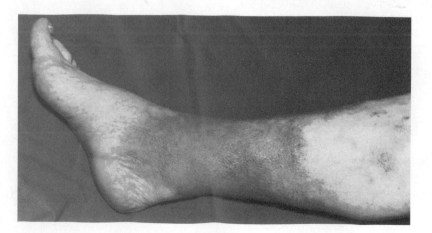

Figure 1.4. Erysipelas

the "butterfly rash" pattern sometimes seen with *lupus* (see chapter 5, page 241). One hallmark of erysipelas is a sharp margin between involved and uninvolved skin; the red edges are usually very clear.

When the infection has thoroughly engaged the lymph system, symptoms will include fever, chills, and systemic discomfort. Facial infections are particularly dangerous because of the risk of intracranial spreading through lymphatic nodes. If erysipelas is left untreated, the bacteria may move past the lymph system and enter the circulatory system, leading quickly, and perhaps fatally, to septicemia, or blood poisoning.

TREATMENT

Not so long ago, streptococcus was streptococcus. A person was diagnosed with an infection like strep throat or erysipelas, given penicillin, and sent home. But those days are gone forever. As good as penicillin is, strep bacteria are smarter, and they have mutated into myriad different drug-resistant forms faster than new antibiotics have been created to kill them. If a person is diagnosed with a strep infection now, prescriptions of antibiotics are likely to take a catch-as-catch-can approach, shooting bullets until one of them finds the target. That is why doctors sometimes change prescriptions in midstream if a patient is not seeing results; her own special brand of streptococcus is simply unaffected by whatever drug she's been taking, and she needs to find one that works better.

MASSAGE?

Here's a condition involving a highly contagious bacterial infection, skin damage, and the risk of blood poisoning if it should find its way into the circulatory system. Massage is systemically contraindicated.

Fungal Infections

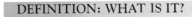 *Derma-skin*

DEFINITION: WHAT IS IT?

The nomenclature for the range of fungal infections people can get is dizzying. Fungal infections of human skin, also called *mycoses*, can involve several different types of fungi (*dermatophytes*). *Dermatophytosis*, then, is another term for mycosis. The lesions the infections create are called *tinea*. And to top it all off, the generic term *ringworm*, although it is misleading because there are no worms involved at all, is frequently used to refer to several types of tinea.

ETIOLOGY: WHAT HAPPENS?

Dermatophytes live on a diet of perspiration and dead skin cells. They thrive in warm, moist places such as skin folds between toes or around the groin. They tend to infect people with depressed or sluggish immune systems. Fungal infections are transmitted via touch: either skin to skin or skin to anything that has some fungus on it, including massage sheets, locker room benches, or the family hairbrush. They can also be communicated by dogs and cats. It takes anywhere from 4 to 14 days for the signs to appear, and during that time the carrier is infectious, which makes this condition very hard to control.

FUNGAL INFECTIONS IN BRIEF

What are they?
Fungal infections of human skin, also called *mycoses*, are caused by fungi called *dermatophytes*. When there is a fungal infection caused by dermatophytes, the characteristic lesions are called *tinea*. Thus, within this heading several different types of tinea are listed.

How are they recognized?
Most tinea lesions begin as one reddened circular itchy patch. Scratching the lesions will spread them to other parts of the body. As they get larger they tend to clear in the middle and keep a red ring around the edges. Athlete's foot, another type of mycosis, will involve moist blisters and cracking between the toes. If it affects the nails they will become yellow, thickened, and pitted.

Is massage indicated or contraindicated?
Massage is at least locally contraindicated for fungal infections in all phases. If the affected areas are very limited—for instance, only the feet are involved or only one or two small, covered lesions appear on the body—massage may be administered to the rest of the body. If there is a large area involved, and especially if the infection is acute (i.e., not yet responding to treatment), then massage is systemically contraindicated.

SIGNS AND SYMPTOMS

There are several varieties of tinea; here are descriptions of the most common ones.

- Tinea corporis, or body ringworm, is relatively common and *very* contagious, so it deserves special attention. It generally begins as one small round, red, scaly, itchy patch of skin on the trunk. Scratching spreads the fungus to other parts of the body, and so other lesions appear. They heal from the center first, and they soon take on the appearance of red circles, or rings, that may gradually increase in size as the fungus spreads out for new food sources. (See Figure 1.5, Color Plate 4.)

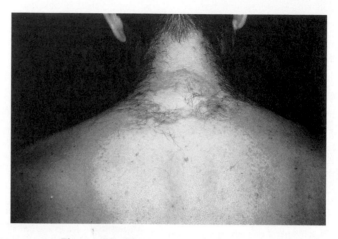

Figure 1.5. Tinea corporis: body ringworm

RINGWORM

Delores G.

Around June of 1994, I was working hard in massage school. I was living in a house where some stray kittens were close by. I wanted to pet them, so I brought them some food. They came out, and I got to pet them while they were eating.

I was sitting down next to them with my knees up. I had shorts on. I was petting them with my left hand, then I held my legs with the same hand when I was done. I also folded my arms, so my left hand touched my right bicep.

About nine days later, specific round red spots developed—the size of a half-dollar—on my left calf and then on my right arm. It wasn't until I remembered petting the kittens that I realized what it came from. About a week after the spots appeared, they started to burn and keep me awake.

Having ringworm was awful. It turns out that I had massaged only two people between being exposed and being diagnosed, so it didn't spread through the class, but I had to wait until I was cleared up before I could work again. I sat out of practices, which was really depressing, *plus* it was spreading all over me, from my right arm to my right breast, and on my other calf.

I treated it by showering and then putting tea-tree oil and antifungal vaginal cream all over me. I did that for two or three weeks before it started to clear up. It was all cleared up in four weeks. We waited an extra week just to be sure, so I missed a total of five weeks of massage.

When I got ringworm, I was extremely run down from school, which probably made me susceptible. My teacher said it was interesting that my body chose ringworm as the thing that would slow me down, but it worked!

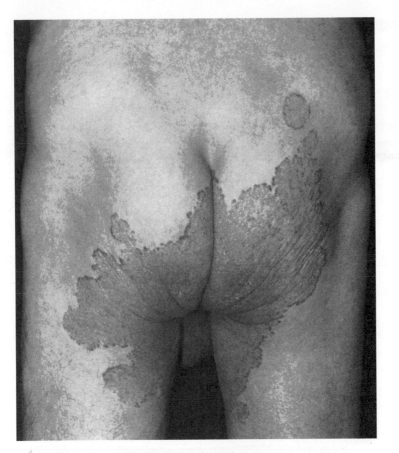

Figure 1.6. Tinea cruris: jock itch

- Tinea capitis, or head ringworm, inhabits the scalp. Lesions here result in typical itchiness and flaking (similar to serious dandruff), and if scratching and secondary infection result in scar tissue, temporary or permanent hair loss may occur. This variety is as contagious as body ringworm.
- Tinea pedis, or athlete's foot, focuses its attention on the skin between the toes. Athlete's foot affects about 20% of the population to some degree. It burns and itches and carries the additional complication of weeping blisters, cracking and peeling skin, and the possibility of infection; athlete's foot can even lead to *lymphangitis* (see chapter 5, page 227) or *erysipelas* (this chapter, page 6). This fungal infection can be particularly hard to get rid of because it can live under the toenails. It thrives in the growth medium provided by closed shoes. If a person has athlete's foot, it is especially important to make sure his feet are always as dry as possible, since these fungi, like most others, love warm, dark, moist places.
- Tinea cruris, or jock itch, is probably the least contagious of the group, but it doesn't stick exclusively to the groin. It can also be found on the upper thigh and buttocks, and lesions may well exist that a client won't be aware of, but which massage therapists must avoid carefully. (See Figure 1.6, Color Plate 5.)

TREATMENT

Treatment for fungal infections can actually be very difficult. Dermatophytes, like some viruses and bacteria, have mutated into many different incarnations of the originals, each one more resistant to standard fungicides than the last. What's more, they somewhat resemble the body's own proteins, which makes it difficult for the immune system to tag it, and slow to fight it. External applications of fungicide are the normal treatment.

PREVENTION

Where any kind of dermatophytosis is concerned, an ounce of prevention is worth a pound of cure. The best way for a massage therapist to avoid getting ringworm is to know what it looks like and to stay away from it. It's also particularly important to maintain one's own health. This gives the body every chance of fighting off any fungal attack.

MASSAGE?

Fungal infections contraindicate massage in every phase (including the invisible two-week gestation period, which is difficult to determine). However, if it's a small infestation (just one or two lesions), it can be considered a *local* caution as long as the lesions are covered and the therapist does a 10% bleach rinse afterward. For clients with athlete's foot that shows blistering, weepy skin, the feet are a local contraindication. The decision might also depend on the therapist's own state of health; if the therapist is feeling run down and vulnerable, this may not be the week to work on someone with ringworm.

Herpes Simplex

DEFINITION: WHAT IS IT?

Among the seven different viruses in the herpes family that affect humans, two distinct, yet closely related types are herpes simplex viruses. The type I virus usually causes the cold sores or fever blisters that are associated with oral herpes, while type II is usually responsible for outbreaks of similar blisters on the genitals, buttocks, and thighs.

DEMOGRAPHICS: WHO GETS IT?

An astounding 30 million people in the United States are affected annually by some variant of the herpes simplex virus. One-half million new infections are expected this year. Men and women are affected equally.

HERPES SIMPLEX IN BRIEF

What is it?
Herpes simplex is a viral infection resulting in cold sores or fever blisters on the face or in the mouth (type I) or around the genitals, thighs, or buttocks (type II).

How is it recognized?
Herpes outbreaks are often preceded by two to three days of tingling, itching, or pain. Blisters then appear, which gradually crust and disappear, usually within two weeks.

Is massage indicated or contraindicated?
Massage is locally contraindicated for any kind of herpes in the acute stage, and systemically contraindicated if the client is showing any systemic signs of infection. The sheets of clients with herpes must be isolated and sterilized. For clients with histories of herpes but no active symptoms, massage is indicated.

COMMUNICABILITY

The herpes virus is famous for communicability. Unlike the AIDS virus and almost every other kind of pathogen, the herpes virus can remain dormant and healthy outside of a host body for hours at a time; exactly how long is a matter of some debate. This means that the face pad that an infected client used can now infect another client. Face cloths and towels are also potentially dangerous. Even leaving aside the strong possibility of infecting other people, herpes is notorious for spreading to other parts of the body. Type I is responsible for causing about 15% of the cases of type II herpes infections. Touching a cold sore and then touching the eye can also result in a painful and dangerous herpetic infection of the cornea (herpes keratitis).

One of the most dangerous aspects of a herpes infection is that a patient could be shedding the virus even from skin that has no visible lesions. This means that all it takes to catch herpes from another person is skin-to-skin contact with live virus. *No sore or break in the skin is necessary.*

SIGNS AND SYMPTOMS

Whether oral or genital, herpes simplex usually presents itself in the same way: the affected area may experience

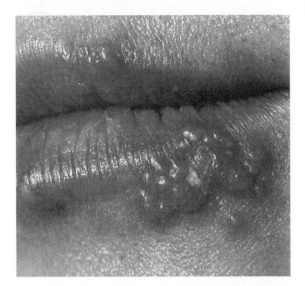

Figure 1.7. Herpes simplex

some pain or tingling a few days before an outbreak (the "prodomic" stage), then a blister or cluster of blisters appears. They erupt and ooze virus-rich liquid all around the area. (See Figure 1.7, Color Plate 6.) The blisters scab over after a week or so, ending the most dangerous phase for spreading the disease. Altogether the outbreak generally lasts about two to three weeks.

Here are some differences in the ways genital and oral herpes present themselves:

- Oral herpes tends to erupt when immunity is otherwise depressed (they are called "cold sores" or "fever blisters" because they often occur when a person is fighting off some other infection), during hormonal changes as in pregnancy or menstruation, after prolonged exposure to sunlight, or during or after any emotional stress. They appear most often on the lips, on the tongue, inside the mouth, and on the skin around the mouth. They may be a lifelong affliction.

- Herpes simplex type I lesions usually appear in or around the mouth, but it is possible for them to appear elsewhere on the body as well. Of special concern to massage therapists is a variety called *Herpes Whitlow*, which is an outbreak of lesions around the nailbeds of the hands.

- Genital herpes outbreaks also correspond to depressed immunity and general stress levels, but they do seem to run a course of appearing with less and less frequency until finally they simply never come back. As stated above, these blisters will appear on the genitals, but they can also be found on the thighs, buttocks, and even on the skin over the sacrum. People who have herpes and are immune-depressed tend to experience outbreaks over larger areas of the body than those with better immunity. The lesions are usually quite painful, but if they are inside the vaginal canal, a woman may be unaware of them, which has important implications for communicability. Genital herpes outbreaks are sometimes accompanied by systemic symptoms: fever, muscle aches, swelling in the inguinal lymph nodes, and difficult or painful urination.

COMPLICATIONS

Secondary infection is a common complication of herpes lesions. Immune-suppressed people (especially AIDS and organ transplant patients) are especially susceptible to infections. Vaginally delivered newborns of mothers with active genital herpes may suffer blindness or even brain damage. Genital herpes has also been statistically connected with higher rates of cervical cancer, so infected women are wise to have frequent Pap smears performed. The herpes simplex virus has also been linked to *encephalitis* (chapter 3, page 143) and *meningitis* (chapter 3, page 146).

TREATMENT

Herpes is a viral infection, which means little can be done for it but wait for it to be over. Acyclovir is one antiviral drug that may suppress viral activity, but it won't prevent future outbreaks. Prevention is the main thrust for treatment of this condition; this means isolating towels, bedding, and clothing, and avoiding sexual contact while lesions are present. Keeping as healthy as possible between outbreaks is an important way to reduce the frequency and severity of herpes episodes.

MASSAGE?

Obviously, massage is contraindicated for clients who have acute herpes outbreaks. If a client has a history of herpes, it's important to explain why it's a bad idea to receive a massage during an outbreak and request that she reschedule if she has blisters on her appointment day. If a client is having systemic symptoms like fever or general achiness, she is systemically contraindicated. Even after a lesion has scabbed over, herpes is, at the very least, a local contraindication. Because this virus can survive outside of a host for hours at a time, consider the sheets of any client with herpes as "hot." Isolate them in a closed container and either have them professionally sterilized or add extra bleach to their wash cycle.

Clients who have active herpes outbreaks are not good candidates to receive massage. Likewise, massage therapists who have active herpes outbreaks need to respect their clients' health by not exposing them to the virus. Scabbed-over cold sores may be very itchy. Massage therapists need to take special care not to inadvertently brush their face with their sleeves, wrists, or hands and then touch a client with a contaminated surface.

Impetigo

DEFINITION: WHAT IS IT?

Impetigo is a bacterial infection that is especially prevalent in children. Lesions usually occur around the nose and mouth, sometimes appearing inside the nostrils or ear canals. Although it usually begins somewhere on the head, impetigo can infect the skin anywhere on the body.

This infection is caused by both staphylococcus and streptococcus bacteria.

SIGNS AND SYMPTOMS

Impetigo begins as a rash with small blisters or pustules filled with clear or murky fluid. These often occur where the skin has been damaged by some other injury. When the blisters pop, a characteristic honey-colored crust forms. (See Figure 1.8, Color Plate 7.) Impetigo is itchy, and is most common in hot, humid climates and in areas with dry, cold winters, when lips and noses become chapped and vulnerable to infection.

TREATMENT

Mild impetigo can be treated with topical antibiotic creme. But if the blisters have spread over much of the

---

IMPETIGO IN BRIEF

What is it?
Impetigo is a bacterial (staphylococcus or streptococcus) infection of the skin.

How is it recognized?
There is a rash with fluid-filled blisters and honey-colored crusts. It usually begins somewhere on the face, but can appear anywhere on the body.

Is massage indicated or contraindicated?
Until the lesions have completely healed, massage is systemically contraindicated for this highly contagious condition.

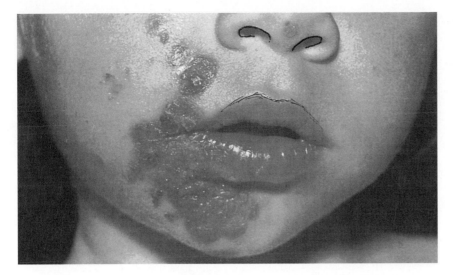

Figure 1.8. Impetigo

body, and especially if there are other signs of systemic infection (i.e., fever and chills), then oral antibiotics are prescribed. Very rarely the infection can complicate into *erysipelas* (this chapter, page 6) or *glomerulonephritis* (chapter 8, page 309).

PREVENTION

Impetigo often appears where the skin has already been damaged, for example, at the site of scabbed-over mosquito bites, cuts, and sores. The first step in prevention is to stop any kind of infection from developing at these sites. Chapped lips and noses should be treated with lubricant to prevent skin damage. All other wounds should be cleaned thoroughly and treated with antibacterial ointment.

This is an extremely contagious condition, and since it is both very itchy and most common in children, special precautions are recommended to prevent its spread. First, the patient must be discouraged from touching or scratching his lesions; impetigo can be spread easily to other parts of the body this way. The lesions must be kept clean and dry, and crusts removed as soon as possible, since they harbor bacteria in the moistness underneath. The patient's bedding and towels must be strictly isolated while he is infected. Children with impetigo are encouraged to stay home from school and avoid contact with other children for one to three days after they begin treatment.

MASSAGE?

This is a contagious bacterial infection of the skin involving very virulent pathogens that can be drug resistant. Massage is systemically contraindicated until the lesions have completely healed.

Lice and Mites

Mites

DEFINITION: WHAT ARE THEY?

Microscopic mites that are invisible to the naked eye cause skin lesions called scabies. (See Figure 1.9.) The female mites burrow under the skin in warm, moist spots where they drink blood, defecate, and urinate, and lay eggs so the next generation can carry on. The

IMPETIGO
This comes from the Latin words *im* and *peto*, which mean "to rush up, attack." This may refer to the invasive and extremely infectious nature of this type of staph infection.

LICE AND MITES IN BRIEF

What are they?

Lice and mites are tiny arthropods that drink blood. They are highly contagious and spread through close contact with skin or infested sheets or clothing.

How are they recognized?

The mites that cause scabies are too small to see, but they leave itchy trails where they burrow under the skin. They prefer warm, moist places such as the axillae or between fingers.

Head lice are easy to see, but they can hide. A more dependable sign is their eggs: nits are small, white, rice-shaped flecks that cling strongly to hair shafts.

Pubic lice look like tiny white crabs.

All three of these parasites create a lot of itching.

Is massage indicated or contraindicated?

Massage is contraindicated for all three infestations, until the infestation has been completely eradicated. If a massage therapist is exposed to any of these parasites, every client he or she subsequently works on will also be exposed even before the therapist shows any symptoms.

Parasitic infestations are something every massage therapist fears. Therapists are so very vulnerable to whatever is crawling around on clients' skin. But here, as for all things fearful, the best defense is information.

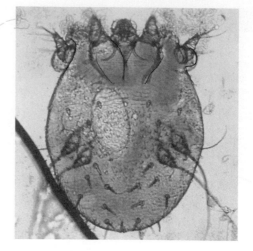

Figure 1.9. Scabies mite

mites' waste is highly irritating, which causes a lot of itching. If scratching damages the skin, a strong possibility exists for secondary infection.

HOW DO THEY SPREAD?

Mites spread readily through close personal contact, as well as through contact with something someone else has worn or lain on—like massage sheets.

SIGNS AND SYMPTOMS

Scabies-causing mites are too small to see with the naked eye, so a visual diagnosis is based on the trails they leave behind. Sometimes their burrows are visible. They look like reddish or grayish lines around the areas scabies favor: the groin, the axilla, the inside of the elbows, between fingers. They like skin folds, although they also colonize the skin around the belt line. Another sign of mite infestation is the irritated blisters and pustules that arise from reactions to their waste and secondary bacterial infection. This condition is itchiest at night, when the mites are most active.

DIAGNOSIS

Scabies lesions can sometimes be hard to diagnose. It's common to find people who are so miserable with their infestation that they can't eat or sleep. Still, the skin tests don't always catch an actual bug, so a definitive diagnosis is difficult to make. It is typically based on the nature of the rash, the client's history, and the possibility that she might have been exposed.

TREATMENT

Mites, like other parasitic infestations, are treated by bathing with a pesticidal shampoo. The mites die within a week of being separated from human contact, so isolating bedding, towels, and clothing for that length of time will help to prevent further outbreaks.

MASSAGE?

Massage is out of the question. If a massage therapist thinks she might have been exposed to mites by accident, she should consider those sheets "hot" (isolate them from other

SCABIES

Valerie

Valerie was a massage student. She worked with a variety of people, including fellow students, friends, and her student internship group—people with AIDS.

One day Valerie noticed that she had some areas on the outsides of her elbows that were slightly but persistently itchy during the day. They gradually developed red bumps. Ironically, this occurred while Valerie was studying skin conditions in her massage course. "It's natural to convince yourself that you have symptoms for a lot of things. I knew something was going on, and it seemed like it *could* be scabies, but my symptoms were different from anything I'd seen described," she said. The itching was not particularly worse at night, and no tracks or typical signs of infestation were noticeable. Even the site of infestation was unusual: scabies mites usually go for warm, moist, protected areas like skin folds on the *insides* of elbows, but not the outsides.

Eventually Valerie went to her general practitioner, who pronounced her condition a "mystery rash" and suggested a corticosteroid creme to limit the itchiness. In a way, Valerie was relieved by this diagnosis: "You never want to think you have scabies," she said. When her husband also developed symptoms, however, he went straight to a dermatologist who immediately diagnosed scabies, and prescribed enough pesticidal soap for the both of them.

The creme was applied all over the body up to the chin; evidently scabies do not infest the head or face. "That night after I washed off the creme, I was really, really, *really* itchy, and then for four or five weeks my skin was raw and uncomfortable." Corticosteroid creme itself can create symptoms that mimic a scabies infestation for weeks at a time. This can lead to a condition called "scabiosis" in which a person is convinced that they need to medicate for scabies again and again, although they are not really infested. Scabiosis can become a life-threatening condition if the patient repeatedly self-medicates.

Six to eight weeks passed between the onset of Valerie's symptoms and a final diagnosis. During this time, Valerie had continued to work on friends and clients as well as to receive massage from other students. Two other classmates were finally infested and diagnosed. "The first few days (after we knew it was scabies) were full of panic and fear. Within a couple of days of people getting over their fear and paranoia, there was a lot of support. People had the attitude that this is just one of the things that can happen when you're a bodyworker."

sheets and wash them with extra bleach) and see a doctor about treating herself right away. The symptoms of scabies sometimes don't show up for days or weeks; it takes that long for a buildup of toxins to become irritating. But the therapist is certainly contagious the whole time; anyone she works on could become infested too. This caution holds true for the next two parasites as well.

Head Lice

DEFINITION: WHAT ARE THEY?

This condition is also called *pediculosis,* and the animal is an arthropod that lives in head hair and sucks blood from the scalp. They are quite a bit larger than mites, and can be

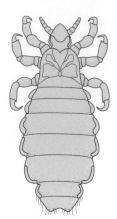

Figure 1.10. Head louse

seen easily without a microscope. (See Figure 1.10.) Their saliva is very irritating, which causes itching and the accompanying complication of possible infection.

HOW DO THEY SPREAD?

Lice jump. They also like hats. They thrive in classrooms and in batters' helmets that are shared by little league teams. A person doesn't need close contact to someone who's infected to catch lice; *no* contact is needed. All he needs to do is try on a hat at the local hat store, or hang his coat on the same hook that an infested person used.

SIGNS AND SYMPTOMS

If a client has lice, the actual parasites may or may not be obvious; they are quite mobile and can hide. But they lay eggs called *nits*. (This is the source of the term "nitpicky.") Nits cling to hair shafts and look like tiny grains of rice. They adhere quite strongly, which is a prime diagnostic feature for pediculosis. Anything else of that size and color, such as dandruff, would brush out easily.

TREATMENT

Again, repeated applications of pesticidal shampoo to kill adults and eggs is the first step in treating lice. Nit combs are used to remove eggs. Sterilizing bedding, towels, and clothing may be necessary, as well as thoroughly cleaning hats, hairbrushes, combs, and anything else that comes in contact with the head.

MASSAGE?

As is true for other parasitic infestations, massage for a client who knows he or she has head lice is contraindicated. If a therapist suspects that he has been exposed, precautionary measures should be taken at once.

Pubic Lice

DEFINITION: WHAT ARE THEY?

Pubic lice are a breed apart from their head-hair-loving relatives. They are tiny arthropods that look a lot like their nickname: crabs. (See Figure 1.11) "Crabs" are a bit less discerning in their tastes; they like pubic hair in the groin best, but they'll also live in armpit hair and body hair. They even can be found in eyebrows and eyelashes.

HOW ARE THEY SPREAD?

Pubic lice are usually spread through sexual contact, but infested massage sheets can spread them as well. They don't jump, however, and they don't spread as easily as head lice. Of all the parasites being discussed, these are the hardest to catch.

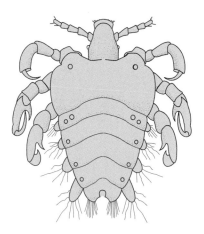

Figure 1.11. Pubic (crab) louse

SIGNS AND SYMPTOMS

Pubic lice look like tiny white crabs, about a millimeter across. They also leave nits, but they are so small they are just barely visible. Like all of the infestations being discussed, the primary symptom is itching.

TREATMENT

Pubic lice, like head lice and mites, are treated with pesticidal shampoos. Pubic lice are the least contagious of the animals discussed here, but they can be spread through contact with infested sheets. The sheets of any client suspected of a crab infestation should be isolated from all others and sterilized as soon as possible.

MASSAGE?

Massage is contraindicated for infestations of pubic lice, as for head lice, mites, and any other parasitic infestation of the skin.

Parasitic infestation carries a powerful social stigma that is negatively associated with poverty and poor hygiene. Remember that *anybody* (including massage therapists) could have this problem, and people in touch professions are in a prime position to cause many outbreaks. So be respectful, and remember that it could happen to anyone.

Warts

DEFINITION: WHAT ARE THEY?

Warts are fascinating. Most warts are small, benign neoplasms caused by the papilloma virus, which targets the keratinocytes, the same cells affected by squamous cell carcinoma. These protein-producing cells then produce extra keratin, which is the material that makes our epithelial cells hard and scaly. The result: *verruca vulgaris*.

ETIOLOGY: WHAT HAPPENS?

Warts affect young children occasionally, adults rarely, and teenagers mercilessly. Most adults who get warts are probably somehow immune-suppressed. Warts can be contagious if the edges are roughened; the virus is contained in the blood and in the shedding skin cells. They are usually self-limiting, that is, they tend to go away on their own. In that sense, they are a viral infection in slow motion: the virus slowly enters the body; it slowly takes over a few skin cells, and they slowly respond. And, slowest of all, the body finally vanquishes this not-very-threatening invader, and that's the end of it. In very healthy people, they usually clear within a year. For others, it can take longer.

SIGNS AND SYMPTOMS

Warts look like hard, cauliflower-shaped growths on the skin. (See Figure 1.12, Color Plate 8.) They are usually more of a nuisance than anything else, but when they occur on the bottom of the feet (*plantar warts*), they can seriously impair function. In this case (and sometimes when they occur on

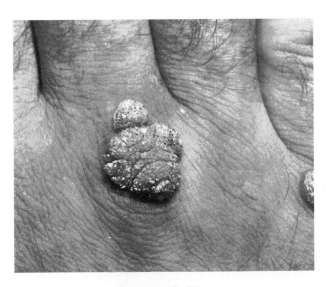

Figure 1.12. Wart

WARTS IN BRIEF

What are they?
Warts are neoplasms that arise from the keratinocytes in the epidermis; they are caused by extremely slow-acting viruses.

How are they recognized?
Typical warts (verruca vulgaris) look like hard, cauliflower-shaped growths. They usually occur on the hands. They can affect anyone, but teenagers are especially prone to them.

Is massage indicated or contraindicated?
Massage is locally contraindicated for warts. The virus is contained in the blood and shedding skin cells, and it is possible to get warts from another person.

the palm of the hands), the warts grow *inward*, creating a sensation of always stepping on something hard that never goes away. (See Figure 1.13, Color Plate 9.)

Plantar warts are distinguishable from corns and calluses because they tend *not* to be bilateral, and they tend to have a speckled appearance from blood in their dilated capillaries. Corns and calluses have no blood source, so they are white.

Verruca vulgaris is the most common kind of wart, but it's worth looking at some of the other types. Sixteen different subtypes of warts exist; only a few will be discussed here.

- Plane warts. These are small, brown, smooth warts that are most often seen on the faces of children.
- Flat warts. These are similar to vulgaris, but they are much smaller and tend to occur in exposed places. Flat warts on the face can be spread by nicks and cuts with shaving.
- Molluscum contagiosum. This is also a children's malady, involving small white lumps.

TREATMENT

If warts are not going away fast enough on their own (which can sometimes take years), medical intervention may be necessary. Any drug store carries chemical preparations that claim to be effective, but they must be used with great caution to avoid damage to surrounding tissues. A standard medical approach is to freeze warts off with liquid nitrogen, but if any of the virus remains in the body, they will probably recur. There are other options, including electrosurgery, carbon dioxide lasers, injections, and excision. These interventions will be particularly important for someone struggling with plantar warts that make it difficult to walk.

One of the best made-up remedies I have heard for warts came from a student who said, "Take a potato and cut it in six pieces. Bury each of the pieces in a different place, and *don't tell anyone where you hid them*. The wart will go away in a couple of weeks. Mine did."

MASSAGE?

Warts locally contraindicate massage. As stated above, the virus is found in the shedded skin cells around the lesion. Further, warts are often caught and torn around the edges, and if the skin is not intact, the client is a walking invitation for infection.

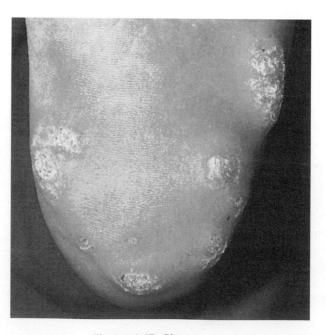

Figure 1.13. Plantar warts

Noncontagious Inflammatory Skin Disorders

Acne

DEFINITION: WHAT IS IT?

Acne is a condition in which a person becomes susceptible to small localized staphylococcus infections, usually on the face, neck, and upper back.

DEMOGRAPHICS: WHO GETS IT?

Many people have painful, awkward memories of adolescence thanks to this condition. When individuals make the transition from childhood to adulthood, their bodies start to secrete the hormones (some estrogen, but mostly testosterone) that are responsible for sexual maturity, mood swings, teenage rebellion, and excess sebum production. Adults can get acne, too, though not necessarily because of excess testosterone production.

ETIOLOGY: WHAT HAPPENS?

As the sebaceous glands go into hyperdrive, it is especially important that their ducts to the surface of the skin stay clear. If any tiny particle, like a flake of dead skin, is caught anywhere in the duct, sebum rapidly accumulates behind it. This pooling of oil is an invitation to the colonies of staphylococcus that grow on the skin. Soon a painful, acute, localized infection creates a whitehead, a pustule, a *pimple*. Blackheads are not pimples with larger-than-usual dirt particles stuck in them, but whiteheads in which the sebum has been trapped long enough to oxidize and turn black. These blemishes usually occur on the face, upper neck, and upper back, in the sebaceous glands that lubricate tiny, almost invisible hair shafts. Acne lesions that go deep into the skin are called *sebaceous cysts*. Their walls tend to become very thick and tough and they take a long time to heal. (See chapter 10, page 362.)

Stress can upset endocrine balance and slow the activity of immune system cells. ("Stress" and "adolescence" are also practically synonymous.) If those macrophages stationed in the superficial fascia are sluggish, they won't be able to fight off the staphylococcus bacteria that want to colonize the sebaceous glands. Furthermore, once the infection has subsided, those same macrophages are going to be slower to consume the residual dead bacteria and white blood cells, which means it takes longer for pimples to fade.

When acne affects adults, it's often because liver congestion makes it difficult to neutralize the normal amounts of testosterone in the system, leading to excess sebum production, and so on. What causes liver congestion? It varies from person to person, but generally high-fat diets, smoking, drugs, and chemical pollutants are the most common culprits for most people. *Hepatitis* (see chapter 7, page 296) and other disorders also severely compromise liver function. Hormonal upsets that accompany birth control pills will often produce acne in mature women as well.

SIGNS AND SYMPTOMS

The symptoms of acne are probably familiar to most people. It looks like small, red, inflamed pustules that may

---

ACNE

The root of this word is probably the result of a copyist's error. The original Greek word, *akme*, means "point of efflorescence." This describes a process in which a crystalline substance gradually changes to a powder as it dries.

ACNE IN BRIEF

What is it?

Acne is a bacterial infection of sebaceous glands usually found on the face, neck, and upper back. It is closely associated with adolescence, or liver dysfunction that results in excess testosterone in the system.

How is it recognized?

It looks like raised, inflamed pustules on the skin, sometimes with white or black tips.

Is massage indicated or contraindicated?

Massage is locally contraindicated for acne because of the risk of spreading infection, causing pain, and exacerbating the symptoms with the application of an oily lubricant.

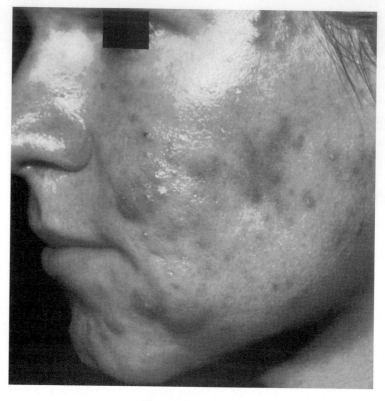

Figure 1.14. Acne

have white or black tips. It can be locally painful, but it is not generally associated with systemic infection. (See Figure 1.14, Color Plate 10.)

TREATMENT

Working with diet and other life habits to cleanse the liver and make its filtering job easier will often result in clearer skin, as well as a host of other benefits. Massage of the abdomen and liver can sometimes help in this process, but it's erroneous to claim that massage will reliably clear up acne—too many other factors need to be considered.

For teenagers with acne, the best advice is the most difficult to follow: *don't touch the face.* Touching, scratching, and popping acne lesions do little except to spread the bacteria and open the possibility of permanent scarring.

When medical help is requested for acne, interventions usually take a two-pronged attack: topical steroids are applied for their anti-inflammatory properties, and antibiotics are administered internally to attack the bacteria. The disadvantage here is that being on a long-term course of antibiotics can play havoc with intestinal flora and the immune system. One alternative is a line of drugs called retinoids, which are effective for acne, but have a list of troubling side effects including joint pain and hair loss. Retinoids are also contraindicated if the patient may be pregnant during treatment, as they are highly implicated in birth defects.

MASSAGE?

Massage of the abdomen and liver can sometimes yield good results. But massage on the lesions themselves is out of the question. Pimples are *infections* and they involve a compromised shield. The skin is no longer intact, which means massage can make the infection worse. Also, the excellent blood supply to the skin creates at least the possibility, if not the likelihood, that the infection could spread. And finally, the lubricant can also block sebaceous glands, further aggravating an already irritable situation.

Giving a client who is prone to acne a wipe down with alcohol after an oily treatment would seem to make some sense because it can cut right through and remove *all* the oil from the skin. But the human body has a habit of lashing back from such extreme changes in environment: it will work overtime to replace (and more) all the natural oils the alcohol just removed. If a client is concerned about the lubricant, the best options are to use a water-based lotion instead of oil, or to recommend that she showers with an astringent soap as soon as possible after her treatment.

Dermatitis/Eczema

DEFINITION: WHAT IS IT?

Dermatitis is an umbrella term for "skin inflammation," which is about as nonspecific as it gets. Many of the conditions in this chapter could be called dermatitis. Contact dermatitis is a skin inflammation caused by an *external* irritation. This separates it from other inflammatory skin conditions that arise from an *internal* source, such as bacterial infection (see *erysipelas*, this chapter, page 6) or *psoriasis* (this chapter, page 26). Atopic dermatitis results from an allergy to some substance to which the skin is exposed. Eczema generally falls under this category.

DEMOGRAPHICS: WHO GETS IT?

Statistics on contact dermatitis are unavailable, since this is such a general kind of problem and it can accompany many other disorders. Eczema, or atopic dermatitis, affects about 3% of the U.S. population. Children are affected as well as adults.

ETIOLOGY: WHAT HAPPENS?

Many types of dermatitis result from an overreaction in the immune system to some irritating substance. These *hypersensitivity reactions* are discussed in detail in the introduction to Lymph and Immune System Conditions (chapter 5, page 219), but it's useful to include an encapsulated version here.

The two types of hypersensitivity reactions that create skin symptoms are Type I allergic reactions and Type IV delayed reactions.

Contact dermatitis is a Type IV response, mediated by a complex organization of immune system agents. Poison oak, poison ivy, and local skin reactions to metals, soaps, dyes, or latex are examples of contact dermatitis.

Atopic dermatitis, or eczema, is an example of a Type I reaction. These are short-term immune system responses to nonthreatening stimuli. In this situation, mast cells in the exposed area release vasodilating chemicals, including histamine, which create an almost immediate inflammatory response.

There are several different forms of eczema, some of which are age specific, but there are two varieties common to adults with significantly different presentations.

Seborrheic Eczema. This is the most common variety. It seems to be genetic in origin, and it is irritated by

ECZEMA
The root of this word is the Greek *ekzeo*, which means "to boil over." This is a very apt description of many types of eczema.

DERMATITIS/ECZEMA IN BRIEF

What is it?
Dermatitis is an umbrella term for inflammation of the skin. Eczema is a type of *atopic* dermatitis, a noncontagious skin rash usually brought about by an allergic reaction. Contact dermatitis is a related but slightly different type of hypersensitivity reaction.

How is it recognized?
Dermatitis presents itself in various ways, depending on what type of skin reactions are elicited. Exposure to poison oak or poison ivy results in large inflamed wheals; metal allergies tend to be less inflamed and more isolated in area.

Eczema usually appears as one of two varieties: very dry and flaky skin (seborrheic eczema) or blistered, weepy skin (dyshidrotic eczema).

Is massage indicated or contraindicated?
The appropriateness of massage depends completely on the source of the problem and the condition of the skin. If the skin is very inflamed or has blisters or other lesions, massage is at least locally contraindicated until the acute stage has passed. If signs indicate a rash could spread (e.g., with poison oak), massage is systemically contraindicated while the irritation is present. Dry, flaky eczema indicates massage. If the skin is not itchy and the affected area is highly isolated, as with a metal allergy to a watch band or earrings, massage is only locally contraindicated.

STRESS, ALLERGIES, AND CORTISOL

Stress can ripple through the body in a number of different chemical ways. Massage therapists study some of these effects because they, too, will have some influence over what chemicals are being released, and that influence should be informed and intentional.

For people who are prone to allergies, long-term stress creates some special problems. Cortisol is the hormone that is specifically related to long-term stress. When it's secreted over a long period of time, cortisol does some things that can damage the body, such as systemically weakening the connective tissues. But cortisol does one thing that is very, *very* good: it is a powerful anti-inflammatory agent. When people undergo long-term stress, their cortisol supplies can become depleted. When cortisol is depleted, very limited resources exist within the body to quell the inflammatory reaction. And for the person subject to allergies, this translates into a difficult time de-inflaming from immune system attacks against nonthreatening stimuli like wheat, pollen, cat dander, or anything else. If the immune reaction takes the form of a skin rash, it may be called dermatitis or eczema.

This is not to say stress is the only cause of allergies, or even the most important one; it's just to point out that stress can often make allergies *worse*.

stress. Occasionally it will present as moist, weepy, blistering skin, but seborrhea eczema is usually red, flaky, and dry, occurring in the creases on the sides of the nose, the knees, the elbows, and the hands. (See Figure 1.15, Color Plate 11.) If it occurs on the scalp, seborrheic eczema has another name: dandruff. As long as the skin is dry, intact, and not puffy or itchy, massage is indicated for seborrheic eczema. Be cautious, though, about making sure there are no breaks in the skin, and use a nonirritating lubricant that won't tend to exacerbate the situation.

Dyshidrosis. This is a rarer form of eczema, but it's still fairly common. In this condition, blisters fill with fluid, occurring mostly on the hands and feet. It is sometimes described as looking like a combination of *fungal infection* (this chapter, page 7) and a contact allergy. Dyshidrosis can be very difficult to treat and sometimes requires systemic steroids. Like seborrheic eczema, dyshidrosis is noncontagious, but *unlike* the dry presentation of eczema, this one includes the danger of blisters being broken, which exposes the client to infection. Therefore, it locally contraindicates massage.

SIGNS AND SYMPTOMS

The symptoms of contact dermatitis vary according to the causative factors. Acute situations typically include local redness, swelling, and itchiness or tenderness. (See Figure 1.16, Color Plate 12.) Long-lasting, low-grade reactions may not show signs of inflammation, although mild itchiness is common.

The symptoms of eczema differ according to what type is present. Specific symptoms are listed in the descriptions above.

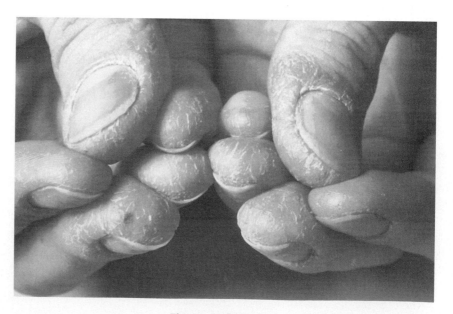

Figure 1.15. Eczema

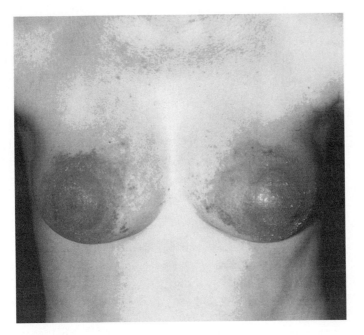

Figure 1.16. Dermatitis

TREATMENT

The medical treatment of choice for dealing with contact dermatitis and eczema is corticosteroid cream. Cortisol, among other things, is a powerful anti-inflammatory (see sidebar), but corticosteroid creams must be used *exactly* as prescribed because . . .

- Steroid creams can cause their own "steroid rash," or they can quell macrophage action, causing users to be prone to *boils*. (This chapter, page 4.)
- There can be a "backlash" effect; after the use of steroidal creams is stopped, the original complaint can come back in a more extreme version.
- If steroid creams are used over a long period of time (several months), permanent changes will be brought about by exposure to a substance that melts connective tissue. The skin can become thin, delicate, and easily damaged. (Of course, massage would be inappropriate in a case like this.)
- Finally, in a worst case scenario, the adrenal glands can suffer damage, which can be life threatening.

Massage practitioners must emphasize the importance of using medications *exactly* as they are prescribed. Above all, a person must make the effort to get to the *root* of the problem, rather than just patching over the symptoms. After all, if a person is allergic to her bath soap, what makes more sense: applying steroid cream daily for months, or changing brands?

MASSAGE?

The appropriateness of massage depends entirely on the causes and severity of a client's dermatitis. If the skin is red, hot, puffy, and itchy from a morning walk through poison oak, massage is *not* appropriate. For one thing, the inflammation will be exacerbated by extra blood in the area, and in addition, the irritating substance (the poison oak oils) can be distributed over more of the client's body, spreading the inflammation. Consider massage for this person, and all other persons with acute dermatitis, systemically contraindicated until the inflammation has subsided.

If, on the other hand, a client is displaying a small, slightly reddened, flaky, circular area on the back of her left wrist (about the place where a wristwatch would usually be

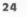

HIVES IN BRIEF

What are they?

Hives are an inflammatory skin reaction to an allergen or emotional stressor.

How are they recognized?

They can be small red spots or large wheals that are warm to the touch and itchy. They generally subside within a few hours.

Is massage indicated or contraindicated?

Massage is systemically contraindicated in the acute stage and locally contraindicated in the subacute stage of hives. By bringing even more circulation to the skin, massage would only make a bad situation worse.

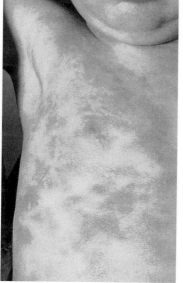

Figure 1.17. Hives

worn), it may be possible to pursue a line of questioning that will determine that massage will not aggravate or spread the irritation, which is probably being caused by an allergy to nickel.

The appropriateness of massage for eczema depends on the type that is present, and whether or not the skin has been compromised to the point where a danger exists for infection. For more details, see the individual descriptions above.

Hives

DEFINITION: WHAT ARE THEY?

Hives, also called *urticaria*, are the result of emotional stress or an allergy. They are an immune response to a substance that is not necessarily threatening to the body.

ETIOLOGY: WHAT HAPPENS?

Let's consider someone who is allergic to shellfish. Somehow, a shrimp finds its way into his lemongrass soup. Within moments, his immune system cells will launch a full-scale attack . . . but they don't quite know where to go. In the confusion, specialized cells called *mast cells* freely distributed in the superficial fascia release histamine. This causes local capillary dilation, extra cell permeability, and *lots* of edema. Hives are an example of a Type I hypersensitivity reaction, or a true "allergic" reaction.

Histamine release causes a localized inflammatory response (redness) and the edema presses on nerve endings (causing itching). Some people need an unexpected encounter with an allergen to make this happen, but for others all it takes is an unfamiliar or threatening situation. Hives are very common. It is estimated that up to 20% of all people will experience them at some point, although they are more frequent with people who suffer from other allergies. Sometimes students break out in hives when they take a test; some may while reading about diseases. Some clients who have never had massage before will get hives the first time they get on a massage table.

SIGNS AND SYMPTOMS

Hives begin as small, raised, reddened areas called wheals that may join to become larger, irregular patches. (See Figure 1.17, Color Plate 13.) The lesions are red around the outside and are sometimes paler in the middle. They are itchy and hot to the touch. They are not contagious, but are usually brought about by a food allergy, an insect bite or sting, a reaction to medication, or emotional stress.

TREATMENT

Hives are always annoying but seldom serious. If they require treatment, it's usually in the form of an antihistamine, to quell histamine release. The one exception is a condition called *angioneurotic edema*. In this case, the hives generally occur on the face and neck, and the tissue under them swells up to the point that breathing becomes difficult. It is rare, but angioneurotic edema can be life threatening, requiring an immediate injection of steroids to bring down the swelling and restore ease of breathing.

MASSAGE?

Hives are systemically contraindicated in the acute phase, and locally contraindicated in the subacute; there's no benefit to bringing more blood into an area that's already too full.

If a client has a history of this kind of problem, it is a good idea to take extra precautions to use an oil or lotion that won't initiate an attack.

Neoplastic Skin Disorders

Moles

DEFINITION: WHAT ARE THEY?

Moles, or *nevi*, are just one among several classes of birthmarks. Where freckles (*epheli*) are groups of melanocytes that become hyperreactive with exposure to UV light, and *lentigos* are simply areas where there are a large number of melanocytes that are not light sensitive, moles are benign neoplasms, or areas where melanocytes replicate on site, although without threatening to invade surrounding tissues. Moles differ from freckles and lentigos by tending to be larger, darker, slightly raised, and by having a different texture from the surrounding area. (See Figure 1.18, Color Plate 14.)

TREATMENT

A mole is not inherently dangerous, but that can change. Risk factors for moles becoming cancerous are determined by how many there are (more than six is reason to be cautious) and how big they are (anything bigger than 5 mm bears watching). About 42% of all large moles appear on the back, where clients can't see them, but *therapists* can. A doctor may suggest removing large moles, just as a precaution. Some doctors recommend tracing a large nevus and then comparing the tracing to the real thing a few times a year, in order for the patient to keep an accurate record of any changes.

MASSAGE?

Massage will neither hurt nor help moles (unless they become irritated or torn), but massage practitioners are in a unique position to see what clients may not be able to; the practitioner may be the one to spot the transition from harmless nevus to life-threatening melanoma. (See *skin cancer*, this chapter, page 28.)

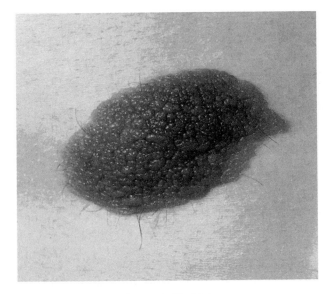

Figure 1.18. Mole

MOLES IN BRIEF

What are they?
Moles are small isolated areas where the pigment cells in the epidermis have produced excess melanin.

How are they recognized?
Moles are usually black or brown (not mixed). They tend to be raised from the skin.

Is massage indicated or contraindicated?
Massage will not help or hurt moles, but massage therapists may be able to see changes in a mole of which the client may be unaware. See more in *skin cancer*, this chapter, page 28.

PSORIASIS IN BRIEF

What is it?

Psoriasis is a noncontagious, nonspreading chronic skin disease with occasional acute episodes.

How is it recognized?

Psoriasis occurs in pink or reddish patches, sometimes with a silvery scale on top. It occurs most frequently on elbows and knees, but it can also be found on the trunk or scalp.

Is massage indicated or contraindicated?

Massage is locally contraindicated in the acute stage of psoriasis, because the extra stimulation and circulation massage provides can make a bad situation worse. But in subacute stages, as long as the skin is intact, massage is a good idea.

PSORIASIS

Psora comes from the Greek word for "the itch."

Psoriasis

DEFINITION: WHAT IS IT?

The introduction to this chapter discusses how the readiness of epithelium to repair itself is a double-edged sword. On the one hand, the body can heal quickly and thoroughly from most insults to the skin. On the other hand, sometimes the ease of replication in skin cells can cause problems, as with this condition. Psoriasis is a chronic skin disease with occasional acute episodes in which epithelial cells in isolated patches replicate too rapidly. Normal skin cells replace themselves every 28 to 32 days; in contrast, psoriatic skin cells divide every 2 to 4 days. The result is a pileup of excess cells that are itchy, red or pink, and scaly. This condition comes and goes, but at present there is no permanent cure.

DEMOGRAPHICS: WHO GETS IT?

Psoriasis affects 5 million Americans; between 150,000 and 260,000 new cases are reported every year. It seems to run in families, and it is most common in individuals between ten and forty years old. (Older and younger people get it too, but not as often.) Psoriasis affects men and women equally.

ETIOLOGY: WHAT HAPPENS?

There are several theories about why psoriasis happens. Recent research indicates that an autoimmune mistake causes T cells in the skin to stimulate inflammation and excess cell production. Vitamin D deficiencies have been observed; one treatment for psoriasis is a topical application of Vitamin D that slows skin cell replication. Genetic predisposition for the disease is another possibility, although no specific genetic marker has been identified.

Psoriatic attacks can be triggered by a number of things: physical or emotional trauma, skin damage, sunburn, hormonal changes, some prescription drugs, or a state of immune suppression. The "repair impulse" makes sense as a response to events that damage the skin, such as sunburn or other infections, but the pathway from emotional upset to psoriasis is indistinct.

SIGNS AND SYMPTOMS

This is a very common condition; most people have at least seen it. It usually takes the form of raised red or pink patches that, if they are present for a long time, develop a white or silvery "scale" on top; they also have sharply defined edges. (See Figure 1.19, Color Plate 15.) The patches, or "plaques," are sometimes slightly itchy, but seldom uncomfortable unless they are in an acute stage, when they can itch and burn severely. Plaques are usually on the knees or elbows, but they can be found on the scalp, trunk, palms, and soles as well. Psoriasis can also get under fingernails and toenails, where it can cause pitting, infection, and sometimes results in the loss of the nail altogether.

In its subacute or nonactive phase, a slight discoloration on the skin will sometimes be seen where the lesions tend to appear. This is especially true on the trunk.

COMPLICATIONS

Although rarely a life-threatening condition, psoriasis can be extreme and uncomfortable in the acute stages. If the patient is very young or very old, the condition may be more difficult to handle. In some severe cases, psoriasis causes profound drying and cracking of

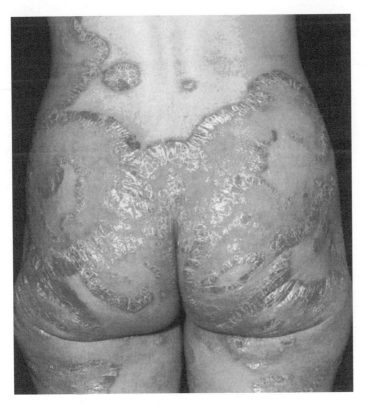

Figure 1.19. Psoriasis

the skin that can lead to infection. The only other complication of psoriasis is a fairly rare condition called *psoriatic arthritis*. This is a type of joint inflammation that affects approximately 10 to 20% of psoriasis patients. The symptoms are very similar to *rheumatoid arthritis* (chapter 2, page 80). If a client has psoriatic arthritis, follow the same rules as for rheumatoid arthritis.

TREATMENT

For such a common skin condition, psoriasis can be surprisingly resistant to treatment. Treatment strategies differ according to the severity of the condition. Three main avenues are pursued: topical applications, phototherapy, and systemic medications.

Topical medications include anything from coal tar extract to steroid creams. The drawbacks of long-term steroid applications are spelled out in the *eczema* section (this chapter, page 21).

Phototherapy stimulates Vitamin D production, which in turn will inhibit skin cell replication. *Some* exposure to UV light can be helpful, but too much will tend to aggravate the outbreaks.

Systemic medications, including steroidal drugs or even cytotoxic drugs (such as chemotherapy), may be used to limit the activity of those skin cells that have run amok. Psoriasis and cancer actually share the trait of uncontrolled replication, and this option is occasionally successful.

Sometimes therapies may be combined for extra effect. The best example of this is PUVA. This is a combination of a special drug and UV light exposure, and it has had considerable success. Unfortunately, it is also linked to increased chances of contracting basal cell or squamous cell carcinoma.

Although there are many types of treatment for psoriasis, none of them has shown to be a permanent solution. The skin will tend to acquire resistance to various treatments, so patients with very severe cases of psoriasis must frequently change strategies.

SKIN CANCER IN BRIEF

What is it?

Skin cancer is cancer in the stratum basale of the epidermis (basal cell carcinoma or BCC); cancer of the keratinocytes in the epidermis (squamous cell carcinoma or SCC); or cancer of the melanocytes (pigment cells) of the epidermis (malignant melanoma).

How is it recognized?

For BCC and SCC, look for the cardinal sign: sores that never heal. These are the clearest indication of BCC or SCC. For malignant melanoma, look for a mole that exhibits the ABCDEs of melanoma discussed on page 32.

Is massage indicated or contraindicated?

For BCC, which does not tend to metastasize, massage is locally contraindicated, as long as the lesion has been diagnosed by a dermatologist. For SCC or malignant melanoma, circulatory massage, which moves material (including malignant cancer cells) into the lymphatic system, is systemically contraindicated until the client has been cleared by a doctor.

SKIN CANCER STATISTICS

Here's the bad news:

- By the time a person has reached 18 years of age, he will have received half or more of his lifetime's exposure to the sun.

- One serious sunburn can increase the risk of skin cancer by up to 50%.

- It is estimated that 1 out of every 7 people in the United States will develop some form of skin cancer sometime in their life.

- Of all people in the United States who reach the age of 65, 40 to 50% will have some kind of skin cancer at least once.

- About 800,000 new cases of squamous cell and basal cell carcinoma are reported every year.

- About 34,000 cases of malignant melanoma presently occur each year, but since 1973, the incidence level has increased by 4% every year.   *(continued)*

MASSAGE?

In ancient Greece, massage with olive oil was the prescribed treatment for psoriasis. It is now recognized that massage *on* the lesions during an acute outbreak will probably only aggravate the situation by stimulating circulation in an area where too much activity is already occurring. Consider this a local contraindication in the acute phase, but otherwise massage is appropriate. (Of course, first it's necessary to be sure drying or cracking of the skin hasn't occurred to make the client vulnerable to infection.) Psoriasis won't be spread by massage, it's not contagious, and massage indirectly may be able to help deal with some of the internal and external stress factors that can stimulate an outbreak.

Skin Cancer

DEFINITION: WHAT IS IT?

Cancer is the uncontrolled replication of cells into tumors. These tumors can damage surrounding tissues, spread throughout the body, and can sometimes be fatal. The cells that replicate in cancer are often cells that have to tolerate a lot of wear and tear: skin cells, the epithelium of the lungs, and the inner layer of the colon are some good examples. These cells heal easily and rapidly, but sometimes that feature backfires, and a situation develops like skin cancer, in which cells that have endured a lifetime of abuse start "healing" in a way that could quite possibly kill.

DEMOGRAPHICS: WHO GETS IT?

Some people wish that sleep could be cumulative—that a person could sleep an extra fourteen hours on a weekend, and then not be tired for all of the following week. Well, in a certain way, sunlight *is* cumulative. Picture a person playing on the monkey bars when he's five, rollerblading when he's ten, hiking in the mountains when he's fifteen, sailing when he's forty, and snorkeling when he's fifty. His skin cells are keeping accurate records of exactly how much and how often he's insulted them with too much sun. And one day, those skin cells may respond to all that exposure by simply going into hyperdrive production. This is a particular risk if a person . . .

- has pale skin that burns but doesn't tan.
- lives in a place with a lot of sunshine.
- spends a good deal of time outside.
- is in any way immune-suppressed.
- is mature and has built up a lifetime of exposure to the sun in his skin cells.

ETIOLOGY: WHAT HAPPENS?

Four basic types of skin cancer have been identified, and each will be discussed in detail.

Actinic Keratosis: Precancerous Lesions

DEFINITION: WHAT IS IT?

This is a precancerous condition that can lead to squamous cell carcinoma.

SIGNS AND SYMPTOMS

Brown or red scaly lesions usually appear on the forehead or other areas subject to a lot of exposure to sun. These sores will form a crust, but don't heal normally. The crust falls off and forms over again. (See Figure 1.20, Color Plate 16.) This pattern is the single most important sign of nonmelanoma skin cancer. It is estimated that one person in every six will have actinic keratosis (AK) lesions at some time, and 10 to 20% of all AK lesions develop into squamous cell carcinoma.

TREATMENT

AK lesions are usually frozen off with liquid nitrogen. They may also be injected with medication, or a topical ointment may be applied. Very large lesions may be excised.

MASSAGE!

Any undiagnosed skin condition contraindicates massage. If a client has AK lesions presently, he should consider having them removed promptly. If he has a history of AK, but nothing more serious has developed, massage is appropriate.

Basal Cell Carcinoma

DEFINITION: WHAT IS IT?

This is by far the most common type of skin cancer; it accounts for about 75 to 90% of all skin cancer cases. Fortunately, it is also the least serious. It is a slow-growing, nonmetastasizing tumor of epithelial cells in the stratum basale of the epidermis. It is not usually

> ### SKIN CANCER STATISTICS, cont.
>
> - Approximately 9,300 deaths from skin cancer were recorded in the United States in 1995.
>
> The good news is that education and vigilance make a big difference in the mortality rates for this disease. Studies done in Queensland, Australia, where melanoma is more common than anywhere else in the world, show that early intervention in the development of malignant melanoma dramatically improves the chances of survival. All types of skin cancer are 100% survivable, if they are caught early enough.

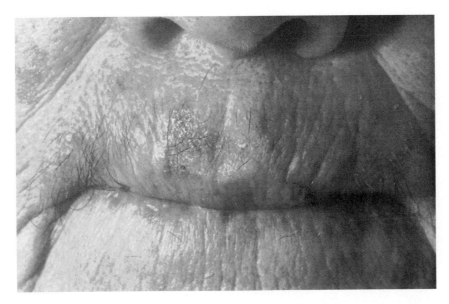

Figure 1.20. Actinic keratosis

dangerous, although if the tumor is left untreated for years, it can become life threatening because other tissues are eroded by the tumor's growth, for example, nearby arteries.

SIGNS AND SYMPTOMS

Basal cell carcinoma (BCC) can be tricky to identify, because it looks like all sorts of different things. Typically it appears on the face, around the bridge of the nose or the eyebrow. It looks like a small, hard, pearl-colored lump, with rounded edges, and a soft, sunken middle. The borders are often hard, and they may bleed and form crusts. The middle of the lump is usually soft, with an open sore that may scab but never permanently heals (an ulceration). BCCs are sometimes called "rodent ulcers." (See Figures 1.21–1.23, Color Plates 17–19.)

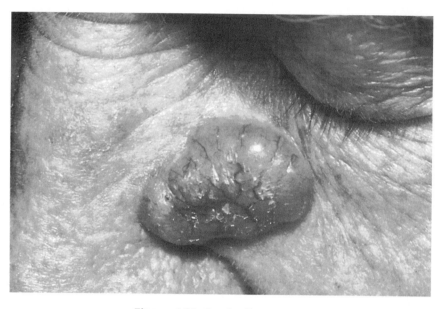

Figure 1.21. Basal cell carcinoma

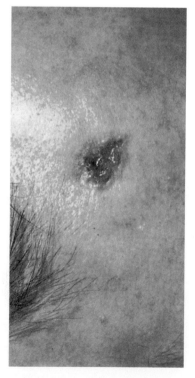

Figure 1.22. Basal cell carcinoma

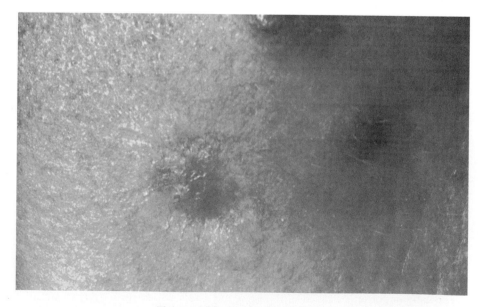

Figure 1.23. Basal cell carcinoma

Another type of BCC is particularly common for elderly fair-skinned people who have spent a lot of time in the sun. This variety looks like flat sores, not on the face, but on the back and trunk. Similar to typical facial BCCs, these sores do not heal, but simply crust, shed the scab, and crust again. This variety of BCC is easily mistaken for seborrheic keratosis, a nonmalignant condition, which is why it's essential for massage therapists to refer any client with suspicious lesions for further diagnosis.

TREATMENT

Basal cell carcinoma, because it grows so very slowly and does not metastasize, responds very well to simply being excised: cut out with a knife or a laser. The tumor-producing cells can also be killed off with liquid nitrogen or with radiation. Occasionally BCC recurs, so it is wise to keep a close watch for any nonhealing sores after an episode.

MASSAGE?

Of course, the ulcer itself locally contraindicates massage (if it is diagnosed as basal cell carcinoma). This isn't something that will spread through the body or that massage will make worse in any way. If a client fits the profile for the flat sore on the trunk, the practitioner may be the one to spot it in the first place. But if there are suspicious lesions on the skin, it is necessary to have a diagnosis *before* the client is safe to receive massage.

Squamous Cell Carcinoma

DEFINITION: WHAT IS IT?

This is a malignancy of keratinocytes in the epidermis. Keratinocytes are the cells that produce keratin, the protein that fills up the epithelial cells migrating toward the surface of the skin.

SIGNS AND SYMPTOMS

Squamous cell carcinoma, or SCC, can occur anywhere there is epidermis —on the skin, usually, but occasionally on mucous membranes too. It is especially common on ears, hands, and lower lips, but it can also happen *inside* the mouth, often as a response to pipe smoking or chewing tobacco and the constant irritation that those habits incur. SCC accounts for about 22% of all skin cancers. It is significantly more dangerous than BCC, since it *can* metastasize through the lymph system, and the tumors can infiltrate deeper tissues far more quickly than BCC.

SCC tumors often happen on preexisting lesions on sun-exposed skin. In other words, they happen where the skin has had to repair itself before. They generally start as hard, firm lumps resembling a wart. The sores appear and *don't heal*. The borders of SCCs are often less distinct than the more self-contained basal cell tumors. (See Figures 1.24 and 1.25, Color Plates 20 and 21.)

Actinic keratosis and squamous cell carcinoma bear one key feature in common with BCC: an open sore that never quite heals. Often a crust forms, but it doesn't hold on; inevitably the crust falls off, and starts to form again. All the while, the sore is ulcerating, and the cancer cells are getting a deeper and deeper grip on the underlying tissues. So people who are experiencing this cycle with a sore *anywhere* on the body, they should *run, not walk* to their nearest dermatologist.

TREATMENT

As with BCC, squamous cell carcinomas are frozen and/or excised. With SCC, however, it is especially important to be sure that all the affected tissue is removed, because if any "hot" cells should find their way into the lymphatics, the cancer could spread elsewhere

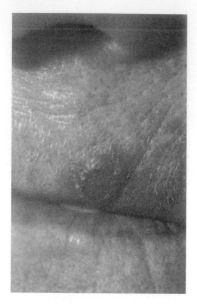

Figure 1.24. Squamous
cell carcinoma

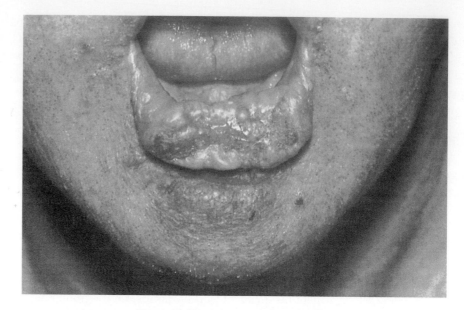

Figure 1.25. Squamous cell carcinoma

in the body. Therefore, excess tissue is often also taken, which may require postoperative skin grafts. The area also may be radiated, to make doubly sure all of the cancer-causing cells are dead.

MASSAGE?

Squamous cell carcinoma contraindicates massage. If a client has had SCC in the past, get approval from his doctor before proceeding. This condition spreads through the lymph system; massage can make it worse. If a client is showing signs of SCC in the present, he should postpone his massage appointment and consult a dermatologist.

Malignant Melanoma

DEFINITION: WHAT IS IT?

Melanocytes are the pigment cells that give skin its color. They are located deep in the epidermal layer. Melanin protects us, as much as it can, from harmful UV radiation from the sun. As in the other cancers discussed here, if these cells get *too much* activity, they can start replicating without control. This is malignant melanoma.

Melanoma is the leading cause of death from skin diseases, and the cause of 75% of all deaths from skin cancer. Fortunately, it is also the least common variety of skin cancer, accounting for about 3% of skin cancer cases (although those statistics are expected to climb).

SIGNS AND SYMPTOMS

Melanoma often starts from a preexisting mole that later in life begins to change; it lightens, darkens, thickens, becomes elevated. Sometimes it is itchy, or bleeds around the edges. (See Figure 1.26, Color Plate 22.)

Here is a simple mnemonic to remember the key diagnostic features for melanoma:

- A: Asymmetrical. Most benign moles are circular or oval. A melanoma will have an indeterminate shape.
- B: Border. The borders of melanomas are irregular and may be indistinct as they blend into the skin.

- C: Color. The colors of most moles are consistent: they are brown or black, but not both. Melanomas are typically multicolored, with brown, black, and even purple all mixed together.
- D: Diameter. Melanomas are large. Any mole that is bigger than 5 mm across should be examined by a dermatologist.
- E: Elevated. Melanomas are usually at least partly elevated from the skin. They may even be big enough to snag on things and bleed.

Because melanoma is a disease of *cumulative* sun exposure, it rarely occurs in young people. Large moles that develop *after* adolescence, however, are highly suspect. Moles in areas that are subject to a lot of irritation are at especially high risk of becoming cancerous.

Men most often get melanoma on the trunk, neck, or head. Women tend to get it on the arms or legs.

TREATMENT

Treatment for melanoma is generally radical; because this cancer spreads very rapidly, there is literally no time to lose. Once a lesion has been positively identified and staged (evaluated for how far it has progressed), it is usually attacked with every weapon in the book: surgical excision, radiation, and removal of all the nearby lymph nodes. Even then the prognosis is entirely dependent on how completely the rogue cells have been removed, and if they were caught before metastasizing to nearby lymph nodes or other organs.

Melanoma does not presently respond to available chemotherapy medications. A promising new aspect of melanoma treatment is emerging with the advent of a variety of "melanoma vaccines." One of these is not a vaccine in the proper sense of the word, that would stimulate the immune system to attack an invader. Rather, it is a drug that serves to *sensitize* the patient to other anticancer drugs. In other words, it makes the cells more receptive, and the drugs work better. Other new treatments work with immune system agents to help the body identify and attack tumors. These are not preventatives for melanoma, but they show promise for stopping the growth of cancerous tumors.

MASSAGE?

Massage is contraindicated for malignant melanoma. The key feature of this disease is how quickly it spreads through the lymph system to create tumors in other parts of the body.

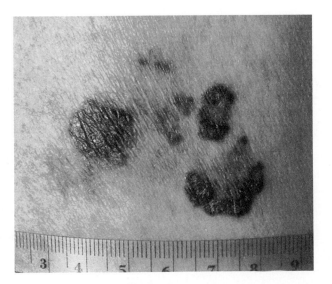

Figure 1.26. Malignant melanoma

Massaging someone with melanoma will help to metastasize his cancer much more efficiently than if it had been left alone.

In situations in which a cancer patient is terminally ill, massage can sometimes be a valuable part of care. In hospice situations, when the patient is aware of the risks and is more interested in the quality of life than the quantity, massage is often taught to family members and friends who are caring for the dying person.

Skin Injuries

Burns

DEFINITION: WHAT ARE THEY?

In discussing burns, most people think about touching a hot iron, or brushing a hand across a broiler rack. But the world of burns goes beyond household appliances. A person can sustain burn damage from dry heat (e.g., irons and broilers), wet heat (e.g., hot liquids or steam), electricity, friction (e.g., "rug burn"), radiation, and corrosive chemicals. Any one of these can destroy the proteins in the exposed skin cells, which causes the cells to die. If a significant amount of skin is affected, it will be unable to accomplish its protective tasks—it *won't* provide a shield from microbial invasion, it *won't* help to maintain a stable temperature, and, perhaps most important, it *won't* provide protection from fluid loss. This opens the door to a number of complications including loss of water, plasma, and plasma proteins, which will lead to shock.

ETIOLOGY: WHAT HAPPENS?

The severity of burns is determined by how deep they go and how much surface area they cover. Three layers form the skin. Three degrees of burn severity exist. This is not entirely coincidence.

First-degree Burns.   This is a sometimes quite painful but relatively mild irritation of the superficial epidermis, characterized by redness but no blistering. Mild sunburn is the most common example. Overexposure to the sun damages cells in the epithelium, creating an inflammatory response. This leads to pain, heat, redness, and swelling. (See Figure 1.27, Color Plate 23.) Sunburns generally heal

BURNS IN BRIEF

What are they?
Burns are caused by damage to the skin that causes the cells to die. They can be caused by fire, overexposure to the sun, dry heat, wet heat, electricity, radiation, extreme cold, and toxic chemicals.

How are they recognized?
First-degree burns involve mild inflammation. Second-degree burns include blistering and damage at the deeper levels of the epidermis. Third-degree burns penetrate the dermis itself and will often show white or black charred edges. In the postacute stage, serious burns will often develop shrunken, contracted scar tissue over the area of affected skin.

Is massage indicated or contraindicated?
Massage is locally contraindicated for all burns (except, perhaps, mild sunburns) in the acute stage. In the subacute and postacute stages, massage may be performed around the damaged area within pain tolerance of the client.

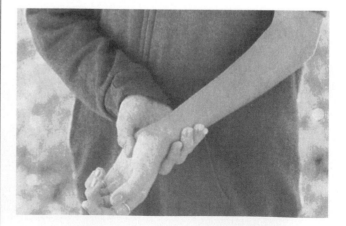

Figure 1.27. First-degree burn (sunburn)

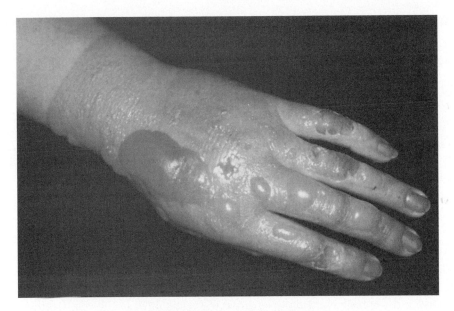

Figure 1.28. Second-degree burn

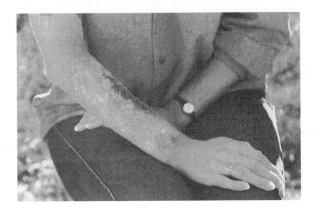

Figure 1.29. Third-degree burn with scar tissue

in two to three days, sometimes with flaking and peeling. If the sunburn is more severe, it will lead to blistering, which is a sign of . . .

Second-degree Burns.   This is damage that involves all layers of the epidermis, and possibly some of the dermis too. Symptoms include redness, blisters, edema, and a lot of pain. Still, if the burn area is fairly small, it will heal in a week (or maybe within a month, if it involves the dermis). Usually the hair shafts and glands do not sustain permanent damage, although some superficial scarring may occur. Second-degree burns can result from sun exposure, as well as from many other things, such as steam under pressure, toxic chemicals, or hot glue guns. (See Figure 1.28, Color Plate 24.)

Third-degree Burns.   These go right down to the bottom of the dermis or beyond, destroying hair shafts, sebaceous glands, erector pilae muscles, sweat glands, and even nerve endings, which paradoxically makes third-degree burns less painful than second-degree burns. Symptoms include whiteness and/or charring. Third-degree burns are dangerous for all the reasons mentioned above: risk of infection, fluid loss, and shock, especially if a significant percentage of the body surface has been affected. In addition to all this, one of the special problems with third-degree burns is the habit they have of contracting quickly and forming a very confining web of scar tissue, even with quickly applied skin grafts. (See Figure 1.29, Color Plate 25.)

SIGNS AND SYMPTOMS

The symptoms of burn damage depend on what level of skin has been affected. Details on symptoms by degree of damage are listed above.

MASSAGE?

The *only* kind of burn that is appropriate for circulatory massage in the acute stage is a very mild sunburn, and of course even then one must work within the client's pain tolerance. By sloughing off dead cells, massage can speed the healing process along, but it's not something to do without a client's permission.

Other burns may be approached in the *subacute* stage as a local contraindication; it's all right to work around the edges *within pain tolerance* to improve elasticity and minimize scar tissue, taking care not to expose the client to infection. In this situation, it is important to work with a doctor to establish when the burn is in a subacute stage and to rule out any other tissue trauma that may contraindicate massage. Manual Lymph Drainage, a technique that specializes in working reflexively to stimulate lymph flow, may also be used with recent burn victims.

Lastly, if the burns are obviously long past the acute and subacute stages—that is, the client feels no pain and all that's left is residual scar tissue—massage is safe. The only caution here is that in serious cases, the client may suffer permanent nerve damage. If that is the case, she won't be able to feel if the massage is doing any damage.

Decubitus Ulcers

DEFINITION: WHAT ARE THEY?

This condition, which is also known as *bedsores*, *pressure sores*, and *trophic ulcers*, is one massage therapists would most likely see when working in a hospital, a hospice, or some other setting with bedridden patients. The problem stems from chronic inadequate blood flow to the skin that stretches over bony or otherwise prominent areas. It almost always occurs in some area that has had constant contact with a surface—usually a bed, but sometimes a cast or a splint.

DEMOGRAPHICS: WHO GETS THEM?

The risk factors for decubitus ulcers include being elderly, underweight, male, nonambulatory, and incontinent.

ETIOLOGY: WHAT HAPPENS?

Imagine looking microscopically into the skin of an immobilized person whose circulation is not regularly stimulated by themselves or anyone else. Capillaries are squeezed between bone and bed, and new epithelial cells are starving for nutrition. The cells close to the surface of the skin died long ago, but now the cells in the deeper layers of the epidermis are dying, too. Small lesions appear at the surface. Bacteria take advantage of the opportunity, and they begin to attack the already weakened skin cells. Capillaries are too narrow to let anything through, including the white blood cells that would otherwise limit the intruders. Gradually, the tissue dies, and along with it the possibility of regeneration. If left unchecked, the ulcer

---

DECUBITUS ULCERS IN BRIEF

What are they?
Decubitus ulcers, or bedsores, are ulcers caused by impaired circulation to the skin. Lack of blood supply leads to irreplaceable tissue death.

How are they recognized?
Unlike other sores, ulcers don't crust over; they remain open wounds that are highly vulnerable to infection.

Is massage indicated or contraindicated?
Once the tissue has been damaged, massage is *strictly* locally contraindicated until the sores have completely healed over.

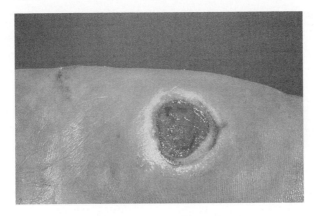

Figure 1.30. Decubitus ulcer

can destroy the dermis, the superficial fascia, and proceed down to the bone. (See Figure 1.30, Color Plate 26.)

SIGNS AND SYMPTOMS

When bedsores first start, they produce slightly reddened, irritated areas on the skin. Soon they turn purple, and then *necrosis*, or tissue death, begins. Ulcers on the skin (and anywhere else on the body) differ from other types of sores because they don't go through a normal healing process. They won't form a crust to cover the regenerating epithelial tissue as ordinary cuts and sores will. Of course, eventually they *can* heal, but not in a normal way; if circulation to the affected area is finally restored, the lesion will close with scar tissue grown over the area, but a permanent dip will remain where the dead tissue will never grow back.

Bedsores can start in a surprisingly short amount of time. They can be a real danger for people with spinal injuries who may have to travel for hours strapped to a back-board. Bedsores and joint and muscle degeneration are the primary reasons comatose people are moved and turned frequently. Heels, buttocks, the sacrum, and elbows are the most common places for bedsores to appear.

TREATMENT

The biggest danger for someone with bedsores is the possibility of infection, which can be life threatening for someone who is bedridden and already immune suppressed. The latest treatment protocols outlined by the Agency for Health Care Policy and Research include good nutrition (extra high protein calories and minerals), avoidance of pressure of any kind, and proper cleaning and dressing of the wound.[1]

Public attention to this problem has been aroused recently as the number of elderly patients rapidly rises, and the cost of treating bedsores is topping $8.5 billion dollars a year. Consequently, more efforts are being made to find ways to prevent these injuries, since preventing bedsores costs only a fraction of what it takes to treat them.

MASSAGE?

Bedsores occur because circulation is interrupted for a long enough period to kill cells. It would make sense that massage, with its wonderful influence over circulatory flow, would be an appropriate way to deal with this problem. But because of the peculiar open-sore nature of ulcers, and because it's virtually impossible to sterilize hands, massage is *not* appropriate for bedsores. If a client is at risk for developing bedsores (and is not otherwise

---

[1] Sandy Rovner. Treating bedsores with a new approach. Washington Post, January 31, 1995.

OPEN WOUNDS AND SORES IN BRIEF

What are they?
These include any injury to the skin that has not healed and that is vulnerable to infection if exposed to bacteria or other microorganisms. Skin injuries are vulnerable as long as there is a visible crust or scab.

How are they recognized?
A crust or scab appears at the site of the injury.

Is massage indicated or contraindicated?
Massage is locally contraindicated for any unhealed skin injury with which bleeding has occurred. When the underlying epidermis has been completely replaced, the scab will fall off and the wound will no longer be at risk for infection.

Massage may be systemically contraindicated if the skin injury is connected to a contraindicated underlying condition such as diabetes.

contraindicated for massage), the improved skin nutrition massage provides could be an excellent preventative measure. But if the sore has already begun to fester, a significant danger of infection exists. The latest research shows that even working around the edges of bedsores is risky, so bedsores locally contraindicate massage.

Open Wounds and Sores

DEFINITION: WHAT ARE THEY?

Many different technical names are listed for all the different ways skin can be damaged: lacerations (rips and tears), incisions (cuts), punctures (any kind of hole), avulsions (something has been ripped off, like a finger or an ear), abrasions (scrapes), vesicles (blisters), pustules (blisters filled with pus), and ulcers (sores with dead tissue that don't complete a normal healing process). Knowing these technical terms is important, but not as important as knowing that massage is inappropriate for any condition in which skin is not entirely intact.

For more information on the specifics of the healing process, see *scar tissue*, this chapter, page 38.

MASSAGE?

Only one rule governs this situation: *if the intactness of the skin has been compromised in any way, the client is a walking invitation for infection.* Usually these injuries are just local contraindications. The exception would be if the open wounds or sores were caused by some other contraindicated condition such as *diabetes* (chapter 4, page 210) or *mites* (this chapter, page 13). But if the client is otherwise healthy, and if he's showing no signs of infection at the site of the wound, massage elsewhere on the body is appropriate.

Scar Tissue

The body's ability to heal itself is one of the wonders of nature. This section deals with superficial scar tissue rather than the internal scarring that accompanies soft tissue injuries, so discussion will be limited to what's happening on the skin.

SCAR TISSUE IN BRIEF

What is it?
It is the growth of new tissue, skin or fascia, after injury.

How is it recognized?
Scar tissue on the skin often lacks pigmentation and hair follicles.

Is massage indicated or contraindicated?
Massage is locally contraindicated during the acute stage of any injury in which the skin has been damaged. In the subacute stage, massage may improve the quality of the healing process.

ETIOLOGY: WHAT HAPPENS?

The skin, because it is subject to a lot of wear and tear, has cells with special properties not found anywhere else in the body. If there is a scrape or abrasion, some basal cells will actually detach themselves from the basement membrane and begin to migrate in a single-layered sheet across the wound. When they reach the other side and touch other epithelial cells, an internal code makes them stop moving. (The absence of this internal code, which is called *contact inhibition*, makes cancer cells so dangerous; nothing ever tells them to *stop*.)

Meanwhile, back at the original site, stationary basal cells are duplicating in order to build up the ranks of migrating cells. When the whole wound has been covered, the new sheet of basal cells will begin dividing to form new strata. After enough bulk has accumulated, the crust (or scab) will fall off and the cells on the surface will become keratinized. Then the wound is healed; it is no longer vulnerable to infection. The whole process generally takes 24 to 48 hours, depending on the size and location of the lesion.

If the injury goes deeper than the dermis, the healing process is more complicated. All the fibroblasts in the area are summoned to the site, so beneath all that basal cell activity, a lot of fibroblastic activity also takes place. This "fill-in" connective tissue is called *granulation tissue*. Eventually, it will change to become an accumulation of collagenous scar tissue, meant to knit up the fascia, but which may intrude on the superficial layers as well. If the scar tissue doesn't stay within the boundaries of the original injury, it is called a *hypertrophic* scar. Sometimes the fibroblasts get much too active and produce much more collagen than is necessary. The scar overflows the injury, resulting in a permanently raised mass of tissue. This is called a *keloid* scar, which can be a very annoying, but seldom dangerous complication of surgery or deep-wound healing.

Scar tissue differs from normal skin in some important ways. The collagen fibers are much denser and they don't lay down in the same patterns as uninjured tissue; no epidermis is on the top; fewer blood vessels are present; and the tissue will probably be missing hair follicles, normal skin glands, and possibly even sensory neurons.

TREATMENT

If hypertrophic scar tissue doesn't recede within a few months of the injury, it may be injected with cortisone to dissolve the excess collagen. Keloids are frozen with liquid nitrogen and then treated with cortisone, but they may still recur.

When a large surface area of skin has been damaged, it is important to control the amount of scar tissue that accumulates. Gene therapy for skin healing is being developed, which involves "shot gun" blasts of genes for the production of a hormone called *epidermal growth factor*. This treatment, which will be useful for very deep wounds, skin diseases, and ulcers, has been shown to speed healing by about 20%. Interestingly, a similar approach is being developed to *slow* healing, which would minimize the accumulation of unsightly scar tissue.

MASSAGE?

Obviously, massage is only appropriate in the subacute stage of healing. Why? Because if the skin is not intact, the client is prone to infection. If someone is healing from a deep wound, such as one occurring with a surgery, they will often benefit from work *around* the area, which will keep the skin supple and seems to inhibit the buildup of keloid-type scars. (See *postoperative situations*, chapter 10, page 367). If a client has old, old scar tissue on the skin, know that sensation in those areas may be reduced, and be extra solicitous of feedback.

Other Skin Conditions

Ichthyosis

DEFINITION: WHAT IS IT?

Ichthyosis is a rare disorder in which the skin is pathologically dry. It creates distinctive diamond-shaped plates on the skin that resemble fish scales—hence its name.

ICHTHYOSIS IN BRIEF

What is it?
Ichthyosis is pathologically dry skin—much more severe than average dry skin.

How is it recognized?
Ichthyosis creates distinctive diamond-shaped "scales" on the skin, usually on the lower legs.

Is massage indicated or contraindicated?
Massage is definitely indicated for this condition. It probably won't be a permanent solution to this congenital problem, but it can certainly make it better in the short run. Take care to avoid areas where cracking exposes the blood to the possibility of infection.

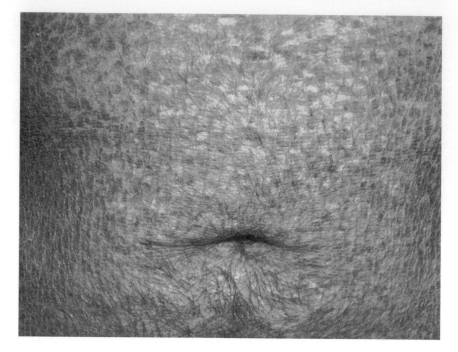

Figure 1.31. Ichthyosis

ICHTHYOSIS

Ichthys is Greek for "fish." Ichthyosis means, literally, "fish condition." Other terms for this condition are equally descriptive: "alligator skin," "sauriasis" (*sauros* is from the Greek for "lizard," as in *dinosaur*), "sauroderma," and "sauriosis."

Sometimes the affected area may become darker than the surrounding areas. (See Figure 1.31, Color Plate 27.)

There are several types of ichthyosis. It can be congenital and associated with birth defects. Other cases are associated with a variety of other diseases, including *Hodgkin's disease* (see chapter 5, page 225) and leprosy.

MASSAGE?

This is one of the few skin conditions that, in the absence of underlying contraindications, massage can really help; it does so by adding nonirritating oil to the skin and by stimulating the sebaceous glands to become active, too. Be cautious, however, of skin that is *so* dry it cracks down to the capillary level, whereupon it becomes, like all compromised skin, susceptible to infection.

CHAPTER REVIEW QUESTIONS: INTEGUMENTARY SYSTEM CONDITIONS

1. Describe the relationship between cortisol depletion and allergies.

2. A client has eczema on her hands that is extremely dry and flaky. Does this condition indicate or contraindicate massage? Why?

3. A client has severe ichthyosis that is cracked and oozing. Does this condition indicate or contraindicate massage? Why?

4. What does psoriasis have in common with cancer?

5. When working with a client who is prone to acne, is it a good idea to follow massage with an alcohol rinse to remove the oil? Why?

6. A client has white flakes that cling to hair shafts and don't brush out. What condition is probably present?

7. A client has a circle-shaped, reddish-pink mark on the back of his upper thigh. What condition may be present?

8. What should be done with this client's massage sheets?

9. In what stage of the development of a decubitus ulcer is massage appropriate?

10. In what situation would an open sore be a systemic rather than simply a local contraindication?

BIBLIOGRAPHY, INTEGUMENTARY SYSTEM CONDITIONS

General References, Integumentary System

1. Carmine D. Clemente, PhD. Anatomy: A regional atlas of the human body. 3rd ed. Baltimore: Urban & Schwarzenburg, 1987.
2. I. Damjanou. Pathology for the health-related professions. Philadelphia: Saunders, 1996.
3. Giovanni de Dominico, Elizabeth Wood. Beard's massage. Philadelphia: Saunders, 1997.
4. Deane Juhan. Job's body: A handbook for bodywork. Barrytown, NY: Station Hill Press, Inc., 1987.
5. Jeffrey R. M. Kunz, MD, Asher J. Finkel, MD, eds. The American Medical Association family medical guide. New York: Random House, Inc., 1987.
6. Elaine M. Marieb, RN, PhD. Human anatomy and physiology. Redwood City, CA: Benjamin/Cummings Publishing Co., Inc., 1989.
7. Ruth Lundeen Memmler, MD, Dina Lin Wood, RN, BS, PhN. The human body in health and disease. 5th ed. Philadelphia: JB Lippincott Co., 1983.
8. Mary Lou Mulvihill. Human diseases: A systemic approach. 2nd ed. Norwalk, CT: Appleton & Lange, 1987.
9. Stedman's medical dictionary. 26th ed. Baltimore: Williams & Wilkins, 1995.
10. Taber's cyclopedic dictionary. 14th ed. Philadelphia: F.A. Davis Company, 1981.
11. Gerard J. Tortora, Nicholas P. Anagnostakos. Principles of anatomy and physiology. 6th ed. New York: Biological Sciences Textbook, Inc.; A&P Textbooks, Inc.; and Elia-Sparta, Inc., Harper & Row Publishers, Inc., 1990.
12. Janet Travell, MD, David G. Simons, MD. Myofascial pain and dysfunction: The trigger point manual. Baltimore: Williams & Wilkins, 1983.

Fungal Infections

1. MedicineNet: Power points about athlete's foot. Information Network, Inc., 1995–1997. URL: http://www.medicinenet.com. Accessed fall 1997.

Herpes Simplex

1. Bruce Bartholomew. Herpes life cycle. In Life Energy Systems, 1995. URL: http://www.herpeszone.com/GENINFO.HTM. Accessed fall 1997.
2. Genital herpes. National Institute of Allergy and Infectious Diseases, August 1992. URL: http://www.niaid.nih.gov/factsheets/stdherp.htm. Accessed fall 1997.
3. MedicineNet: Sexually transmitted diseases in women. Information Network, Inc., 1995–1997. URL: http://www.medicinenet.com. Accessed fall 1997.
4. Jay Siwek, MD. Herpes infections. Washington Post Health (Consultation), July 19, 1994.
5. Rick Weiss. Should herpes drugs be sold over-the-counter? Washington Post Health, May 17, 1994, p. 7.

Impetigo

1. Impetigo. Copyright 1998 ADAM Software, Inc., all rights reserved. Copyright 1998 CommuniHealth. URL: http://www.healthanswers.com. Accessed winter 1998.

Lice and Mites

1. It's a lousy job: Head lice require proper treatment and persistant nit-picking. Mayo Foundation for Medical Education and Research. Mayo Health O@sis: March 6, 1996. URL: http://www.mayo.ivi.com/mayo/9603/htm/head_lic.htm. Accessed fall 1997.

Warts

1. Viral warts. A Medical Education Service for the Public by National Skin Centre. National Skin Centre (Singapore), 1995. URL: http://medweb.nus.sg/nsc/nsc.html. Accessed fall 1997.

Acne

1. Acne vulgaris (pimples). A Medical Education Service for the Public by National Skin Centre. National Skin Centre (Singapore), 1995. URL: http://medweb.nus.sg/nsc/nsc.html. Accessed fall 1997.
2. MedicineNet: Power points about acne. Information Network, Inc., 1995–1997. URL: http://www.medicinenet.com. Accessed fall 1997.

Dermatitis/Eczema

1. Hand eczema. A Medical Education Service for the Public by National Skin Centre. National Skin Centre (Singapore), 1995. URL: http://medweb.nus.sg/nsc/nsc.html. Accessed fall 1997.
2. Sally Squires. New cream effective in itching of eczema. Washington Post Health, November 8, 1995.
3. Treatment for eczema /atopic dermatitis. National Jewish Medical and Research Center, 1995. URL: http://www.njc.org/MFhtml/ECZ_MF.htm. Accessed fall 1997.

Hives

1. Urticaria. Copyright 1998 ADAM Software, Inc., all rights reserved. Copyright 1998 CommuniHealth. URL: http://www.healthanswers.com. Accessed winter 1998.
2. Urticaria. A Medical Education Service for the Public by National Skin Centre. National Skin Centre (Singapore), 1995. URL: http://medweb.nus.sg/nsc/nsc.html. Accessed fall 1997.
3. Urticaria-Hives. American Academy of Dermatology, 1983, Revised 1991, 1992, 1993. URL: http://tray.dermatology.uiowa.edu/PIPs/Urticaria.html. Accessed fall 1997.

Moles

1. Mole patrol. Washington Post Health, October 11, 1994.

Psoriasis

1. Psoriasis statistics. National Psoriasis Foundation, Inc., Portland, Oregon, 1997. URL: http://www.psoriasis.org/stat.html. Accessed fall 1997.
2. Questions and answers about psoriasis. National Institute of Arthritis and Musculoskeletal and Skin Diseases, January 1997. URL: http://www.nih.gov/niams/healthinfo/psoriafs.htm. Accessed fall 1997.

Skin Cancer

1. MedicineNet: Power points about skin cancer. Information Network, Inc., 1995–1997. URL: http://www.medicinenet.com. Accessed fall 1997.
2. What is actinic keratosis? Originally published by The Skin Cancer Foundation, Northeast Dermatology Associates, PA, 1996, 1997. URL: http://www.nedermatology.com/skincancer/ak/index.html. Accessed fall 1997.
3. What is melanoma? Northeast Dermatology Associates, PA, 1996, 1997. URL: http://www.nedermatology.com/skincancer/mm/index.html#what. Accessed fall 1997.
4. What is melanoma? National Cancer Institute. URL: http://cancernet.nci.nih.gov/clinpdq/pif/Melanoma_Patient.html. Accessed fall 1997.

Burns

1. MedicineNet: Burns. Information Network, Inc., 1995–1997. URL: http://www.medicinenet.com. Accessed fall 1997.

Decubitus Ulcers

1. Robert C. Kohnle, DC. Pressure sores: The problem. Dermasafe Systems. URL: http://www.dermasafe.com/dermstdy.html. Accessed fall 1997.
2. Sandy Rovner. Treating bedsores with a new approach. Washington Post, January 31, 1995.
3. Treatment of pressure ulcers. The Agency for Health Care Policy and Research, AHCPR Publication No. 95-0652, 1994. URL: http://text.nlm.nih.gov/ahcpr/put/www/putctxt.html. Accessed fall 1997.

Scar Tissue

1. Can you make a scar less noticeable? Originally published in Mayo Clinic Health Letter, October 1993. Mayo Foundation for Medical Education and Research. Mayo Health O@sis: 1996. URL: http://www.mayo.ivi.com/mayo/9310/gtm/scar_qa.htm. Accessed fall 1997.
2. Rick Weiss. Wound-healing gene may soon repair skin. Washington Post Health, October 11, 1994.

Musculoskeletal System Conditions

After reading this chapter, you should be able to tell . . .

- What the disorder is.
- How to recognize it.
- Whether massage is indicated or contraindicated for that condition.
- Whether a contraindication is local or systemic, or refers to a specific stage of development or healing.
- Why those choices for massage are correct.

In addition to this basic information, you should be able to . . .

- List three differences between osteoarthritis and rheumatoid arthritis.
- Name what Paget's disease and osteoporosis have in common.
- Name the leg muscles most involved with pes planus and pes cavus.
- Name four types of fractures.
- Name the medical emergency situation associated with shin splints.
- Name two causes for patellofemoral syndrome.
- Describe the difference between structural and functional problems in postural deviations.
- Name three possible causes of thoracic outlet syndrome.
- Name two diseases associated with advanced gout.
- Name three structures the brachial plexus passes through, around, or under on the way to the arm.

INTRODUCTION

This chapter will discuss disorders and injuries involving muscles, bones, and joint structures, including ligaments, tendons, tendinous sheaths, and bursae. Together these structures are the tools that provide humans with shape, strength, and movement. They are composed almost entirely of the material that binds people together and permeates every part of the body: connective tissue.

Injury to any of the connective tissue structures (except bone and sometimes cartilage) can be tricky for many medical professionals to identify. Magnetic Resonance Imaging (MRI) can be useful, but at present the ability to identify soft tissue damage is extremely limited. A thorough clinical exam will still yield the most comprehensive information

CONNECTIVE TISSUE FIBERS

Connective tissue comes in all shapes and forms in the body. It's difficult to accept that the loose, jiggly deposits of fat in the subcutaneous layer of the skin are technically in the same class of tissue as bones, but it's true. The unifying feature in all types of connective tissue (except blood and lymph) is the presence of particular types of protein fibers. The two that will be examined here are *collagen* and *elastin*.

Elastin is a protein fiber that lives up to its name. It is stretchy, and has good potential for rebound; in other words, it will snap back to its original size after being stretched out. But elastin is low in tensile strength; it is relatively easy to break fibers to pieces.

Collagen is another protein fiber, but it is quite different in most qualities from elastin. It has little ability to stretch, and poor rebound potential; once collagen has been stretched out, it tends to stay loose rather than go back to its original length. But collagen does have tremendous tensile strength: it takes a great deal of force to stretch collagen, and even more force to physically tear or fray the fibers.

One other property of collagen is that under certain circumstances it tends to bind things together. If general circulation to an area is impaired, the collagen-based connective tissue membranes that are intended to be slick and slippery for freedom of movement will instead become thick and gluey. Collagen fibers from one structure may even fuse with fibers from a neighboring structure. This can happen at any level within muscle groups or individual muscles. Muscle sheaths can stick to each other so that individual muscles can no longer contract independently; fascicles can stick together within muscle bellies; even individual myofibers can stick together. These sticky places, or *adhesions*, can greatly impair mobility and flexibility, while increasing the chances for injury when they are stressed to the point of tearing.

about injury to muscles, tendons, ligaments, and other connective tissues. Massage therapists, with their in-depth understanding of the musculoskeletal system (particularly with the formation of adhesions and scar tissue), are in a unique position to help persons suffering from these types of injuries.

BONES

BONE STRUCTURE

The arrangement of living and nonliving material in bone is quite fascinating. The collagen matrix on which solid bone is built is arranged as circles within circles. The calcium and phosphorus deposits grow on this scaffolding in a similarly circular pattern, leaving holes for a generous blood supply. In addition, most long bones in the body grow in a gently spiraled direction, much like tree trunks. And the shaft—or diaphysis—of long bones is hollow, filled with red marrow in youth and yellow marrow in adulthood. All these design features give bone some remarkable properties: terrific resilience, support, and strength combined with a relatively lightweight construction.

The commands to move the rock-like calcium and phosphorus salts around the collagen matrix are carried out by specialized cells. *Osteoblasts*, or "bone builders," help to lay new deposits, while *osteoclasts*, or "bone clearers," break them down. These cells are located both in the periosteum around the outside of the bone and the endosteum on the inside of the shafts. They can alter the shape of the bones from interior and exterior aspects.

Osteoblasts and osteoclasts perform their duties under the orders of two hormones. *Calcitonin*, produced in the thyroid, *lowers* blood calcium by telling osteoblasts to pull calcium out of the blood and put it wherever the bones need it most. *Parathyroid hormone*, or PTH, *raises* blood calcium by telling the osteoclasts to dismantle calcium deposits and send the valuable mineral back into the bloodstream. There it is available to help with muscle contractions, nervous transmission, blood clotting, and so on. So the health and shape of the bones depends not only on a person's physical activity, but on whatever other chemical demands the body may be making on its calcium banks.

This is, in essence, Wolff's law, which states that, "Every change in the form and the function of a bone, or in its function alone, is followed by certain definite changes in its internal architecture and secondary alterations in its external conformation."[1] In other words, bone is living tissue and will remodel according to the stresses that are placed upon it.

---

[1] Stedman's Medical Dictionary. 26th Edition. Baltimore: Williams & Wilkins, 1995:943.

BONE FUNCTION

The skeleton provides a bony framework, protection for vulnerable organs, and leverage for movement. It also produces new red blood cells and stores calcium and phosphorus for future use. For young people, bone is definitely not a mass of stone-like inert material; in fact, osteoblasts and osteoclasts will easily remodel bone to accommodate whatever stresses are put on it. The younger the body, the higher a percentage of living material exists within bones. Gradually, over years, however, the ratio of inert material to living material shifts; in elderly people, bone has little remaining living tissue, and the density of its mineral stores has decreased, hence its brittleness and slowness to heal.

MUSCLES

MUSCLE STRUCTURE

Muscles are composed of specialized thread-like cells that, with electrical and chemical stimulation, have the power to contract while bearing weight. These cells run the full length of the muscle. They are composed of tiny fibers called *myofibrils*. Muscle cells are individually encased in a connective tissue envelope, the *endomysium*. Packets of wrapped cells are encased in another connective tissue envelope, the *perimysium*. These bundles are called *fascicles*. The fascicles are bound together by yet another connective tissue membrane, the *epimysium*. (See Figure 2.1.) Finally, some large muscle groups are further bound by an external connective tissue membrane, which then blends into the subcutaneous layer of the skin, or the deep fascia (which is—surprise!—another connective tissue membrane).

MUSCLE FUNCTION

When muscles work, they consume fuel and produce both energy (the pulling together of their bony attachments) and wastes. What wastes are produced depends on how much work is done, how fast and how long it's being done, and what kind of fuel is available to do it. Muscles that work when adequate supplies of oxygen are easily accessible burn very cleanly (*aerobic metabolism*); the waste products they produce are carbon dioxide and water. But when they work without adequate oxygen (*anaerobic metabolism*), a variety of

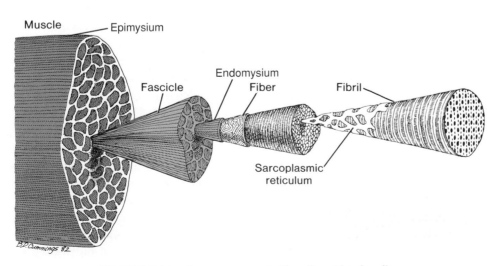

Figure 2.1 Muscles are composed of bundles within bundles,
all enveloped by connective tissue membranes

other wastes are produced. Among these is lactic acid, a byproduct of anaerobic combustion that is also a nerve irritant.

This begs the next question: What causes muscle soreness? This is a controversial issue that is the subject of ongoing debate. One factor is probably the accumulation of lactic acid, which will irritate nerve endings in overused muscles. Another theory is that there may be some calcium leakage from *sarcomeres*—segments of myofibrils where chemical reactions take place. This leakage can then cause microspasms. Soreness may also involve tiny microscopic tears of muscle cells. With microscopic injuries such as these, microscopic pockets of inflammation will accompany them. Swelling and tearing stimulate nociceptors (specialized nerve endings designed to transmit messages about tissue damage), which give the brain information about pain and injury. Massage can influence the processing of chemical residues and minor inflammations by moving fresh, highly oxygenated blood into sore areas, while flushing old, toxic, stagnant interstitial fluid out. Imagine rinsing an old, dirty, smelly sponge in a stream of clean running water. Every time the sponge is squeezed, out flows dirty, discolored liquid. Each time the sponge is released, clean fresh water fills it up again. This is what vigorous, well-applied circulatory massage does for sore, tired muscles suffused with waste products.

JOINTS

Three different classes of joints are found in the body: synarthroses ("immovable" joints, such as those between the cranial bones—although even these joints aren't *completely* immovable), amphiarthroses ("slightly movable" joints, such as those between the bodies of the vertebrae), and diarthroses ("freely movable" joints). Of these classes of joints, the diarthrotic, or *synovial* joints, are by far the most vulnerable to injury. For this reason, it is worth briefly reviewing synovial joints in preparation for a discussion of what happens when they're injured.

JOINT STRUCTURE

Look at Figure 2.2. Note that the whole unit is constructed so no rough surfaces ever have to touch, even in joints that bear an enormous amount of weight, like knees and ankles. Articular cartilage, made of densely formed collagen fibers around chondroitin sulfate (very slippery material) and water, cap the ends of bones where they meet. Maintaining the slickness of that cartilage is key to maintaining the health of the joint. Fortunately, each synovial joint has a synovial membrane that produces synovial fluid, creating a generally synovial ("egg-like") environment. As long as the membrane and cartilage stay wet and smooth, the joint will not suffer any internal damage. It takes only a very small amount of synovial fluid to lubricate the inside of a joint space.

JOINT FUNCTION

It is a bit redundant to discuss joint function here; this isn't a kinesiology text that will define flexion as opposed to extension, or rotation versus circumduction. Suffice to say that the function of synovial joints is to allow movement between bones, providing the fulcrum bones use for leverage.

Joints, like most other structures in the body, are designed for use. With healthy use, the joint structures will stay smooth, slick, and well lubricated. Movement of the joint capsule stimulates the production of synovial fluid, which then circulates through the joint space for the health of all joint components. Lack of movement will result in a shortage of synovial fluid; too much movement, especially too much *irritating* movement, can

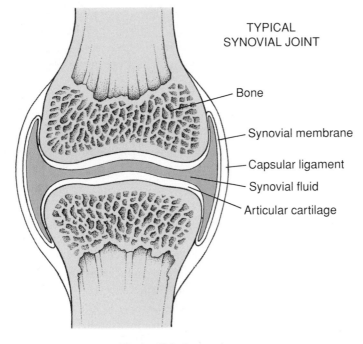

TYPICAL
SYNOVIAL JOINT

Bone

Synovial membrane

Capsular ligament
Synovial fluid
Articular cartilage

Figure 2.2 Synovial joint

damage articular cartilage, or cause the bones of the joint to change shape in such a way that smooth surfaces are made rough, thus opening the door to irreversible arthritis. Other factors that can influence joint health are trauma, calcium metabolism, and nutrition.

OTHER CONNECTIVE TISSUES

Structures outside of the joint capsule (tendons, tendinous sheaths, ligaments, bursae) are very susceptible to damage. Tendons connect muscle to bone, and they are an early line of defense when a joint undergoes traumatic stress. Depending on the force of the trauma, ligaments are also quick to suffer injury, although the medial and lateral stabilizers outside the joint capsule and the internal stabilizers are generally damaged before the specialized capsular ligament that comprises the joint capsule itself. Bursae, little fluid-filled sacks that cushion areas where two bones might otherwise collide or allow tendons to slide over sharp corners, tend to be irritated by repetitive stress. The body grows new bursae anywhere it needs a little extra protection, and these new bursae can also become irritated and painful.

GENERAL CONNECTIVE TISSUE PROBLEMS

Every part of the body is supported by connective tissue. It wraps around muscle cells and neurons; it supports blood vessels and the tubes of the digestive tract. It is the framework on which bones grow. Connective tissue provides the structure for the functioning cells of most organs. It gives strength and elasticity to most of the body's membranes. Indeed, connective tissue is such a large proportion of the entire human body, it can be said that a person's general health can be determined by the strength, resiliency, and power held in his or her connective tissues.

So what happens when a person's connective tissues become systemically weak? Most people know someone who seems to get injured at the drop of a hat. Some people twist their ankles getting out of cars or they wrench their backs when they pick up a chair. It seems as though pain and injury follow them where ever they go. Very often the culprits in situations like these are complicated interconnected problems involving long-term stress, poor nutrition, high levels of chronic muscle contraction, elevated cortisol levels in the blood, sleep disorders, and incomplete healing.

The hormone most closely linked to long-term stress is cortisol. This important and beneficial chemical helps to limit inflammation and redirects metabolism away from fast-burning glucose and toward slower-burning proteins. This is a fine mechanism for dealing with the threat of long-term hunger or famine, but for people with elevated cortisol levels who are *not* suffering from life-threatening food shortages this means that cortisol will systemically weaken all types of connective tissue, increasing the chances for injury and ongoing pain.

When injury occurs, long-term stress, coupled with pain, will interfere with sleep cycles enough to significantly inhibit secretions of somatotropin (growth hormone), as well as the neurotransmitters that moderate pain sensation. This makes it difficult to heal from simple injuries, and reinforces a pain-stress-sleeplessness cycle similar to the pain-spasm-ischemia cycle seen with many muscular problems.

The point of all this is that, contrary to how many people view the body, it is not made of a series of interchangeable parts. When a car has a tire that keeps going flat, the owner replaces the tire, and the problem is solved. But when a person has an ankle that keeps getting sprained, or a back so fragile it interferes with leading a normal life, or headaches that intrude upon day-to-day functioning, the answer isn't just in the ankle, or the back, or the neck muscles. The answer is found in the totality of how a person's mental and emotional states are echoed in his or her physical body; it's in how one's eating habits support or don't support one's healing; it's in whether the individual gets adequate amounts of high-quality sleep. Massage therapists who specialize in helping people with musculoskeletal problems need to address all these issues when clients have recurring, ongoing, or stubborn injuries that don't follow what is usually considered a normal healing process.

The convenient thing about musculoskeletal problems, as far as massage therapists are concerned, is that most are *not* related to an infectious agent; a person can't catch or distribute an epidemic of sprained ankles. Nor do these problems usually lead to permanent damage that massage can make worse; for example, increasing circulation will *not* spread tendinitis throughout the body. But skillful, careful, knowledgeably applied massage administered in the appropriate stage of healing can help many musculoskeletal conditions to improve. Sometimes the improvement is only a temporary cessation of pain (which is a noble purpose in itself), but often this work can bring about the lasting changes that make structurally based massage an important factor in the healing process.

MUSCULOSKELETAL SYSTEM CONDITIONS

Muscular Disorders
   Contractures
   Fibromyalgia
   Myositis Ossificans
   Shin Splints
   Spasms, Cramps
   Strains

Bone Disorders
   Fractures
   Osteoporosis
   Paget's Disease
   Postural Deviations

MUSCULOSKELETAL SYSTEM CONDITIONS, cont.

Joint Disorders

Ankylosing Spondylitis

Chondromalacia/Patellofemoral

Syndrome

Dislocations

Gout

Osteoarthritis

Rheumatoid Arthritis

Septic Arthritis

Spondylosis

Sprains

Temporomandibular Joint Disorders

Other Connective Tissue Disorders

Baker's Cysts

Bunions

Bursitis

Dupuytren's Contracture

Ganglion Cysts

Hernia

Pes Planus

Plantar Fasciitis

Tendinitis

Tenosynovitis

Torticollis

Whiplash

Neuromuscular Disorders

Carpal Tunnel Syndrome

Herniated Disc

Sciatica

Thoracic Outlet Syndrome

Muscular Disorders

Contractures

DEFINITION: WHAT ARE THEY?

Contractures are permanently shortened muscles or muscle groups that either have been immobilized or have sustained neurological damage.

ETIOLOGY: WHAT HAPPENS?

Consider for a moment what goes on inside an unused muscle: the lymph becomes stagnant, circulation diminishes, connective tissue starts to thicken. (You will find more on this in the introduction to the "Lymph and Immune System Conditions" chapter.) If the immobilization occurs because of nerve damage, the degeneration happens even faster than with simple immobility. This, then, is the setup for a contracture: shrinking, atrophying muscle fibers, and growing, thickening fascia. If it continues to its logical conclusion, the muscle bulk will actually reduce and all the connective tissue fascia will shrink to fit—a contracture. (See Figure 2.3.)

SIGNS AND SYMPTOMS

Principally, a muscle or group of muscles is permanently shortened. For some reason this happens in flexion more often than in extension. Because connective tissue does not stretch or give like muscle tissue, the area will feel hard and unyielding. Some contractures occur with long-term

CONTRACTURES IN BRIEF

What are they?

Contractures are permanently shortened muscles or muscle groups that are surrounded by thick, contracted fascia.

How are they recognized?

Contractures usually happen in flexion rather than extension. The muscles lose bulk and the tissue is hard and unyielding.

Is massage indicated or contraindicated?

Massage is indicated for contracture in which sensation is present, although it may do little to reverse the process if it's gone too far. Massage can be a good preventative measure for contractures.

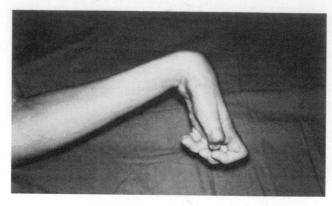

Figure 2.3 Contracture

[handwritten margin note] caused by stress, chemical imbalance; sleep imbalance who do not reach REM sleep depression

casting. They may also be a result of neurologic trauma, for instance, a spinal cord injury. In these cases, the tissue involved will probably also be sensory impaired.

MASSAGE?

If the contracture is due to nerve damage and is accompanied by sensory paralysis, massage is contraindicated. The prognosis for such tissue is that it will continue to atrophy, and eventually will be replaced with fat. However, if the contracture is caused by temporary immobilization, the tissue health may be reclaimed if it hasn't degenerated too far. Deep, specific connective tissue–oriented work can help to soften and unbind some of the fascial prison in which the muscle cells find themselves. Movement and stretching to align the collagen fibers in appropriate directions will also be a key part of this rehabilitation (see *scar tissue*, chapter 1, page 38). In general, however, massage is better at *preventing* contractures than it is at reversing them.

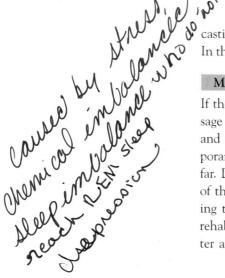

FIBROMYALGIA IN BRIEF

What is it?
Fibromyalgia is a condition that involves chronic muscle pain, trigger points, tender points, and nonrestorative sleep.

How is it recognized?
Fibromyalgia is diagnosed when other diseases have been ruled out, and seven to ten active trigger points are identified.

Is massage indicated or contraindicated?
Massage is indicated for fibromyalgia. Care must be taken not to overtreat, however, because patients are extremely sensitive to pain and may have accumulations of waste products in the tissues that are difficult to flush out adequately.

Fibromyalgia

DEFINITION: WHAT IS IT?

Fibromyalgia is a combination of signs and symptoms that incapacitates up to 3% of the population of the United States. Women affected by this condition outnumber men by about 7 to 1.

ETIOLOGY: WHAT HAPPENS?

Fibromyalgia is very different from most other muscle problems. It is not a viral or bacterial or fungal infection that causes the problem, nor is it an autoimmune mistake, nor a direct result of injury. Rather, some suggest it is related to a person's emotional state, sleep disorders, and possible chemical imbalances.

A number of contradictory theories and opinions exist to describe what actually causes fibromyalgia. From a massage therapist's point of view, this is just one condition that falls under the broad umbrella of stress-related chronic pain syndromes. It is closely tied to other stress-related problems, such as *irritable bowel syndrome* (chapter 7, page 288), *migraine headaches* (chapter 3, page 154), fatigue, including *chronic fatigue syndrome* (chapter 5, page 229), and depression. *Myofascial pain syndrome* is a related disorder with signs and symptoms similar to fibromyalgia. All of these conditions are exacerbated by stress, so just dealing with the problems of living with fibromyalgia can make the symptoms worse. Looking for a specific cause is a bit like wondering which came first, the chicken or the egg.

Two theories about sources for fibromyalgia will be considered here. These theories are not mutually exclusive; in fact, they fit well together.

Sleep Disorder. One theory states that fibromyalgia begins as a sleep disorder. Persons with fibromyalgia may receive adequate hours of sleep, but they don't reach Stage IV sleep, wherein the body's tissues are healed and rejuvenated. This leads to chemical imbalances in the central nervous system, the muscles, and the blood. These imbalances will slow healing and decrease pain tolerance. In essence, poor sleep makes a person vulnerable to the syndrome of fibromyalgia. A study in which normal subjects who were sleep-deprived quickly developed the signs and symptoms of fibromyalgia is compelling evidence for this theory.[2]

A Trigger Point Is Born. Another approach to this condition begins by looking microscopically at how the muscles develop trigger points. Consider the stereotype of a postal worker. She puts in eight long hours every day reading illegible zip codes and routing pieces of mail to the correct destinations. She *hates* her job. By nine-thirty every morning, her shoulders are beginning their day-long journey up to her ears, and her trapezius is doing all the work. Furthermore, her head juts forward and downward in order to read the envelopes. No other muscles keep the head from slumping down onto her chest, so it falls to the trapezius, again, to do the work. It's no great surprise that a few muscle fibers are beginning to microscopically fray. They don't get the opportunity to relax and exchange waste products for nutrients, and because every muscle fiber in the area is similarly stressed, the blood flow to the area is severely limited.

The combination of mechanical stressors and emotional state has now created an injury. Blood components such as histamine and prostaglandins may leak into the area, causing more pain. Any normal muscle's response to injury is to *tighten up*, both as a reaction to pain, and as a splinting mechanism against even further injury. Under normal circumstances, this would be followed by a typical inflammatory response: edema, fibroblastic activity, scar tissue, and finally a healed muscle. But in *this* case the inflammatory response is not complete and the trapezius gets stuck in a pattern of pain, which leads to spasm, which leads to local ischemia, which reinforces the pain, which creates more spasm, ad infinitum. And the tiny area where those myofibers first began to fray has now become a trigger point.

Satellite Points. Manual pressure on the postal worker's trigger point creates a surprising amount of pain, both locally, and, mysteriously, up over the back of her head, causing headaches. If this situation has been ongoing for a matter of weeks or months, movement patterns to compensate for the sore shoulder will redistribute stress throughout the back and neck muscles. The splenius cervicis may experience more stress than it can handle, and *another* trigger point, a *satellite* trigger point is formed. The satellite point can refer pain to yet another area, around the pectoralis major or minor, for instance. Now an area is constantly being told, erroneously, that it is in *pain*. What is the body's reaction to pain? *Tighten up!* That chest muscle may form its own trigger point simply because it has been told that it's hurting, even though there's no mechanical force being exerted on it. And the cycle goes on, and on, and on.

---

[2] David A. Nye, MD. Fibromyalgia: A guide for patients. Eau Claire, WI: Midelfort Clinic.
http://Prairie.lakes.com/~roseleaf/fibro/pt-faq.html. Accessed fall, 1997.

FIBRO·MYO·ALGIA
This simply means muscle pain. "Fibromyalgia," "fibrositis," "myofibrositis," and "fibromyositis" are all terms that have been used to put a name to a bewildering set of signs and symptoms that no one has ever completely defined.

[Handwritten margin notes:]

Theory - sleep disorder, never reach Stage 4. Creates chemical imbalance. Mechanical stressor creates edema

To be definate of the disease take meds, TrP therapy - goes away.

Trigger points that have not been irritated will sometimes go into a latent state. They are not painful, nor do they refer pain. But it will take very little stimulus to turn a latent trigger point into an active one. These sore spots have palpable "knots" or sometimes taut bands that send pain shooting in predictable directions. The pain from these chronically irritated areas will prevent a patient from getting the rest she needs. She might sleep for eight hours, but she wakes up tired, sometimes feeling as if she'd worked all night.

The relationship between fibromyalgia and sleep disorders is very close. Which one precedes the other is a moot point, as far as massage is concerned.

Much still is not understood about trigger points and fibromyalgia. It's unknown why the whole inflammatory process doesn't complete the healing process and turn the affected area to scar tissue. In fact, it's clear that scar tissue *doesn't* form because biopsies of affected tissues show no such change.

Also, although different people have different "hot spots," the referred pain pattern from specific trigger points is consistent from one person to another. Yet, at the same time, it doesn't follow nerve supply pathways, energy meridians, or any other pattern ever observed. (See Figure 2.4.)

Finally no one knows why the location of various trigger points is so predictable from one person to the next. It may be that some of the common ones, in the trapezius for example, are culturally specific. It seems likely that Australian bushmen have a whole different trigger point map than American postal workers.

DIAGNOSIS

No definitive means exists to diagnose for fibromyalgia. When a certain criteria of signs and symptoms have been observed, a battery of tests may be run to rule out several diseases that mimic fibromyalgia. If these tests are negative, a positive diagnosis can be made.

Here are some of the signs and symptoms that characterize fibromyalgia:

- Palpable nodules or bands in muscles that may twitch and are highly sensitive and that tend to "melt" or disappear with applied pressure and stretching of the tissue. (See Figure 2.5.) These trigger points are consistent from person to person. The presence of seven to ten or more trigger points is the medical convention for a positive diagnosis.
- Widespread pain in shifting locations that is extremely difficult to pin down. The intensity of the pain may vary widely (in other words, there are good days and bad days).
- Stiffness after rest.
- Low stamina.
- Sensitivity to cold, especially to damp cold.
- Low pain tolerance.

TREATMENT

Fibromyalgia is a disorder unlike most others, and it tends to confound the usual medical approach to disease. A typical disease, treated in a typical, i.e., medical, way would be diagnosed and then prescribed a course of drugs to ameliorate the symptoms, attack the invading microorganisms, or both. Of course, with fibromyalgia no microorganisms are present, so the drugs usually recommended are mainly palliative: analgesics to start, followed by stronger muscle relaxants and painkillers if symptoms persist. These are administered with sleeping aids to help break the cycle of nonrestorative sleep and pain.

What seems to work best is a course of therapy that gives the patient control of her own healing process. The first priority is to educate her as completely as possible about her condition, emphasizing that though she may feel incapacitated this is *not* a permanently crippling disease. Second, the responsibility for healing must be entirely in the patient's

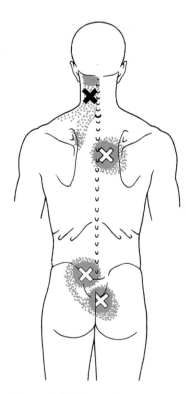

Figure 2.4 Fibromyalgia common trigger points and referred pain patterns

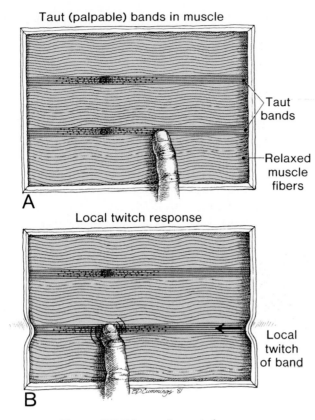

Taut (palpable) bands in muscle

Figure 2.5 Fibromyalgia twitch response

hands, through nutrition, sleep, exercise, stretching, and reducing emotional stress. This may be accomplished through psychological counseling, support groups, or any combination of the two. Massage fits well into both the stress-reducing and muscle-stretching parts of the healing process. Finally, the fibromyalgia patient must be trained to move and work in ways that don't create new injury. If the movement and postural patterns that create the trigger points in the first place aren't addressed, no amount of intervention will make them disappear forever.

MASSAGE?

Let's consider our postal worker, who's in a tremendous amount of muscular pain—debilitating pain. She doesn't have an inflammatory condition and she's not contagious. But she does have chronically tight muscles that literally are unable to relax; the pain-spasm cycle doesn't ever let go. Inside those muscles, her tissues are suffused in metabolic waste, blood flow is blocked, and nerve endings are irritated. If the pain-spasm cycle could be broken with a little pressure and gentle stretching, her condition would improve. Clearly fibromyalgia indicates massage, but with some specific cautions.

Fibromyalgia patients *live* in pain. Some moments are more severe than others, but constant, ongoing, uninterrupted pain is a hallmark of this condition. Their tissues are drowning in irritating chemicals and they lack the neurotransmitters that block some of the pain transmission. In other words, these people are extremely hypersensitive and very easy to overtreat. A good massage therapist will aim for trigger point release and toxic flushing, a little with each session. Ice is contraindicated for fibromyalgia; any kind of cold can exacerbate symptoms.

It usually takes a long time to become incapacitated by fibromyalgia; it can also take a long time to recover. But if a client experiences being pain free, even for just a short time

MYOSITIS OSSIFICANS IN BRIEF

What is it?
This is the growth of a bony deposit in soft tissues. It usually follows trauma that involves significant leakage of blood between fascial sheaths.

How is it recognized?
An x-ray is the best way to see this problem, but it is palpable as a dense mass where, anatomically, no such thing should be.

Is massage indicated or contraindicated?
Massage is always locally contraindicated for myositis ossificans, but work around the edges of the area—within pain tolerance—may stimulate the reabsorption of the bone tissue without doing further damage.

after each massage, she will feel more able to take control of her own healing process, which is the most important step toward recovery.

Myositis Ossificans

DEFINITION: WHAT IS IT?

Myositis ossificans means "muscle inflammation with ossification." Actually, this is a misnomer because it can occur in any kind of soft tissue, not just muscle, and it is not always associated with inflammation.

ETIOLOGY: WHAT HAPPENS?

In this condition, an internal injury occurs with a lot of bleeding, usually between fascial sheets where the capillary supply is practically nil. The blood pools between layers of connective tissue, often the fascial sheaths around muscles, where it quickly coagulates, becoming thick and jelly-like. If the blood is never broken up and reabsorbed into the body, the liquid will disperse, leaving behind a calcium/iron formation that will look and feel like a bone.

Myositis ossificans is identified by a specific bony pattern: within weeks of the injury, an outside border of mature bone forms around an inside area of cellular material. This condition most often affects adolescents and young adults between the ages of 10 and 30.

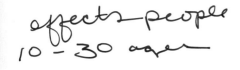
affects people 10 - 30 ages

SIGNS AND SYMPTOMS:

Myositis ossificans comes in all shapes and sizes. Usually x-rays will show a clearly visible growth adjacent to a long bone. Occasionally it will be less dense and well defined, appearing as a veil-like thickening in the soft tissues. It generally occurs after a significant injury with internal bleeding, but it also follows infections, burns, intramuscular injections (as with drug abuse), and other more obscure conditions. In the acute stage the area will feel bruised; later it will feel harder, crusty, and locally tender. Eventually little or no local pain may remain, but a dense, unyielding mass will exist where nothing hard should be.

TREATMENT

Most often the medical approach to this problem is to immobilize the area and let time take care of it. This is good advice for an already hardened leakage, to prevent further irritation and bleeding in surrounding tissues. In many cases, the growth will decrease in size within four to six months. It may disappear altogether within one or two years.

MASSAGE?

locally contraindicated

Myositis ossificans is always locally contraindicated. If the injury is acute, it is unwise to increase the bleeding or impair the healing process by stimulating and stretching the affected tissue. If the leakage has begun to coagulate but has not yet calcified, massage may be instrumental in stimulating reabsorption, but it is still necessary to work only around the edges of the injury because working in the middle of it can aggravate it and lead to more bleeding. If the injury is old, it is *still* a local contraindication; massage may impale soft tissues on the bony growth and cause more internal bleeding. Working within tolerance around the edges, however, can stimulate the body's own mechanisms to reabsorb this old, useless deposit.

Shin Splints

DEFINITION: WHAT IS IT?

"Shin splints" is an umbrella term used to describe a variety of lower leg problems including muscular strains and hairline fractures of the tibia. The tibialis anterior and posterior are frequently involved. Occasionally they'll both be injured at the same time, which is especially miserable.

ETIOLOGY: WHAT HAPPENS?

A few features make the lower leg more than usually susceptible to certain injuries. Before discussing what goes wrong, let's take a brief look at the construction of the lower leg and foot.

Many muscles in the body are almost entirely separate from their attaching bones, touching only at the ends of their tendons. Tibialis anterior and posterior, however, attach to the tibia from beginning to end, and almost along the entire length of the muscle bellies. The tibialis anterior actually blends directly into the periosteum along the whole bone (see Figure 2.6); the connective tissue

SHIN SPLINTS IN BRIEF

What are they?

Shin splints are lower leg problems involving some combination of an injury to the anterior or posterior tibialis and possible hairline fractures of the tibia. They are usually brought about by overuse or misalignment in the ankle. *ie: running, soccer,*

How are they recognized?

Pain along the tibia may be superficial or deep, mild or severe. It is often made worse by resisted dorsiflexion for anterior tibialis or resisted plantarflexion for posterior tibialis.

Is massage indicated or contraindicated?

Massage is indicated for mild shin splints, but is advised only with caution for periostitis or stress fractures and is contraindicated entirely for anterior compartment syndrome.

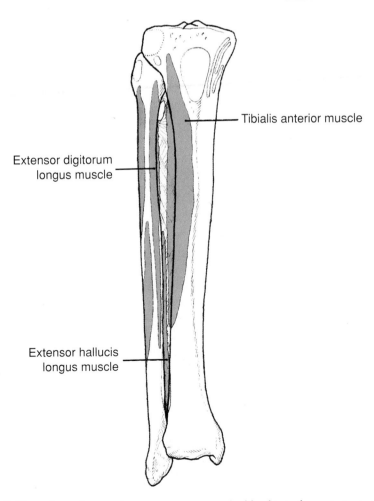

Tibialis anterior muscle

Extensor digitorum longus muscle

Extensor hallucis longus muscle

Figure 2.6 Shin splints: the anterior compartment muscles blend into the periosteum on the tibia

membrane (endomysium) around each muscle is seamlessly woven into the connective tissue wrapping (periosteum) of the tibia. The muscles themselves are wrapped in tough fascial sheaths, and those sheaths along with the ones belonging to the other anterior leg muscles (extensor digitorum longus and extensor hallucis longus), are wrapped together in yet another layer of fascia. The tibialis posterior attaches to the posterior aspect of the tibia in a similar way; the myofiber sheaths blend directly into the periosteum and interosseus ligament of the tibia and fibula.

Feet are designed to spread out and rebound with each step. When that doesn't happen all kinds of things can go wrong. If there is inadequate shock absorption—from flat feet (see *pes planus*, this chapter, page 101); bad shoes; bad surfaces to walk, run, or jump on; or any combination of the above—the tibia and the muscles in the lower leg, especially tibialis anterior and posterior, will absorb a disproportionate amount of the shock. They're not designed for this job, however, and ongoing stress will cause the bone to crack and the muscles to fray and become inflamed.

With chronic overuse or misalignment, the lower leg muscles become irritated, inflamed, and possibly suffer some internal microtearing. The periosteum of the injured tibia may do the same. The difficulty with inflammation in this area is that there simply isn't room within all those fascial sheaths to allow for excess fluid retention. Even a small amount of edema will put pressure on nerve endings and limit blood flow, which, in typical vicious circle fashion, will make it hard for excess fluid to leave the area.

Causes for inflammation in the lower leg include exercising with inadequate foot support or on bad surfaces; unusual amounts of exercise followed by a period of rest (continued gentle movement would help the fluid to keep moving out of the area); or running mostly uphill or downhill or on uneven surfaces.

SIGNS AND SYMPTOMS

Pain from shin splints can be mild or severe, and the location will vary according to which of the structures has been damaged. It will become worse with whatever actions the affected muscles do: dorsiflexion, inversion, or plantarflexion. Shin splints are rarely visibly or palpably inflamed. If the tibia is red, hot, and puffy, suspect a more severe injury than shin splints to the lower leg.

RELATED CONDITIONS

Muscle strains are the first step in a series of lower leg injuries. Here are the conditions that may follow, if the irritation is not resolved and the activity that caused it continues unabated:

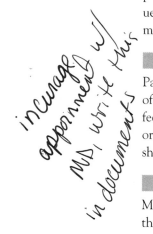

encourage client to approach w/ MD, write this in documents

- Periostitis. This is an inflammation of the periosteum, which may happen with damage to either the anterior or posterior tibialis muscles. The seamless connection of membranes begins to rip apart, and the fibers of the muscles pull away from the bone. This condition sometimes may leave the bone feeling bumpy or pitted; that's where scar tissue has knit the connective tissue membranes back together.
- Stress fractures. These are small, hairline fractures of the tibia. They are extremely painful, and nothing will heal them except time. They are frequently the result of "running through the pain." They are best diagnosed by bone scan, which will look for heightened areas of circulatory activity. Stress fractures of the tibia don't usually show up well on x-rays.
- Anterior compartment syndrome. This is a culmination of the vicious circle of edema that limits blood flow, which limits the exit of excess fluid. It can affect the tibialis anterior, extensor digitorum longus, and the extensor hallucis. Because the external fascia on the lower leg is such a tough container, the swelling can actually cause tissue death if it's not resolved naturally, with steroid injections, or with surgi-

cal intervention. Anterior compartment syndrome is an emergency situation and should be treated as soon as possible.

TREATMENT

The typical approach to shin splints is to reduce activity and to alternate applications of heat and cold. If the situation has worsened to become anterior compartment syndrome, steroid injections may be suggested, or surgery may be performed to split the fascia and allow room for those compressed blood vessels that were unable to do their jobs.

MASSAGE?

As long as the problem is not too advanced, massage is absolutely indicated. The lower leg muscles are impossible to thoroughly stretch out and clean up with exercise alone, but massage can give them a luxurious inch by inch stretching and broadening that will cleanse the tissues more efficiently than anything else. In fact, massage is an excellent way to *prevent* shin splints and periostitis from complicating into anterior compartment syndrome.

For really hot, inflamed, painful cases, however, it is necessary to wait until the pain and inflammation has subsided. Obviously, if someone has too much fluid in a closed area, the last thing they need is massage to exacerbate it. What they really need, if the pain isn't *much* better in two or three days, is to see a doctor. Stress fractures and anterior compartment syndrome are serious problems that require medical attention.

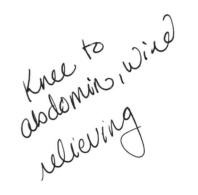

Knee to abdomin, wire relieving

Spasms, Cramps

DEFINITION: WHAT ARE THEY?

A spasm is an involuntary contraction of a muscle. Clonic spasms are marked by alternating cycles of contraction and relaxation, while tonic spasms are sustained periods of hypertonicity. (It's also worth pointing out at this point that *spasm* is different from *spasticity*.) The difference between *spasms* and *cramps* is somewhat arbitrary; cramps are strong, painful, usually short-lived spasms. So one could say that tight, painful paraspinals are in *spasm*, while a charleyhorsing gastrocnemius is a *cramp*. The severity of these episodes will depend on how much of the muscle is involved. "Spasms" and "cramps" are sometimes used in reference to visceral muscle, too (e.g., *spastic constipation*), but this discussion will be restricted to the involuntary contraction of skeletal, or so-called voluntary, muscle.

ETIOLOGY: WHAT HAPPENS? ★

Three of the most common situations will be addressed here.

Nutrition. Calcium and magnesium deficiencies, in addition to causing all sorts of problems later in life, can also make one prone to cramping, especially in the feet.

Ischemia. When a muscle or part of a muscle is suddenly or gradually deprived of oxygen, it can't function properly. Rather than becoming loose and weak, it becomes tighter and tighter. Often this is a gradual process, but sometimes it is a sudden and violent reaction to oxygen shortage.

SPASMS, CRAMPS IN BRIEF

What are they?
Spasms and cramps are involuntary contractions of skeletal muscle. Spasms are considered to be low-grade, long-lasting contractions, while cramps are short-lived, very acute contractions.

How are they recognized?
Cramps are extremely painful with visible shortening of muscle fibers. Long-term spasms are achy and cause inefficient movement, but may not have acute symptoms.

Is massage indicated or contraindicated?
Massage is locally contraindicated for acutely cramping muscle bellies, though origin/insertion work can trick the proprioceptors into letting go. Subacute cramps respond well to massage, which can reduce residual pain and clean up chemical wastes. Underlying cramp-causing pathologies must be ruled out before massage is applied.

Massage is indicated for long-term spasm because it can break through the ischemia-spasm-pain cycle to reintroduce circulation to the area, as well as reduce muscle tone and flush out toxins.

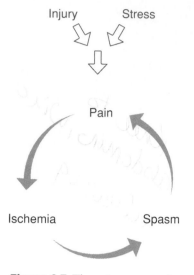

Figure 2.7 The pain-spasm cycle

What causes this oxygen deprivation? Anything that impedes blood flow into the affected areas. Consider a typical tight, painful iliocostalis—one of the paraspinal group of muscles that holds the back erect. This muscle is tight, hard, and a little achy, but most of all, overworked. The fibers are shortened and thickened with the effort of keeping the spine upright, and this makes it harder for the supplying capillaries to deliver the goods—namely, oxygen. In protest, the iliocostalis draws up even tighter, which further inhibits the influx of oxygen: a vicious circle of ischemia causing spasm, causing pain, which leads to spasm, and so on. Furthermore, muscles forced to work without oxygen will accumulate the chemical by-products of anaerobic combustion. These metabolic wastes are irritating to nerve fibers, and will further reinforce the spasm. And the whole picture is complicated by the fact that as postural habits develop, the brain comes to interpret these sensations as normal, and the proprioceptors will actually reinforce the patterns that cause the problem. This situation can exist for years at a time without any real relief, until the circle of ischemia-spasm-pain is interrupted. (See Figure 2.7.)

Pregnancy may be another cause of ischemic pain. As the fetus lays on the femoral artery (just where it splits off from the abdominal branch), it can interfere with blood flow into the leg, prompting a violent contraction of the gastrocnemius. This is a classic example of an acute cramp or charley horse. Other kinds of circulatory interruptions or nervous system problems can cause them, too, so when making a decision about whether massage is appropriate, it's important to be sure that no underlying pathology—such as cardiac weakness, for example—is creating an oxygen deficiency.

Splinting. The last variety of cramps and spasms discussed here is a reflexive reaction against injury. Consider an acute whiplash. The interspinous and intertransverse ligaments have been severely wrenched, and the body senses a potentially dangerous instability in the cervical spine. Of *course* the postural neck muscles will contract; as far as they're concerned, they are literally keeping the head from falling off. This kind of spasm is an important protective mechanism. It keeps the injured person from moving in such a way as to cause further injury. The muscles create an effective splint; the range of motion of affected joints is generally very small. The proprioceptors say, "You can move this far; no further." See more on this situation under *whiplash*, this chapter, page 108.

MASSAGE?

Ischemic cramps indicate massage, as long as the ischemia isn't related to a contraindicated condition. But even when underlying pathology has been ruled out, massage must be used with caution. If a therapist tries to "fluff up" a cramping gastrocnemius, he or she can damage the fibers. A better strategy is to stretch the tendons and antagonists of the affected muscle to gently but quickly persuade the proprioceptors that there is no real crisis and they may safely allow the muscle to let go. When the problem has moved out of the acute stage, it is possible to go back and clean up some of the toxic waste left behind, always at the tolerance of the client.

In regards to splinting, massage therapists should not interfere with this protective mechanism. If they do, the client will probably get up off the table with his newly loosened scalenes, and those muscles will clamp right back down, maybe even tighter than before.

Days or weeks later, the ligaments will be ready to take on some weight-bearing stress, but the muscles may no longer be able to let go spontaneously. *Now* massage can do some real good. By working to soften the hardened muscle tissue, we can reduce toxicity, improve blood flow, and speed healing. Spasm with the need for splinting is to be highly respected. When the injury moves into a subacute stage, massage is indicated and will contribute to a healing process with a minimum of scar tissue, fibrosis, and permanent shortening.

Strains

leave 48hrs untill massage

DEFINITION: WHAT ARE THEY?

Strains are a subject of semantic debate. Some people will say that the word "strain" refers only to tendon tears; others will insist it refers only to muscle tears. In this book, it will refer to an injury to the muscle-tendon unit, with an emphasis on muscles. *Tendinitis*, or inflammation of tendons due to tears, is addressed in a later section.

SIGNS AND SYMPTOMS

What happens when a muscle is injured? The same thing that happens when a tendon or ligament is injured: fibers are torn, the inflammatory process begins, and fibroblasts flood the area with collagen to knit the injury back together. Symptoms of this process include mild or intense local pain, stiffness, and pain on resisted movement or stretching. Unless it is a *very* bad tear, no palpable heat or swelling will be present. The distinction is that muscles, unlike tendons and ligaments, are *not* made exclusively of connective tissue, and while this is a good thing in terms of blood flow, an accumulation of excess scar tissue in muscles acts differently than it does in tendons and ligaments.

Impaired Contractility.   Scar tissue can seriously impede the contractility of uninjured myofibers. When the muscle tries to contract, it bears the weight not only of its bony insertion, but of the fibers that are disabled due to the mass of collagen that is binding up uninjured fibers. This significantly increases the chance for repeated injury, more scar tissue, and further weakening of the muscle.

Adhesions.   All the collagen that is manufactured around an injury doesn't lay down in alignment with the muscle fibers. Randomly arranged collagen fibers will tend to bind up different layers of tissue that are designed to be separated. The result of one thing getting stuck to another is called an *adhesion*. Adhesions may be *within* the muscle, as is frequently seen with the paraspinals, or *between* muscles, when muscle sheaths stick to other muscle sheaths. Hamstrings are a common place to see this phenomenon. Wherever they occur, adhesions limit mobility and increase the chance of injury. (See Figure 2.8.)

TREATMENT

People rarely seek medical treatment for muscular injuries unless they are so painful that they interfere with normal functioning. In those cases, medication may be administered to deal with pain and inflammation, possibly along with muscle relaxants to address secondary spasm. While these can be useful tools, none of them really address the problem, which is how well are these injured fibers going to heal?

STRAINS IN BRIEF

What are they?
Strains are injured muscles.

How are they recognized?
Pain, stiffness, and occasionally palpable heat and swelling will be present. Pain is exacerbated by stretching or resisted exercise of the injured muscle.

Is massage indicated or contraindicated?
Massage is indicated for muscle strains, to influence the production of useful scar tissue, reduce adhesions and edema, and reestablish range of motion.

STRAINS

Acute injuries. The general rule for massage and soft tissue injuries is that massage therapists *must respect the acute stage of injury*. Important things are happening during this time, and therapists ought not to interfere. It is during this stage that the inflammatory reaction begins with the release of chemicals that . . .

1) set up edema, which limits movement;
2) call in white blood cells to eat up the debris; and
3) irritate nerve endings so that the person feels pain and takes the injury seriously.

Some types of massage are appropriate with *some* types of acute injuries, but they are highly specialized and not appropriate for casual experimentation.

How long is an acute injury acute? It depends on the injury, but the most commonly accepted guideline is 48 hours.

Subacute injuries. This is where massage therapists can be most effective. As they strum over the newly formed scar tissue in an injured tendon or ligament, they are fulfilling their ultimate goal: creating an internal environment that is conducive to the best possible healing. The tension and stretch massage creates will help determine the orientation of new collagen fibers. Massage will flush out the irritating chemicals that interfere with the inflow of fresh blood. Massage therapists are instrumental in the rehabilitation of an injured structure so that it will end up looking and behaving as though it never was hurt at all.   (continued)

STRAINS, cont.

Chronic injuries. In this stage, massage therapists can still be major contributors to the healing process, but their effectiveness will be determined by how big, how old, and how accessible the injury is, as well as other variables, such as the diet and lifestyle of the client. These are the situations where therapists have to use their most powerful tools—cross fiber friction, ice, stretching, movement recommendations—everything that is at their disposal to rework that gnarled up old scar tissue inside and out.

MASSAGE?

Skillful, knowledgeable massage can make the difference between a one-time muscle strain that takes a few weeks to resolve and a painful, limiting, chronically recurring condition that makes it impossible to participate in an activity a client used to love. Special techniques involving very specific frictions with no oil have been developed to significantly improve the healing process. By applying skills to the proper formation of scar tissue, the reduction of edema, the limiting of adhesions, and the improvement of circulation and mobility, massage can turn an irritating muscle tear into a trivial event.

Bone Disorders

Fractures

DEFINITION: WHAT ARE THEY?

Fractures include any variety of broken bone, from a hairline crack to a complete break with protrusion through the skin.

Fractures come in all shapes and sizes. The three basic classes are *simple*, wherein the bone is completely broken but there is little or no damage to the surrounding soft tissues; *incomplete*, in which the bone is cracked but not completely broken; and *compound*, wherein the bone is completely broken and a great deal of soft tissue is damaged—in fact, the bone protrudes through the skin and is susceptible to infection. Several variations on these themes can be found, including *stress* fractures and *compression* fractures; a variety called a *march* fracture occurs in the metatarsals. *Greenstick* fractures involve bending and partial breakage of the bone; *comminuted* fractures involve shattering of the broken bone; and an *impacted* fracture is a break with the end of one bone wedged into the other. (See Figure 2.9.) *Mal-union* fractures are fractures that heal in a nonanatomic position. Many others, named for the doctors who first described them or the special joints they affect, won't be discussed here.

DEMOGRAPHICS: WHO GETS THEM?

About 5.6 million people in the United States will experience a broken bone this year. It happens to children often because they engage in the risky behaviors that invite that sort of accident. But childrens' bones have a much higher proportion of living cells and flexible cartilage to inert mass than adults' bones do. In fact, bones don't complete their calcification until the end of puberty. Children also have more growth hormone, which allows them a faster and more complete recovery than most adults can anticipate. Elderly people, while not doing much tree climbing and skateboarding, have bones that are quite a bit more brittle and less resilient than young people's, and it takes a great deal less stress to lead to a fracture for them.

FRACTURES IN BRIEF

What are they?
A fracture is any kind of broken or cracked bone.

How are they recognized?
Most fractures are painful and involve loss of function at the nearest joints, but some may be difficult to diagnose without an x-ray.

Is massage indicated or contraindicated?
Massage is locally contraindicated for acute fractures, but work done on the rest of the body can yield reflexive benefits. Massage is indicated for people in later stages of recovery from fractures.

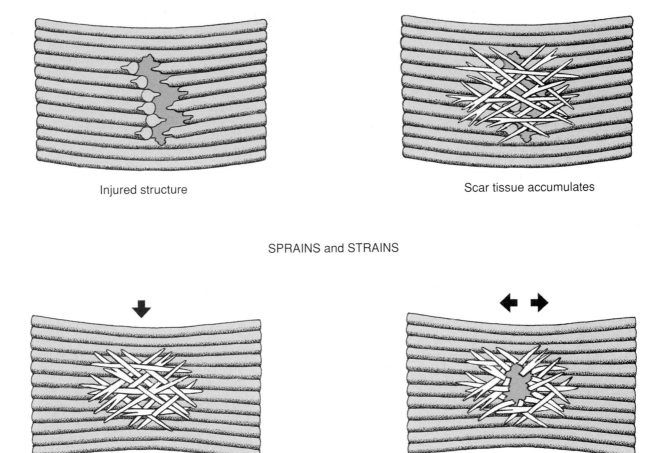

Injured structure

Scar tissue accumulates

SPRAINS and STRAINS

Scar tissue contracts: Structural weak spot

New injury at site of scar tissue

Figure 2.8 Strains, sprains, tendinitis: the injury-reinjury cycle

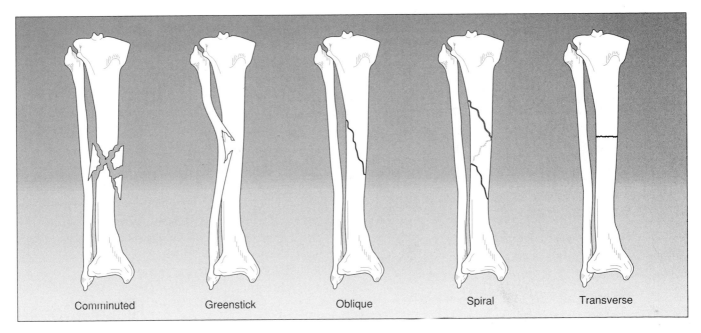

Comminuted   Greenstick   Oblique   Spiral   Transverse

Figure 2.9 Different types of fractures

DIAGNOSIS

Big bone breaks are usually obvious: they are painful, they usually follow a specific traumatic event, and they severely limit the function of the affected joints. But some fractures can be difficult to identify without an x-ray or bone scan, particularly if they are accompanied by a lot of soft-tissue trauma. *Sprained ankles* (this chapter, page 87) and *shin splints* (this chapter, page 55) are two conditions that frequently hide bone fractures.

TREATMENT

Most fractures will heal well if they are casted to immobilize the bones. Fibroblasts immediately infiltrate the area and build a framework of collagen. Next, osteoblasts lay down the framework for bone tissue that later will become dense and hard.

Some fractures need more support than a standard cast can offer, especially if the break involves a joint, as in the wrist or ankle. Pins or plates may be introduced to further stabilize the joint, but these carry a small risk of introducing infection to the site.

Occasionally, broken bones fail to grow together; the gap fills with fibrous tissue instead of new bone. This is a condition called "non-union fracture" and is most common among smokers and adults with very severe fractures. Treatment options for this kind of situation include bone grafts, electromagnetic stimulation, ultrasound, and, possibly in the near future, "bone paste": a substance that can be injected into the area of a fracture. It mimics real bone, hardens in a matter of hours, and gradually dissolves as new regenerated bone takes its place.

MASSAGE?

The rules for working with fractures are guided by common sense: acute or unset broken bones obviously contraindicate massage. But casted fractures will result in stasis and edema that can be very much improved by massage, if there is adequate access. Even if there is no access to a broken leg, for instance, reflexive benefits may be gained by working on the other limb. In addition, massage can improve how movement compensation patterns may affect the rest of the body.

OSTEOPOROSIS IN BRIEF

What is it?

This is loss of bone mass and density brought about by endocrine disorders and poor metabolism of calcium.

How is it recognized?

Osteoporosis in the early stages is identifiable only by x-ray and bone-density tests. In later stages, compression or spontaneous fractures of the vertebrae, wrists, or hips often result. Kyphosis brought about by compression fractures of the vertebrae is a frequent indicator of osteoporosis.

Is massage indicated or contraindicated?

Very gentle massage is indicated for persons with osteoporosis. Massage will not affect the progression of the disease once it is present, but may significantly reduce associated pain. Massage for acute fractures, however, is contraindicated (see this chapter, page 60).

Osteoporosis

DEFINITION: WHAT IS IT?

Osteoporosis means, literally, "porous bones." In this condition, calcium is pulled off the bones faster than it is replaced, leaving them thinned, brittle, chalky, and prone to injury.

DEMOGRAPHICS: WHO GETS IT?

This disease affects an estimated 25 million Americans. It affects women about five times more often than men because they have lower bone density to begin with, and they bear children, which is an enormous drain on calcium reserves. Small-boned, thin women get it more often than others, especially those who are postmenopausal and/or anorexic. Caucasian and Asian women are more likely to develop this condition, but African-American and Hispanic women are also at risk.

Although a genetic marker for osteoporosis has been identified, other risk factors are major contributors to this disease. Therefore, bone density is determined only about 60% by heredity, and 40% by controllable factors such as diet, smoking, exercise, and stress levels. Chronic secretions of cortisol have recently been shown to be extremely destructive to bone density.[3]

ETIOLOGY: WHAT HAPPENS?

Before discussing the bones, it's worthwhile to point out a few things about calcium. First of all, the bones are not the only part of the body that needs calcium. They happen to be a convenient storage medium, but calcium is consumed in nearly every chemical reaction that results in muscle contraction and nerve transmission. Calcium is also essential to blood clotting and pH balance. These are very important functions, and the body has a strict prioritizing system: chemical reactions that are crucial to moment-to-moment survival are more important than maintaining the density of the vertebrae.

Second, calcium requires an acidic stomach environment in order to be absorbed into the body. If calcium enters the body in a form that impedes its contact with hydrochloric acid (e.g., in dairy products or "calcium rich" antacids), the body actually may not be able to absorb very much of the calcium that is available. Similarly, if natural secretions of hydrochloric acid are reduced, as in postmenopausal women, the result is less access to ingested calcium.

Finally, calcium is constantly lost through sweat and urine. Some substances, specifically meat-based proteins, will cause higher levels of calcium to be excreted in urine. So although a person may take in ample supplies of calcium, she will tend to lose it if she also eats a lot of meat. This may help to explain why vegetarians have a statistically lower rate of osteoporosis than the general population and why, although the United States is a leading consumer of milk, it also has higher osteoporosis rates than other countries with average diets that are lower in animal proteins.

COMPLICATIONS

Complications of osteoporosis center around pathologically weak bones. Thinned vertebrae lead to a loss of height and the characteristic rounded "widow's hump" of kyphosis. There can be chronic and/or acute back pain in this stage as the vertebrae continue to degenerate. People with osteoporosis are also prone to other fractures with little or no cause; these are called *spontaneous* or *pathological* fractures. Hips, vertebrae, and wrists are particularly vulnerable to breakage. And since in advanced age people are naturally low on both living osteocytes and growth hormone to induce the healing process, it is particularly difficult to recover from any injury of this severity.

DIAGNOSIS

Osteoporosis is a virtually silent disease until it's too late to do anything about it. In the early stages, only x-rays and bone-density tests will yield any conclusive information. (See Figure 2.10.) In the later stages, however, the disease is often identified by compression fractures in the vertebrae.

TREATMENT

Once osteoporosis has been identified, a number of treatment options are available to keep it from getting worse. Among these are *estrogen replacement therapy* (ERT). Estrogen influences calcium absorption. Postmenopausal women secrete this hormone only in very small amounts, so replacing it can improve calcium uptake. Unfortunately, estrogen supplements are also associated with breast and uterine cancers, so ERT isn't for everybody. *Calcitonin*, a manmade version of a different hormone, is another option, as are *biophosphates*, which inhibit bone breakdown and increase bone density.

---

[3] Mary Anne Dunkin, ed. Bones and depression. Arthritis Today 1995 (Nov–Dec). Arthritis Foundation. http://www.arthritis.org/at/archive/1995/11_12/08sf.shtml.

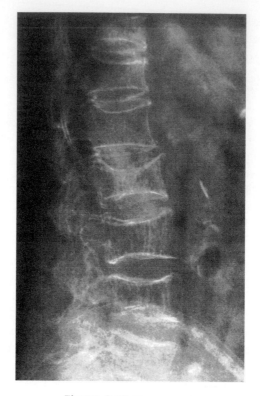

Figure 2.10 Osteoporosis

Exercise is almost always a part of the osteoporosis treatment strategy. Since bone will remodel according to the stresses placed on it, weight-bearing stress will ensure that maintaining healthy mass is a high priority. For someone with this condition, exercises such as gentle weight training or walking are more beneficial than cardiovascular exercises like swimming or cycling. Diet also plays an important part of dealing with osteoporosis. Specific vitamins and other substances may improve calcium uptake, even for postmenopausal women, but this book is not the place to discuss them.

PREVENTION

This disease is easy to prevent, feasible to slow down or halt, and difficult to reverse. The causes of it are many and varied, but center around one main theme: the time to build up calcium reserves is in youth and early adulthood. The skeleton grows in height until about age 20, but it continues to accumulate *density* until about age 35. After that point, it tends to progressively demineralize. Studies show that today many Americans get only half or even less of the recommended daily allowance of calcium;[4] this doesn't bode well for future osteoporosis statistics.

Diet is not the only preventive measure to take against osteoporosis. Bone is living tissue that will remodel according to stresses placed upon it, and one of the best things anyone can do to prevent osteoporosis is to give the skeleton regular weight-bearing stress, in the form of exercise. This makes the maintenance of bone density a high priority, and ensures the activity of osteoblasts to keep those calcium deposits coming in.

MASSAGE?

In the treatment of clients with osteoporosis, the appropriateness of massage will vary from person to person. The only way massage could worsen the situation would be to ex-

[4] National Osteoporosis Foundation. How can I prevent osteoporosis? Washington, DC: author. http://www.nof.org/PreventOsteo.html.

ert undue mechanical force, which could lead to the possibility of fractures. On the other hand, consider the condition of the muscles of someone with osteoporosis—massage can offer a lot of symptomatic relief, even if it can't reverse the degeneration of the bone tissue. In any case, caution is the key with this condition. Don't look for miracles; taking someone out of their pain for a few hours is miracle enough.

Paget's Disease

DEFINITION: WHAT IS IT?

Paget's disease is a condition in which normal bone is reabsorbed at abnormally high rates. It is replaced with fibrous connective tissue, which never mineralizes completely. This leaves the affected bones badly weakened and distorted.

DEMOGRAPHICS: WHO GETS IT?

This is one of the most common metabolic bone diseases, second only to *osteoporosis* (this chapter, page 62). It affects approximately 3% of people over 40 and 10% of people over 80 in the United States. Twice as many men have Paget's disease as women, and though African Americans can develop it, it is especially prevalent in Caucasians of Northern European descent. It is very rare in Asians.

ETIOLOGY: WHAT HAPPENS?

Every day, microscopic amounts of calcium in the bones are constantly being dissolved into the bloodstream, only to be replaced by new supplies. The osteoclasts, which break down bone, and osteoblasts, which build it up, keep each other in balance, and the bones adapt to available nutrition and weight-bearing stress. But if both the osteoclasts and osteoblasts become hyperactive, the reshaping process of the bones doesn't function correctly. In Paget's disease, new deposits are laid down faster than old ones are dissolved.

Typically this disease occurs in two stages. In the vascular stage, bone is broken down and replaced—not with high-quality calcium deposits, but with new blood vessels and fibrous tissue. Then, in the sclerotic stage, the new material hardens and becomes brittle, but not strong. This shows up as a characteristic mosaic pattern on x-rays. The bones most often affected by this disease are the ilium, cranial bones, the spine, clavicle, and femur.

CAUSE

The cause of Paget's disease is unknown at present, but research is leaning toward the idea of a very slow-acting virus that may live in the system for years before causing any damage. A genetic component is definite, since Paget's disease often runs in families, but this may simply indicate a susceptibility to the particular virus involved.

SIGNS AND SYMPTOMS

Bone pain is the major symptom of Paget's disease. This probably happens as the periosteum (the nerve supply for the bones) is stretched with new growth. In later stages, the bones may be tender and visibly deformed. The joint pain of *osteoarthritis* (this chapter, page 77) is also an indicator for Paget's disease, as the bony deformations will frequently disrupt joint function.

PAGET'S DISEASE

Sir James Paget was an English surgeon who lived from 1814 to 1899. He was the first to document the bony disorder described here, as well as two types of rare malignancies: extramammary Paget's disease and mammary Paget's disease.

PAGET'S DISEASE IN BRIEF

What is it?

This is a bone disorder in which healthy bone is rapidly reabsorbed and replaced with fibrous connective tissue.

How is it recognized?

Bone pain is the primary symptom. X-rays are used for a definitive diagnosis.

Is massage indicated or contraindicated?

Due to the lack of knowledge about the actual causes of Paget's disease, massage is systemically contraindicated in all but the mildest cases, and those should be massaged under a doctor's supervision.

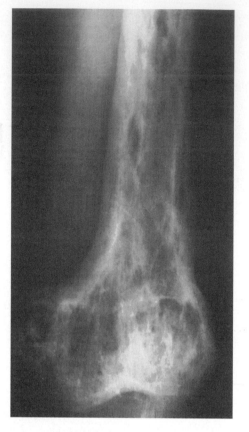

Figure 2.11 Paget's disease

COMPLICATIONS

Paget's disease has several serious complications brought about by changes in bone size and strength. There is a high risk of *fractures* (this chapter, page 60) in the affected bones. If the cranial bones begin to put pressure on parts of the central nervous system, deafness or brain damage could result. *Congestive heart failure* (chapter 4, page 206) may occur because the heart is pumping blood not only through healthy, normal vessels, but also through whole new networks of useless vessels in the new fibrous tissue. And finally, Paget's disease is associated with various kinds of bone cancer.

DIAGNOSIS

This condition is diagnosed primarily by x-ray or bone scan, which is a test to detect heightened circulation and activity in bone tissue (See Figure 2.11). A blood test to identify alkaline phosphatase (an enzyme produced by over-active osteoblasts) may confirm the diagnosis.

TREATMENT

Treatment for Paget's disease is surprisingly similar to that of osteoporosis; the two conditions have in common the unwanted breakdown of healthy bone tissue. Exercise is the first recommendation for Paget's disease, in order to maintain function and healthy bone mass as much as possible. Aspirin and anti-inflammatories may be suggested for pain relief. And finally, calcitonin or biophosphates may be prescribed to inhibit osteoclast activity.

MASSAGE?

No definitive information is available on this topic. But since this is a disease involving inflammation, impaired circulation, and weakened bones, massage is not appropriate for

contraindicated

any but the very mildest cases of Paget's disease. And even then, it would be wise to work under the supervision of a medical professional.

Postural Deviations

DEFINITION: WHAT IS IT?

Although it is tempting to think about the spine in terms of a ship's mast, a column, or a tent pole held erect by muscular tension, it is actually much stronger than any of those. The curvatures in the cervical, thoracic, and lumbar regions give the spine ten times the resistance it would have if it were perfectly straight. Sometimes, though, these natural curvatures are overdeveloped, which reduces resiliency and strength, rather than enhancing it. Kyphosis ("humpback"), lordosis ("swayback"), and scoliosis ("S," "C," or "Reverse- C" curve) are the specific problems to be addressed here. (See Figure 2.12.)

ETIOLOGY: WHAT HAPPENS?

It is sometimes convenient to think about the spine in only two dimensions at a time. In other words, scoliosis would be simply an S-shaped curve from left to right, and

> ### POSTURAL DEVIATIONS IN BRIEF
>
> **What are they?**
> Postural deviations are overdeveloped thoracic or lumbar curves (kyphosis and lordosis) or an S-curve or a C-curve in the spine (scoliosis).
>
> **How are they recognized?**
> Extreme curvatures are visible to the naked eye, although x-rays are used to pinpoint the exact places where the problems begin and end.
>
> **Is massage indicated or contraindicated?**
> Massage is indicated for all postural deviations as long as other underlying pathologies have been ruled out. Massage may or may not be able to reverse any damage, but it can certainly provide relief for muscular stress.

10 X risistance

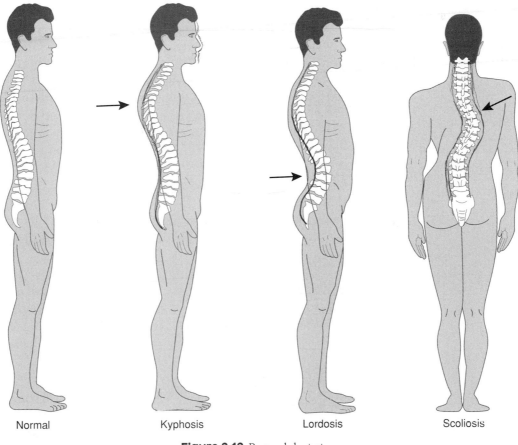

Normal   Kyphosis   Lordosis   Scoliosis

Figure 2.12 Postural deviations

lordosis and kyphosis would be exaggerated forward and backward curves. The truth is not nearly so simple. With any imbalance in the stacking of the vertebrae, rotations will occur in one direction or another to complicate the issue. Thus scoliosis is not merely a left-right aberration, but involves a spiral twisting of the vertebral column as well. Similar lateral imbalances will be observed with most cases of lordosis and kyphosis.

One important thing to remember with postural deviations is the difference between a *functional* problem and a *structural* one. In the early stages of any of these conditions, it may be the soft tissues that are pulling the spine out of alignment: a *functional* problem. At this point the condition is probably at its most treatable: muscles, tendons, and ligaments can be exercised, stretched, and manipulated into new holding and movement patterns. Functional deviations can also be brought about by structural problems elsewhere in the body: unequal leg length, for instance. But if the soft tissues are left untreated and the bones are constantly pulled in one direction or another, they will actually change shape to adapt to those stressors. At this point, the condition becomes a *structural* dysfunction, and is much harder to reverse.

SIGNS AND SYMPTOMS

Postural deviations can range from being painfully obvious to quite subtle. A visual exam will yield a lot of information about kyphosis and lordosis, and even mild scoliosis may be visible with a forward-bending test. Clients' complaints will often include muscular tension and sometimes nerve impairment along with chronic ache and loss of range of motion.

Scoliosis.   Scoliosis is a problem for approximately 2% of all teenagers. It affects girls seven times more frequently than boys, and almost always involves a bend to the right. It usually appears during the rapid-growth years of late childhood and early adolescence. Mild scoliosis, which is any curve less than 30° to 40°, is treated, if at all, with exercise, chiropractic, a corrective brace, and/or electromuscular stimulation to strengthen the muscles of the stretched side of the spine. If the scoliosis measures at over 40° in childhood, the chances that it will worsen are very great. It typically progresses at 1° every year.

The cause of most cases of scoliosis is unknown. Some situations can be traced to polio, tuberculosis, tumors, or a congenital birth defect. Others are related to unequal leg length or problems in the pelvic bones. But the vast majority of cases (80%) have no known source.

Complications of scoliosis include *neuritis* (chapter 3, page 157), as misshaped bones press on nerve roots; *spondylosis* (this chapter, page 84); and heart and lung problems from a severely restricted rib cage.

Surgery for scoliosis involves inserting rods that straighten and fuse the affected vertebrae. This limits spinal mobility but it can definitely improve the quality of life for people with advanced scoliosis.

Kyphosis.   Kyphosis is an overdeveloped thoracic curve. In young people it is very often a result of muscular imbalance, and may be treated with physical therapy. Kyphosis in older people may be due to muscular imbalance, but it could also be a complication of *osteoporosis* (this chapter, page 62) or *ankylosing spondylitis* (this chapter, page 69). A kyphotic curve of 20° to 40° is considered normal. Surgical intervention isn't usually suggested for anything under a 75° curvature.

Lordosis.   Lordosis or swayback is an overpronounced lumbar curve. The architecture and musculature of the low back makes it particularly vulnerable to this kind of imbalance. It can often be much improved by exercise and physical therapy (including massage). Lordosis, although not dangerous in itself, can lead to more serious low back pain. (See *sciatica*, this chapter, page 118, and *herniated disc*, this chapter, page 114.)

TREATMENT

Treatment options for different kinds of postural deviations are outlined in the descriptions above.

MASSAGE?

As long as there is no underlying pathology, massage is indicated for all kinds of postural deviations. In the early stages of these conditions, a situation of chronic soft-tissue (that is, muscular, tendinous, and ligamentous) stresses are pulling on the bones and changing the architecture of the spine. Caught early enough, many bad postural habits can be reversed without permanent damage. But bone is living, adaptable tissue, and left untreated, the vertebrae will eventually remold themselves to permanently imprint a postural pattern.

Massage certainly won't make any of these conditions any worse, and could quite possibly offer a lot of relief by simply reducing some of the tension that both causes and accompanies spinal imbalance. If a therapist is very skilled and the circumstances are just right, massage may set the stage for a permanent change in bony alignment.

Joint Disorders

Ankylosing Spondylitis

DEFINITION: WHAT IS IT?

Ankylosing spondylitis (AS) is a spinal inflammation leading to stiff joints. And this means very stiff—these joints can become permanently fused. This is a progressive inflammatory arthritis of the spine, sometimes called rheumatoid spondylitis.

DEMOGRAPHICS: WHO GETS IT?

Ankylosing spondylitis is an inherited autoimmune disorder that tends to affect men between 16 and 35. A gene has been identified that seems to increase the tendency to develop this disease, but it is not a definitive factor; many people with the AS gene never have symptoms. About 1%, or 2.5 million, people in the United States have some degree of ankylosing spondylitis; 90% of them are males.

ETIOLOGY: WHAT HAPPENS?

The disease typically starts at the sacroiliac joint on one or both sides. Though it generally sticks to spinal joints, the hips, shoulders, toes, and sternoclavicular joints also may be affected. The joints become inflamed in the acute stage and when the inflammation subsides, the bony surfaces inside the joint have become roughened. Eventually they fuse together. The pattern of inflammation and damage proceeds up the spine leaving in its wake a trail of injured vertebrae that tend to freeze in slight or sometimes extreme flexion. (See Figure 2.13.) If the progression reaches all the way up to the neck, the cervical vertebrae may fuse with the head in a permanently flexed position as well. There can also be fusions at the vertebral-costal joints, resulting in a locked ribcage and difficulty with breathing.

ANKYLOSING SPONDYLITIS

"Ankyle" comes from the Greek *ankylos*, meaning bent or crooked, and *ankylosis*, meaning stiffening of the joints. "Spondylitis" means spinal inflammation. Ankylosing spondylitis: inflammatory stiffening of the spine in a bent position.

ANKYLOSING SPONDYLITIS IN BRIEF

What is it?

Ankylosing spondylitis (AS) is a progressive arthritis of the spine.

How is it recognized?

It generally begins as stiffness and pain around the sacrum, with occasional referred pain down the back of the buttocks and into the legs. It has acute and subacute episodes. People with advanced AS are locked in a flexed position.

Is massage indicated or contraindicated?

Massage is indicated in the subacute stages of AS only, and then only under a doctor's supervision. During acute episodes, massage is at least locally contraindicated in areas of pain and inflammation.

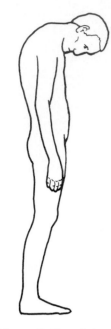

Figure 2.13 Ankylosing spondylitis

SIGNS AND SYMPTOMS

Ankylosing spondylitis usually starts as chronic low back pain. Often pain is felt in the buttocks, and sometimes all the way down into the heels. This can sometimes lead to a misdiagnosis of herniated disc. The spine and hips feel stiff and immobile; this is usually much worse in the morning or after prolonged immobility. The condition has acute and subacute stages. During acute episodes, the person has a general feeling of illness, a slight fever, and the eyes may become dry, red, and uncomfortable. Pain and stiffness gradually spread higher and higher up the spine. Usually the disease will limit itself to the low back, but occasionally it proceeds right up into the neck.

COMPLICATIONS

Loss of lung capacity is the major complication for this disease. If a person is bent over and his ribs can't expand, it is very difficult to get an adequate supply of oxygen into the body, or to dispel carbon dioxide. This results in constant shortness of breath, low stamina, and reduced resistance to chest infections such as pneumonia from which, depending on posture, it can be very difficult to recover.

Spinal fusions and loss of mobility will increase the risk of spinal fractures. If the disease progresses all the way up the neck, the jaw will also be stiff, so that talking and eating become difficult.

The inflammatory nature of AS is not restricted to joints around the spine. The inflammation may spread to other organs, including the eyes, lungs, heart, and kidneys.

DIAGNOSIS

Ankylosing spondylitis is identified by observable symptoms, blood tests, and x-rays. It can be difficult to diagnose in the early stages, since many disorders can cause diffuse back pain and stiffness. It sometimes takes years to confirm a diagnosis of AS.

One feature that can assist in a diagnosis of AS is that it often appears along with other disorders. Particular red flags are chronic prostatitis, Crohn's disease, *ulcerative colitis* (see chapter 7, page 290), and *psoriasis* (see chapter 1, page 26). Also, people in the immediate family of an AS patient show statistically higher rates of psoriatic arthritis, Reiter's Syndrome (a systemic inflammatory condition), Crohn's disease, and ulcerative colitis.

TREATMENT

The first, best option for dealing with ankylosing spondylitis (which has no known cause, and therefore, no cure) is exercise. Physical therapy is recommended to develop a series of exercises that will, as much as possible, preserve the suppleness of the spine and the strength of the paraspinals, without aggravating the condition. Maintaining correct posture for as long as possible is the primary goal, since the vertebrae tend to fuse in a flexed position.

If exercise alone is not helping, painkillers and anti-inflammatories may be prescribed. In very extreme cases, surgery may be suggested: an osteotomy is a procedure which will cut through the fused joints and re-fuse them in a straightened position. If the knees, shoulders, or hips have been impaired, joint replacement surgery may also be suggested.

MASSAGE?

Little is well understood about this disease, and virtually nothing is known about how massage might affect it. But because it is an inflammatory condition, and because it does spread, a massage practitioner would have to proceed with extreme caution. Always work with this condition in conjunction with a doctor. Only work when the inflammation is subacute; reschedule an appointment rather than working on someone whose spinal joints are inflamed. If a client is in the early stages of this disease, massage may help to preserve that precious mobility of the spine. If a client is more advanced, massage will probably have little effect except pain relief, since the muscles are being stretched over immobile joints.

Chondromalacia/Patellofemoral Syndrome

DEFINITION: WHAT IS IT?

Chondromalacia is a condition in which the patellar cartilage becomes damaged as it contacts the femoral cartilage. This situation is sometimes a precursor of *osteoarthritis* at the knee (see this chapter, page 77).

Chondromalacia is almost always associated with overuse, although it may be precipitated by a specific injury or trauma. PFS, a collection of signs and symptoms that indicate damage to the patellar cartilage, is a term that is sometimes used interchangeably with chondromalacia.

ETIOLOGY: WHAT HAPPENS?

There are two main ways to wear down the cartilage on the back of the patella. One is by simple overuse. Unfortunately, one person's "I've overused it" is another person's "I barely got started." That's because everyone is born with a different amount of cartilage on the patella. People with "thick cartilage" genes may never get PFS, but for people with "ridiculously thin cartilage" genes, it will take only a small amount of use to wear through it and land with a textbook example of overuse PFS.

The other way to wear down patellar cartilage is something, unlike genetic structure, that people have some control over: the alignment of the knee. If the patella is pulled slightly to one side or the other, the wear on the cartilage will be uneven, and will leave the client vulnerable to cartilage damage.

SIGNS AND SYMPTOMS

Symptoms of PFS include pain that is usually felt deep in the knee, stiffness after long immobility, difficulty walking down stairs, and a characteristic crackling, grinding noise on movement.

DIAGNOSIS

PFS can be difficult to diagnose, especially in the early stages before damage to the bones is visible. The problem is that what is often called chondromalacia or PFS may actually be another condition, *patellar tendinitis*. This is significant because while chondromalacia is largely unaffected by massage, patellar tendinitis responds beautifully, for a possibly virtually pain-free resolution. (See *tendinitis*, this chapter, page 103.) So it's important to have a clear idea of what a client really has. One useful clue is that patellar tendinitis often hurts going *up* stairs (resisted extension of the leg) while chondromalacia may hurt more going *down* stairs (the weight of the femur pushing on the patella). However, only a doctor with an arthroscope can give an absolutely definitive diagnosis.

TREATMENT

The long-term prognosis for someone with PFS depends entirely on what they do with it. It seldom gets to the point of requiring a joint replacement. But this condition is badly

CHONDROMALACIA/ PATELLOFEMORAL SYNDROME IN BRIEF

What is it?
Chondromalacia is a pathological softening of the patellar cartilage. Patellofemoral syndrome (PFS) is an overuse syndrome that can lead to this sort of damage.

How is it recognized?
Chondromalacia causes pain at the knee, stiffness after immobility, and discomfort in walking down stairs.

Is massage indicated or contraindicated?
Massage is indicated for chondromalacia and PFS, assuming the knee is not acutely inflamed. Massage may or may not be useful to correct these problems, but it will certainly do no harm.

CHONDROMALACIA

"Chondro" comes from the Greek word *chondrion*, which refers to groats, a type of coursely ground meal. Essentially it means a gritty substance, and can refer to gristle as well as to cartilage. "Malacia" comes from the Greek word *malakos*, for "softening." Chondromalacia, then, is a softening of cartilage.

irritated by jarring, jouncing, bouncing kinds of exercise. If one kind of activity becomes prohibitive (running and aerobics are not great choices for someone with PFS), it can probably be replaced with something else, like swimming, walking, cycling, or skating. Patients may have to experiment, under a doctor's supervision, to find the exercise activities that work best.

MASSAGE?

If the knee is inflamed and painful, massage is locally contraindicated. But chondromalacia and PFS are more often chronic, low-level irritations that interfere with normal activity, and massage certainly won't make the situation any worse. Whether massage can be instrumental in *improving* knee function depends on the situation. The quadriceps and other muscle-tendon units that cross the knee are likely to be stiff and tender if there is chronic pain, and massage can address that. If massage is included in a treatment strategy to retrain the knee extensors to track the patella appropriately over the joint, it can be a useful part of an effort to slow down or stop permanent cartilage damage.

Dislocations

DEFINITION: WHAT ARE THEY?

When the bones in a joint are separated so that they no longer articulate, the joint is said to be dislocated. It's hard to imagine this happening without damage to most of the surrounding tissues as well; muscles, tendons, blood vessels, and nerves are generally also injured in a traumatic dislocation. (See Figure 2.14.) Bursae will probably also become in-

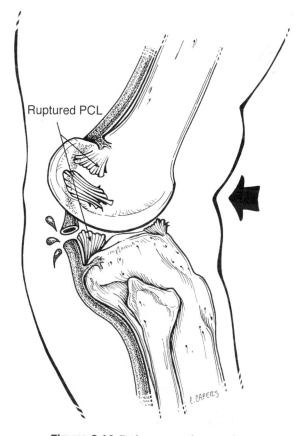

Ruptured PCL

Figure 2.14 Dislocations often involve extensive soft tissue damage

DISLOCATIONS IN BRIEF

What are they?
Dislocations are traumatic injuries to joints in which the articulating bones are forcefully separated.

How are they recognized?
Acute (new) dislocations are extremely painful. The bones may be visibly separated and a total loss of function occurs at the joint.

Is massage indicated or contraindicated?
Massage is indicated in the subacute stage for dislocations, as long as work is conducted within pain tolerance. As the area heals, massage may be useful for managing scar tissue accumulation and muscle spasm around the affected joint.

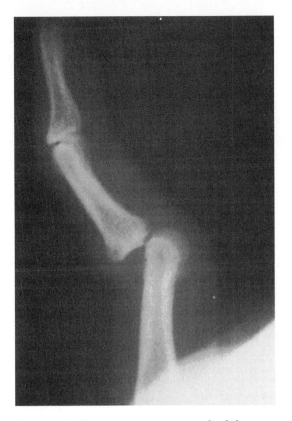

Figure 2.15 Fingers are common sites for dislocations

flamed. Dislocations are most often due to trauma, but some are brought about by congenital weakness of the ligaments, and others by diseases such as rheumatoid arthritis, which may involve degenerated bone tissue inside joints, raising the risk of having the joint literally fall apart.

SIGNS AND SYMPTOMS

Most of the joints in the body will not dislocate without huge amounts of force. The shoulder, because of the shallowness of the glenoid fossa, and the fingers are the joints most at risk for dislocation. (See Figure 2.15.) The TMJ, or temporal-mandibular joint is another common site. (See *TMJ Disorders*, this chapter, page 89.) Symptoms of a newly dislocated joint include swelling, discoloration, loss of function, and, most obviously, a lot of pain.

COMPLICATIONS

Uncomplicated traumatic dislocations are painful, and take a long time to heal, but they are not usually serious. Fibrosis or *contractures* (this chapter, page 49) may develop after prolonged splinting. Occasionally a nerve will be severely damaged by the bone, but this is the exception rather than the rule.

If, however, the ligaments supporting the damaged joint have become stretched, they may lose some of their ability to do their job. The ligaments may even rupture and detach from the bone altogether. In this case, the joint may become unstable and prone to reinjury: "subluxation" if the bones move out of alignment, "spontaneous dislocation" if the bones completely separate. These mishaps are especially common in the shoulder and jaw. The muscles that cross over these unstable joints are likely to be much tighter than is ideal, because the ligaments aren't doing their job. This can lead to *fibromyalgia* (this chapter, page 50) or *tendinitis* (this chapter, page 103). But the most serious long-term consequence of ligament laxity is the possibility of developing *osteoarthritis* (this chapter, page 77).

TREATMENT

Acute dislocations require immediate attention. If large joints are not relocated within about fifteen minutes, the tissues will swell up so much and the muscles will contract so tightly that it will be difficult to move the joint without a general anesthetic. After the joint is relocated, an x-ray is usually taken to rule out the possibility of a *fracture* (this chapter, page 60). The joint will then typically be splinted for two or three weeks until the capsular ligament and other supportive ligaments are ready to carry their weight again. Physical therapy is prescribed to strengthen and retrain the muscles surrounding the joint.

If the ligaments have ruptured or are simply too lax to properly support the joint capsule, surgery may be recommended. Typically this involves shortening and/or reattaching the damaged ligaments to the bone using stitches or staples. Arthroscopic surgery for dislocated shoulders is a new field that may be able to improve joint function without the complications of major surgery.

An alternative to surgery for chronically lax ligaments is a highly specialized series of injections of substances called *proliferants*. They are designed to stimulate the growth of new collagen fibers, which, with appropriate stretching and exercise, will lay down in alignment with the original fibers. This procedure can actually tighten stretched-out ligaments, thus reducing the chance of future injury.

MASSAGE?

Obviously, massage is out of the question for an acute injury of this type. In the subacute stage, massage may help untangle the muscular and tendinous scar tissue that is likely to develop as a result of dislocations, as long as the basic rules about working within tolerance, following up with ice, and monitoring results are followed.

If a client has an *old* dislocation that occasionally subluxates or even entirely dislocates without trauma, massage will do no harm as long as care is taken be sure the client is positioned in a way that feels safe and comfortable.

Gout

DEFINITION: WHAT IS IT?

Gout is one of the oldest diseases in recorded medical history. In 580 AD, Alexander of Tralles wrote, "Gout sufferers should eat little meat, drink no alcohol and eat the underground stems of calchium (autumn crocus)."[5] One of the drugs in use today for the treatment of gout is colchicine, a synthetic version of autumn crocus.

Gout has been known as the "disease of kings," associated with rich diets and decadent living. This is illustrated by a list of some of gout's most famous victims: Alexander the Great, Henry VIII of England, Charles V of Spain and his son Phillip II, Dr. Samuel Johnson, Wolfgang von Goethe, and Benjamin Franklin.

Gout is a type of inflammatory arthritis with a chemical cause, rather than a result of wear and tear or immune system mistakes.

DEMOGRAPHICS: WHO GETS IT?

Gout affects men more than women, by a wide margin: 80% of gout sufferers are men (the prime age to develop the disease is 75 years); 20% are women, and most of those are postmenopausal. The United States has about one million gout patients.

[5] Thomas DiBacco. The pain of gout. Washington Post, October 11, 1994:Z19.

ETIOLOGY: WHAT HAPPENS?

With gout, the body is unable to shed enough uric acid (sodium urate). This substance, a relatively heavy by-product of digestion, will tend to collect in the feet and precipitate out of the blood, forming little crystals. These collect in interstitial spaces, and diffuse into joint capsules. The sharp, pointy, irritating crystals of sodium urate will grind on joint capsules and aggravate them into an inflammatory response. It takes a lot of uric acid to create acute gouty arthritis, or AGA, but once it accumulates, it doesn't go away.

In later stages of the disease, deposits of sodium urate called *tophi* will develop inside joints. These tophi will progressively erode all of the joint structures, leading to a complete loss of function. Tophi also grow along tendons and in subcutaneous tissues. They have been found in myocardium, pericardium, aortic valves, and even the pinna of the ear!

GOUT IN BRIEF

What is it?
Gout is an inflammatory arthritis caused by deposits of sodium urate (uric acid) in and around joints, especially in the feet.

How is it recognized?
Acute gout causes joints to become red, hot, swollen, shiny, and extremely painful. It usually has a sudden onset.

Is massage indicated or contraindicated?
Massage is systemically contraindicated for gout in the acute stage, and locally contraindicated for gouty joints at all times.

RISK FACTORS

Sodium urate, the substance that forms gout crystals, is a by-product of uric acid. Uric acid is a waste product from the metabolism of a certain component of nucleic acids called *purines*. A diet that is high in purines will tend to produce more uric acid in the body than a diet that is not. What's high in purines? Red meat, organ meats, fish, foul, lentils, alcohol, mushrooms, and some vegetables, including peas, asparagus, and spinach. Where does all the uric acid go? To the kidneys, to be excreted. Here is where the problems may start.

- Metabolic gout: In this situation the kidneys may be functioning normally, but the body is producing too much uric acid for them to keep up. This is the case for someone with a particularly high protein/alcohol intake.
- Renal gout: In this case the uric acid load may be normal, but the kidneys aren't functioning well. They can't handle the job of excreting all the uric acid, and so it ends up in the bloodstream, and eventually, in the feet. This kind of kidney insufficiency may be hereditary or related to other problems, such as *diabetes* (chapter 4, page 210) or lead poisoning.
- Both: Here the kidneys are compromised and the purine intake is high. This is gout, waiting to happen.

There is a clear connection between elevated levels of uric acid (*hyperuricemia*) and gout, but the two things are not always identical. Many people have hyperuricemia without ever having gout. Conversely, some people with gout show normal or even below normal levels of uric acid in the blood.

Other risk factors for gout besides a high purine diet include obesity, sudden weight gain, moderate to high alcohol consumption, high blood pressure, and certain blood disorders that can raise uric acid levels.

Once some combination of these risk factors is in place, it may take a very little push to precipitate an attack of gout. There is very often a specific event that triggers an episode. Some dependable triggers are episodes of especially heavy eating or alcohol consumption, sudden illness, dehydration, surgery, or injury to the foot.

SIGNS AND SYMPTOMS

AGA has some very predictable patterns. It has a sudden onset, and almost always happens in the feet first, especially at the joints of the great toe. (See Figure 2.16.) It may also appear in the ankles, knees, wrists, and fingers.

Sometimes a person will have just one attack of gout, and then never be bothered by it again. Usually the second attack will come several years later. The third attack will happen after a shorter interval, and the fourth one, shorter still. Each event resolves itself in a few days or weeks. After 10 to 20 years, a patient may end up with almost constant acute attacks of this disease, but often by that time the associated problems of this condition may make toe pain the least of his worries.

The acute gouty joint will show all the signs of extreme inflammation. The joint may swell so much that the skin becomes hot, red, dry, shiny, and exquisitely painful. This phase of inflammation is often accompanied by a moderate fever (up to 101° or so) and chills.

COMPLICATIONS

The complications of gout are actually complications of having too much uric acid in the bloodstream, which indicates kidneys that are not functioning at adequate levels. Uric acid crystals don't cause only gout; they can also cause *kidney stones* (chapter 8, page 310). If the kidneys become sufficiently clogged by kidney stones, the result will be *renal failure* (chapter 8, page 314). Impaired kidneys can't process adequate fluid. This stresses the rest of the circulatory system, causing *high blood pressure* (hypertension), (chapter 4, page 199), the end result of which can be *coronary artery disease* (atherosclerosis) (chapter 4, page 193) or *stroke* (chapter 3, page 161). All of these problems—hyperuricemia, kidney insufficiency, gout, high blood pressure, and cardiovascular disease—are closely related.

DIAGNOSIS

Gout is usually easy to recognize by its specific pain profile: sudden onset with long intervals between attacks. However, it sometimes mimics a few other conditions, including *rheumatoid arthritis* (RA) (this chapter, page 80), *septic arthritis* (this chapter, page 83), psoriatic arthritis, or pseudogout, another chemically based arthritis in which crystals of an entirely different type are deposited in and around joints. The only conclusive diagnosis for gout is an examination of aspirated fluid from an affected joint to look for uric acid crystals.

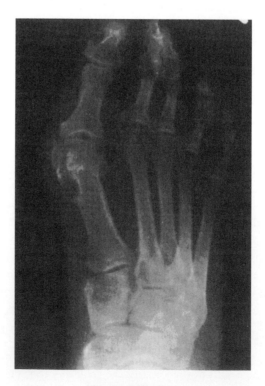

Figure 2.16 Gout

TREATMENT

A standard medical approach to gout takes three paths: pain relief (with analgesics *other* than aspirin, which inhibits uric acid excretion), anti-inflammatory drugs, and, finally, drugs that will modify metabolism. Preventive measures include increasing fluid intake (other than caffeine or alcohol, which act as diuretics), losing weight, and limiting purine-rich foods.

MASSAGE?

Gout, at the very least, locally contraindicates massage of the affected joints at all times. The last thing this client needs is to have someone grind those little crystals any deeper into his flesh. In its acute stage, gout systemically contraindicates massage, but it's unlikely that anyone in a full-blown attack would try to keep a massage appointment. Any client who is prone to gout is a good candidate for other circulatory or excretory problems; he should receive medical clearance before receiving massage.

Osteoarthritis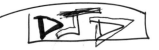

DEFINITION: WHAT IS IT?

Osteoarthritis is a condition in which synovial joints, especially weight-bearing joints, are irritated and inflamed. This condition is distinguished from other types of arthritis by being directly related to wear and tear of the joint structures.

DEMOGRAPHICS: WHO GETS IT?

Also called *degenerative joint disease*, this is by far the most common type of arthritis in the world. Osteoarthritis affects close to 16 million Americans, and is responsible for 7 million doctor visits each year. It's also an occupational hazard for massage therapists, who may get it at the saddle joint of the thumb because it's easy to put too much pressure on this joint if good body mechanics aren't employed.

ETIOLOGY: WHAT HAPPENS?

Joints, especially knees and hips, endure tremendous weight-bearing stress and repetitive movements; their design is a marvel of efficiency and durability. But the environment inside a joint capsule is actually very precarious. Any imbalance can have cumulative destructive impact. And once the path toward arthritis has begun, it's possible to slow the process, but there is no turning back.

All synovial joints have five features in common: the articular bones, the cartilage that covers them, a ligamentous joint capsule, a synovial membrane that lines it, and the synovial fluid to lubricate the cartilage. In weight-bearing joints, it's important to remember that the articulating layers of cartilage are almost always touching; one layer of cartilage rests directly on top of the other.

Progression

- Step One: Cartilage Damage. After years of use or repetitive injury, the cartilage in a knee or hip may begin to flake, just the tiniest bit. If the cartilage on one side of the joint is even slightly roughened, it

---

OSTEOARTHRITIS IN BRIEF

What is it?
This is joint inflammation brought about by wear and tear causing cumulative damage to articular cartilage.

How is it recognized?
Affected joints are stiff, painful, and occasionally palpably inflamed. Osteoarthritis most often affects knees, hips, and distal joints of the fingers.

Is massage indicated or contraindicated?
Massage is locally contraindicated in the acute stage and indicated in the subacute stage, when it can contribute to muscular relaxation and mobility of the affected joint.

will act like sandpaper on the cartilage of the opposite side, instead of being smooth for easy, gliding movement. Then the *other* cartilage gets rough and further damages the first side. Once cartilage damage inside the joint occurs, the downhill slide has begun. The only question is, how far will it go? (See Figure 2.17.)

- Step Two: Bony Adaptation. The cartilaginous surfaces of two articulating bones become rough instead of smooth. Each time one moves, the other gets irritated. An inflammatory reaction may ensue. Since the cartilage is no longer doing its job, the bones (which are living tissue and will respond to stresses put upon them) will begin to adapt. But bones can't replace damaged cartilage. Instead of making a new, smooth surface inside the joint capsules, bones will have a tendency to thicken at the condyles, and make small spurs on the ends, where they sense the most stress. This will further limit freedom of movement and increase pain.

- Step Three: The Muscles React. Any muscles that cross a stiff, painful, and constantly aggravated joint will tend to tighten up. That's what muscles do when they are in areas of constant pain (see *spasms, cramps,* this chapter, page 57). It's also likely that they would develop some trigger points in the process, because they won't really get to relax as long as that joint is in pain. And the tension they cause will compress the joint, making it even more painful, which will reinforce the spasm, and so on. (See *fibromyalgia,* this chapter, page 50.)

- Step Four: Atrophy. Eventually the arthritis sufferer will want to stop using the injured joint, because it hurts so much. Lack of use may lead to atrophy: wasting away. The surrounding muscles will weaken, the synovial membranes will stop functioning, and the joint fluid will dry up. It could progress to the point where even if the patient wanted to move again, she wouldn't be able to because the muscles and the joint structures will have degenerated too far.

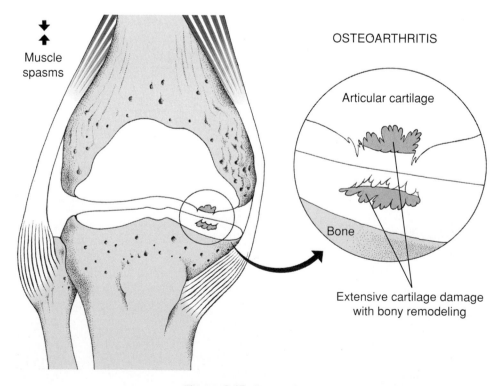

Figure 2.17 Osteoarthritis

CAUSES

Many changes in the body may begin the process of joint degeneration. When the ligaments that surround joints become chronically loose, the joint can become unstable, raising the risk of arthritis (see *dislocations*, this chapter, page 72). Repetitive pounding stress, such as running or jumping with inadequate support, also opens the door to problems. Hormonal imbalances and nutritional deficiencies, including inadequate calcium metabolism, may compromise the health of joint structures. Age itself will tend to change the quality of articular cartilage, making it drier and more prone to injury.

In determining the source of the problem, many experts distinguish between primary or idiopathic osteoarthritis, which has no discernible cause, and secondary osteoarthritis, which develops as a result of injury or cumulative wear and tear.

SIGNS AND SYMPTOMS

The symptoms of osteoarthritis all revolve around inflammation of the joint capsule. In the acute stage the joints will be hot, painful, and swollen. In the subacute stage the joints will have milder pain and stiffness. Osteoarthritis can be completely debilitating when it occurs at the hip or knee because the pain and limitation are badly exacerbated by walking.

DIAGNOSIS

Osteoarthritis is identified by physical examination and patient history. Tests may be conducted to rule out other conditions, but no blood test will absolutely confirm the presence of osteoarthritis. Even x-rays can be misleading. They may be used to back up a diagnosis, but a surprisingly high percentage of people who show osteoarthritis-like bony deformations on x-ray experience no pain at all. This is because different people are blessed with different thicknesses of cartilage, which doesn't show on x-rays. A person with thin cartilage will be more likely to feel pain from arthritis than a person with thicker cartilage. (See *chondromalacia/patellofemoral syndrome*, this chapter, page 71.)

RELATED CONDITIONS

Degenerative joint disease almost always affects the big weight-bearing joints like knees, hips, and the spine. In the spine it is called *spondylosis* (this chapter, page 84). Its tendency to damage these joints is one of the features that distinguishes it from rheumatoid arthritis. Like RA, osteoarthritis can affect the fingers, but osteoarthritis usually happens in the distal interphalangeal joints (DIPs), while RA is more common in the proximal interphalangeal joints (PIPs) and hand joints. Another difference is that RA tends to be bilaterally symmetrical, while osteoarthritis will simply follow the pattern of most use.

Finally, RA, *lupus* (chapter 5, page 241), and other types of inflammatory arthritis will create systemic reactions in the body: fever, deposits in other types of tissues, etc. Osteoarthritis limits its damage exclusively to synovial joints. It is *not* a systemic disease.

TREATMENT

Osteoarthritis is seldom curable or reversible. Caught in early stages, proliferant injections inside the affected joint may stimulate the growth of new cartilage, while similar injections to the surrounding ligaments can help them to tighten up and do a better job of stabilizing the joint. But most treatment strategies are geared for preparing a patient to live with this condition for a long, long time. Pain relieving and anti-inflammatory medicines may be suggested or prescribed, and moderate exercise and activity is highly recommended to keep the affected joints as mobile and healthy as possible.

If these methods are ineffective and the arthritis is bad enough to seriously limit someone's activity, the next step is to consider joint replacement. Although this is a major operation, some remarkable things are being accomplished with it, and the speed of recovery can be surprisingly short. A new surgical technique that shows promise involves growing some of the patient's own cartilage cells in a laboratory, and then "patching" them over the damaged areas of the joint. This may be significantly less stressful and easier to recover from than a complete joint replacement.

MASSAGE?

Acute arthritis, like other acute inflammatory conditions, contraindicates massage. Massage is indicated for osteoarthritis in the subacute stage, when goals would be to reduce pain through release of the muscles surrounding the affected joints, and to maintain range of motion through gentle stretching and passive gymnastics.

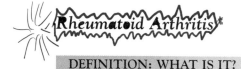

DEFINITION: WHAT IS IT?

This condition is sometimes called "crippling arthritis," which is a misnomer. *Rheumatoid* means "of the nature of rheumatism." *Rheumatism* means "pain in muscles or joints." In short, the name of this disease tells very little except that it involves pain and inflammation of the joints.

DEMOGRAPHICS: WHO GETS IT?

This disease affects 2.1 million Americans, and women are affected about three times more frequently than men. Statistics indicate that it is most common among 20 to 40 year olds, but it can strike anyone, including children and adolescents. It tends to run in families, and a genetic marker has been identified. This marker, however, only identifies persons at risk for the disease. Most people who bear the gene do *not* develop RA.

ETIOLOGY: WHAT HAPPENS?

RA is an autoimmune disease. This condition is brought about by a mistake in the vastly complex and usually very effective immune system. Normal, healthy tissues are misidentified as threatening invaders, and are attacked by immune system agents. Autoimmune diseases are triggered by pathogens that closely resemble some part of the body's own proteins. A pathogen's protein coat needs to have only five amino acids in the same order as some normal, healthy part of the body to trigger an autoimmune disease response.

In rheumatoid arthritis, an immune system attack is targeted for a specific protein, but that protein *isn't* on an invading microbe; it's in the synovial membranes. This leads to all the cardinal signs of inflammation: heat, pain, redness, swelling, loss of function. In later stages the antibodies may also attack the heart, blood vessels, lungs, and fascia.

Several pathogens that may initiate rheumatoid arthritis have been identified. They include a variety of streptococcus bacterium, borellia (the same bacterium that causes Lyme disease), and some retroviruses. Contracting and sustaining damage from rheumatoid arthritis begins with exposure to one of these pathogens. Here is an example of a typical progression of rheumatoid arthritis:

RHEUMATOID ARTHRITIS IN BRIEF

What is it?
Rheumatoid arthritis (RA) is an autoimmune disease in which synovial membranes, particularly of the joints in the hands and feet, are attacked by immune system agents. Other structures, such as muscles, tendons, and blood vessels, may also be affected.

How is it recognized?
In the acute phase, affected joints are red, swollen, hot, and painful. They often become gnarled and distorted. It tends to affect the body symmetrically, and it is not determined by age.

Is massage indicated or contraindicated?
Massage is systemically contraindicated during acute episodes of RA. Massage is indicated in the subacute stages when it may be used to reestablish mobility and to reduce the stresses that can trigger another flare.

- A person has a bout with strep throat. She goes through the usual process of producing T cells, B cells, and antibodies. She wins the fight, and the bacterium is vanquished, but now she has a regiment of memory cells and antibodies in circulation, looking for any remnants of the invading microorganisms.
- Her antibodies get confused. The proteins in synovial membranes have enough in common with the proteins in the strep molecules that her immune system raises the alarm and launches a full-scale attack. This is where genetics may play a role; this person's antibodies are actually programmed to be "auto-antibodies."
- The synovial membrane thickens and swells. Fluid inside the joint capsule begins to accumulate, which causes pressure and pain.
- The inflamed tissues release enzymes that erode cartilage, eventually right down to the bone. This is the process that causes the tell-tale deformation of the joint capsules and "gnarled" appearance accompanying RA. (See Figure 2.18.)
- Fibrous scar tissue develops to connect the raw ends of the bones.
- The scar tissue ossifies, and the joint is permanently fused.

Actually, the disease doesn't always progress all the way to the final two steps. As serious a condition as RA could be, it seldom fulfills the worst of its promises. After coping with the disease for 10 to 15 years, approximately 20% of affected people are in remission. Most are able to retain full-time employment. After 15 to 20 years of living with RA, only about 10% of affected people are permanently disabled.

SIGNS AND SYMPTOMS

Symptoms of RA vary considerably at the onset of the disease. Many people experience a period of weeks or months during which they experience a general feeling of illness: lack of energy, lack of appetite, low-grade fever, and vague muscle pain, which gradually becomes sharp, specific joint pain. About 10% experience a sudden onset with joint pain alone. Rheumatic nodules—small, painless bumps that appear around fingers, elbows, and other pressure-bearing areas—are also common indicators of the disease.

In the acute stage, the affected joints are red, hot, painful, and stiff, although they improve considerably with moderate amounts of movement and stretching. The joints RA most often attack are the knuckles in hands and toes. RA can also appear in ankles and

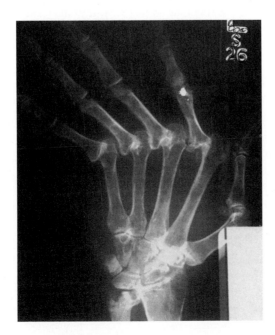

Figure 2.18 Rheumatoid arthritis

wrists; knees are less common, and one of the rarest (and most serious) places to get it is in the neck. It generally affects the body bilaterally, although it sometimes will be worse on one side than the other.

COMPLICATIONS

If someone has rheumatoid arthritis, it means her immune system is confused about what it should be fighting. Synovial membranes are just one of the types of tissue that may be attacked. Other possibilities lead to the following related conditions:

- Rheumatic nodules on the sclera ("whites") of the eyes.
- Sjogren's syndrome (pathologically dry eyes and mouth).
- Pleuritis, which makes breathing painful and increases vulnerability to lung infection.
- Pericarditis, or inflammation of the pericardial sac around the heart.
- Vasculitis, or inflammation of blood vessels. This complication carries another set of risks: *Raynaud's syndrome* (chapter 4, page 202), *skin ulcers* (chapter 1, page 36), bleeding *intestinal ulcers* (chapter 7, page 278), and internal hemorrhaging.
- *Bursitis* (this chapter, page 95) and *anemia* (chapter 4, page 178) are also common complications of RA, especially when onset of the disease occurs in childhood.

Advanced structural damage also brings a set of complications. Deformed and bone-damaged joints may dislocate or even collapse, rendering them useless. The tendons that cross over distorted joints sometimes become so stretched that they snap. If the disease causes a collapse at the C1–C2 joint, the resultant injury to the spinal column may even result in paralysis.

DIAGNOSIS

Many clues help to differentiate RA from *osteoarthritis* (this chapter, page 77). RA is not a result of age and joint wear and tear; it does not target the weight-bearing joints; it tends to act symmetrically on the body, rather than simply where the most use has worn down a joint. Nonetheless, it can be difficult to distinguish between the two conditions.

Rheumatoid arthritis is typically diagnosed through a description of symptoms, x-rays, and a blood test to check for rheumatoid factor, a substance that is present in most, but not all, cases. Even then the diagnosis is sometimes not considered conclusive until the patient has been under observation for a long while.

TREATMENT

Once the presence of rheumatoid arthritis has been confirmed, the first step is to try to prevent the disease from progressing. New drug therapies have been developed toward this goal. Emotional and physical trauma have also been known to exacerbate RA attacks, as if the body gets ready to defend itself against *something*, but it can't figure out what. Therefore, keeping the patient as healthy and stress free as possible is important; rest and moderate exercise are key parts of the program.

Other treatment strategies revolve around the goals of minimizing pain and retaining maximum muscle health and joint function. Physical therapists are sometimes recommended to set up exercise programs. Medications may include drugs for pain relief and anti-inflammatories. If the disease continues to get worse, cytotoxic drugs are sometimes used in an effort to reduce white blood cell and antibody activity.

Surgery is seldom considered anything but a last resort for RA patients. If just one joint has been damaged, and if the damage is quite severe, a *synovectomy*, or removal of the synovial membrane, is sometimes performed. Joint replacements are sometimes performed. One fairly new and radical procedure, called *plasmapheresis*, is being used for very extreme cases of RA. This procedure was originally developed to aid in the removal of heavy metals and other toxins from the bloodstream; now it has a broader application. Blood is continually drawn, the aggravating factors (in this case antibodies) removed, and then the blood is replaced in the body. The procedure takes several hours at a time and has a list of serious side effects and complications, so it is seldom used except in the most serious cases.

MASSAGE?

In its acute phase, RA is an inflammatory condition caused by agents in the circulatory system. Anything that increases circulation will also increase the chance that the disease will spread to other joints in the body. In its subacute phase, RA leaves the joints stiff but not inflamed, and the muscles and tendons around them stressed and tight from chronic pain. Rheumatoid arthritis indicates massage only in the subacute stage. Massage can improve mobility and the health of the soft tissues surrounding the joints. In addition to the structural benefits it offers, massage can also be an important part of the keep-healthy-and-stress-free part of prevention strategy. If massage can help to balance the autonomic nervous system, it may also help to reduce the incidence of attack.

Septic Arthritis

DEFINITION: WHAT IS IT?

This is a form of arthritis brought about by a bacterial infection. Puncture wounds that penetrate the joint capsule, introducing staphylococcus or streptococcus, are one source. The infiltration could also result from a surgical procedure or a nearby infection, or the bacteria could have traveled from elsewhere in the body. Six out of every 100,000 people will contract septic arthritis sometime in their life.

ETIOLOGY: WHAT HAPPENS?

It's not easy for an infection to penetrate a joint. No blood vessels go in; unless something contaminated violently penetrates the joint capsule, it's largely a matter of random diffusion through a very tough, thick capsular ligament. But once a bacterial colony is established inside a joint capsule, it will probably thrive. It's warm, it's dark, it's moist, there's plenty to eat and not a white blood cell in sight. Septic arthritis can become very serious in a matter of hours as the bacteria feast on the tissues, filling the joint space with fluid and pus. Permanent damage to the joint will occur if the infection is not treated promptly.

One special variety of septic arthritis is caused by the gonorrhea bacterium. Babies are particularly susceptible to this condition, especially in the hip joint. Another type of bacteria-caused arthritis, called *migratory arthritis*, is brought about by the tick-borne spirochete *Borrelia burgdorferei*, which is also responsible for Lyme disease.

SIGNS AND SYMPTOMS

The symptoms are redness, pain, heat, swelling, and mild to high fever, sometimes hitting 104°, which is quite extreme for adults. Usually just one joint is affected; knees and hips are the most common sites.

Septic arthritis due to gonorrhea has a slightly different pattern. It starts around the sacroiliac joint and progressively moves up the spine much in the manner of *ankylosing spondylitis* (this chapter, page 69), but it shares the same inflammatory symptoms as standard septic arthritis.

SEPTIC ARTHRITIS IN BRIEF

What is it?
Septic arthritis is joint inflammation caused by infection inside the joint capsule.

How is it recognized?
This condition shows the cardinal signs of inflammation: pain, heat, redness, and swelling. It is often accompanied by fever.

Is massage indicated or contraindicated?
Massage is systemically contraindicated for septic arthritis until the infection is completely gone from the joint. At that time, massage may be useful to help restore function.

TREATMENT

Fluid is withdrawn from the joint for diagnosis. If it is found to be full of living and dead bacteria along with whatever white blood cells squeezed their way through the capsular ligament, the joint is then *aspirated* or drained. Antibiotic drugs are administered orally, as an injection into the joint, or both. After the infection has subsided, the joint is set up for rehabilitation to prevent, or at least limit, permanent loss of function.

MASSAGE?

Absolutely not, under any conditions, should massage be given to someone with septic arthritis. Think about what a full range-of-motion gymnastic would do to the bacteria hiding in a corner of an ankle joint: not only could the infection spread more thoroughly through the joint capsule, the infection could get into another part of the body altogether. And because this condition often goes hand-in-hand with a high fever, it strictly systemically contraindicates massage, until the infection is gone.

Once the possibility of infection is past, however, massage can be beneficial to help restore range of motion and suppleness to the joint and surrounding structures.

Spondylosis

DEFINITION: WHAT IS IT?

Spondylosis is the term used to describe osteoarthritis occurring specifically in the spine. Another term for the same condition is *degenerative joint disease*.

ETIOLOGY: WHAT HAPPENS?

Spondylosis usually occurs in the most mobile parts of the spine: the lumbar and cervical regions. Bony remodeling of the vertebral bodies and joints will lead to inflammation and restricted range of motion. One possible cause of this damage is thinned discs that are no longer elastic or resilient. The soft part of the disc calcifies with the aging process. Spondylosis is also a frequent complication of *herniated discs* (this chapter, page 114). Chronic misalignment is another causative factor. This situation will signal bones that *should* be touching to thicken in a peculiar pattern that is exclusive to spondylosis. The bony growths, called *osteophytes*, can also grow inside joint capsules or in the intervertebral foramen, putting pressure on the nerve roots that live there. (See Figure 2.19.) Eventually, arthritic vertebrae may fuse together completely. (See Figure 2.20.)

SIGNS AND SYMPTOMS

Sometimes spondylosis has no symptoms whatever. If the bony changes are not pressing on nerve roots, but growing somewhere that impedes movement, the main symptom will be a slow, painless but irreversible stiffening in the neck.

When the osteophytes *do* press on a nerve root, the symptoms will be very much like those discussed for herniated discs. They include shooting pain, tingling, pins and needles, numbness, and specific muscle weakness. One difference between disc pain and osteophytic pain is that discs, because they are more elastic and flexible than bone spurs, will tend to create pain acutely but intermittently. Osteophytes, on the other hand, do not come and

---

SPONDYLOSIS IN BRIEF

What is it?
Spondylosis is osteoarthritis of the spine.

How is it recognized?
It is identifiable by x-ray, which shows a characteristic thickening of the affected vertebral bodies, facets, and ligamentum flava. Symptoms will be present if pressure is exerted on nerve roots. These will include pain, numbness, paresthesia, and specific muscle weakness.

Is massage indicated or contraindicated?
Massage is indicated for spondylosis, with caution. Muscle splinting, which protects the joints against movement that may be dangerous, is often a feature of this condition; massage therapists should not interfere with this mechanism.

go; if they are in a place to create pain when a person is in a certain position or posture, that pain will be dependable, and it will probably get worse over time instead of better.

COMPLICATIONS

Spondylosis itself is a slowly progressing arthritis that mostly affects middle-aged and elderly people who have accumulated the kind of wear and tear in their spine that would

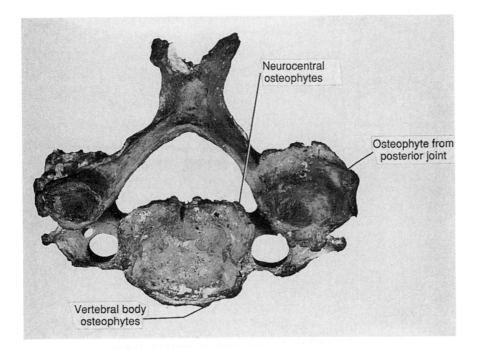

Figure 2.19 Osteophytic growths with spondylosis

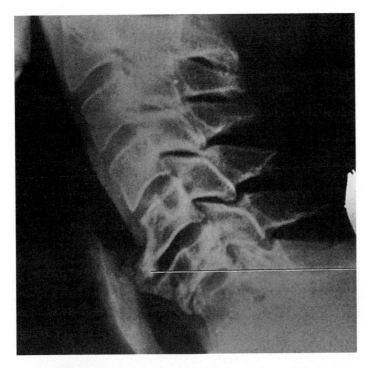

Figure 2.20 Fusion of vertebral bodies with spondylosis

make them vulnerable to this kind of condition. What makes spondylosis more dangerous is the seriousness of the complications that can arise from it.

- Spreading problems in the spine. This is not a progressive disease that travels through the blood. But if two vertebrae become fused through bony remodeling, that puts much more stress on the joints above and below the fusion to provide mobility. Those joints can then become unstable, develop arthritis, and experience the same bony remodeling that created the first problem. Or, the stress of hypermobility may cause disc problems. Herniated discs can be both a *predisposing factor* and a *complication* of spondylosis.
- Nerve pain. This is the consequence of having osteophytes grow where they put pressure on nerve roots in the foramina. (See *neuritis*, chapter 3, page 157).
- Secondary spasm. This will accompany the nerve pain. Muscle spasm may be confined to the paraspinals, where it will exacerbate the problem by compressing the affected joints, or it may follow the path of referred pain. Muscles may also go into spasm to protect the spine from movement that would otherwise be excruciatingly painful.
- Blood vessel pressure. Osteophytes in the neck are sometimes situated to press on the vertebral arteries as they go up the transverse foramina. If the head is turned or bent in a certain position, the patient may feel dizzy, have headaches, or double vision from impaired blood flow into the head.
- Spinal cord pressure. This is a rare and extremely serious complication of spondylosis in the neck. Osteophytes will very occasionally grow in a place to put pressure not on the nerve roots, but in the spinal cord itself. This will be felt as progressive weakening down the body, possible loss of bladder and bowel control, and even eventual paralysis. The surgery for this condition involves creating a larger foramen for the spinal cord to pass through and permanently fusing the involved vertebrae.

    Another possibility is that once these joints have weakened, any minor trauma that involves hyperextension of the neck may also lead to spinal cord pressure.

DIAGNOSIS

The characteristic thickening or hypertrophy of the vertebral bodies that accompanies spondylosis is easily identified by x-ray. Also a predictable distortion of facet joints in the lumbar spine occurs, and the ligamentum flava, the ligaments that cover the joint capsules, will often visibly thicken and buckle with spondylosis.

It's important to point out that x-rays of 25 to 50% of all people over 50 years old will show signs of spondylosis.[6] X-rays of 75% of people over 75 years old will be positive for spondylosis—and most people will never experience arthritic pain! Therefore, if a mature person complains of low back or neck pain, an x-ray is likely to point toward spondylosis, while the pain may actually be something completely different, such as an inflamed disc or injured spinal ligaments.

TREATMENT

Treatment will depend on which (if any) complications present themselves. Anti-inflammatories are the usual first recourse. Movement and exercise can limit progression once the damage has begun.

If symptoms get worse, a variety of surgeries can create more space for nerve roots or the spinal cord. These often involve spinal fusions, however, and they work best for younger patients who have not been having arthritic symptoms for a long time or in more than one joint.

---

[6] Richard Kim, MD, MS. Cervical spondylosis. http://mcns10.med.nyu.edu/spine/spine_surgery_p5.html. Accessed January 27, 1997.

MASSAGE?

Massage for spondylosis is appropriate, with caution. If the joints are acutely inflamed, the surrounding muscles will tend to splint them against painful movement. This splinting mechanism is important, and must be respected by massage therapists. For this reason, and because of the other serious complications of spondylosis, in this situation it is highly recommended to work with a primary caregiver who has a complete set of x-rays.

Sprains

DEFINITION: WHAT ARE THEY?

Sprains are tears to ligaments: the connective tissue strapping tape that links bone to bone throughout the body.

ETIOLOGY: WHAT HAPPENS?

Sprains, strains, and tendinitis are all injuries to structures that are composed largely of connective tissue fibers arranged in linear patterns. They have a lot in common including symptoms, healing mechanisms, and treatment protocols. Thus much of the information in this segment is applicable to all three conditions. Their differences will be emphasized here, as well as guidelines for how they may be seen in the same light.

Linearly arranged structures such as muscles, tendons, and ligaments are injured when some of their fibers are ripped. The severity of the injury depends on what percentage of the fibers are affected. First-degree injuries involve just a few fibers; second-degree injuries are much worse; and third-degree injuries are ruptures: the entire structure has been ripped through and no longer attaches to the bone.

The process of repairing muscle, tendon, or ligament tears involves the laying down of new collagen fibers, not in alignment with the injured structure, but whichever way the fibroblasts happen to deposit them. (See *inflammation*, chapter 5, page 237.) The perfect combination of movement, stretching, and weight-bearing stress in the subacute phase of recovery will help to reorient the fibers in alignment with the injured structure. If this happens in the best possible way, the new scar tissue actually becomes part of the muscle fascia, tendon, or ligament. But in a sedentary rather than a mobile situation, scar tissue seldom resolves itself so neatly.

Distinguishing Features. What makes sprains unique? A few things distinguish sprains from strains and tendinitis, which will be dealt with in other sections.

- Sprains are injured ligaments, not muscles or tendons. Ligaments are the connectors that hold the bones together. Structurally they are a little different from tendons; the dense linear arrangement of collagen fibers affords little stretch and almost no rebound. If a ligament is stressed enough to become injured, it will tend to tear before it stretches. And if it does get stretched, it won't rebound to its original length, and it won't stabilize the joint as well as it did before the injury.
- Sprains are more serious than strains and tendinitis. Because tendons and muscles tend to be more elastic and less densely arranged than ligaments, they will stretch before a ligament does. The "lines of defense" in joint injuries are: muscles, tendons, ligaments, joint capsule—so a sprain is one step away from a *dislocation* (this chapter, page 72). Furthermore, ligaments don't have the same rich blood supply as muscles, and they are denser than tendons. This means they don't have the same access to circulation, which makes them slower to heal than muscles or tendons.

SPRAINS IN BRIEF

What are they?
Sprains are injured ligaments.

How are they recognized?
In the acute stage, symptoms include pain, redness, heat, swelling, and loss of joint function. In the subacute stage, these symptoms will be abated, although perhaps not entirely absent. At all stages pain will be present on passive stretching of the affected ligament.

Is massage indicated or contraindicated?
Massage is indicated for subacute sprains. It can influence the healthy development of scar tissue and reduce swelling and damage due to edematous ischemia. Care must be taken to rule out bone fractures.

- Sprains tend to swell. With a few exceptions, acute sprains swell much more than muscle strains or tendinitis; it's one way to differentiate between injuries. Swelling is a protective measure that martials the body's healing resources and limits movement, which prevents further injury. Ligaments are sometimes contiguous with the joint capsules of the joints they cross over, so an injury to them will sometimes signal the joint to swell, too. Ligaments that are not attached to joint capsules swell much less than those that are.

SIGNS AND SYMPTOMS, ACUTE STAGE

Acute sprains will show the usual signs of inflammation: pain, heat, redness, and swelling, with the added bonus of loss of function because the rapid swelling splints the unstable joint and makes it extremely painful to move. Sprains in any stage will be especially painful with passive stretches of the structure.

Sprains can happen at almost any synovial joint, but the anterior talo-fibular ligament of the ankle is probably the most commonly sprained ligament in the body. Ligaments overlying the sacro-iliac joint are also very commonly injured, as are various ligaments around the knees and fingers.

SIGNS AND SYMPTOMS, SUBACUTE STAGE

In the subacute stage, signs of inflammation may still be present, but they will have subsided and the joint will have begun to regain some function. The physiological processes are no longer geared toward blood clotting and damage control; they have shifted toward clearing out debris and rebuilding torn fibers. The amount of time that passes between acute and subacute stages will vary with the severity of the injury, but the 24-to-48-hour rule is usually dependable. Remember, though, that some injuries can waver back and forth between acute and subacute, especially in response to certain kinds of activity or massage.

COMPLICATIONS

In a few situations, injured ligaments can lead to more serious problems. A sprain is such a common injury that it is important for massage therapists to be familiar with all its repercussions.

- Masking symptoms. An acute sprain may mask the symptoms of a bone fracture, especially in the foot. It is important to have clients get an x-ray to rule out fractures before beginning to work with a sprained ankle.
- Repeated injury. Internal scar tissue (scar tissue that accumulates within a specific structure) that never remodels just lies there in a big, gummy mass. It can interfere with the function of undamaged fibers. It can weaken the integrity of the whole structure, which, along with the increase in ligament laxity (see below), makes repeated injury a very common complication of sprains. This pattern is present with strains and tendinitis, too. (See Figure 2.8.)
- Ligament laxity. A ligament that has been injured, in addition to having some torn fibers, will often be looser than uninjured ligaments. This is because it has been asked to stretch further than it could go, and ligaments have almost no rebound capability. When a joint becomes unstable because of loose, lax ligaments, excessive movement of the bones occurs. The bones may rock around and knock together, causing *osteoarthritis* (this chapter, page 77) and a host of other problems.

TREATMENT

A long time ago, the recommendations for sprains included hot soaks and total immobilization. Clearly both of these strategies were ineffective at creating a good healing environment. The heat would increase edema and the accumulation of scar tissue, while immobilization would prevent the fibers from becoming aligned with the injured structure. These days *ICE therapy* (ice, compression, elevation) is considered the norm, with an emphasis on moving the joint within range of pain tolerance absolutely as soon as possible. The potential benefits are clear: ice keeps edema at bay, limiting further tissue damage from ischemia; compression does the same; elevation also encourages lymph flow *out* of an already impacted area. And introducing movement capitalizes on exactly what bodies are designed to do to help form scar tissue that strengthens, rather than weakens, an injured ligament.

If exercise is overdone, it will cause more tearing and more scar tissue. If it's done too little, the scar tissue will glue itself in its original random arrangement and bind up the undamaged ligament fibers as well, increasing the risk of future injury. But if it's done *just right*, exercise and stretching will "teach" the new collagen fibers which way to lay, and they will remodel themselves according to the stresses put upon them.

MASSAGE?

Massage is *great* for sprains. It can reduce adhesions and influence the direction of new collagen fibers in the healing process. It can address edema and toxic accumulations from secondary muscle spasm. Massage will also help with stiffness from the temporary loss of joint function. But massage must be done *after* the acute stage has subsided. There *are* modalities for dealing with acute sprains, but it's a highly technical field and not for casual experimentation.

Temporomandibular Joint Disorders

DEFINITION: WHAT ARE THEY?

The term "temporomandibular joint disorders" (TMJ) refers to a multitude of problems in and around the jaw. This collection of signs and symptoms is usually associated with malocclusion (a dysfunctional bite), bruxism (teeth grinding), and loose ligaments surrounding the jaw that cause excessive movement between the bones, damage to the internal cartilage, and possible dislocation of the joint. (See *dislocations*, this chapter, page 72.)

ETIOLOGY: WHAT HAPPENS?

When chronic misalignment, trauma, or muscle tension affect the highly specialized joints at the jaw, a person may find it difficult to open or close his mouth without pain. Chewing and swallowing become problematic, and pain in the jaw can reverberate systemically throughout the body.

The temporal-mandibular joint is like no other in the body. Far from being a simple hinge joint, the TMJ moves up, down, forward, back, and side to side. The jaw is unusually mobile, and the shape of the joint will actually stretch with the position of the mouth. (See Figure 2.21.) A fibrocartilage disc is meant to cushion the two bones (the temporal bone and the condyle of the mandible) but, like the menisci in the knee, this disc is sometimes pulled awry or injured, which can lead to problems in the joint. Lastly, a muscle is involved in this joint—the lateral pterygoid, which attaches directly to the fibrocartilage disc. The lateral pterygoid doesn't act like other muscles: it doesn't relax by order of the central nervous system.

TEMPOROMANDIBULAR JOINT DISORDERS IN BRIEF

What are they?
TMJ disorders arise when constant strain, stress, and malocclusion of the jaw lead to arthritis, inflammation, and dislocation of the temporomandibular joint.

How is it recognized?
Symptoms of TMJ disorder include head, neck, and shoulder pain, ear pain, mouth pain, clicking or locking in the jaw, and loss of range of motion in the jaw.

Is massage indicated or contraindicated?
Massage can be useful for TMJ problems, especially before arthritic irritation begins. However, this condition must be diagnosed by a physician.

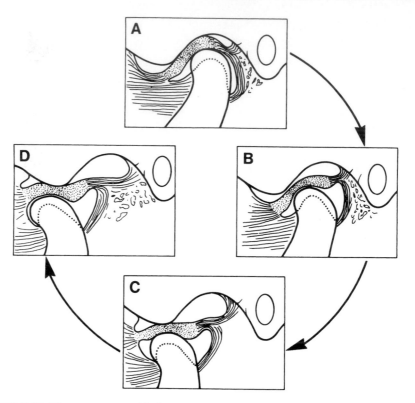

Figure 2.21 The temporomandibular joint allows great mobility as the jaw moves forward

Instead, it constantly pulls on the disc, acting as a kind of spring. This constant tension makes the lateral pterygoid especially prone to trigger points, which can both mimic and precipitate true TMJ syndrome.

CAUSES

The American Dental Association estimates that 44% to 99% of TMJ problems are precipitated by some kind of trauma.[7] This may be direct impact to the face or head, or indirect repercussions of trauma elsewhere in the body. For instance, a childhood fall could set up imbalances in the spine that may culminate in neck and jaw problems.

TMJ disorder may also be a frequent consequence of car wrecks. A whole scenario of the progression of "jaw-lash" has been developed to explain the whiplash-like results seen after this kind of acceleration-deceleration accident. (See *whiplash*, this chapter, page 108.)

Precipitating trauma aside, this is often a "circular" disorder. That is, the things that make TMJ problems worse can also be the symptoms. This is true of teeth grinding, muscle tightness, and *osteoarthritis* (see this chapter, page 77). Rheumatoid arthritis occasionally strikes here, but osteoarthritis is a far more frequent cause for TMJ problems. Other causes include misalignment of the bite and congenital malformations of the bones. Some sources suggest that TMJ syndrome is entirely a muscular disorder, but this is contradicted when the problems progress to arthritis and bony adaptation. Travell and Simons point out that when the jaw flexors, especially the lateral pterygoid, are overengaged, the constant pulling will mechanically displace the internal disc, thus starting the downward slide toward arthritis. In other words, *fibromyalgia* (this chapter, page 50) that is linked to chronic muscle spasm is both a cause and a complication of this disorder.

---

[7] Wesley E. Shankland, II, DDS, MS, PhD. Causes of TMJ. American Academy of Face, Head, and Neck Pain. http://www.netset.com/~docws/page4.html.

According to Travell and Simons's findings, about 70% of the people who complain of TMJ symptoms show some disc displacement.[8]

It is impossible to ignore the emotional component of TMJ disorders. If one looks at the body as a physical expression of the emotional state, it is easy to see how closely chronic emotional stress and chronic jaw stress are linked together. Regardless of whether a precipitating injury occurred or not, people who chronically clench their teeth are setting themselves up for jaw problems in the future.

SIGNS AND SYMPTOMS

The signs and symptoms of TMJ syndrome are these:

- Jaw, neck, and shoulder pain. This can be from actual deterioration of bony structures inside the capsule (arthritis), or it can be local and referred pain generated by tight, trigger-point laden muscles.
- Limited range of motion. Deformation or displacement of the cartilage inside the joint can make it difficult or impossible to open the mouth all the way.
- Popping in the jaw. This is usually attributed to the disc or bone being out of alignment, which then interferes in jaw opening. A similar "clicking" sensation is sometimes felt by people with knee problems that involve the discs there.
- Locking of the joint. Again, this is a result of having the fibrocartilage disc interfere with normal joint movement.
- Grinding teeth (bruxism). Like many things about this disorder, this symptom is also a possible cause of the problem. A chronically shortened set of jaw flexors will lead to clenching and grinding of teeth, especially during sleep, when the joint should be as relaxed as possible.
- Ear pain. Because of the location of the joint, pressure may be exerted directly on the eustachian tubes. Symptoms in this case would include a feeling of stuffiness in the ears and loss of hearing.
- Headaches. Two thousand pounds per square inch of pressure are placed at the second molar when the teeth are clenched. It is no surprise that the cranial bones would be stressed if this happens all night long. Headaches can also be related to trigger points of muscles in spasm and to cervical subluxation.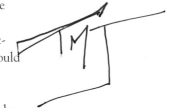
- Chronic misalignment of cervical vertebrae. This is probably a result of the muscular hypertonicity that is generated by this problem. As pain refers from the jaw to the neck and shoulders, the muscles there will tighten up and pull asymmetrically on the neck bones. No matter how often the neck is adjusted, or how brilliantly the neck muscles are massaged, this pain-spasm cycle will not abate until the jaw situation is addressed.

DIAGNOSIS

Many conditions present signs and symptoms similar to TMJ disorder, but they won't respond at all to the most advanced kinds of interventions. Therefore, it is critically important to differentiate between true TMJ disorder, which involves bony or cartilaginous deformation inside the joint capsule, and the other diseases and conditions that can cause head, neck, and shoulder pain.

First among these is fibromyalgia. More than any other condition, this one is both a precursor and a complication of TMJ disorder. Jaw surgery won't resolve trigger points, but resolving trigger points could eliminate the need for future jaw surgery. It is important to remember, though, that true TMJ disorder can (and probably will) be present

---

[8] Janet Travell, MD; David G. Simons, MD. Myofascial pain and dysfunction: The trigger point manual. Baltimore: Williams & Wilkins, 1983:176.

simultaneously with fibromyalgia. Other conditions that cause head, neck, and shoulder pain include:

- Sprain of the ligament that attaches the stylomandibular joint to the base of the skull. This is also called *Ernest Syndrome*.
- *Trigeminal Neuralgia*, also called *Tic Douleroux*, is an extremely painful result of damage to the trigeminal nerve (see chapter 3, page 164).
- *Occipital Neuralgia* is damage to the greater or lesser occipital nerves.
- *NICO (Neuralgia Inducing Cavitational Osteonecrosis)* is a recently recognized problem in which tissue death occurs at the site of extracted teeth, which causes pain in the face. Another term for this is *osteomyelitis*.

Some diagnostic tools that identify TMJ disorder include MRIs, which can show whether or not the internal cartilage is chipped or subluxated; x-rays of the jaw and head; and electromyography, which will show muscle function around the joint. A trained clinician can also feel a subluxation when fingers are inserted in the ear of the patient during chewing.

TREATMENT

Treatment for TMJ disorder is divided into surgical and nonsurgical options. In most cases, nonsurgical options are tried first. These include applying heat to painful areas, physical therapy, ultrasound and massage for jaw muscles, anti-inflammatory medicine, and local anesthetics. Special splints that reduce bone-to-bone pressure may be prescribed, although some specialists feel that ill-fitting splints will make matters worse rather than better. Proliferant injections to tighten the ligaments that surround the jaw may also be effective. If these noninvasive techniques are successful, the TMJ disorder may be averted before permanent bony distortion or cartilage damage inside the joint occurs.

In some situations the onset of symptoms may be very fast, for instance, with a car wreck or a fall. If such a patient has been severely debilitated, or if noninvasive techniques have been unsuccessful and other problems have been ruled out, surgery may be considered. Several different surgeries have been developed. These range from an outpatient procedure in which scar tissue and adhesions inside the joint are dissolved to arthroscopic surgery to manipulate the cartilage to full prosthetic joint replacement.

MASSAGE?

Massage can be especially useful in the early teeth-clenching stages of TMJ problems, not only by addressing the jaw flexors, but by helping to increase the client's awareness of this habit. It's surprising how often people grit their teeth without realizing it; again, the proprioceptors can adapt to assume that this is *normal*, even if it's not *optimal*. And of course, in addition to helping reduce excessive muscle tone, massage can also deal with some of the referred pain patterns that can be such a problem with this condition.

Other Connective Tissue Disorders

Baker's Cysts

BAKER'S CYSTS
Dr. William Baker was a British surgeon who lived from 1839 to 1896. He was the first to notice and document the odd, usually painless swellings some people have in the popliteal fossa.

DEFINITION: WHAT ARE THEY?

Baker's cysts are posterior extensions of the joint capsule of the knee.

ETIOLOGY: WHAT HAPPENS?

Some Baker's cysts are probably genetic anomalies; others may be formed when the strength of the synovial membrane is compromised, as in *rheumatoid arthritis* (this chapter, page 80). Baker's cysts may go undetected for years until there is some local injury or disruption that causes the pouch to fill up with synovial fluid, creating a sac that moves slightly under the superficial fascia in the back of the knee. (See Figure 2.22.)

Baker's cysts are not usually dangerous. The only risks they pose is that a cyst could become big enough to press on nerves or impair blood flow through the lesser saphenous vein in the back of the leg. If that is the case, a hazard may exist of blood clots forming distal to the cyst.

TREATMENT

Draining the cyst is one option, but it is not always a permanent solution; it will fill up again if the cause of the swelling is not identified and treated. Surgery to remove the cyst is another possibility, although even in this case, if the area is irritated again, another cyst may form.

MASSAGE?

It is possible, though unlikely, that massage could rupture a Baker's cyst, but a therapist would have to be working much deeper in the popliteal fossa than good sense allows. Because of the possibility of blood clotting if the sac is big enough to put pressure on the lesser saphenous vein, Baker's cysts are considered local contraindications for massage. Also, massage anywhere distal to the cyst requires the utmost caution. Watch for signs of fluid accumulation and poor blood return below the knee: coldness, clamminess, edema that is more pronounced on the cysted side than the uncysted side. (See Figure 2.23.) These are all signs that the cyst is big enough to cause a problem. If that's the case, consider it and everything distal to it, a local

BAKER'S CYSTS IN BRIEF

What are they?
Baker's cysts are fluid-filled extensions of the synovial membrane at the knee. They protrude into the popliteal fossa.

How are they recognized?
Baker's cysts are usually painless sacs that are palpable deep to the superficial fascia in the popliteal fossa.

Is massage indicated or contraindicated?
Massage is locally contraindicated in the popliteal fossa anyway, and especially if the client has a Baker's cyst. In addition, if any signs of circulatory disruption (coldness, clamminess, edema) are distal to the cyst, that whole area is a contraindication, and the client needs to be cleared of the possibility of thrombosis.

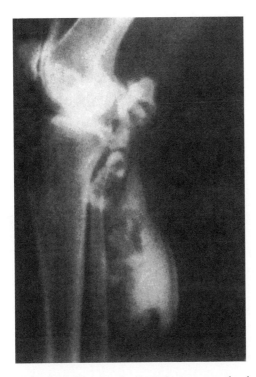

Figure 2.22 The pouch of a Baker's cyst is clearly visible posterior to the knee joint

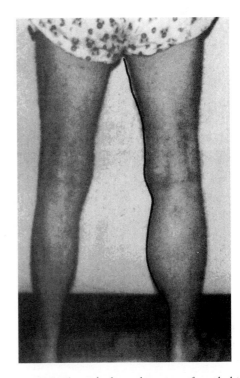

Figure 2.23 The right lower leg is significantly bigger than the left, due to the presence of a Baker's cyst

contraindication, and recommend that the client visit a doctor to rule out the possibility of *deep vein thrombosis* (see chapter 4, page 187).

> ### BUNIONS IN BRIEF
>
> **What are they?**
>
> A bunion is a protrusion at the metatarsal-phalangeal joint of the great toe that occurs when the toe is laterally deviated.
>
> **How are they recognized?**
>
> Bunions are recognizable by the large bump on the medial aspect of the foot. If they are inflamed, they will be red, hot, and possibly edematous.
>
> **Is massage indicated or contraindicated?**
>
> Vigorous massage is locally contraindicated at the point of a bunion regardless, and especially when or if it is inflamed. Massage elsewhere on the foot or body is very much indicated within pain tolerance to help with compensation patterns that occur when it is difficult to walk.

BUNIONS

This term comes from an Old French word, *buigne*, which means a bump on the head. Its synonym, "Hallux Valgus," comes from the Latin for "big toe turned outward."

Bunions

DEFINITION: WHAT ARE THEY?

This condition is also known as *hallux valgus*, which means "laterally deviated big toe." The joint capsule is stretched, and a callus grows over the protrusion. A smaller version of the same problem sometimes appears at the base of the little toe; this is called "tailor's bunion."

DEMOGRAPHICS: WHO GETS THEM?

Bunions occur approximately ten times more often in women than in men. Anyone can get them, but the condition is linked to a habit of wearing high-heeled, narrow-toed shoes. A genetic weakness in the toe joints may predispose one to bunions regardless of footwear, but anyone can get bunions.

ETIOLOGY: WHAT HAPPENS?

What's happening is actually a bony misalignment, wherein the proximal phalanx of the great toe is laterally deviated. This misalignment can be the result of an overarched foot, which places excessive pressure on the medial aspect of the foot. This in itself can cause erosion inside the joint, but the acute pain of bunions is more often related to a variety of *bursitis* (this chapter, page 95).

Bursae can spontaneously generate in places subject to considerable wear and tear—the bump formed by a bunion is a natural spot for that protective impulse. And if that new bursa should get irritated and inflamed, it will become a case of friction bursitis, which can be extremely painful, even debilitating. Ultimately if this badly misaligned weight-bearing joint is not somehow corrected or supported in a way that limits erosion of the joint structures, the bunion patient can also develop bone spurs and/or degenerative joint disease, also known as *arthritis* (this chapter, page 77) at that joint, which can make it chronically painful to do anything with it, including walking.

SIGNS AND SYMPTOMS

Most people have at least seen bunions; they look like an enormous lump on the medial side of the metatarsal-phalangeal joint of the great toe. (See Figure 2.24.) If it happens to be inflamed, the area will be red, hot, and painful. If the bunion is present but not irritated, a simple protrusion will show up, often covered with a thick layer of callus.

TREATMENT

The first steps in treating a bunion are to remove whatever irritants are making it happen, or making it worse. This usually means switching footgear, or even cutting holes in shoes to make room for the protrusion. Other noninvasive techniques include the use of massage and ultrasound to reduce internal adhesions and inflammation. Elevating the heel to an appropriate height can diminish pain, and a corticosteroid injection can reduce inflammation. But if irreversible damage has occurred inside the joint, and if the bunion is causing enough pain to significantly limit the patient's activity, surgery may be recommended to realign and fuse the joint. This will eradicate the bunion, but it can also eradicate any movement at the joint, so surgery is considered a "last ditch" option.

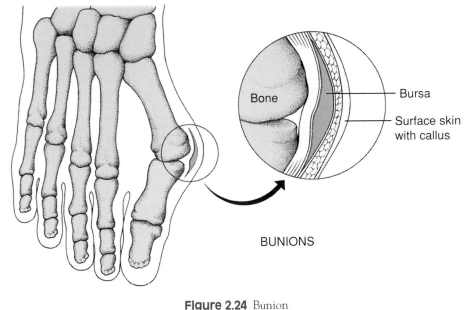

Bone

Bursa

Surface skin
with callus

BUNIONS

Figure 2.24 Bunion

Acutely inflamed bunions are a local contraindication; massage elsewhere on the body is perfectly safe. If no acute bursitis is present, massage is appropriate, although the bump itself is still a local contraindication because of the risk of irritating a bursa or osteophyte. Massage will *not* make bunions go away. Therapists don't have access to genetic patterning, nor to the inner workings of the affected joint. The best massage can do is work with the compensation patterns that will ripple through a body that is forced to move differently because of foot pain. This can mean concentrating on the intrinsic muscles of the affected foot, and it can mean working with the extrinsic muscles for gross movement everywhere else on the body.

Bursitis

DEFINITION: WHAT IS IT?

Bursae are small closed sacks made of connective tissue. They are lined with synovial membrane, and they are filled with synovial fluid. In fact, they resemble joint capsules in every way except that they lack the cartilage, bones, and capsular ligaments that all diarthrotic joints have. Bursitis is inflammation of the bursae: these fluid-filled sacks, when inflamed, generate excess fluid, which causes pain and limits mobility. Most bursae are very small, but the ones that surround the knee and shoulder can be quite large.

Bursitis comes in all shapes and forms, some of which have descriptive names, like *housemaid's knee* and *student's elbow*, which occurs on the point of the olecranon. (See Figure 2.25.) *Weaver's bottom* is bursitis on the ischial tuberosity. Trochanteric, or hip bursitis, is another common variety. The most common type of bursitis, at the pad between the humerus and the acromion, is called subacromial bursitis, but could be labeled "*jackhammerer's shoulder.*"

What is it?

A *bursa* is a fluid-filled sack that acts as a protective cushion at points of recurring pressure, eases the movement of tendons and ligaments moving over bones, and cushions points of contact between bones. Bursitis is the inflammation of a bursa.

How is it recognized?

Acute bursitis is painful and will be aggravated by both passive and active motion. Muscles surrounding the affected joint will often severely limit range of motion. It may be hot or edematous.

Is massage indicated or contraindicated?

Massage is locally contraindicated in the acute phase of noninfectious bursitis. Massage elsewhere on the body during an acute phase, and directly on the muscles of the affected joint (within pain limits) in a subacute phase, is perfectly appropriate.

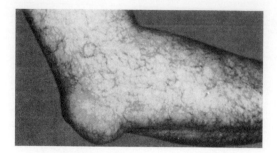

Figure 2.25 Bursitis: student's elbow

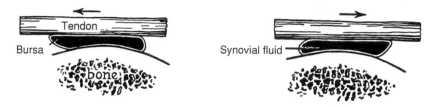

Figure 2.26 Bursae allow tendons to move freely over bony prominences

ETIOLOGY: WHAT HAPPENS?

Imagine stretching a rubber band over the sharp edge of a table. Now imagine moving it back and forth for several minutes at a time. It wouldn't be long before that rubber band would fray and then break. But if a small water balloon is inserted between the rubber band and the edge of the table, the rubber band (i.e., tendon) has freedom to move without the friction caused by the table (i.e., bone). The water balloon (i.e., bursa) has protected it from damage. Bursae serve to ease the movement of tendons over bony angles. (See Figure 2.26.) They also cushion the bones where they would otherwise bang against each other. Bursae pad people's sharpest corners: they are found on elbows, knees, heels, ischial tuberosities, and between layers of fascia. Bursae can grow anywhere the body experiences extra wear and tear around a joint.

Without bursae, several tendons would fray and rupture in short order. Some bones that are not meant to touch *would* touch, with great force. Exposed corners, like elbows or hallux valgus (*bunions*, this chapter, page 94) would have no protection.

CAUSES

Repetitive stress is usually the culprit behind bursitis. Performing the same movement or rubbing the same spot over and over, day after day, will sooner or later irritate that fluid-filled sack. Then the inflammatory process will try to pack a tangerine's worth of fluid into a sack the size of a grape, which *hurts*. In response to the pain, the muscles that surround the joint will go into spasm, splinting the injury. This drastically limits the range of motion of the affected joint. Sometimes the muscles can actually aggravate and prolong an attack of bursitis by compressing the joint and the bursa at the same time. (See *spasm*, this chapter, page 57.)

Bursitis often occurs in concert with other inflammatory conditions. It tends to accompany general area inflammation, so if a person has shoulder tendinitis, bursitis will often be present as well. (Unfortunately, it's hard to treat the tendinitis if the bursitis is in the way.) It will also attend *rheumatoid arthritis*, (this chapter, page 80) and some chronic infections, especially syphilis and *tuberculosis* (chapter 6, page 257).

SIGNS AND SYMPTOMS

The symptoms of bursitis include pain on any kind of movement, passive or active, along with heat, edema, and extremely limited range of motion because of the muscular splinting reaction to pain.

DIAGNOSIS

Bursitis isn't usually caused by an infectious agent, and bursae don't show up on x-rays. Therefore, its diagnosis largely depends on ruling out anything else it could be, which includes tendinitis, arthritis, ligament sprains, and any other problems specific to the joint or area being affected.

TREATMENT

Opinions vary about the duration of the average bursitis episode. Some orthopedists predict several weeks; others suggest it will usually clear up in about two. For some people bursitis can last much longer; untreated bursitis can become a chronic situation that lasts several months or even years. Obviously, a lot depends on which bursae are inflamed, and what the precipitating factors are. Treatment strategies range from warm, moist applications (cold is too intense for this inflammation; the muscles seize up and make it worse) to aspiration of excess fluid to corticosteroid injections. One or two injections generally clear away even chronic inflammation, and since the chemical is being injected into a closed cavity, one doesn't have to deal with the same side effects that a systemic dose of steroids involves.

As a last resort, some doctors suggest the possibility of a *bursectomy* to simply remove a badly inflamed bursa. But the only way to be sure that the bursitis is permanently cured is to get rid of the aggravating factors that caused it. No matter how often or how effectively bursitis is treated, if the stimulus that irritated the bursa to begin with is not removed, no treatment will be permanently successful. Even removing the bursa may eventually backfire, because the body can grow new ones! What does removing the irritating stimulus mean? It means learning some new movement patterns that don't put so much stress in just one spot. It means strengthening the muscles that surround the affected joint. It means finding a different way to do a job, or possibly even finding a new line of work.

MASSAGE?

This is a local contraindication, especially in an acute phase. It is tempting to try to release the muscles around an inflamed bursa. Resist it: although the muscles are likely to be tight, working to loosen them will not solve any problems until the inflammation itself has subsided. Bursitis usually doesn't involve a pathogen that can spread, so massage is certainly indicated for the rest of the body. (If the bursitis is caused by an infectious agent, the client is systemically contraindicated until the infection has completely subsided.)

In the subacute stage, a skilled massage therapist can address the muscles that cross over the affected joint, and may well have some success at decompressing the bones that are re-irritating the affected bursa. And, as with any condition that involves prolonged pain and immobility, it's a good idea to look for compensation patterns that may cause pain.

Dupuytren's Contracture

DEFINITION: WHAT IS IT?

This condition, also called *palmar fasciitis*, is an idiopathic thickening and shrinking of the palmar fascia that constricts the movement of the fingers. Usually it's the ring

---

DUPUYTREN'S CONTRACTURE IN BRIEF

What is it?
Dupuytren's contracture is an idiopathic shrinking and thickening of the fascia on the palm of the hand.

How is it recognized?
It usually affects the ring and little fingers, pulling them into permanent flexion.

Is massage indicated or contraindicated?
Massage is indicated for Dupuytren's contracture as long as sensation is present, although it may do little to reverse the process if it's gone too far.

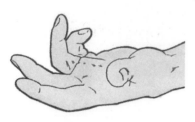

Figure 2.27 Dupuytren's contracture

DUPUYTREN'S CONTRACTURE

Baron Guillaume Dupuytren (1777–1835) was a French surgeon and pathologist who documented this condition as well as other specific diseases and conditions. He also put his stamp on several surgical procedures, including Dupuytren's suture, Dupuytren's amputation, and Dupuytren's tourniquet.

and little fingers that are most severely affected, although the index and middle fingers may also be bent. (See Figure 2.27.)

DEMOGRAPHICS: WHO GETS IT?

No one knows exactly *why* the fascia shrinks in this way, although some think it may have to do with repetitive micro trauma, and a genetic connection does seem to be at least partially responsible. This condition strikes mostly middle-aged white men and statistically it shows some links to alcoholism and epilepsy.

TREATMENT

If this condition is left untreated, the affected fingers will eventually lose all function. It's as though the connective tissue simply strangles the muscles and nerves until nothing is left of them. If it is caught before too much atrophy sets in, corticosteroid injections to reduce fascial buildup can be an effective treatment. Surgical intervention may also stop the progression, and physical or occupational therapy can help to restore the use of the fingers. The surgery slices through the palmar fascia, releasing the underlying tissues from their constricting blanket. Naturally, a lot of scar tissue is generated in recovery from this kind of surgery, and care must be taken to avoid ending up with worse fibrotic buildup than before the surgery. Even when surgery is successful, Dupuytren's contracture sometimes recurs.

MASSAGE?

Dupuytren's contracture does not stem from nerve injury, and sensation is present in the hand, at least before the progression has gone too far. Therefore, massage is appropriate in early stages. But connective tissue is very tough. Massage will certainly not make the condition any worse, but it may not make it better either. Massage is a good preventative measure for contractures, but if this condition is already present it may not be possible to reverse it.

Ganglion Cysts

DEFINITION: WHAT ARE THEY?

Ganglion cysts are small (about pea-sized) connective tissue pouches filled with fluid. They grow on joint capsules or tendinous sheaths. Sometimes they are attached to a ligament or directly to the periosteum. They usually appear on the wrist or the top of the foot.

Ganglion cysts are not dangerous unless their growth interferes with nearby nerves. They're not even usually painful, except that they have a habit of growing in places where they can get snagged a lot. This can put them in a state of chronic irritation, which can make it difficult for them to heal and subside.

TREATMENT

Generally the treatment for ganglion cysts is to leave them alone. It may take a while, but they usually cycle through by themselves. They may be aspirated to relieve internal pressure. The traditional "home remedy" for ganglion cysts is to smash them with a Bible; the surgical equivalent of this procedure is called a "Bible treatment." Ganglion cysts tend to grow back, though, so surgery isn't typically recommended.

GANGLION CYSTS IN BRIEF

What are they?
Ganglion cysts are small fluid-filled connective tissue sacks that are attached to tendons, tendinous sheaths, ligaments, or periosteum.

How are they recognized?
Ganglion cysts are small bumps that usually appear on the wrist or ankle. They are not usually painful, unless they are in a place to be injured by normal wear and tear.

Is massage indicated or contraindicated?
Massage is locally contraindicated for ganglion cysts. It cannot make them better, and may irritate them through excess fluid flow.

MASSAGE?

This is a *local contraindication*. Massage certainly will not make ganglion cysts bigger, worse, or more painful, *unless* they are over stimulated. Massage can't make them go away either, so massage therapists should leave them alone. If a client has a mysterious small bump on the wrist, foot, or anywhere else, it is necessary to get a diagnosis before working anywhere in the area.

Hernia

DEFINITION: WHAT IS IT?

"Hernia" means hole. Specifically in this case, it means "hole through which contents that are supposed to be contained are protruding." There are hernias of muscles through fascia, of vertebral discs, even of the brain through the cranial wall. This section discusses the most common types of hernias, which occur in various places around the abdomen.

ETIOLOGY: WHAT HAPPENS?

Hernias can be caused by a number of different factors, from congenital weakness of the muscular wall to childbirth to abnormal straining that increases the internal abdominal pressure. They can go undetected for a long time if they have a slow onset and the hole is large enough that the intestine isn't impaired in any way. Most hernias are *reducible*, which means the contents can be easily put back where they belong manually. Generally, though, they'll get worse and worse, bulging more and more often, and perhaps creating a bigger and bigger hole. Therefore, once a hernia has been identified, surgery to tighten up or close the hole is recommended sooner rather than later. Where a hernia will happen and what it will feel like depends a lot on gender and what makes the abdominal contents push against the walls.

SIGNS AND SYMPTOMS

The signs and symptoms of hernias will depend on what part of the abdominal wall has been compromised.

Hiatal Hernia. This is a hole in the esophageal opening of the diaphragm through which the stomach protrudes upward. The main symptom is heartburn from the gastric juice splashing up into the esophagus, where it can cause irritation, ulcers, and even perforations. This condition is not gender specific, except that pregnant women sometimes get it. The most common subjects for hiatal hernias are elderly, overweight people whose diaphragms are worn and stretched.

Epigastric Hernia. This is a bulging above the stomach. In this condition, the linea alba is split, and a portion of the omentum pushes through. The symptoms, besides a visible lump protruding above the belly button, may include a feeling of tenderness or heaviness in the area, but seldom extreme pain. This hernia is seen in women and men, but it is more common in men.

Paraumbilical Hernia. This is another split of the linea alba, this time right at the navel. It is sometimes a complication of childbirth. The symptoms are the same as the epigastric type, but the bulge is lower. This type of hernia is almost always experienced by women.

GANGLION CYSTS

"Ganglion" comes from the Greek word for swelling or knot. It is used to describe the small fluid-filled sacs that can develop around hand and feet joints, but the term is also used in reference to the nervous system, where clusters of nerve cell bodies are also referred to as ganglia.

HERNIA IN BRIEF

What is it?
A hernia is a hole or rip in the abdominal wall or the inguinal ring through which the small intestines may protrude. A hiatal hernia forms where the diaphragm opens to allow the esophagus to pass; when this hole becomes wider, the stomach protrudes upwardly.

How is it recognized?
Abdominal hernias usually show some bulging and mild-to-severe pain, depending on whether or not a portion of the small intestine is trapped. Hiatal hernias are usually distinguished by the presence of chronic heartburn.

Is massage indicated or contraindicated?
Massage is locally contraindicated for unreduced hernias, and systemically contraindicated for unreduced hernias that show signs of infection. For recent surgeries, *postoperative situations* (chapter 10, page 367) should be observed. For old hernia surgeries, massage is indicated.

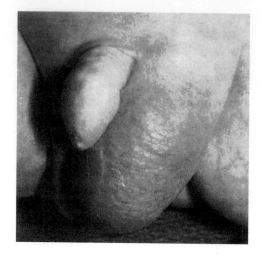

Figure 2.28 Inguinal hernia

Femoral Hernia. This is the female equivalent to the inguinal hernia. In this case, the abdominal contents are protruding through the femoral ring just below the inguinal ligament. Femoral hernias usually happen only in women, and they can be hard to detect. They can be very dangerous, however, because the hole around the intestine is usually quite small, which increases the chance of strangulation or obstruction of the intestine.

Inguinal Hernia. This is the most common variety of hernia. Inguinal hernias are holes in the abdominal wall at the inguinal ring. This opening—for the spermatic cord to exit the abdomen—is a structurally weak spot. A sudden change in internal abdominal pressure, such as coughing, sneezing, or heavy lifting, may force a section of small intestine right through at this point.

There are actually two types of inguinal hernias: **direct,** which is what has just been described, and **indirect,** in which the intestines are pushed into the inguinal canal. This type of hernia is most often experienced by infant boys. (See Figure 2.28.)

COMPLICATIONS

The seriousness of a hernia is determined by how big it is. Paradoxically, the bigger the better, at least for the short term. Small holes, as seen with femoral hernias, have a much greater chance of trapping the intestine in such a way that it cannot function. Either it becomes obstructed, in which case the patient will experience abdominal pain, nausea, and vomiting, or it will become strangulated—cut off from its blood supply. In this case, the area rapidly becomes red, enlarged, and extremely painful. If medical intervention does not occur quickly, the strangulated loop of intestine will become infarcted, and possibly gangrenous.

TREATMENT

Surgery is frequently recommended even for mild hernias, because they will tend to get worse as time passes. Sewing up a small stretch of abdominal fascia is a lot easier than repairing a big rip. A relatively new surgical technique involves inserting a small piece of mesh at the site of the tear. This helps to distribute the force of abdominal pressure more evenly than do stitches or staples alone. Sometimes special corsets or trusses are recommended to prevent sudden changes in abdominal pressure, but these days those are considered only temporary measures, not a solution to the problem.

MASSAGE?

If a client has been diagnosed with a hernia but has not had surgery, consider that part of the body locally contraindicated for any kind of deep massage. Stretching the fascia around an already weakened area could have disastrous results. If, on the other hand, they *have* had surgery, follow the guidelines for postoperative cautions. If their hernia surgery is ancient history, and they're having no pain, massage does not pose a danger in any way.

Pes Planus

DEFINITION: WHAT IS IT?

This is the medical term for feet that lack the medial arch between the calcaneus and the great toe, the lateral arch between the calcaneus and the little toe, and the transverse arch that stretches across the ball of the foot. In other words, pes planus means *flat feet*.

CAUSES

The cause of pes planus may be a congenital problem in the shape of the foot bones or the strength of the foot ligaments. Occasionally it can be caused by an accident leading to the rupture of the posterior tibialis tendon. Or it may arise from the unending battle between the deep flexors and everters, combined with footwear that offers little or no support to the intertarsal ligaments that are supposed to hold the arches up. (See Figure 2.29.) Interestingly, these factors may also lead to the exact opposite of flat feet—jammed arches, aka, *pes cavus*.

COMPLICATIONS

Whichever direction the tarsal bones go—to the floor or to the roof—if they lack mobility, a critical feature of foot architecture is missing: shock absorption. Each time the foot hits the ground, thousands of pounds of downward pressure should be softly distributed through the tarsals, which flatten out and then rebound in preparation for the next step. If the arches are somehow compromised and the bones lose their bounce, all that force must reverberate through the rest of the skeleton. This is how flat feet or jammed arches can lead to *plantar fasciitis* (this chapter, page 102), knee problems, hip problems, back problems, and even headaches. The biggest idea that should echo throughout good anatomy training is *everything in the body is connected to everything else*. Pes planus is an excellent example of how an "insignificant" problem in one place can create *very* significant problems elsewhere. These problems are, by the way, very hard to track down and correct unless a therapist knows where to look.

MASSAGE?

Massage is indicated for pes planus. If the problems are congenital, massage won't have much lasting effect, but even temporary relief from pain is better than nothing. Furthermore, massage can ameliorate some of the distant effects of flat feet: knee strain, hip rotation, and so on.

If the flat feet are due to muscular or ligamentous stresses, on the other hand, massage may have some success at equalizing the tensions between antagonistic muscles and

---

PES PLANUS IN BRIEF

What is it?
This is the medical term for flat feet.

How is it recognized?
The feet lack arches. Pronation of the ankle will probably also be present.

Is massage indicated or contraindicated?
Massage is very much indicated. In some cases, the health of intrinsic foot muscles and ligaments can be improved to the point where alignment in the foot is also improved. In other cases, where the ligaments are lax through genetic problems, massage may not correct the situation, but neither will it make it worse.

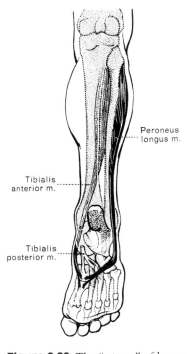

Peroneus longus m.

Tibialis anterior m.

Tibialis posterior m.

Figure 2.29 The "stirrup" of lower leg muscles that support the medial arch of the foot

PLANTAR FASCIITIS IN BRIEF

What is it?
Plantar fasciitis is the pain and inflammation caused by injury to the plantar fascia of the foot.

How is it recognized?
Plantar fasciitis is acutely painful after prolonged immobility. Then the pain recedes, but comes back with extended use. It feels sharp and bruise-like just at the anterior calcaneus or deep in the arch.

Is massage indicated or contraindicated?
Massage is indicated for plantar fasciitis. It can help release tension in deep calf muscles that put strain on the plantar fascia; it can also help to affect the development of scar tissue at the site of the tear.

stimulating the ligaments. Ligaments and tendons are nourished by a very meager blood supply. Deep, specific massage tips the scales, drawing lots of fresh blood to ligaments that otherwise wouldn't get it.

Plantar Fasciitis

DEFINITION: WHAT IS IT?

This is a condition involving pain and inflammation of the plantar fascia, which stretches from the calcaneus to the metatarsals on the plantar surface of the foot.

DEMOGRAPHICS: WHO GETS IT?

This is a common problem; 95% of all heel pain is diagnosed as plantar fasciitis. It affects men and women equally and though children can get it, adults are far more susceptible because their plantar fascia has generally lost some of its youthful elasticity.

ETIOLOGY: WHAT HAPPENS?

When the plantar fascia is overused or stressed by misalignment, its fibers will tend to fray. This is essentially the same thing as a tendon or ligament tear. (See Figure 2.30.) Very frequently, an x-ray will show that a bone spur has developed at the attachment to the calcaneus. It was once assumed that these bone spurs caused the pain of plantar fasciitis. It's

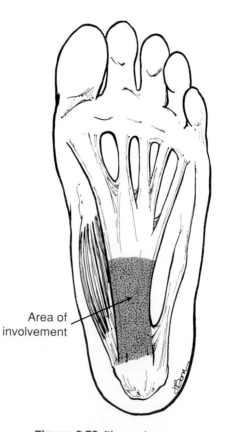

Area of involvement

Figure 2.30 Plantar fasciitis

now understood that although up to 40% of all adults have some level of bone spur growth on the foot, the vast majority have no pain at all.

The pain that accompanies plantar fasciitis occurs when the foot has been immobile for several hours, and then is used. The fibers of the fascia begin to knit together during rest, and are constantly retorn each time the foot goes into even gentle weight-bearing dorsiflexion.

CAUSES

Causes of plantar fasciitis are varied, but most boil down to overuse or alignment stresses. Being overweight can predispose someone to plantar fasciitis, as can wearing shoes without good arch and lateral support. Flat or pronated feet are associated with this problem. Very tight calf muscles are also contributing factors, especially for runners. Plantar fasciitis also may occur as a secondary complication to an underlying disorder such as *gout* (this chapter, page 74) or *rheumatoid arthritis* (this chapter, page 80).

SIGNS AND SYMPTOMS

Plantar fasciitis follows a distinctive pattern that makes it easy to identify: it is acutely painful for the first few steps every morning. Then the pain subsides or disappears altogether, but becomes a problem again with prolonged standing, walking, or running. Often, a sharp "bruised" feeling appears either just anterior to the calcaneus on the plantar surface or deep in the arch of the foot.

TREATMENT

The first, best thing to do for plantar fasciitis is to remove the tensions that cause it to be reinjured every morning when the foot first hits the floor. Orthotics are an important strategy; these should be in all shoes, including bedroom slippers. Someone with plantar fasciitis should *never* go barefoot. A fairly new device that's getting good reviews is a specially designed night splint that holds the foot in a slightly dorsiflexed position. This allows the plantar fascia fibers to knit back together in a way that won't be stressed and retorn so easily.

Anti-inflammatory drugs, ice, stretching, and deep massage of the calf muscles and the site of the tear are frequently prescribed for plantar fasciitis. Corticosteroid injections are sometimes given to reduce inflammation, but they may weaken the collagen fibers, so they are used only sparingly. As a last ditch option, surgery may be performed to sever the plantar fascia altogether. This may eradicate pain, but will also create more instability in the foot, which can lead to problems in the rest of the body.

MASSAGE?

Massage is often suggested both to release the deep calf muscles and to have an organizing influence on the growth of scar tissue on the plantar fascia itself.

Tendinitis

DEFINITION: WHAT IS IT?

Tendinitis involves injury and inflammation in tendinous tissues. It has a lot in common with strains and sprains, and in fact, it may sometimes be difficult to delineate one injury from another. (See Figure 2.8.)

TENDINITIS IN BRIEF

What is it?

Tendinitis is inflammation of a tendon, usually due to injury at the tenoperiosteal or musculotendinous junction.

How is it recognized?

Pain and stiffness will be present, as well as, in acute stages, palpable heat and swelling. Pain is exacerbated by resisted exercise of the injured muscle-tendon unit.

Is massage indicated or contraindicated?

Massage is locally contraindicated for acute tendinitis. Massage is indicated for tendinitis in the subacute stage, to influence the production of useful scar tissue, reduce adhesions and edema, and reestablish range of motion.

ETIOLOGY: WHAT HAPPENS?

Tendinitis can occur anywhere in the tendon, but tears happen most frequently at the tenoperiosteal junction or the musculotendinous junction. These areas mark the shift of one tissue type into another, and though the transition may be gradual, a weak point still exists in the structure that is vulnerable to injury.

SIGNS AND SYMPTOMS

The symptoms of tendinitis are very similar to strains, though they may be more intense. The acute stage may show some heat and swelling, depending on which tendons are affected. Most tendon swelling is not visible, but there are a few exceptions, particularly in the achilles tendon and the posterior tibialis tendon at the medial ankle, both of which may swell a lot with injury.

In all stages of tendinitis, stiffness and pain will be present on resistive movements and in stretching. The main difference between tendinitis and muscle strains is that it is easier to get a bad tendon tear than it is to get a bad muscle tear; muscles are a lot more elastic than tendons are. This condition will have a more distinct acute and subacute stage than muscle strains.

TREATMENT

As with muscle and ligament tears, standard medical approaches to this kind of injury focus on symptom abatement rather than scar tissue management. Unfortunately, this can create a stubborn, serious problem out of a potentially very minor one, as the unresolved scar tissue weakens rather than strengthens the tendon. Fortunately, recent advancements in the understanding of how scar tissue develops have begun spreading into more mainstream applications, so the "take these painkillers and don't move it for two weeks" kinds of treatment strategies for soft tissue injuries are becoming less and less common.

MASSAGE?

Massage is certainly indicated for tendinitis. But again, this condition is more serious than a simple muscle tear, and the acute phase must be respected to allow the body to begin the process of cleaning up debris and laying down new fibers in peace. In the subacute stage, however, massage will be valuable not only for the mechanical action it can have on badly placed collagen fibers, but for the circulatory turnover it will stimulate in the area of nonvascularized tendons.

Sprains, strains, and tendinitis all respond best to massage in a subacute phase, as soon as the acute symptoms have passed. This is when massage can have the most profound influence over the quality of healing. The sooner it's treated, the more complete resolution a client is likely to have. But even years-old injuries respond well to massage if the circumstances are right. It may not be possible to completely reverse 10-year-old tendinitis, but any amount of improvement is significant, and for a client who has been living with pain and limitation, any improvement is a lot better than nothing.

Tenosynovitis

DEFINITION: WHAT IS IT?

Tenosynovitis is a situation in which tendons that pass through a synovial sheath become irritated and inflamed.

TENOSYNOVITIS IN BRIEF

What is it?
Tenosynovitis is the inflammation of a tendon and/or surrounding synovial sheath. It can happen wherever tendons pass through these sheaths, but is especially common in the forearm, particularly in the extensor muscles.

How is it recognized?
Pain, heat, and stiffness will be present in the acute stage. In the subacute stage, only stiffness and pain may be present. The tendon may feel or sound creaky (crepitis) as it moves through the sheath. It is difficult to bend fingers with tenosynovitis, but even harder to straighten them.

Is massage indicated or contraindicated?
Massage is locally contraindicated for tenosynovitis in the acute stage, and very much indicated in the subacute stage.

ETIOLOGY: WHAT HAPPENS?

Some tendons have to pass through very narrow, crowded passageways or around sharp corners to reach their bony attachments. Without any lubrication, those tendons and their neighbors would soon be worn to a frazzle. But they do have lubrication, provided by special sheaths made of connective tissue and lined with synovial membrane. As the tendon or group of tendons pass through the sheath, synovial fluid is secreted to provide lubrication and ease of movement. (See Figure 2.31.)

Repetitive stress, percussive movement, or constant twisting can cause the tendons inside synovial sheaths to become irritated. The sheath may become inflamed and then shrink around the tendons in such a way that it inhibits freedom of movement. A cycle

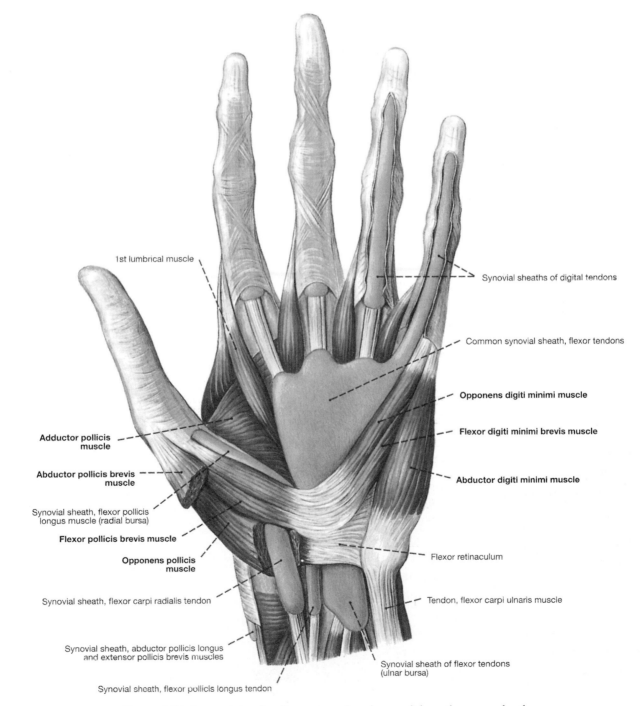

1st lumbrical muscle

Synovial sheaths of digital tendons

Common synovial sheath, flexor tendons

Opponens digiti minimi muscle

Flexor digiti minimi brevis muscle

Adductor pollicis muscle

Abductor pollicis brevis muscle

Abductor digiti minimi muscle

Synovial sheath, flexor pollicis longus muscle (radial bursa)

Flexor pollicis brevis muscle

Opponens pollicis muscle

Flexor retinaculum

Synovial sheath, flexor carpi radialis tendon

Tendon, flexor carpi ulnaris muscle

Synovial sheath, abductor pollicis longus and extensor pollicis brevis muscles

Synovial sheath of flexor tendons (ulnar bursa)

Synovial sheath, flexor pollicis longus tendon

Figure 2.31 Synovial sheaths allow groups of tendons to slide easily over each other

of stiffness followed by irritating movement that creates more stiffness, pain, and inflammation may develop.

CAUSES

Tenosynovitis is usually caused by trauma, repetitive movement, or excessive exercise. It can happen anywhere synovial sheaths are: the wrist, the ankle, the long head of the biceps, or near the thumb, which has a special name: "De Quervain's tenosynovitis." Occasionally it can be caused by a local infection that inflames the synovium, but it is usually brought about by mechanical stress. Tenosynovitis also occurs as a complication of other inflammatory wrist problems including *rheumatoid arthritis* (this chapter, page 80) and *fractures* (this chapter, page 60).

SIGNS AND SYMPTOMS

Symptoms of tenosynovitis are predictable: local pain, sometimes with swelling and heat. In the case of "trigger finger" it may be difficult to bend the joint, and unbending it is even harder; excessive force must be applied to slide the tendon through its sheath, and the joint usually extends with a sudden "pop." There is often a grinding noise or feeling called "crepitis" when the affected joint is moved. Movement of the tendon through the sheath will tend to exacerbate the problem, but lack of movement will decrease the production of synovial fluid. It can be a very frustrating condition, because nothing seems to make it better.

TREATMENT

If the synovium is inflamed because of infection, the obvious course is to treat it with antibiotics. Noninfectious tenosynovitis is typically treated with anti-inflammatory drugs, then injected with steroids; if this treatment protocol fails, the synovium is surgically split.

MASSAGE?

This is an inflammatory condition, and what's worse, the inflammation is confined to a very small, crowded space. This makes it counterproductive to massage, since massage will only make it hotter and more swollen. During the acute phase, tenosynovitis locally contraindicates massage.

During the subacute stage, however, massage is indicated because of its ability to reduce inflammation, flush out toxins, and create very specific movements of structures against each other to prevent the accumulation of scar tissue and/or adhesions. Massage may or may not actually be able to solve the problem of irritation inside the synovial sheath, but it can improve the nutrition and freedom of movement available to the affected structures.

Torticollis

DEFINITION: WHAT IS IT?

This is an umbrella term for any condition that causes the head to be pulled to one side. A unilateral spasm of a neck muscle or muscles causes the head to become stuck in flexion and rotation.

TORTICOLLIS IN BRIEF

What is it?
Torticollis is a unilateral spasm of neck muscles. The spasm may be related to a variety of causes.

How is it recognized?
Flexion and rotation of the head are the main symptoms. Torticollis may also refer pain into the neck, shoulders, and back.

Is massage indicated or contraindicated?
This depends on the cause of the problem. One variety, called simple wryneck, resulting from trigger points, cervical misalignment, ligament sprain, or trauma may be appropriate for massage if no acute inflammation is present. Spasmodic torticollis patients may benefit from pain relief offered by massage, but work should be done under supervision. If symptoms don't improve or if any signs of systemic infection occur, a more thorough diagnosis should be sought.

ETIOLOGY: WHAT HAPPENS?

A spasmed sternocleidomastoid is usually the culprit in torticollis, but the trapezius, scalenes, splenius cervicis, or capitis and levator scapulae may be involved. Any attempt to move the head and neck out of their position may cause significant pain. Under this umbrella, several variations are linked to whatever forces have caused the problem:

- Congenital Torticollis: In this situation a genetic abnormality results in the development of only one sternocleitomastoid muscle. Because there are so many other muscles that rotate and flex the head, this problem may be overcome by exercise. (See Figure 2.32.)
- Infant Torticollis: In the late stages of pregnancy, the fetus may lie with the head twisted to one side. This can create a shortened or weakened sternocleitomastoid, as well as cranial bone distortion. This condition is usually successfully treated with exercise and special helmets designed to reshape the cranial bones.
- Spasmodic Torticollis: This condition is an idiopathic spasm of the neck muscles. The spasms may be tonic (sustained contractions), clonic (tremors), or both. Spasmodic torticollis affects adults, creating chronic pain in the neck, back, and shoulder. It has a slow onset that peaks within two to five years. Occasionally it will spontaneously resolve, but may occur again in later years.
- Wryneck: This is a simple stiff neck, often caused by irritation of the intertransverse ligament at C_7. A cervical misalignment may also create the problem, which will not be relieved until both the muscles and the bony alignment have been addressed. Trigger points and spasm in the splenius cervicis are another possible cause. Short-lived cases of wryneck may be brought about by sleeping in a bad position, or some other event or trauma that might cause irritation in the neck muscles.
- Other: Torticollis can, on rare occasions, be the earliest presenting sign of a more serious condition. Cases have been documented where it was the first symptom of bone cancer in the spine (the tumor may affect the motor and/or sensory neurons), bone infections, and even a bad infection of the adenoids: lymph nodes in the neck, which can get so filled with pus that they irritate and cause spasm in the nearby muscles.

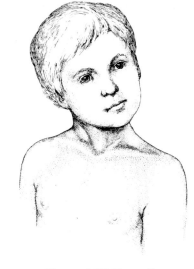

Figure 2.32 Torticollis

T O R T I C O L L I S

This comes from the Latin, *tortus*, "twisted," and *collum*, "neck." Torticollis is a general term for a twisted neck, which its synonym, "wryneck," implies.

SIGNS AND SYMPTOMS

Symptoms of torticollis vary according to the predisposing causes. For specific information, refer to the types of torticollis described above.

TREATMENT

Treatment for torticollis depends on the underlying cause. For congenital or infantile situations, exercise to strengthen the auxiliary muscles is called for. For spasmodic torticollis, special drugs or even surgery to limit the spasms may be recommended. Wryneck from subluxated vertebrae can be addressed by bony manipulation. Wryneck caused by ligament irritation may be resolved by specific frictions to the lesion; if the scar tissue is very old and difficult to access, corticosteroid injections to limit inflammation and reduce scar tissue may be helpful. Torticollis related only to muscle spasm and trigger points will respond well to massage.

MASSAGE?

Chiropractic or manipulation with massage for uncomplicated wryneck is a powerful combination because both the hard and soft tissues will receive the attention they need. Remember, though, that torticollis can be an early symptom of some other more serious problems, so if the client is not improving, or is showing any other signs of infection, a more complete diagnosis is necessary.

WHIPLASH IN BRIEF

What is it?

Whiplash is an umbrella term referring to a series of injuries that may occur with cervical acceleration/deceleration. These injuries include sprained ligaments, strained muscles, misaligned or fractured vertebrae, herniated or ruptured discs, TMJ problems, and central nervous system damage.

How is it recognized?

Symptoms of whiplash will vary according to the nature of the injuries. Pain at the neck and referring into the shoulders and arms along with headaches are the primary indicators.

Is massage indicated or contraindicated?

Massage is contraindicated for acute stages of whiplash, and very much indicated for the subacute stage, when in conjunction with chiropractic or manipulation, it can contribute to a thorough resolution of the problem.

Whiplash

DEFINITION: WHAT IS IT?

Whiplash, or CAD (cervical acceleration-deceleration), is a broad term used to refer to a mixture of injuries, including sprains, strains, and possibly bone fractures and herniated discs. These injuries are usually, but not always, associated with car accidents in which the head "whips" forward and back in rapid succession. (See Figure 2.33.)

ETIOLOGY: WHAT HAPPENS?

In a whiplash accident, the cervical muscles (especially the scalenes and splenius cervicis; muscles that attach to the spinous processes are not so prone to tearing) are frequently injured (see *strains*, this chapter, page 59). Spinal ligaments may also be damaged (see *sprains*, this chapter, page 87). Two frequently injured ligaments massage can't touch are the anterior and the posterior longitudinal ligaments. But the ligaments that *are* accessible are the supraspinous and the intertransverse ligaments. Any combination of these ligaments may be affected, depending on the trauma. Other structures that are injured with CAD include discs, which may herniate or even rupture; vertebrae, which can come out of alignment or fracture; the temporomandibular joint; the spinal cord, which may get stretched and then become edematous; and even the brain, which can become bruised and damaged in concussion.

SIGNS AND SYMPTOMS

A lot of crossover exists between what may be considered a symptom of whiplash, and what is a complication, or resulting disorder, so here is a list of both.

- Ligament sprains. The supraspinous and intertransverse ligaments that connect the vertebrae to each other are very vulnerable to injury in a whiplash-type of accident. These ligaments can refer pain up over the head, into the chest, and down the arms. It's important to know about these structures because referred pain from ligaments can often be misdiagnosed as pain from nerve damage.

    Ligament sprains often take a long time to heal and they tend to accumulate a lot of excess scar tissue. They may be the most common cause of lasting pain and dysfunction when a whiplash injury occurs.

- Misaligned cervical vertebrae. This will generally show clearly on an x-ray. Vertebrae may be displaced to the front, back, side, or rotated one way or another. In some very extreme cases there may even be cracks, or *fractures* (this chapter, page 60) in the vertebrae. Left untreated or incompletely treated, misaligned vertebrae with their lax ligaments and lack of structural support, will often develop *spondylosis* (this chapter, page 84).

- Herniated disc. This is not inevitable, but it frequently happens that the neck ligaments are so stressed in a trauma of this force that the annulus cracks, too, allowing the nucleus pulposis to seep into spaces where it doesn't belong. Car wrecks and other major traumas of this type are the easiest way to cause a herniation in the cervical region. (See this chapter, page 114.)

- Spasm. In the acute stage, the paraspinals and other neck muscles will go into spasm to "splint" or give extra support to the stretched neck ligaments. But this reaction

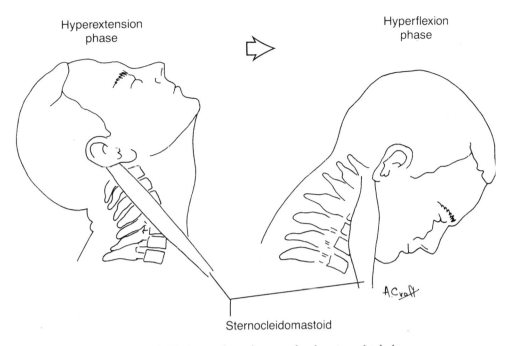

Hyperextension phase

Hyperflexion phase

Sternocleidomastoid

Figure 2.33 Cervical acceleration-deceleration whiplash

WHIPLASH

Client X

The Sneezer

A massage therapist met with a first-time client approximately one year after that person had been involved in a car accident. The client was still in considerable pain. He was diagnosed with whiplash and was seeking massage under prescription from his doctor.

The therapist worked slowly and carefully, and was encouraged by the client to go deeper into his neck muscles, all the way down to the transverse processes of the neck vertebrae. He felt better after the massage: his muscles were looser and he had an improved range of motion.

Several hours later, the client sneezed. The force of the motion wrenched his neck and reinjured the tissues so that he felt greater pain, more spasm, and had much less range of motion than he had *before* his massage. He returned for another session, but it was ineffective at reducing his pain and dysfunction. He never sought massage again.

What is the moral here? It is utterly unclear whether the first massage put the client at risk of reinjuring himself simply by sneezing. The therapist followed all the rules of good sense, worked under medical supervision, and let the client guide her into how much pressure he felt comfortable to receive. Yet, it is necessary to entertain the possibility that the massage somehow *did* put the client at risk, even though the therapist was well informed and made what seemed to be the right decisions. The point is that no two people will go through the same kind of healing process, and no two people will respond to massage the same way. Massage therapists must weigh the benefits and risks of their work on a case-by-case basis. It's impossible to rely only on books and rules to make decisions about whether to give massage.

has a tendency to outlive its usefulness. Spasm of neck muscles will also significantly limit range of motion. (See this chapter, page 57.)

- Neurological symptoms. These can include dizziness, blurred vision, abnormal smell or taste, tinnitus, and loss of hearing. These signs indicate cranial trauma: the brain has been bruised and may have some internal bleeding. This is usually the result of a specific blow—hitting the head on the steering wheel, for instance—but post-concussion syndrome can also happen without direct impact.

- TMJ disorders. Again, direct impact of the jaw on a steering wheel or dashboard can obviously damage the TMJ, but some research suggests that the joint can be traumatized just by the rapid acceleration/deceleration that accompanies whiplash injuries. TMJ disorders often go unaddressed until the more critical, acute aspects of whiplash have passed. (See this chapter, page 89.)

- Headaches. These will arise for a variety of reasons, including but not limited to referred pain and trigger points from spasming muscles in the neck; sprained ligaments that refer pain up over the head; cranial bones that may be out of alignment; stress and its autonomic action on blood flow; muscle tightness in the neck; and head, TMJ problems, and concussion. (See chapter 3, page 153.)

DIAGNOSIS

Some assumptions can be made about which precise structures have been injured based on whether the car wreck was a direct head-on or a rear-end collision. But these assumptions will not hold true if the accident occurred at any kind of angle, or if the patient's head was turned in any direction at the moment of impact. A good clinical exam that tests for injured ligaments and muscles will yield very precise information about whiplash injuries. MRIs can show if and where discs are bulging, while x-rays will show vertebral subluxations and fractures. Care must be taken, however, to delineate between what these tests show and what patients report: very frequently MRI or x-ray pictures will show problems that actually don't create symptoms for the patient.

TREATMENT

Neck collars are used for acute whiplash patients to take the stress off their wrenched ligaments, and to try to reduce muscle spasm. But the sooner the injured structures are put back to use, the less scar tissue will accumulate. Therefore, collars are strictly for short-term use, as this kind of immobilization can create more long-term problems than benefits.

Further treatment for whiplash will depend on the type and severity of specific injuries that have occurred.

MASSAGE?

Mechanical massage in the acute stage of this injury is contraindicated. This is an important phase of healing with which massage therapists must not interfere. Gentle reflexive work with the intention to balance the autonomic nervous system rather than to make changes in the tissue may ameliorate the emotional trauma and shock such an injury often incurs. As long as it doesn't disrupt the cellular activity at the site of the injury, this type of work is a fine idea.

If it has been established that no other serious disorder exists, such as a herniated disc or spinal fracture, chiropractic or manipulation alone can be sufficient to undo the damage done to the cervical vertebrae in a whiplash injury. But if muscle spasm is not addressed, bony adjustments will be difficult to perform, and probably won't hold for long because the muscles will simply pull the bones out of alignment again. Furthermore, in the absence of the circulation that can be stimulated by massage, the injured ligaments will have little access to nutrition. They will tend to accumulate masses of scar tissue, which will bind to other ligaments and other muscles sheaths, thus turning a temporary loss of range of motion into a permanent one.

Chiropractic or manipulative therapy *with* massage can yield good results, blending the best of soft tissue work (to prevent or reduce muscle spasm, scar tissue accumulation, adhesions, fibrosis, and ischemia) with the best of bony alignment. It is not unheard of for someone to emerge from a whiplash recovery with this kind of care in better shape than before they began.

Neuromuscular Disorders

Carpal Tunnel Syndrome

DEFINITION: WHAT IS IT?

Carpal tunnel syndrome (CTS) is a set of signs and symptoms brought about by the entrapment of the median nerve between the carpal bones of the wrist and the transverse carpal ligament that holds down the flexor tendons. (See Figure 2.34.) The median nerve supplies sensation to the thumb, forefinger, middle finger, and one half of the ring finger. (See Figure 2.35.) If it is caught or squeezed in any way, it will create symptoms in the part of the hand the nerve supplies.

DEMOGRAPHICS: WHO GETS IT?

This is an occupational hazard for massage practitioners and anyone else who performs repetitive movements for several hours every day: people who work with keyboards, string musicians, bakers, check-out clerks. The chances are excellent that any massage therapist will encounter it in his or her practice.

ETIOLOGY: WHAT HAPPENS?

Knowing that the median nerve is being impeded does not give a complete picture of the problem. Pressure on the median nerve may arise from several sources. In order to develop a treatment strategy (and to assess the appropriateness of massage), the aggravating factors must be determined. Here are some possible causes, with basic medical treatment strategies attached:

- Edema. Fluid retention, which is common for overweight people as well as menopausal and pregnant women, will create extra pressure in an area where there's no room to spare. The wrist is particularly susceptible because of its normal gravitational position; it's easy for fluid to pool here. CTS due to edema is usually bilateral, and is quite common. It is most often treated with diuretics or other methods designed to help get rid of excess fluid.
- Subluxation. Sometimes the carpal bones, especially the capitate bone in the center of the distal row of carpal bones, subluxate toward the palmar side. This can put mechanical pressure on the median nerve that cannot be removed by diuretics, anti-inflammatories, or any other drugs. This type of CTS is almost always unilateral. Manipulation is the treatment of choice, although the bones often move back into place without intervention. Waiting for that to happen can be something of a gamble, though, because the longer the irritation goes on, the higher the chances of

> ### CARPAL TUNNEL SYNDROME IN BRIEF
>
> **What is it?**
> Carpal Tunnel Syndrome (CTS) is irritation of the median nerve as it passes under the transverse carpal ligament into the wrist. It has several different causes.
>
> **How is it recognized?**
> CTS will cause pain, tingling, numbness, and weakness in the part of the hand supplied by the median nerve.
>
> **Is massage indicated or contraindicated?**
> Massage is indicated with extreme caution for CTS. Work on or around the wrist must stop immediately if any symptoms are elicited, but some types of CTS will respond well to massage. It is necessary to get a medical doctor's diagnosis in order to know which type of CTS is present.

sustaining nerve damage, and the less likely it is that the problem will spontaneously resolve.

- Fibrotic buildup. The human body simply wasn't designed to perform the same movements for eight hours a day, five days a week. In an attempt to keep up with demands, the body will tend to *hypertrophy*, or grow bigger and thicker wherever we are using it most. This is true of muscles and bones, and it also happens with the tendons and supportive connective tissues at the wrist. If they thicken because of overuse, they will press on anything soft trying to get through tiny "tunnels" between the carpal bones, namely, the median nerve. The transverse carpal ligament may also swell with chronic irritation, adding to the pressure on the median nerve.

TREATMENT

Treatment for this situation begins with a wrist splint to require less work from those supportive tissues, and anti-inflammatories, oral or injected. Corticosteroid injections into the wrist may also be recommended to de-inflame the area and melt excess connective tis-

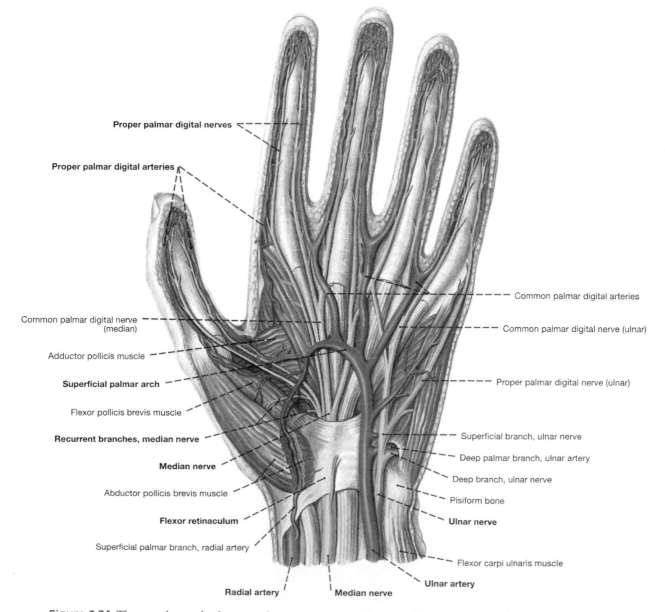

Figure 2.34 The carpal tunnel is between the transverse carpal ligament (flexor retinaculum) and the carpal bones

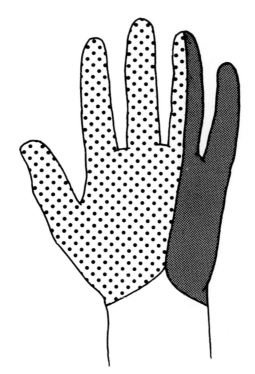

Figure 2.35 CTS affects the thumb, index, middle, and half the ring finger

sue. If the ligaments surrounding the wrist have become loose enough to allow nearby structures to become irritated, proliferant injections may be recommended to tighten them up. CTS treatment culminates with surgery: cutting open the transverse carpal ligament, and scraping down some of the accumulated connective tissue. Unfortunately, scar tissue from surgery will often bind up the same area that was scraped clear, thus resulting in a recurrence of symptoms.

It is important to point out that CTS is one of several conditions brought about by repetitive stress (RSIs, or "repetitive stress injuries"). The physical stress of repeating the same movements hour after hour, day after day is one part of this picture, but nutritional deficiencies, poor alignment, fatigue, and the resulting risk for trauma and accidents are also contributing factors.

SIGNS AND SYMPTOMS

Depending on the source and severity of the problem, CTS can manifest as tingling, pins and needles, burning, shooting pains, intermittent numbness, and weakness as innervation to the hand muscles is interrupted. It is often worse at night when people may sleep on their arm or turn their wrist into awkward positions. It is painful enough to wake some people out of a deep sleep. Logically it shouldn't, but often it does involve pain going proximally up the forearm from the wrist. (Nerves generally only refer distally.) If pressure is taken off the nerve promptly, no lingering symptoms will remain. But the worst case scenario involves permanent damage to the median nerve, resulting in some loss of muscle function and sensation in the hand.

DIAGNOSIS

Carpal tunnel syndrome is generally diagnosed by a nerve conduction test that measures the strength of nerve impulses passing through the wrist into the hand. It is important to get a very solid diagnosis before attempting to treat this problem because many other disorders can cause similar problems.

Lots of things can cause pain or reduced sensation in the wrist and hand. The possibilities include but are not limited to . . .

- Neck injuries: Herniated discs and irritated neck ligaments will refer pain distally. The worse the irritation, the further the pain will refer.
- Shoulder injuries: Some rotator cuff tendons also refer pain down the arm. The worse the injury, the further it refers. So again, *very* bad shoulder injuries can actually cause pain in the wrist and hand.
- Thoracic outlet syndrome: Nerve and vascular entrapment at the pectoralis minor and/or scalenes can create pain in the wrist. (See *thoracic outlet syndrome*, this chapter, page 120.)
- Other wrist injuries: These can include arthritis, tendinitis, and ligament sprains, all of which can cause pain in the wrist and hand, and none of which will be affected by any of the standard treatments for CTS.

The difficult thing about CTS is that injuries often run in combinations. In other words, wrist and hand pain can be caused by any blending of real CTS factors and factors that mimic CTS, but that don't respond to typical CTS remedies or interventions.

TREATMENT

The treatment options for CTS depend entirely on what the causes are. Treatments may range from vitamin therapy to bony manipulation to surgery. For more details, review the Causes in this section. Various kinds of carpal tunnel syndrome and other nerve impairment problems often respond well to acupuncture, which seems to have a positive affect on nerve conduction in general. If a client is reluctant to consider surgery, this may be a viable alternative.

MASSAGE?

The appropriateness of massage absolutely depends on which kind of CTS the client has, and that determination should not be made by the massage therapist. So what can a responsible therapist do? Be sensible: work conservatively, check with the client's doctor, monitor results. Edematous CTS responds well to massage that focuses on draining the forearm. Fibrotic CTS may or may not improve with massage, depending on how thick and where the fibrosis is. CTS due to a subluxation may respond to massage and traction, but wrist adjustments are not in the scope of practice of massage.

If work on or around the wrist creates any symptoms, stop immediately! If, on the other hand, a client experiences some improvement, the therapist may be on the right track. Proceed slowly, have a clear image of what needs to be accomplished, and work with a doctor for a definitive diagnosis.

Herniated Disc

DEFINITION: WHAT IS IT?

A herniated disc is a disc in which the soft nucleus pulposis or the annulus fibrosis protrudes beyond its normal borders. If the bulge puts pressure on the spinal cord or spinal

---

HERNIATED DISC IN BRIEF

What is it?
A herniated disc is a situation in which the nucleus pulposis or the surrounding annulus fibrosis of an intervertebral disc protrudes in such a way that it puts pressure on nerve roots or on the spinal cord itself.

How is it recognized?
The symptoms of nerve root pressure include referred pain along the dermatome, specific muscle weakness, paresthesia, and numbness.

Is massage indicated or contraindicated?
Massage is indicated in the subacute stage of herniated discs.

nerve roots, it will cause pain. If the bulge doesn't interfere with nerve tissue, most likely no symptoms will be present.

ETIOLOGY: WHAT HAPPENS?

A typical intervertebral disc is quite a complex package, with an outer wrapping of very tough, hard material called the annulus fibrosis, which envelopes a soft, gelatinous center called the nucleus pulposis. Ideally, the shape of the nucleus should be roughly spherical, with the harder annulus layers forming flat surfaces above and below the ball. This combination of textures gives the disc the advantages of strength and resiliency, which it needs to do its job of separating and cushioning the vertebrae. (See Figure 2.36.) The spine is capable of bearing a great deal of weight, partly thanks to the arrangement of the discs.

The outer ring of annulus fibrosis is an arrangement of concentric circles of collagen fibers. These fibers resemble Chinese handcuffs: the tighter they're pulled, the stronger they become. On the other hand, the closer the vertebrae are, the looser (and weaker) the collagen fibers are. This has great implications for the nucleus pulposis, which depends on a very tight, solid exterior wall for support.

The annulus fibrosis is very strong, but studies show that it starts to degenerate at about 25 years. It will sustain multitudes of micro-traumas, but they all contribute to future trouble. At the same time, the nucleus pulposus tends to shrink and dry with age. By the time most people are in their fifties, the nuclei of their discs are no longer soft and gelatinous; they have hardened and thinned.

CAUSES

When the nucleus pulposis protrudes through a hole or crack in the annulus (the hernia), it can press on nerve tissue and cause very severe problems. This scenario is generally the case for people under 45 or 50. For older people the annulus itself may crack and exert pressure on nerve tissue. Of course, if these protrusions don't happen to press on nerve roots or the spinal cord, no pain will be present.

Causes of disc injury may vary according to the general health of the connective tissues of the person involved. For some people it takes a major trauma like a car accident to damage the tissues enough to cause pain. For people with weak, loose intervertebral ligaments the spine is less stable and the risk of disc damage from ordinary, everyday activity is higher. The classic scenario for this kind of disc damage is an incident that involves simultaneous lifting and twisting.

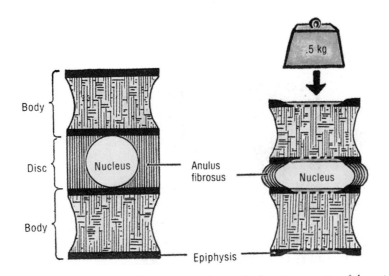

Figure 2.36 Intervertebral discs increase the weight-bearing capacity of the spine

PROGRESSION

When an intervertebral disc is injured and puts pressure on nerve tissue, it's often because of a certain sequence of events on top of a lifetime of normal wear and tear. Here is a typical example of how a lumbar disc may herniate:

- A person bends over to pick up something heavy—a basket full of laundry, for example. Going into trunk flexion flattens the anterior portion of the nucleus, and opens up a posterior space while stretching the posterior fibers of the annulus.
- The person jerks into an erect posture, possibly twisting at the same time, while carrying a heavy load. Sudden return to extension, especially while carrying something heavy, quickly redistributes the nucleus, and shoots it into that posterior space with great force.
- The protruding section of nucleus presses against the weakest part of the posterior annulus and breaks through, which then puts pressure on nerve roots. Or, the force of the motion, combined with the brittleness of the annulus, causes the annulus to crack and put pressure on nerve tissue.

Many variations on this theme exist. Discs that cause pain usually bulge posterolaterally, because that's the path of least resistance in the tight space they inhabit, but they can also go to the left or the right side. (See Figure 2.37.) A "mushroom" disc may bulge in both directions. Occasionally one will bulge directly posteriorly, which puts pressure on the spinal cord rather than nerve roots. This is a very serious situation that can lead to permanent damage. But usually the protrusion is on nerve roots rather than the spinal cord, and the amount of herniated material is very small. It will dry up and take pressure off the nerve roots within a few days or weeks. This leaves the disc permanently thinned, but doesn't necessarily lead to long-lasting problems.

L4 and L5 herniations are the most common with the kind of lifting or lifting-and-twisting injury described here. Cervical herniations are a common problem for car crash survivors; many similarities can be seen between the action of a *whiplash* (this chapter, page 108) and the injury described here. Thoracic herniations are possible, but rarer since the ribs make the thoracic spine much more stable than its cervical and lumbar counterparts.

It won't make a great deal of difference to the applicability of massage to specific cases, but it is useful to be able to recognize the terminology for different types of disc problems that may turn up in a diagnosis.

- bulge: This refers to a situation where the entire disc protrudes beyond the normal boundaries of the vertebral body.

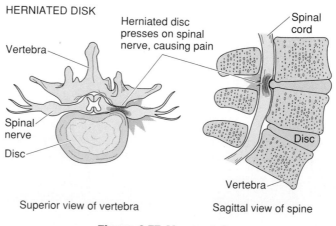

Figure 2.37 Herniated disc

- protrusion: In this case, a focal point exists where the nucleus pulposus extends out of the annulus. If it protrudes postero-laterally, it will tend to put pressure on nerve roots. If it protrudes straight back, it could put pressure on the spinal cord itself.
- extrusion: This is a protrusion of a small piece of the nucleus with a narrow connection back to the body of the nucleus. In some cases the protrusion can separate from the nucleus altogether.
- rupture: The nucleus pulposis has burst and leaked its entire contents into the surrounding area. Ruptures are less painful than other disc problems, because the pressure has been removed from the nerve roots.

SIGNS AND SYMPTOMS

No direct nerve or blood supply connects to discs, so the only symptoms elicited are from the pressure exerted on surrounding ligaments and nerve fibers. The pressure can come and go as the patient's position and alignment shifts, and so the symptoms may be intermittent. This is very important: it is appropriate to work on someone with a herniated disc when their symptoms are abated; it is not appropriate to work when the affected disc is irritated and painful. Symptoms of an acute situation include . . .

- Local and referred pain. There will be pain at the disc from the local inflammation and ligament irritation, as well as pain felt along the dermatome for the affected nerve roots. A dermatome chart is a critical piece of equipment for a massage therapist working with this population.
- Specific muscle weakness. It is important to clarify the difference between *general* weakness, which will occur after a length of time of disuse or injury to whole muscle areas, and *specific* weakness, which will occur very quickly, and *only in the muscles supplied by the affected nerve*.
- Paresthesia. "Pins and needles"—this will happen along the affected dermatomes.
- Numb-likeness. Numb-likeness is a feeling of reduced sensation, but not completely absent sensation. It is a common symptom of ligament damage (which may frequently accompany disc damage).
- Numbness. Total numbness is one distinguishing factor between disc problems and ligament injuries. A disc protrusion can completely cut off sensation to areas within a particular dermatome.

DIAGNOSIS

It's important to get a solid diagnosis for herniated discs because many of the signs and symptoms listed above may be caused by other disorders entirely. Many neurologists agree that herniated discs account for less than 2% of all neck and back pain.

Discs are generally diagnosed by a combination of x-rays, CAT scans, myelograms, and MRIs. Similar symptoms may be exhibited by two other conditions that require vastly different treatment. *Spondylosis* (this chapter, page 84) may lead to osteophytes, and bone cancer may cause tumors. Both may lead to the same kind of nerve pressure that creates the signs of a herniated disc.

One situation that mimics a disc problem but is actually much less serious is a ligament sprain. Irritated spinal ligaments running between spinous or transverse processes can refer pain along the same dermatomes as the nearby discs. Ligament injuries do not cause total numbness or specific muscle weakness, however, and they respond well to specific types of massage. (See *sprains*, this chapter, page 87.)

TREATMENT

The best of all possible resolutions for a herniated disc is for the bulging nucleus pulposus to be reabsorbed into the center of the disc, and for the annulus to close down behind it.

Chiropractors and osteopaths will work to correct bony alignment to create a maximum of space into which the nucleus may retreat. Medical doctors will recommend strict bed rest for the same reason. If it seems warranted, traction may be used to help. Physical therapy and special classes on correct posture and body mechanics are often recommended to people recovering from disc problems. Drugs that are prescribed for herniated discs are aimed at the muscular tendency to seize up in response to this kind of trauma: muscle relaxants and painkillers. If nothing else is working, cortisone is sometimes injected into the area. This powerful anti-inflammatory helps only about half the time, and is often considered the last resort before surgery.

If bed rest doesn't do the trick and the protrusion doesn't dry up and disintegrate, it may be necessary to consider other kinds of intervention. One option is called *chemonucleolysis*. This procedure involves injecting a preparation of papain, an enzyme from papayas that dissolves proteins (it is also used in meat tenderizer), into the disc. This material will reduce the size of the protrusion, take pressure off the nerve tissue, and so restore the patient to a pain-free state, all without major surgery. *Transcutaneous diskectomies*, the removal of disc material through a tiny incision, are sometimes also possible. Open surgery is generally recommended, though, when the disc is putting pressure directly on the spinal cord. In this procedure, a portion of the posterior arch of the vertebra is cut, and the protruding part of the disc is removed, along with the rest of the nucleus pulposis. Another surgical option is to fuse the affected vertebrae together. This certainly increases stability at the spot, but may lead to hypermobility at the joints above and below the fusion as they compensate for the loss of motion at the fused joint. Hypermobility will then increase the risk of future herniations at the joints above and below the site of the original problem.

MASSAGE?

Most people with herniated discs have good days and bad days. Don't work on the bad days, and on the good days, work with the intention of creating space for the retreat of the bulging tissue. Referred pain and muscle spasms always accompany this condition. Compensation patterns that develop with chronic back pain also demand attention.

It is especially important not to work alone with a herniated disc. Muscle spasm can serve an important protective function for newly damaged discs, and releasing it too soon may put a client in danger. (See *spasms, cramps*, this chapter, page 57.) Working with another professional who can handle the bony and/or medical end of it will help the client get better faster and more completely than she or he would have with either professional alone.

Sciatica

DEFINITION: WHAT IS IT?

This term describes any situation that causes the sciatic nerve to become irritated and inflamed, resulting in pain from the buttocks down to the legs.

ETIOLOGY: WHAT HAPPENS?

The sciatic nerve is the largest nerve in the body, about as thick as a thumb. It runs through the deep lateral rotators and down the posterior aspect of the thigh. (See Figure 2.38.) Irritation of this nerve may begin inside the spinal canal or it may arise from ligamentous or muscular causes. It's important to know the difference, because

---

SCIATICA IN BRIEF

What is it?

Sciatica is inflammation of the sciatic nerve. The source of irritation may be inside or outside the spinal canal.

How is it recognized?

Symptoms of sciatic nerve irritation include shooting pain along the dermatome, numbness, or reduced sensation and paresthesia.

Is massage indicated or contraindicated?

Massage is indicated for sciatica brought about by muscular or ligamentous forces, but for problems that begin in the spinal cord, the guidelines in the *herniated disc* or *spondylosis* sections of this chapter must be followed.

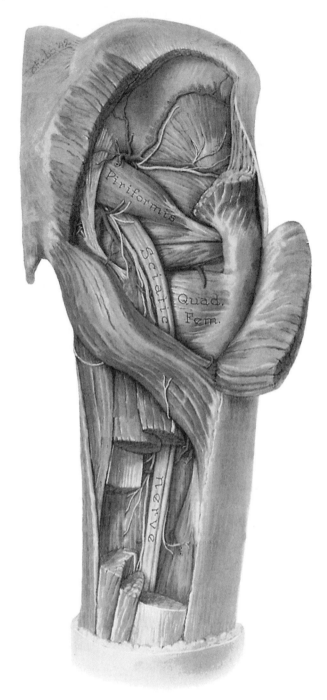

Figure 2.38 The sciatic nerve runs through the deep lateral rotators

while sciatica that begins in the spine must be dealt with medically, most ligamentous or muscular related sciaticas respond well to skillful massage.

The two main culprits for sciatica that begins in the spine are *herniated discs* (this chapter, page 114) and *spondylosis* (this chapter, page 84). In the first case, the disc protrusion is pressing at L4 or L5 (the most frequent sites for herniation). In the second case, osteophytes or bone spurs are growing at those levels. In especially unlucky cases they will grow in exactly the right spot to press against the spinal nerves as they exit the intervertebral foramen. It's not in the scope of practice of massage therapists to diagnose which condition is present, but it is important to find out, because each of these circumstances has different treatment protocols.

Sciatica caused by structures outside the spine can often improve with massage. Some injuries that cause buttock and leg pain include sacro-iliac, sacrotuberous, and sacro-spinous ligament tears (see *sprains*, this chapter, page 87), and spasm of the piriformis or other deep lateral rotators (see *spasms*, this chapter, page 57). Other contributing factors include different leg lengths or foot problems that reverberate up into the hips. (See *pes planus*, this chapter, page 101.)

SIGNS AND SYMPTOMS

Symptoms of sciatica include shooting, burning pains through the buttock and down the back of one leg; tingling; paresthesia (pins and needles); and numb-likeness (reduced sensation). Two additional symptoms that are particular red flags for a problem in the spine (that is, a herniated disc or spondylosis) are *total numbness* and *specific muscle weakness*.

MASSAGE?

Check the guidelines for *spondylosis* (this chapter, page 84) and *herniated disc* (this chapter, page 114). Sciatica due to disc problems or spondylosis is much less common than pain caused by soft tissue injury, so massage will usually be appropriate. But if any doubt arises in the matter, it's important to get a confirmed diagnosis before beginning any work.

Thoracic Outlet Syndrome

DEFINITION: WHAT IS IT?

Thoracic outlet syndrome (TOS) is a neurovascular entrapment: the nerves of the brachial plexus or the blood vessels running to or from the arm (or some combination of both) are impinged or impaired in some way.

ETIOLOGY: WHAT HAPPENS?

The brachial plexus, the tangled network of spinal nerves that supplies the arm with sensation and motor control, is comprised of spinal nerves C5 to T1. These nerves interconnect as they travel a complicated path to get to their final destinations in the arm: they go from intervertebral foramina through the anterior and medial scalenes, between the clavicle and the first rib, under the pectoralis minor and around the humerus. If some part of the plexus is somehow compressed along the way, the client will feel it somewhere along the distance of that nerve.

Pinched nerves are only one part of thoracic outlet syndrome. This is a neurovascular entrapment, and the vessels at risk are the subclavian vein and the axillary artery, which is the distal portion of the subclavian artery. These vessels, while not being vulnerable to osteophytes and herniated discs like the nerves, are equally at the mercy of the compression that can happen when muscles in small spaces get too tight. (See Figure 2.39.)

CAUSES

Thoracic outlet syndrome can be caused by anything that interferes with the functioning of the brachial plexus nerves or the subclavian and axillary blood vessels, or both. Here are some possibilities:

THORACIC OUTLET SYNDROME IN BRIEF

What is it?
Thoracic outlet syndrome (TOS) is a collection of signs and symptoms brought about by occlusion of nerve and blood supply to the arm.

How is it recognized?
Depending on what structures are compressed, TOS will show shooting pains, weakness, numbness, and paresthesia along with a feeling of fullness and possible discoloration of the affected arm from impaired circulation.

Is massage indicated or contraindicated?
This depends on the source of the problem. If it is related to muscle tightness, massage is indicated. TOS due to muscle degeneration or some other disorder such as *spondylosis* (this chapter, page 84) or *herniated disc* (this chapter, pages 114) will not respond well to massage.

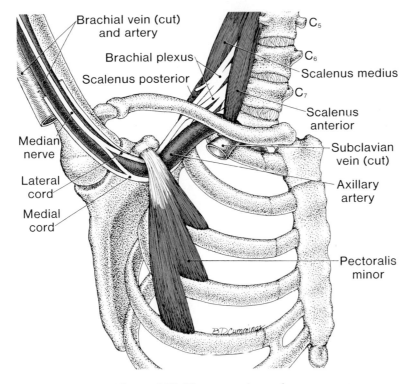

Figure 2.39 Thoracic outlet syndrome

- Cervical misalignment. This could be a subluxation, but would more likely be a rotation with subluxation of any combination of lower cervical vertebrae. Which nerves are affected (and therefore the location of the symptoms) would depend on what level or levels of spinal nerves are being compressed.
- Cervical ribs. Sometimes the transverse processes of the cervical vertebrae grow longer than normal, extending into territory where they don't belong. On an x-ray they actually look like little ribs sticking out into the soft tissues of the neck. They are usually unilateral, and C7 is the vertebra that grows them most frequently.
- Spondylosis. Imagine what a bone spur growing right into the nerve root at C6 (or any other cervical nerve root) would do. *That's* TOS due to spondylosis. (See *spondylosis*, this chapter, page 84.)
- Rib misalignment. The joints that join the ribs to the spine are full synovial joints, called *zygopophyseal joints*. Like the intervertebral joints, the rib joints sometimes subluxate. When this happens to the first rib, problems could arise at either of *two* spots: right under the anterior scalene, or between the coracoid process and the ribs. In both of those locations, the brachial plexus nerves can easily be caught between a bone (the first rib) and a hard place (a tight muscle or another bone).
- Tight muscles. Specifically, the anterior and medial scalenes, and the pectoralis minor.
- Atrophied muscles. Many cases of TOS may be related to muscle atrophy as an outcome of chronic muscle tightness. The pectoralis minor, in a constant battle with the rhomboids and levator scapulae, is especially prone to this phenomenon, particularly for people with a "caved in" kind of posture. Eventually the pectoralis minor becomes shrunken and fibrotic, while its antagonists on the back, especially the rhomboids, become stretched out and hypotonic. If muscles that support the shoulder girdle are abnormally underdeveloped, the clavicle and scapula may collapse onto the ribs, compressing and irritating brachial plexus nerves and the axillary artery.

SIGNS AND SYMPTOMS

Symptoms of TOS include all signs of *neuritis* (chapter 3, page 157): shooting pains; numbness and numb-likeness; weakness; tingling and pins and needles. Add to these the vascular symptoms: a feeling of "fullness" when blood return from a vein is blocked, or coldness and weakness when blood flow to the axillary artery is impaired. The affected arm may even show a different coloration.

DIAGNOSIS

There are several ways to look for the presence of TOS. In the Wright hyperabduction test, the hand is placed over the head and the head is turned toward the affected side. If this exacerbates symptoms or reduces the strength of the pulse of the affected side, impingement to the axillary artery and lower brachial plexus nerves is suspected. For Adson's test, the head is extended and rotated toward the affected side. The client takes a deep breath and the radial pulse on the affected side diminishes or even completely disappears. TOS due to muscle atrophy may show best when a client lies on his affected side and the pulse is diminished from axillary artery compression.

CONFUSING SIGNS

Many, many things cause pain in the shoulders, arms, wrists, and hands. Some of these problems are often missed by standard diagnosis, simply because most soft tissue injuries don't show up on most medical tests. This is unfortunate, because it makes it hard for people to get an accurate diagnosis for their most common and treatable problems. Here are just a few of the things that will cause pain in the shoulder, arm, wrist, or hand, and that can be hard to pin down in an accurate diagnosis.

Causes of Pain in the Shoulder, Arm, Wrist, or Hand

- spondylosis
- vertebral misalignment
- cervical rib pressing on the brachial plexus
- tight scalenes, pectoralis minor
- carpal tunnel syndrome
- wrist tendinitis or sprain
- herniated disc
- costal misalignment
- injured cervical ligaments
- rotator cuff tendinitis
- elbow tendinitis
- arthritis in shoulders, elbows, or wrists

TREATMENT

The treatment for thoracic outlet syndrome will depend entirely on what's causing it, which is why it's important to get an accurate diagnosis of the cause of this problem. Different strategies are more appropriate for spondylosis than for tight scalenes, for instance. TOS due to muscle atrophy responds best to strengthening exercises.

MASSAGE?

If the TOS isn't from a muscular spasm, massage won't make much lasting difference. But if it is related to spasm, it can respond very well to massage. The client should also learn some specific stretches and exercises for pectoralis minor, its antagonists, and the scalenes in order for the massage to have lasting impact.

CHAPTER REVIEW QUESTIONS: MUSCULOSKELETAL SYSTEM CONDITIONS

1. What is the relationship between fibromyalgia and sleep disorders?

2. What does "hernia" mean? Name three kinds of abdominal hernias.

3. Why are herniated discs in the thoracic spine rare?

4. Where do massage therapists often suffer from osteoarthritis?

5. Why are women more prone than men to osteoporosis?

6. Describe how pes planus can lead to headaches.

7. What kind of muscle spasm is actually an important part of the healing process?

8. What is more serious: sciatica from a problem inside the spinal cord or from a problem outside the spinal cord? Why?

9. In which stage of healing do soft tissue injuries generally contraindicate massage? Why?

10. What does ICE stand for?

11. Define "specific weakness."

12. Describe the pain-spasm-ischemia cycle.

13. Describe the differences between strains, sprains, and tendinitis.

13. Describe the relationship between stress and chronic injury.

BIBLIOGRAPHY, MUSCULOSKELETAL SYSTEM CONDITIONS

General References, Musculoskeletal System

1. Ben Benjamin, PhD, Gale Borden, MD. Listen to your pain: The active person's guide to understanding, indentifying and treating pain and injury. Harrisonville, VA: The Viking Press and Penguin Books, 1984.

2. Carmine D. Clemente, PhD. Anatomy: A regional atlas of the human body. 3rd ed. Baltimore: Urban & Schwarzenburg, 1987.

3. I. Damjanou. Pathology for the health-related professions. Philadelphia: WB Saunders, 1996.

4. Giovanni de Dominico, Elizabeth Wood. Beard's massage. Philadelphia: WB Saunders, 1997.

5. Deane Juhan. Job's body: A handbook for bodywork. Barrytown, NY: Station Hill Press, Inc., 1987.

6. I.A. Kapandji. The physiology of the joints: Annotated diagrams of the mechanics of the human joints. Volume one, upper limb. 5th ed. New York: Longman Group Limited, Churchill Livingstone, Inc., 1982.

7. I.A. Kapandji. The physiology of the joints: Annotated diagrams of the mechanics of the human joints. Volume two, lower limb. 2nd ed. New York: Longman Group Limited, Churchill Livingstone, Inc., 1970.

8. I.A. Kapandji. The physiology of the joints: Annotated diagrams of the mechanics of the human joints. Volume three, the trunk and vertebral column. New York: Longman Group Limited, Churchill Livingstone, Inc., 1974.

9 Jeffrey R. M. Kunz, MD, Asher J. Finkel, MD, eds. The American Medical Association family medical guide. New York: Random House, Inc., 1987.

10. Elaine M. Marieb, RN, PhD. Human anatomy and physiology. Redwood City, CA: Benjamin/Cummings Publishing Co., Inc., 1989.

11. Ruth Lundeen Memmler, MD, Dina Lin Wood, RN, BS, PHN. The human body in health and disease. 5th ed. Philadelphia: JB Lippincott Co., 1983.

12. Mary Lou Mulvihill. Human diseases: A systemic approach. 2nd ed. Norwalk, CT: Appleton & Lange, 1987.
13. Stedman's medical dictionary. 26th ed. Baltimore: Williams & Wilkins, 1995.
14. Taber's cyclopedic dictionary. 14th ed. Philadelphia: F.A. Davis Company, 1981.
15. Gerard J. Tortora, Nicholas P. Anagnostakos. Principles of anatomy and physiology. 6th ed. New York: Biological Sciences Textbook, Inc.; A&P Textbooks, Inc.; and Elia-Sparta, Inc., Harper & Row Publishers, Inc., 1990.
16. Janet Travell, MD, David G. Simons, MD. Myofascial pain and dysfunction: The trigger point manual. Baltimore: Williams & Wilkins, 1983.
17. Janet Travell, MD, David G. Simons, MD. Myofascial pain and dysfunction: The trigger point manual. Baltimore: Williams & Wilkins, 1983.

Fibromyalgia

1. Fibromyalgia treatment. The Center for Integrated Therapy. URL: http://www.medhelp.org/www/piic/piic3.htm. Accessed fall 1997.
2. Fibromyalgia: Coping with very real pain. Mayo Foundation for Medical Education and Research. Mayo Health O@sis: September 16, 1996. URL: http://www.mayo.ivi.com/mayo/9609/htm/fibromya.html. Accessed fall 1997.
3. Fibromyalgia: Widespread and difficult to diagnose. Arthritis Foundation, 1997. URL: http://www.arthritis.org/news/release/fibromyalgia.hmtl. Accessed fall 1997.
4. Steven Mann. Cognitive/somatic pain management with fibromyalgia and chronic myofascial pain. Massage Therapy Journal, 1995;34(4):35–45.
5. MedicineNet: Power points about fibromyalgia. Information Network, Inc., 1995–1997. URL: http://www.medicinenet.com. Accessed fall 1997.
6. David Nye, MD. Fibromyalgia: A guide for patients. URL: http://Prairie.lakes.com/~roseleaf/fibro/pt-faq.html. Accessed fall 1997.

Myositis Ossificans

1. Soft tissue calcifications. Michael L. Richardson, MD, 1994. URL: http://www.rad.washington.edu/Books/New Approach/SoftTissueCa.html. Accessed fall 1997.

Shin Splints

1. Daniel J. Hoefer. Periostitis ("Shin Splints"). Radiology Resident Case of the Week, October 17, 1996. The author(s) and the University of Iowa, 1992–1997. URL:http://indy.radiology.uiowa.edu/Providers/TeachingFiles/RCW2/101796/101796.html. Accessed fall 1997.
2. Frederick Matsen, III, MD. Treatment of compartment syndrome. University of Washington, 1995–1997. URL: http://www.orthop.Washington.edu/Bone%20and%20Joint%20Sources/yycctryy1_1.html. Accessed fall 1997.

Strains

1. Jeff Lace, MS, PT. An overview of common injury terminology. John C. Lincoln Sports Medicine and Physical Therapy. URL: http://www.health-net.com/injuries.htm. Accessed fall 1997.
2. Wayne Girdlestone. Tendinitis, paratendinitis and tendinosus. Balance Fitness Magazine; 11(September 1995). The International Communique Ltd., 1995. URL: http//balance.net/95/1_9/sports/therapy/injury/tendons.htm. Accessed fall 1997.

Fractures

1. Treatment methods are tailored to the break. Mayo Foundation for Medical Education and Research. Mayo Health O@sis: April 1996. URL: http://www.mayo.ivi.com/mayo/9604/htm/fracture.htm. Accessed fall 1997.

Osteoporosis

1. Boning up on calcium and osteoporosis. Physician's Committee for Responsible Medicine. URL: http://www.envirolink.org/arrs/essays/calcium.html. Accessed fall 1997.
2. David Brown. Simple genetic test may identify increased risk of osteoporosis. Washington Post, January 20, 1994:A3.
3. How can I prevent osteoporosis? National Osteoporosis Foundation, August 1997. URL: http://www.nof.org/PreventOsteo.html. Accessed fall 1997.
4. How can I tell the health of my bones? National Osteoporosis Foundation, 1997. URL: http://www.nof.org/BoneHealth.html. Accessed fall 1997.
5. Osteoporosis and diet: No bones about it. Mayo Foundation for Medical Education and Research. Mayo Health O@sis: May 1, 1996. URL: http://www.mayo.ivi.com/mayo/9605/htm/osteoca.htm. Accessed fall 1997.
6. Strength training may lower risk of osteoporosis. Mayo Foundation for Medical Education and Research, 1996. Mayo Health O@sis. URL:http://www.mayo.ivi.com/mayo/9310/htm/stren_up.htm. Accessed fall 1997.

7. What if I have osteoporosis? National Osteoporosis Foundation, August 1997. URL: http://www.nof.org/HavingOsteoporosis. html. Accessed fall 1997.

8. What is osteoporosis? National Osteoporosis Foundation, June 1997. URL: http://www.nof.org/Osteoporosis.html. Accessed fall 1997.

9. Who's at risk? National Osteoporosis Foundation. URL: http://www.nof.org/Risk.html#NOF. Accessed fall 1997.

10. MaryAnne Dunkin, ed. Bones and depression. Arthritis Today 11-12/95. Arthritis Foundation. http://www.arthritis.org/at/ archive/1995/11_12/08sf.shtml.

Paget's Disease

1. Abramson NJ, Weissman, BN. Paget's disease. BrighamRAD Teaching Case Database [online collection of case studies], 1994. URL: http://www.med.harvard. edu/brad-bin/create page.py/12/full. Accessed September 10, 1997.

2. Paget's disease of bone. Osteoporosis and Related Bone Diseases Resource Center. URL: http://www.osteo.org/paget.html. Accessed fall 1997.

Postural Deviations

1. Approaches to differential diagnosis in scoliosis. Michael L. Richardson, MD, 1994. URL: http://www.rad.washington. edu/Books/NewApproach/scoliosis.html. Accessed fall 1997.

2. John Albert Odom, Jr., MD. Spinal deformities: The benefits of early detection and treatment. The Colorado Spine Center, PC, 1994. URL: http://www.coolware. com/health/medical_reporter/scoliosis. html. Accessed fall 1997.

Ankylosing Spondylitis

1. Ankylosing spondylitis. Arthritis Foundation Arthritis Medical Information Series 9050/6-85.

2. Frequently asked questions: Ankylosing spondylitis surgery. Adult Spine Surgery Service. The Penn State University, 1997. URL: http://www.ortho.hmc.psu.edu/ spine/FAQs_AS.html. Accessed fall 1997.

3. MedicineNet: Power points about ankylosing spondylitis. Information Network, Inc., 1995–1997. URL: http://www.medicinenet.com. Accessed fall 1997.

Dislocations

1. Thomas A. Dorman, Thomas A. Ravin. Diagnosis and injection techniques in orthopedic medicine. Baltimore: Williams & Wilkins.

Gout

1. Thomas V. DiBacco. The pain of gout: Baffling condition left doctors guessing. Washington Post, October 11, 1994:Z19.

2. Gout fact sheet. Arthritis Foundation, 1997. URL: http://www.arthritis.org/ facts/fs/gout.shmtl. Accessed fall 1997.

3. Frederick Matsen, III, MD. Pseudogout. University of Washington Academic Medical Center, 1995–1997. URL: http://www.orthop.washington.edu/bone-joint/pzzzzzzz1_1.html. Accessed fall 1997.

4. MedicineNet: Power points about gout and hyperuricemia. Information Network, Inc., 1995–1997. URL: http://www.medicinenet.com. Accessed fall 1997.

Osteoarthritis

1. MedicineNet: Power points about osteoarthritis. Information Network, Inc., 1995–1997. URL: http://www.medicinenet.com. Accessed fall 1997.

2. Osteoarthritis fact sheet. Arthritis Foundation, 1997. URL: http://www.arthritis. org/facts/fs/osteoarthritis.shmtl. Accessed fall 1997.

Rheumatoid Arthritis

1. Focus on . . . Rheumatoid arthritis. Reprinted from the December 1994 issue of Medical Sciences Bulletin. Published by Pharmaceutical Information Associates, Ltd. © Vir Sci Corporation. URL: http://pharminfo.com/cgi_bin/print_hit_ bold.pl/pubs/msb/rheumart.html. Accessed fall 1997.

2. MedicineNet: Power points about rheumatoid arthritis. Information Network, Inc., 1995–1997. URL: http://www. medicinenet.com. Accessed fall 1997.

3. Rheumatoid arthritis fact sheet. Arthritis Foundation, 1997. URL: http://www. arthritis.org/facts/fs/rheumatoid.shtml. Accessed fall 1997.

Septic Arthritis

1. Septic arthritis. Copyright 1998 ADAM Software, Inc., all rights reserved. Copyright 1998 CommuniHealth. URL: http://www.healthanswers.com. Accessed winter 1998.

Spondylosis

1. Richard Kim, MD, MS. Lumbar stenosis (spondylosis). URL: http://mcns10.med. nyu.edu/spine/spine_surgery_p3.html. Accessed fall 1997.

2. Richard Kim, MD, MS. Cervical spondylosis. URL: http://mcns10.med.nyu.edu/ spine/spine_surgery_p5.html. Accessed fall 1997.

3. Rick Weiss. Back pain and MRIs: Vivid diagnostic images are a mixed blessing. Washington Post Health, July 19, 1994:7.

Sprains

1. Wayne Girdlestone. Tendinitis, paratendinitis and tendinosus. Balance Fitness Magazine; 11(September 1995). The International Communique Ltd., 1995. URL: http//balance.net/95/1_9/sports/therapy/injury/tendons.htm. Accessed fall 1997.

Temporomandibular Joint Dysfunction

1. Wesley E. Shankland, II, DDS, MS, PhD. Symptoms of TMJ pain. URL: http://www.netset.com/~docws/page3.html. Accessed fall 1997.
2. Wesley E. Shankland, II, DDS, MS, PhD. Causes of TMJ. URL: http://www.netset.com/~docws/page4.html. Accessed fall 1997.
3. Wesley E. Shankland, II, DDS, MS, PhD. Treatment of TMJ. URL: http://www.netset.com/~docws/page5.html. Accessed fall 1997.
4. Wesley E. Shankland, II, DDS, MS, PhD. Pain disorders that are confused with TMJ. URL: http://www.netset.com/~docws/page6.html. Accessed fall 1997.
5. What is temporomandibular joint disease? K. E. Goldman, 1995, 1996, 1997. URL: http://www.calweb.com/~goldman/tmj.htm. Accessed fall 1997.

Baker's Cysts

1. Ben Benjamin, PhD. Understanding Baker's cyst. Massage Therapy Journal; 32(3):20.

Bunions

1. Rick Positano, John Waller. Are other treatments for bunions as helpful as surgery? Washington Post Health, August 24, 1993.
2. Michael L. Richardson, MD, Sigvard T. Hansen, MD, Ray F. Kilcoyne, MD. Hallux valgus tutorial. University of Washington Department of Radiology. URL: http://www.rad.washington.edu/Anatomy/HalluxValgus/HalluxValgus.html. Accessed fall 1997.

Bursitis

1. A patient's guide to common shoulder problems. Medical Multimedia Group. URL: http://www.sechrest.com/mmg/shoulder/index.html. Accessed fall 1997.

2. Bursitis: Common inflammation responds to simple care. Mayo Foundation for Medical Education and Research, 1996. Mayo Health O@sis. URL: http://www.mayo.ivi.com/mayo/9506/htm/bursitis.htm. Accessed fall 1997.

Dupuytren's Contracture

1. DeQuervain's tenosynovitis. Medical Multimedia Group, 1996. URL: http://www.sechrest.com/mmg/ctd/dqt.html. Accessed fall 1997.
2. Trigger finger and thumb. Medical Multimedia Group, 1996. URL: http://www.sechrest.com/mmg/ctd/trigger.html. Accessed fall 1997.

Hernia

1. MedicineNet: Power points about gastrointestinal reflux disease. Information Network, Inc., 1995–1997. URL: http://www.medicinenet.com. Accessed fall 1997.

Plantar Fasciitis

1. Heel pain: It's usually a sign of plantar fasciitis. Mayo Foundation for Medical Education and Research, 1996. Mayo Health O@sis. URL: http://www.mayo.ivi.com/mayo/9607/htm/heelpain.htm. Accessed fall 1997.
2. Eric Lauf, DPM. Prefab orthoses: Treating flatfoot. Biomechanics Magazine 1996; III(4). Miller Freeman, Inc., a United News & Media company, 1997. URL: http://www.biomech.com/archive/1996/apr96/prefab.html. Accessed fall 1997.

Tendinitis

1. Wayne Girdlestone. Tendinitis, paratendinitis and tendinosus. Balance Fitness Magazine, 11(September 1995). The International Communique Ltd., 1995. URL: http//balance.net/95/1_9/sprots/therapy/injury/tendons.htm. Accessed fall 1997.

Torticollis

1. Management of plagiocephaly and torticollis. John Graham, Jr., MD, ScD, 1996. Cedars Sinai Medical Center, UCLA School of Medicine. URL: http://www.csmc.edu/pediatrics/refguide/helmet/helmet.html. Accessed fall 1997.
2. Pongsakdi Visudhiphan, MD, Surang Chiemchanya, MD, Racha Somburanasin, MD, Dhanit Dheandhanoo, MD. Torticollis as the presenting sign in cervical spine infection and tumor. Clinical Pediatrics 1982; 21(2):71–76.

3. There are three different forms or types of ST. National Spasmodic Torticollis Association. URL: http:www.blueheronweb.com/nsta/Forms.htm. Accessed fall 1997.

4. Treatments for ST. National Spasmodic Torticollis Association. URL: http:www.blueheronweb.com/nsta/Treatment.htm. Accessed fall 1997.

Whiplash

1. Post concussion syndrome. Body-Mind Publications, 1997. URL: http://www.olywa.net/bmp/postcon.htm. Accessed fall 1997.

Carpal Tunnel Syndrome

1. A patient's guide to carpal tunnel syndrome. Medical Multimedia Group, 1996. URL: http://www.sechrest.com/mmg/cts/ctsintro.html. Accessed fall 1997.

2. MedicineNet: Power points about carpal tunnel syndrome. Information Network, Inc., 1995–1997. URL: http://www.medicinenet.com. Accessed fall 1997.

Herniated Disc

1. A patient's guide to low back pain. Medical Multimedia Group, 1997. URL: http://www.sechrest.com/mmg/backpain.html. Accessed fall 1997.

2. Georges Y. El-Khoury, MD. Diagnosis of disk disease. Department of Radiology, University of Iowa College of Medicine, the Author(s) and the University of Iowa, 1992–1997. URL: http://www.vh.org/Providers/Textbooks/DiagnosisDiskDisease/DiagnosisDiskDisease.html. Accessed fall 1997.

3. Richard Kim, MD, MS. Cervical disc disease. URL: http://mcns10.med.nyu.edu/spine/spine_surgery_p4.html. Accessed fall 1997.

4. Richard Kim, MD, MS. Lumbar disc disease. URL: http://mcns10.med.nyu.edu/spine/spine_surgery_p2.html. Accessed fall 1997.

5. What's behind back pain and what can you do to prevent it? Mayo Foundation for Medical Education and Research, 1996. Mayo Health O@sis. URL: http://www.mayo.ivi.com/mayo/9402/thm/backcare.htm. Accessed fall 1997.

Sciatica

1. Brent S. E. Rich, MD, ATC, Douglas McKeag, MD. When sciatica is not disk disease. The Physician and Sports Medicine 1992; 20(10):105–115.

2. What's behind back pain and what can you do to prevent it? Mayo Foundation for Medical Education and Research, 1996. Mayo Health O@sis. URL: http://www.mayo.ivi.com/mayo/9402/thm/backcare.htm. Accessed fall 1997.

Thoracic Outlet Syndrome

1. MedicineNet: Power points about thoracic outlet syndrome. Information Network, Inc., 1995–1997. URL: http://www.medicinenet.com. Accessed fall 1997.

2. Rich Phaigh. Tests for thoracic outlet syndrome. Massage Therapy Journal 1995; 34(2):26–27.

Nervous System Conditions

After reading this chapter, you should be able to tell . . .

- What the disorder is.
- How to recognize it.
- Whether massage is indicated or contraindicated for that condition.
- Whether a contraindication is local or systemic, or refers to a specific stage of development or healing.
- Why those choices for massage are correct.

In addition to this basic information, you should be able to . . .

- Know which nerve is involved in Bell's palsy.
- Name three classes of headaches.
- Name two signs that a headache could be indicative of a life-threatening situation.
- Name two types of seizures.
- Know the causative agent for shingles.
- Know the difference between myelin and neurilemma.
- Name three diseases that may be confused with multiple sclerosis.
- Know the target tissue of the polio virus.
- Name six symptoms of stroke.
- Know the difference between transient ischemic attack and stroke.

INTRODUCTION

By the time most massage therapists finish their training, they probably know more about the nervous system than they ever suspected even existed, and they'll probably still feel like rank amateurs on the subject. That feeling is common to most people who study this topic. Fortunately, only a passing familiarity with the structure and function of this system is needed in order to make educated decisions about massage and most nervous system disorders. Most of the conditions considered here affect the peripheral nerves rather than the central nervous system (CNS), so this introductory discussion will focus mainly on the structure and function of the parts of the nervous system massage therapists can touch—which, not coincidentally, are also the parts of the system that are most vulnerable to injury.

FUNCTION

What are nerves? Nerves are bundles of individual neurons: single-celled fibers capable of transmitting electrical impulses from one place to another. At their most basic level, their function is to transmit information from the body to the brain (sensation) and responses from the brain back to the body (motor control). Interconnected neurons in the brain also provide the potential for consciousness, creativity, memory, and other fascinating abilities that are beyond the scope of what massage therapists are qualified to deal with, and so won't be discussed here.

STRUCTURE

Peripheral nerves are composed of bundles of long filaments (neurons) that run from the spinal cord to wherever in the body they supply sensation or motor control. Each neuron is a single living cell. It is a bit boggling to realize that the neuron running from the low back to the skin of the great toe is all one unbroken microscopic fiber, but that's the way it is. Neurons have three parts: the dendrite (which carries impulses *toward* the

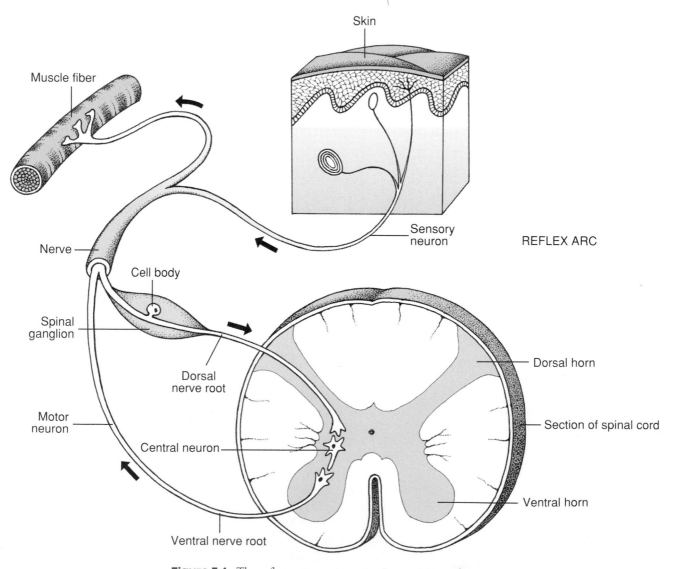

Figure 3.1. The reflex arc connects sensation to motor response

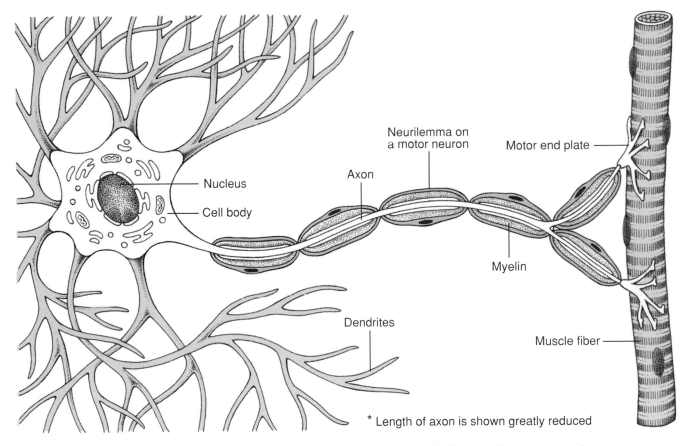

Figure 3.2. Neurons in the peripheral nervous system are covered with Shwann cells, forming *neurilemma*

cell body), the cell body, and the axon (which carries impulses *away* from the cell body). Sensory neurons therefore have exceptionally long dendrites to carry information toward the cell body in the CNS, while motor neurons have very long axons to carry messages from the CNS out to their cell bodies in the muscles and glands. Motor and sensory neurons communicate via synapses in the spinal cord, sometimes by way of some combinations of central, or association, neurons. At the same time that an immediate response is generated at the spinal cord level, the information also travels up the spine into the brain. This immediate reaction is called the reflex arc. (See Figure 3.1.)

Most neurons in the peripheral and central nervous system have a waxy insulating coating called *myelin*. This layer of material speeds nerve conduction along the fiber, and also prevents the jumping of electrical impulses from one fiber to another. In the peripheral nervous system, neurons have another protective feature in *neurilemma*: an outside covering of special cells that can help to regenerate damaged tissue. (See Figure 3.2.)

Peripheral nerves typically run close to the bone, where they are protected from most injuries. In a few places they are vulnerable, however. These spots are *endangerments* for massage therapists, who could potentially cause injury to delicate tissues at these points. (Self defense classes call them *targets*.) For specific information on nerve endangerments, refer to appendix 3, page 389.

It is a convenient analogy to think about nerves as bundles of electrical wires. The similarities are obvious: here are thousands of filaments carrying electrical impulses, each one is wrapped by an insulating layer of myelin, and they are bundled together for efficiency. The analogy stops, however, when one considers the effect of external pressure on nerve fiber transmission. In *Job's Body*, Deane Juhan points out that a piece of electrical cable with a truck parked on it will continue to carry its electrical messages, but a sciatic nerve squeezed by a tight piriformis will have a drastically reduced flow of energy through it.[1] Nerves function with a combination of electrical and fluid flow; fluid flow will be severely limited by external pressure. Consider the implications of that pressure on a femoral nerve that is hugged by a spasmed psoas, or the brachial plexus nerves running through a tangled maze of scalenes and pectoralis minor muscles.

GENERAL NEUROLOGICAL PROBLEMS

Most of the nervous system disorders that massage can affect will involve some kind of mechanical pinching or distortion of peripheral nerves as they wend their ways from the spinal cord to their destinations in the body. Peripheral nerve damage has a generally good prognosis because of the regenerative properties provided by the neurilemma.

Other neurological problems will involve the brain or spinal cord, which have very limited ability to regenerate, and which massage obviously cannot directly access. But even when the spinal cord has been injured, overlapping patterns of innervation created by the twists and turns of the plexi often allow at least partial use of what would otherwise be a totally lost limb. This is a remarkable advantage that begins to explain the benefits of the confusing routes that nerves take through the plexi. The best plan, when faced with a client who has sustained CNS damage, is to address the *symptoms* of these disorders as well as possible, looking for sensation where it is present, and to create as hospitable an internal environment as possible.

Organic and mechanical problems with the central and peripheral nervous systems are one class of neurological problem massage therapists will encounter. Mental illness, which can also be classified as a neurological problem, is another situation altogether. Many people have a bewildering array of mental or physical qualities that set them apart from the arbitrary standards called "normal." Some of these people will seek massage as a way to deal with some of the difficulties that their "abnormalities" create.

Massage therapists can thus be put in the precarious position of deciding whether or not their work is an appropriate part of someone's healing, or even just coping, process. Sometimes the answer will clearly be "no" (for instance, with someone who obviously is in need of psychological counseling instead of or in addition to massage). At other times it will be less clear, and it will be necessary to seek out the opinion of other professionals. Mental health patients who are on heavy, long-term doses of medication are in a particularly vulnerable position in regards to massage. Though massage is usually a good thing, it can change the internal chemistry of the body and brain significantly. When massage elicits a parasympathetic response, the types of neurotransmitters and hormones circulating in the body may shift radically away from "flight or fight" chemicals to substances that allow for relaxation and even sleepiness. If a client is on medication to achieve equilibrium, it is inappropriate for a well-meaning but ignorant massage therapist to throw him off balance. Always consult with the client's medical and healthcare team before proceeding.

Disorders of the nervous system can produce a bewildering variety of startling and sometimes intimidating symptoms. In working with these patients, as with all others, massage therapists must remember that their prime objective must always be, "do no harm."

---

[1] Deane Juhan. Job's body: A handbook for bodywork. Barrytown, NY: Station Hill Press, Inc., 1987:158.

NERVOUS SYSTEM CONDITIONS

Chronic Degenerative Disorders
Amyotrophic Lateral Sclerosis
Chorea
Multiple Sclerosis
Parkinson's Disease
Peripheral Neuropathy

Infectious Disorders
Encephalitis
Herpes Zoster
Meningitis
Polio
Post Polio Syndrome

Nervous System Injuries
Bell's Palsy
Headaches
Hyperesthesia
Neuritis
Spinal Cord Injury
Stroke
Trigeminal Neuralgia

Other Nervous System Disorders
Seizure Disorders

Chronic Degenerative Disorders

Amyotrophic Lateral Sclerosis

DEFINITION: WHAT IS IT?

Also known as *Lou Gehrig's disease*, this is an extremely mysterious condition of the motor neurons of which science is just beginning to catch a glimmer of understanding.

DEMOGRAPHICS: WHO GETS IT?

The three basic types of amyotrophic lateral sclerosis (ALS) include sporadic, which accounts for about 95% of the cases in the United States; familial, which shows a genetic link for about 5% of U.S. cases; and the Mariana Island variety, which is endemic to a specific population in the Western Pacific islands. ALS usually affects people between 40 and 70 years old, although familial ALS tends to have a younger onset than the sporadic type. Between 4,000 and 5,000 new cases are diagnosed in the United States every year; approximately 30,000 people in this country are living with this disease right now. It affects men about twice as often as women.

ETIOLOGY: WHAT HAPPENS?

The cause of ALS is unknown. It involves the degeneration of motor neurons, which leads to the progressive and irreversible atrophy of voluntary muscle.

SIGNS AND SYMPTOMS

ALS presents very different symptoms in different people. The most common pattern is to see stiffness, weakness, and awkwardness in one hand, which slowly spreads to other parts of the body. Fasciculations, or visible muscle twitching, may be present. Sometimes weakness in the legs is the first sign. For other people, the first indication of the disease

---

AMYOTROPHIC LATERAL SCLEROSIS IN BRIEF

What is it?
Amyotrophic lateral sclerosis (ALS) is a progressive disease that begins in the central nervous system. It involves the degeneration of motor neurons and the subsequent atrophy of voluntary muscle.

How is it recognized?
Symptoms of ALS include weakness, fatigue, and muscle spasms. It appears most frequently in men between 40 and 70 years of age.

Is massage indicated or contraindicated?
Massage is indicated for ALS, with caution and under a doctor's supervision.

is difficulty in speaking. Weakness and lack of coordination in the proximal aspects of the extremities—shoulders and thighs—will appear. A gradual onset of weakness, fatigue, and muscle spasms will progress distally. Eventually the semi-voluntary muscles for breathing and swallowing will be affected, and communication can become very difficult.

ALS does not affect sensory neurons or intellectual capacity at all.

DIAGNOSIS

No definitive test exists for ALS. It is typically diagnosed through history, physical exam, nerve conduction studies, and electromyographs, which show loss of muscle function caused by lack of nerve stimulation. Care must be taken to differentiate ALS from other conditions that have some similar symptoms: muscular dystrophy, *multiple sclerosis* (this chapter, page 135), and peripheral nerve damage, for instance.

A common triad of signs, when seen together, form the most dependable diagnosis for ALS. They are: atrophic weakness in the hands and forearms; mild spasticity in the legs; and general hyperreflexia all over the body. The disease may be present without this trio of signs, however, so diagnosis can sometimes take several months or even years to accomplish.

TREATMENT

Up until very recently, treatment for ALS has been strictly palliative, that is, aimed at managing the severity of the symptoms only. Some of these options include moderate exercise and physical and occupational therapy to maintain muscle strength as long as possible. Heat and whirlpools are used to control muscle spasms, and speech therapy helps with difficulties in swallowing and speech. In advanced cases, swallowing may be so difficult that the insertion of a stomach tube (gastrostomy) may be recommended. Since this disease does not impede cognitive or emotional processes at all, psychological therapy for ALS patients and their families is an important part of the treatment plan.

Drug treatment for ALS has traditionally been used only to help combat general fatigue or secondary infections, but recent research focuses on substances that keep nerves functioning longer than before. This is not a cure for ALS, but it may significantly prolong the lives of people affected by this disease.

PROGNOSIS

Once diagnosed, this disease, which has no known cure, will usually result in death within 2 to 10 years. Usually death comes about from complications of paralysis, particularly systemic infections like *pneumonia* (chapter 6, page 252) or *kidney infection* (chapter 8, page 313). One-half of all ALS patients will succumb within three years of diagnosis. Ninety percent will die within six years. Some ALS patients, however, have survived for decades. How? No one knows.

MASSAGE?

This disease is not blood or lymph-borne, it doesn't involve sensory paralysis, and it's not contagious. It is treated with heat, exercise, and physical therapy. Therefore, *within limits*, and in the absence of other contraindicated circumstances, massage may also be appropriate. Massage therapists who get a chance to work with ALS patients should do so under a doctor's supervision, and keep careful notes on their work to make available for others.

Chorea

CHOREA
This word comes from the Greek *choreia*, a "choral dance." It has the same root as the word "chorus," which gives some insight into what those Greek choruses were doing during all those tragedies.

DEFINITION: WHAT IS IT?

This condition refers to involuntary twitching that can be a symptom of a number of different types of central nervous system problems.

ETILIOGY: WHAT HAPPENS?

Chorea or tremors can occur in a variety of ways. The most common versions are discussed below.

- *Essential Tremor* is a chronic tremor that is not secondary to any other pathology. Three to four million people in the United States have essential tremor, which is slowly progressive but not usually debilitating. Onset can occur as early as adolescence, but essential tremor most often shows up at about 45 years of age. It is often an inherited disorder.

  Some medications do treat essential tremor, and moderate alcohol consumption can relieve symptoms. Too much alcohol, however, will make it worse.

- *Huntington's disease* is a hereditary degeneration of nerve tissue in the cerebrum. Symptoms don't usually show until adulthood, when tremors and progressive dementia become irreversible. The average age of onset is between 35 and 50 years. It affects approximately five out of every one million people in the United States.

  Huntington's disease is diagnosed by CT scan, MRI, and DNA marker studies.

- *St. Vitus' dance*, or chorea minor, is a rarer but more famous disorder. This is a problem that begins in childhood, or occasionally during pregnancy. Again, no cure is known, but the prognosis is not so bleak; it usually passes without serious incident, although sedation during convulsive episodes may be recommended.

- *Parkinson's disease* is another CNS disorder involving involuntary movement, but it is dealt with elsewhere in this chapter. (See this chapter, page 139.)

MASSAGE?

If a client has episodes of uncontrolled muscular contraction and has not been diagnosed, it is important to get medical clearance before performing massage. Massage may very likely help to reconnect these patients with their bodies in a way that is beneficial, but it is vital to work under medical supervision.

Multiple Sclerosis

DEFINITION: WHAT IS IT?

Multiple sclerosis (MS) is a condition characterized by the inflammation and then gradual degeneration of myelin sheaths in the spinal cord and brain.

DEMOGRAPHICS: WHO GETS IT?

MS strikes both men and women, but women get it at least twice as often. Two out of three cases are identified between the ages of 20 and 40. The average age of onset overall is 33. It is practically unknown for MS to be first diagnosed during childhood or after the age of 60. Statistically, MS favors people from latitudes far away from the equator both North and South, but no one really knows whether this is an environmental or genetic tendency. About 350,000 cases of MS are known in the United States, and about 8,800 new cases are diagnosed every year.

CHOREA IN BRIEF

What is it?
Chorea is involuntary twitching, usually due to essential tremor, Huntington's disease, or Parkinson's disease.

How is it recognized?
Chorea is identified through uncontrolled gross motor movements.

Is massage indicated or contraindicated?
Massage is indicated for most kinds of chorea, as long as medical clearance has been obtained.

MULTIPLE SCLEROSIS IN BRIEF

What is it?
Multiple Sclerosis (MS) is an idiopathic disease that involves the destruction of myelin sheaths around both motor and sensory neurons in the CNS.

How is it recognized?
MS has many symptoms, depending on the nature of the damage. These can include fatigue, eye pain, spasticity, tremors, and a progressive loss of vision, sensation, and motor control.

Is massage indicated or contraindicated?
Massage is indicated in subacute stages of MS, when the client is in remission, rather than during acute periods, when function is diminishing.

MULTIPLE SCLEROSIS

Tricia, 36 years old

"It takes all the courage I can muster just to stand up in the morning."

Everyone has problems. Everyone gets in their own world so much. Now I look at someone with a disability and I wonder if they have it. You start to watch people walk and wonder if they've got it.

One and a half years ago, we had just moved into a new house and my youngest child had just started school. For the first time in 15 years, I was looking forward to having some time, to getting on with my life.

Then there was a pain in my left heel that felt like a stone bruise. We were just back from a long vacation, so I thought it was from too much walking. Two weeks later there was a lack of sensation in my foot and it traveled up my leg to my knee. It began affecting my right leg, too. Then there was numbness and tingling in my left hand. It felt like I had just had a shot of Novocain, it was that kind of tingling.

Try walking on the balls of your feet for a whole day. Then you'll get an idea of how hard it was. I couldn't put my heels down because there would be a sharp tingling "funny bone" feeling. My walking was so labored, I got to the point where I would rather shimmy on my chest like an army guy to get from room to room. I wasn't crying, I wasn't upset, it was just easier to crawl.

Although I felt stressed about not knowing what was happening to me, I put off going to the doctor. I finally went to my OB for my headaches. He gave me migraine medication, but it didn't work.

He sent me to a neurologist who checked me out and watched me walk. Then, while I was sitting there, he went out into the hall with another doctor and they started speaking in medical jargon that I couldn't understand; it made me really nervous. When he came back he asked me, "Will you come in for a spinal tap?"

"Why?"

"There are some things we want to check out."

"What do you think I have?"

"I think you have MS."

"Excuse me?"

I never *dreamed* it would be something like this.

They started me on IV steroids. The next morning I got up after a bad night, and for the first time in two months I could walk normally. I was so excited, I woke my family and called my mom on the phone. But by the end of that morning, I was already beginning to feel tired. My condition deteriorated in spite of the steroids. By the end of the week I couldn't even get up off the couch to let the home care nurse in.

My neurologist finally sent me to the University Hospital. There they did lots of other tests, more spinal taps, and an MRI. The MRI showed tiny spots in my brain, but nothing like what they were expecting. The spinal taps all came back negative.

They had me talking to teams of doctors. I talked to neurologists, immune specialists, nutritionists, and psychiatrists. The head of the department was prepared to tell my family I had chronic progressive MS, which meant I could be dead in a matter of weeks. I finally decided that I needed to be home, I needed to be with my family, so I checked out even though they didn't want me to.

(continued)

MULTIPLE SCLEROSIS, cont.

I continued physical therapy at a local clinic. At first they would have me sit in a warm pool with jets of water after I exercised, and I would go home feeling so drained and worn out, it was awful. Finally they adjusted that part of it and I did better.

Today I still don't have much sensation below my knees. It takes all the courage I can muster just to stand up in the morning. I never know what kind of day I'll have, whether I'll be able to walk without a cane, whether I'll be tied to the house because my digestive system is unpredictable. I have terrible headaches that begin on the lower half of one side of my face and go up into my ear. I have days when I can't eat at all. I've had episodes of dizziness and double vision. I'm not on steroids now, but I take an antidepressant for the headaches. We're still struggling to find the right dose. My greatest fear, even more than being in a wheelchair, is that I will lose bladder or bowel control, or go blind.

But my doctor says my scenario is good. It's been a year and a half without any exacerbations and he says I'm in remission. The only thing that's worse are my headaches, which are more painful and happen more often.

I think everything depends on your attitude. A major thing for me is to feel needed. If I have a purpose, I feel better. My aunt has MS, and she practically runs her family business. It's just amazing to see her get up and go. She says there are some days that if she didn't have that business to go to, she wouldn't be able to get out of bed. I have a chance now to see what other people have to deal with, and some of them are so much worse off than I am, not just because of physical problems, but other kinds of problems too. I have five wonderful children and a husband who loves me. My doctor thought I was going to die, and here I am in remission. I just feel so lucky to be here.

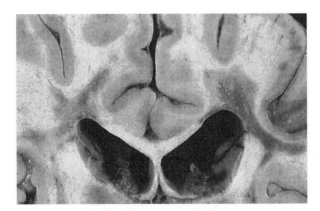

Figure 3.3. Multiple sclerosis: demyelination of white matter in the central nervous system

ETIOLOGY: WHAT HAPPENS?

The word sclerosis means "hardened scar or plaque." In multiple sclerosis, several different areas in the central nervous system often show these plaques where myelin should be. (See Figure 3.3.) As the myelin is replaced, the electrical impulses that should be tying the whole system together literally short circuit. This results in motor and sensory paralysis, instead of coordinated movement and feeling. The signs and symptoms of the disease, like so many disorders of the CNS, depend entirely on where and how much of the nerve tissue has been impaired.

CAUSES

This is one of those mysterious conditions that defies any efforts to pin it down to a single distinct cause. One theory involves an unidentified virus, which may lead to an autoimmune reaction against myelin. The human herpes virus type 6 (HHV-6) has recently been implicated in MS and other demyelinating diseases, but has not been named as a definitive cause. MS does *not* seem to be directly hereditary, although an inherited vulnerability to other MS triggers may exist. People who have a close relative with MS have only a 2 to 5% chance of developing the disease themselves.

SIGNS AND SYMPTOMS

This disease is sometimes called *the Great Imitator* because its initial symptoms can look like anything, depending on what area of nerve tissue has been affected. The earliest symptoms (which are almost never identified as such) generally include temporary tingling or weakness in isolated areas in the extremities, especially after exercise or a hot bath. Other early indicators include eye pain (optic neuritis is considered by some to be a reliable precursor of MS; see *neuritis*, this chapter, page 157), fatigue, and Lhermitte's sign: electrical sensations running down the spine when the neck is in flexion. Later symptoms include clumsiness, spasticity, blurred speech and/or vision, problems with light and color perception, and loss of bladder control. Facial pain (*trigeminal neuralgia*, this chapter, page 164, is also associated with MS), vertigo, tremors, memory loss, and difficulties in concentration may also be present. Many MS patients also experience digestive disturbances that vary greatly from day to day.

The order in which MS symptoms appear can vary widely, which is one reason this condition is so difficult to diagnose.

Most MS patients who are diagnosed at a relatively young age experience periods of diminished function that may last days or weeks, followed by longer periods of remission during which function is partially or totally restored. New plaques are forming on the myelin sheaths during these episodes of degeneration. Many people have only one attack and complete recovery in their lifetime. Persons who show no symptoms until later in life often have a steadily progressive situation with no periods of remission.

DIAGNOSIS

There is as yet no definitive test to diagnose MS. The disease is identified through a description of symptoms, a family health history, a spinal tap to look for raised antibody levels and myelin fragments, and MRIs that can reveal central nervous system lesions. (The lesions shown in MRIs may be from sources other than MS, however, so they are not considered a definitive diagnosis.) Nerve conduction tests to measure the speed of electrical impulses through nerves may also be conducted.

Several conditions can produce MS-like symptoms. Part of a thorough diagnosis is ruling these out:

- Lyme disease
- AIDS
- Scleroderma
- Vascular problems in the brain
- Herniated or ruptured disc
- CNS tumors
- Fibromyalgia

TREATMENT

Different cases of MS respond to vastly different kinds of approaches, ranging from vitamin therapy to hyperbaric oxygen chambers. Therefore, it is quite possible that one day it will be discovered that MS is not a single disease at all, but rather a group of several distinct problems which produce similar symptoms, but which must be treated differently.

Treatment for MS usually takes a two-pronged approach: symptom abatement and inflammation control. Medicines that will modify disease activity, i.e., control the frequency and severity of attacks, are also used.

Symptom control is generally aimed at the most debilitating aspects of MS. Drugs to combat fatigue work well for some patients, but are poorly tolerated by others. Other medications can help with bladder control, constipation, tremors, facial pain, and spasticity. Perhaps the most important symptom or complication of MS to treat is the depression that often accompanies any degenerative disease.

Steroids are sometimes prescribed to limit inflammation during acute MS episodes. These can reduce symptoms in the short run, but have not been shown to have long-lasting benefits, and their side effects can be severe. Therefore, they are usually used only as a temporary measure.

Some of the most exciting research happening in MS treatment is in drugs that can improve the efficiency of electrical transmission even through damaged neurons. While still in the experimental stages now, these medicines may soon become the standard treatment for MS patients.

PROGNOSIS

Even though not much is understood about the cause of this disease, many statistics indicate how it affects the populations of people who have it. For instance, about one third of the people diagnosed with this disease have no lasting debilitation. Seventy percent of people diagnosed with MS are fully functional five years after diagnosis. Half of them are still working 10 years after diagnosis, and 66% of them are fully ambulatory 25 years after diagnosis. That's all on the bright side. The darker side shows that about one-fifth, or 20%, of all patients don't experience the typical relapse-remission cycle. Instead, they suffer a slow, steady degeneration. These patients usually have a late onset of the disease, and they experience the most extreme form of it.

MS is not a terminal disease in itself. People who have MS generally have a life span about six years shorter than average. People who die prematurely from this disease are usually immobile, and they fall prey to an opportunistic disease such as a *kidney infection* (chapter 8, page 313), *urinary tract infection* (chapter 8, page 318), or *pneumonia* (chapter 6, page 252).

MASSAGE?

This disease usually has acute and subacute periods; massage is indicated in the subacute stages. *But* care must be taken not to overstimulate the client, which can result in painful and uncontrolled muscle spasms. Symptoms may also be exacerbated by heat. Clients with MS will present their symptoms and problems differently. If sensation is present, massage can be useful as an agent against stress (which seems to trigger relapses), depression, and spasticity, and it will help to maintain the health and mobility of the tissues. In areas where sensation is not present, nonmechanical types of work (i.e., very light effleurage and energy work) may keep some of the neurons firing.

Parkinson's Disease

ETIOLOGY: WHAT HAPPENS?

In order to discuss this condition thoroughly it will be necessary to review some of the inner workings of the brain.

PARKINSON'S DISEASE

Dr. James Parkinson (1755–1824) was a British physician who first documented this chronic degenerative nervous system disorder.

PARKINSON'S DISEASE IN BRIEF

What is it?
Parkinson's disease is a degenerative disease of the substantia nigra cells in the brain. These cells produce the neurotransmitter dopamine, which helps the basal ganglia to maintain balance, posture, and coordination.

How is it recognized?
Early symptoms of Parkinson's include general stiffness and fatigue; resting tremor of the hand, foot, or head; stiffness; and poor balance. Later symptoms include a shuffling gait, a "mask-like" appearance to the face, and a monotone voice.

Is massage indicated or contraindicated?
Massage is indicated for Parkinson's disease, under a doctor's supervision. Care must be taken for the physical safety of these clients, who cannot move freely or smoothly.

The structures in the brainstem that lead up to the cerebrum help with unconscious homeostatic maintenance. At the lower edges of the cerebrum, the basal ganglia are found: little pockets of gray matter embedded in white matter. The basal ganglia, with the cerebellum, provide learned reflexes and some basic kinds of motor control and coordination. ("Coordination" here means the balance in action between prime movers and their antagonistic muscles.)

Healthy basal ganglia cells are supplied with a vital neurotransmitter, *dopamine*, by another nearby structure, the *substantia nigra* (aka: "black stuff"). In Parkinson's disease, the substantia nigra cells die off, depriving the basal ganglia of dopamine. Without dopamine, the basal ganglia cannot maintain the careful balance between agonists and antagonists in the body, and so coordination degenerates and controlled movement becomes very difficult.

CAUSES

No one really knows what causes the substantia nigra to degenerate in Parkinson's disease. Environmental agents may be one cause; a statistical rise in patients under 50 years of age substantiates that theory. A small percentage of cases can be traced to other specific factors: carbon monoxide poisoning is evidently one cause, as is heavy metal poisoning. It can also follow trauma, neurovascular disease, and exposure to certain drugs or minerals. The drug-induced form is reversible.

Whatever the root cause, current research is focusing on the process of *apoptosis* (cellular "suicide") that occurs in the substantia nigra. One theory holds that immune system agents create a surplus of chemical messengers in the substantia nigra that carry instructions for cells to self-destruct. A similar problem with apoptosis of specific nervous system cells exists in other neurodegenerative diseases, such as *amyotrophic lateral sclerosis* (this chapter, page 133) and Alzheimer's disease.

SIGNS AND SYMPTOMS

Symptoms of Parkinson's disease can be divided into primary and secondary problems. Primary symptoms arise from the disease itself, while secondary symptoms are direct results of primary symptoms.

Primary Symptoms

- Nonspecific achiness, weakness, and fatigue. Parkinson's disease has a very slow onset and is most common in elderly people. Therefore, these early symptoms are often missed, either because they are too subtle to be seen, or because there's an assumption that a certain amount of fatigue and stiffness is just a natural part of growing older.
- Resting tremor. This phenomenon is present in about 75% of all Parkinson's patients, and is often one of the first noticeable symptoms. A rhythmic shaking or "pill rolling" action of the hand is often seen. Tremor may also affect the foot, head, and neck. This tremor is most noticeable when the patient is at rest but not sleeping. It will often disappear entirely when the patient is engaged in some other activity.
- Bradykinesia. This means difficulty in initiating or sustaining movement. It can take a long time to begin a voluntary movement of the arm or leg, and the limb's move-

ment may be halting and interrupted midstream. Parkinson's patients sometimes report feeling "rooted to the floor" when they can visualize moving a leg, but it doesn't happen without sustained effort.

- Rigidity. Gradually the muscles, particularly the flexor muscles, of Parkinson's patients become permanently hypertonic. This can give rise to a characteristically stooped posture as the trunk flexors contract more strongly than the paraspinals. This will be particularly visible when Parkinson's accompanies *osteoporosis* (chapter 2, page 62), as it often does. Rigidity will also make it difficult to bend or straighten arms and legs, and can cause a particular "mask-like" appearance to the face as the facial muscles lose flexibility and ease of movement. (See Figure 3.4.) This also accounts for a reduced rate of eye blinking.

    It's important to point out that the rigidity that accompanies Parkinson's is *not* the same thing as spasticity, which implies a different kind of nerve damage. (See *spinal cord injury*, this chapter, page 158.) Massage is indicated for rigidity (with caution) while generally it is not recommended for spasticity.

- Poor postural reflexes. Disruption in the activity of basal ganglia cells results in uncoordinated movement and poor balance. Parkinson's patients are particularly susceptible to falling.

Secondary Symptoms

- Shuffling gait. Difficulty in bending arms and legs will make walking a special challenge for Parkinson's patients. Often the ability to swing the arm is noticeably diminished on one side. The patient takes small steps, and may then have to stumble forward to avoid falling. This chasing after the center of gravity is called a *festinating* gait.

- Changes in speech. Parkinson's patients will experience gradual rigidity of the muscles in the larynx that control vocalization. Their speech gradually becomes monotone and expressionless, and progresses toward constant whispering. Muscular changes in the mouth and throat also create problems with swallowing and drooling, particularly while laying down.

- Changes in handwriting. The loss of coordination in fine motor muscles will change the ability of a Parkinson's patient to write by hand. "*Micrographia,*" or progressively shrinking, cramped handwriting, is one of the later symptoms of this disease.

- Sleep disorders. Parkinson's patients experience a variety of sleep disorders, from a complete reversal of normal sleeping schedules to sleeplessness because it is difficult or impossible for them to move in bed.

- Depression. The progressive nature of this condition makes anxiety and depression a very predictable part of the disease process. Depression can also be related to insomnia, or it can be a side effect of medication. Sometimes the symptoms of depression can outweigh the symptoms of the disease, and treatment for depression can lessen Parkinson's symptoms as well.

- Mental degeneration. This is a subject of some controversy. Some sources suggest that advanced Parkinson's patients will experience memory loss and deterioration of thought processes. Others suggest that mental problems are side effects of Parkinson's medication and not a part of the disease itself.

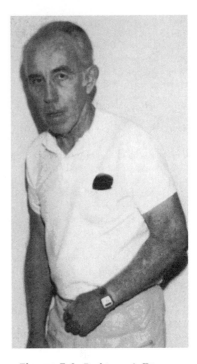

Figure 3.4. Parkinson's Disease: note the stooped posture and "masklike" face.

TREATMENT

In Parkinson's disease, a dopamine deficiency exists in the basal ganglia of the brain. Prescribing large doses of a manmade version of this neurotransmitter called L-dopa is one treatment that has yielded some success, but it is not a permanent solution. Patients seem to build up a resistance to the drug, and it has a number of troubling side effects, including hallucinations and dementia. Some dopamine agonists can be substituted when it becomes necessary. Doctors working with Parkinson's patients must monitor their medications carefully and make frequent adjustments.

Physical, speech, and occupational therapies are often employed to maintain the health and general functioning levels of Parkinson's patients for as long as possible. Psychotherapy and support groups are recommended to cope with the effects of depression.

Several experimental treatments for Parkinson's disease are in development. Among these are drugs that will inhibit the apoptosis of substantia nigra cells. Another is deep brain stimulation, which involves planting an electrode in the basal ganglia which is then manually operated by the patient.

Tissue transplants are also under investigation. Special cells from the adrenal glands can produce dopamine under certain circumstances, but they won't connect to the correct synapses in the brain. Genetically engineered cells can be inserted, but again, they won't produce dopamine exactly when and where it's needed. Experiments with brain cells of aborted human fetuses have yielded good results, but the ethical complications are being debated. The promising findings of these experiments have led to the investigation of whether genetically manipulated nonhuman (e.g., pig) brain cells could produce the same good results.

MASSAGE?

Parkinson's patients experience progressive stiffness and rigidity of voluntary muscles. Massage *under a doctor's supervision* can be a valuable tool not only to maintain flexibility and range of motion, but to reduce anxiety and depression. It is important to work in cooperation with a client's primary physician, because massage may impact the need for antidepressive medication. Be aware, however, that clients with Parkinson's disease do not have the freedom of movement that most other people do, and they may have great difficulty in getting on and off tables safely. Some massage therapists overcome this obstacle by doing their work with these clients on the floor.

Peripheral Neuropathy

PERIPHERAL NEUROPATHY IN BRIEF

What is it?

Peripheral neuropathy is damage to peripheral nerves, usually of the hands and feet, as a result of some other underlying condition such as alcoholism, diabetes, or lupus. *HIV, AIDS, deficient B vit, Arsine, Lead, mercury*

How is it recognized?

Sensory damage, motor damage, or both may be present. Symptoms include burning or tingling pain beginning distally and slowly moving proximally; loss of movement or control of movement; hyperesthesia; and eventual numbness.

Is massage indicated or contraindicated?

Massage is at least locally contraindicated for peripheral neuropathy, because it may irritate a hyperesthesiac condition. Many underlying causes of peripheral neuropathy may contraindicate massage systemically.

DEFINITION: WHAT IS IT?

Peripheral neuropathy, like so many conditions in this chapter, is not a disease in itself, but a symptom or a complication of other underlying conditions.

CAUSES

Most cases of peripheral neuropathy are complications of long-standing bouts with *diabetes* (chapter 4, page 210) or *alcoholism* (chapter 10, page 356). More rarely, this condition will develop because of certain vitamin deficiencies (especially B), tumors, or exposure to toxic substances. The toxins in question include arsenic, mercury, lead, and the organophosphates in insecticides. Peripheral neuropathy can also be associated with various cancers, *HIV/AIDS* (chapter 5, page 233), *lupus* (chapter 5, page 241), *rheumatoid arthritis* (chapter 2, page 80), and other diseases that cause *vasculitis*, or inflammation of the blood vessels.

SIGNS AND SYMPTOMS

Most cases of peripheral neuropathy begin very subtly and slowly. Damage to sensory neurons will produce burning pain or tingling in the hands and feet, which will gradually spread proximally into the limbs and finally the trunk. Extreme sensitivity to touch (see *hyperesthesia*, this chapter, page 156) can follow, but eventually will be replaced by a far more dangerous symptom: numbness. Numbness is dangerous because if a person can't feel something—her toe, for instance—she can't tell if it's been injured or infected. Secondary ulcers and infections are common complications of numbness with any disease.

Motor neuron damage will create weakness and possibly limited or uncontrolled movement. Specific muscle weakening and atrophy will also be a part of advanced peripheral neuropathy.

TREATMENT

Treatment for this condition depends entirely on the underlying pathology that is causing the nerve damage. Generally, once damage to the peripheral nerves is complete, the only course of action is to interrupt the *cause* of the damage. In the most common cases of diabetes and alcoholism, that means treating those problems as aggressively as possible. For people who are suffering from chemical exposure, the treatment is to remove them from the source of the poisons as quickly as possible. If the damage is limited to the outer layers of the neurons, a full recovery may be possible. Otherwise, permanent damage could result.

MASSAGE?

If a client has undiagnosed tingling or numbness, she needs to see a doctor; it could be any number of things, peripheral neuropathy included. Clients with nerve damage are likely to be hyperesthesiac, which contraindicates massage, at least locally. And if a client is numb or has reduced sensation, *these* contraindicate massage, too, since she is unable to give informed feedback about her comfort. Massage is, in most cases, contraindicated for peripheral neuropathy. *Nerve damage*

Contrindicated!

Infectious Disorders

Encephalitis

DEFINITION: WHAT IS IT?

This is a central nervous system disorder on which massage has little, if any, effect. Encephalitis is an inflammation of the brain or meninges.

DEMOGRAPHICS: WHO GETS IT?

The Centers for Disease Control has located several places in the United States where species of encephalitis viruses are endemic. These special types of virus include St. Louis encephalitis, western and eastern equine encephalitis, California encephalitis, and Cache Valley encephalitis.

ETIOLOGY: WHAT HAPPENS?

Encephalitis is usually brought about by a viral infection, but occasionally it stems from something more exotic, such as a paramecium carried by the tsetse fly. The viruses most often responsible for this disease are *herpes simplex* (chapter 1, page 10), mumps, measles, chicken pox (see *herpes zoster*, this chapter, page 144), Epstein Barr, cytomegalovirus,

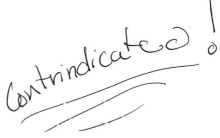

ENCEPHALITIS IN BRIEF

What is it?
Encephalitis is inflammation of the brain usually brought about by a viral infection. *mumps, Chic pox, herpes, exotic places*

How is it recognized?
Signs and symptoms of encephalitis include fever, headache, confusion, and personality and memory changes. Encephalitis is diagnosed through examination of cerebrospinal fluid and analysis of CT or MRI scans. *Double vision, part - full paralysis*

Is massage indicated or contraindicated?
Massage is systemically contraindicated for acute encephalitis, but if a client has had it in her history with no signs of present infection, massage is perfectly acceptable.

and *HIV/AIDS* (chapter 5, page 233). Several varieties of encephalitis can be carried by birds and mosquitoes; in this case, an epidemic outbreak of the disease will occur.

SIGNS AND SYMPTOMS

Symptoms of encephalitis range from being so mild they're never even identified to very, very severe. How the disease will present itself depends on the virus involved and the age and general health of the patient. Infants, elderly, and AIDS patients are most vulnerable to the very extreme forms of the disease while others will only rarely experience any lasting damage from the inflammation.

The mild end of the symptomatic scale includes headaches, drowsiness, irritability, and disordered thought processes. But in more severe cases the drowsiness can progress to stupor and then coma. The patient may also experience fever, double vision, confused sensation, impaired speech or hearing, convulsions, and partial or full paralysis. Changes in personality, intellect, and memory may also occur, depending on which parts of the brain are affected.

DIAGNOSIS

Spinal tap

The presenting symptoms for any central nervous system disturbance are so varied and individualized, it is difficult to make a conclusive diagnosis without a full range of intrusive testing. For encephalitis, this means a spinal tap to look for signs of inflammation in the cerebral spinal fluid, along with a CT scan or MRI to look for signs of inflammation in the central nervous system. This is an improvement over older methods of diagnosis, which required a biopsy of brain tissue!

TREATMENT

Loving Care

Viruses don't respond to antibiotic therapy, which is designed to disable bacteria only. Encephalitis brought about by the herpes simplex virus, however, responds well to acyclovir (an antiviral agent) and interferon, an immune system substance that also fights some kinds of cancers. Other treatments for encephalitis focus on symptom abatement. Sometimes steroids are administered to deal with inflammation, but most cases of encephalitis are treated with little more than tender loving care.

PROGNOSIS

The prognosis for encephalitis depends on the vulnerability of the patient, the virulence of the pathogen, and how early treatment is administered. Very often healthy people can emerge from a short-term infection with no lasting damage. But prolonged inflammation in the central nervous system will eventually cause permanent damage to structures that have little or no capacity to heal. Thus permanent paralysis or personality changes may be the result of a serious bout with this disease.

MASSAGE?

Contraindicate

If a client has a known history of encephalitis and if she is exhibiting any signs of the infection, especially headache, fever, and irritability, *massage is systemically contraindicated*. If, on the other hand, it shows up on her medical history as a past infection and she is otherwise healthy, massage should be just fine.

Herpes Zoster

DEFINITION: WHAT IS IT?

Also known as *shingles*, this condition is a viral infection of the nervous system. In this case the targeted tissues are the dendrites at the end of sensory neurons. Imagine growing painful, fluid-filled blisters on all the nerve endings of a specific dermatome: that is a fair idea of what a bad case of shingles feels like. Shingles affects about 300,000 people in the United States every year. It seldom affects the same person twice.

ETIOLOGY: WHAT HAPPENS?

The virus at fault here is the chicken pox virus, which can be called *varicella zoster virus*. When a person is exposed to chicken pox in childhood, the normal disease process occurs: painful, itchy blisters appear; they fade away; and the patient can go back to business as usual. The difference between other viruses and chicken pox is that although a full complement of anti–chicken pox antibodies will be present, the virus is never fully expelled from the body. Instead, it goes into a dormant state in the dorsal root ganglia (the meeting point for all the sensory neurons in each dermatome). Later in life, the virus may reactivate.

Sometimes the immune response will quell future attacks before any symptoms appear. But if the virus awakens when the immune system is below par for some other reason—stress, old age, other diseases—a person might get chicken pox again, but adults are much more likely to get shingles.

CAUSES

No one is exactly sure what will cause a resurgence of the herpes zoster virus. Contributing factors include the ones listed above: stress, old age, impaired immunity because of other diseases (shingles is notorious for accompanying advanced *tuberculosis*, chapter 6, page 257, or *pneumonia*, chapter 6, page 252). Shingles occasionally occurs after severe trauma or as a drug reaction. And of course, if an adult has never been exposed to chicken pox, that person is vulnerable if they have contact with the varicella zoster virus. Although the fluid in zoster blisters is filled with virus, shingles isn't particularly contagious, unless a person comes in contact with it while his own immune system is depressed or if he has never been exposed to the virus in the first place. In this case, an adult may get either shingles or chicken pox, but shingles is more likely.

SIGNS AND SYMPTOMS

Pain is the biggest symptom of this disease—pain before the blisters break out, pain while they develop, erupt, and scab over, and pain even after they've healed and the skin is intact again. (Post herpetic *neuralgia*, this chapter, page 164, is one complication of this disease.) The blisters may grow along the entire dermatome, but more often they appear along an isolated stretch. It is nearly always a unilateral attack. (See Figure 3.5, Color Plate 28.) Intercostal nerves are the most frequently affected, although the trigeminal nerve is also attacked. The worst kind of situation involves the optic branch of the trigeminal nerve because the risk of corneal ulcers and permanent damage to the eye is very high.

TREATMENT

Herpes zoster is usually treated mainly palliatively. Acyclovir, the antiviral medication used for herpes simplex,

---

HERPES ZOSTER IN BRIEF

What is it?
Herpes Zoster, or shingles, is a viral infection of sensory neurons from the same virus that causes chicken pox.

How is it recognized?
Shingles creates extremely painful blisters along the dermatomes, usually around the ribs, but occasionally of the trigeminal nerve. It is almost always unilateral.

Is massage indicated or contraindicated?
Massage is systemically contraindicated during the acute stage of shingles, because this is such a painful condition. After the blisters have healed and the pain has subsided, massage is appropriate.

A CHICKEN POX VACCINE?

A controversy is rising over the need for a chicken pox vaccine. It is generally such a benign childhood rite of passage that some doctors argue that such a vaccine is really unnecessary. A vaccine is currently available through state health departments, but no statistics are available regarding how it affects the chances of contracting shingles later in life. From the perspective of economic impact, a chicken pox vaccine might well become popular, simply for the amount of money to be saved by employers who pay for sick days while parents stay home with infected children.

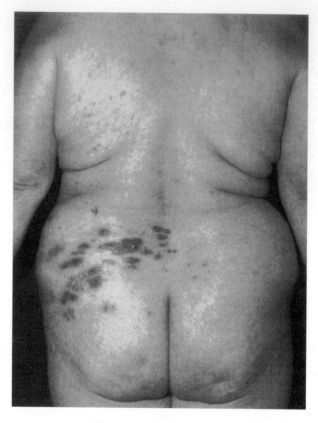

Figure 3.5. Herpes zoster

also has some success with herpes zoster. Beyond that, soothing lotion, steroids for anti-inflammatory action, and painkillers are used.

MASSAGE?

Herpes zoster is the kind of disease that is very kind to massage practitioners: during an acute outbreak of this condition, the last thing a client will look for is someone to *touch* her. Occasionally very mild outbreaks may occur, for which massage may be only <u>locally contraindicated</u>, according to the tolerance of the client. After the infection has past and the lesions have completely healed, <u>massage is perfectly appropriate</u>.

Meningitis

DEFINITION: WHAT IS IT?

"Meninges" + "itis": this is an infection of the meninges, specifically the pia mater and arachnoid layers of connective tissue membrane that surround the brain and spinal cord.

DEMOGRAPHICS: WHO GETS IT?

Over 70% of meningitis infections are in children under five years of age. The infectious agents are probably quite common, but only create problems for people whose resistance is low. An estimated 17,500 people in the United States have meningitis each year.

ETIOLOGY: WHAT HAPPENS?

Meningitis can be caused by a bacterial infection from the middle ear, an upper respiratory or sinus infection, or it can be a viral complication of *polio* (this chapter, page 148), mumps, *herpes simplex* (chapter 1, page 10), or mononucleosis. A skull fracture can also provide a portal of entry. More rarely, meningitis can be related to a tumor or a fungal infection.

COMMUNICABILITY

Meningitis can be contagious. Its mode of transmission is much like the common cold: an infected person sneezes or coughs and then touches some surface such as a doorknob. An uninfected person contaminates her hand, then touches her eye or mouth. In some places in the world, epidemics of meningitis do occur. The "meningeal belt" of subsaharan Africa, for instance, has seasonal outbreaks of the disease.

SIGNS AND SYMPTOMS

The symptoms of an acute meningitis infection include very high fever and chills, a deep red or purple rash, extreme headache, irritability, aversion to bright light, and a stiff, rigid neck. The neck is held tightly because any movement or stretching of the swollen meninges is excruciatingly painful. Drowsiness and slurred speech may also be present. More extreme infections will cause nausea, vomiting, delirium, and even convulsions or coma.

Viral meningitis often presents more extreme symptoms than does bacterial meningitis; however, viral infections seldom leave any lasting damage behind them. Untreated bacterial meningitis can cause permanent CNS damage such as loss of hearing or vision, paralysis, or mental retardation.

A meningitis infection incubates from 2 to 10 days for bacterial infections and up to 3 weeks for viral infections. Symptoms generally peak and then recede over a period of 2 to 3 weeks.

DIAGNOSIS

Meningitis is diagnosed through a spinal tap that examines the cerebrospinal fluid for pus, fragments of pathogens, and reduced glucose levels (the infectious agents consume the glucose that would normally be available to the CNS).

TREATMENT

If the pathogen is identified as a bacterium (*neisseria meningitidis*, or meningococcus is the most serious agent), large doses of antibiotics are administered immediately.

Most people emerge from meningitis infections with no lasting damage.

PREVENTION

In the United States, the HiB (Haemophilus influenzae) vaccine is probably the most effective prevention against meningitis in children. Vaccines against two of the three types of meningococcus bacteria also exist, but they are generally recommended only for people planning to travel to places where epidemics are in progress.

MASSAGE?

Meningitis absolutely contraindicates massage in the acute stage. These people don't just need bed rest; they need hospital care. For clients who have recovered from meningitis

---

MENINGITIS IN BRIEF

What is it?
Meningitis is an infection of the meninges, specifically the pia mater and the arachnoid layers.

How is it recognized?
Symptoms of acute meningitis include very high fever, rash, photophobia, headache, and stiff neck. Symptoms are not always consistent, however; they may appear in different combinations for different people.

Is massage indicated or contraindicated?
Meningitis is strictly contraindicated in the acute phase. People who have recovered from meningitis are perfectly fine to receive massage.

POLIO IN BRIEF

What is it?
Polio is a viral infection, first of the intestines, and then (for about 1% of exposed people) the anterior horn cells of the spinal cord.

How is it recognized?
The destruction on CNS motor neurons leads to degeneration, atrophy and finally paralysis of skeletal muscles.

Is massage indicated or contraindicated?
Massage is fine for postacute polio survivors. Massage can be indicated for post polio syndrome, but only under a doctor's supervision.

POLIO

This is from the Greek word for "gray." Polio denotes damage to the gray matter of the central nervous system. Poliomyelitis indicates damage and inflammation in the gray matter specifically in the spinal cord (*myelos* means "marrow").

POLIO: IT'S ALMOST EXTINCT

The statistics on polio are among the most promising of any infectious disease in the world. The last new case in the entire Western hemisphere was diagnosed in Peru in August of 1991. In 1988, the World Health Organization collected data that reported about 35,000 new cases of polio worldwide. In 1994, that number was down to close to 6,000 cases. Admittedly, the WHO estimates that the number of reported cases is well below the true number of new cases, but nevertheless, it is predicted that by 2005, almost 70 years after Franklin Delano Roosevelt announced his "War on Polio," this disease will be extinct.

with no lasting effects, massage is perfectly appropriate. If there is residual paralysis, follow the guidelines for *spinal cord injury* (this chapter, page 158).

Polio

DEFINITION: WHAT IS IT?

Poliomyelitis, or *infantile paralysis*, as it used to be known, is a viral disease. Most viruses have a target tissue, or a "favorite food," so to speak. Herpes zoster targets sensory neuron dendrites; most cold viruses attack mucous membranes. AIDS goes after helper T cells. The polio virus targets intestinal mucosa first, and anterior horn nerve cells later.

ETIOLOGY: WHAT HAPPENS?

The polio virus usually enters the body through the mouth; contaminated water is the usual medium. It gets past the acidic environment of the stomach, and sets up an infection in the intestine. New virus is released in fecal matter, possibly to contaminate water elsewhere.

For 99% of people exposed to the polio virus, this is the end of the story. Severe flu-like symptoms will appear: headache, deep muscular ache, and high fever. These are followed by an intestinal infection, a bout with diarrhea, and then the infection is over. But in about 1% of people who are infected, the virus will travel into the central nervous system, where it targets and destroys nerve cells in the anterior horns of the spinal cord. This impedes motor messages leaving the spinal cord, which in turn leads to rapid deterioration and atrophy of muscles and motor paralysis.

A couple of interesting facets of polio are worth exploring. First, when people are exposed to this virus in infancy, they seldom get seriously ill. The later the exposure, the more dangerous this virus can be. So although this disease has been identified from as far back as 3000-year-old Egyptian carvings, it didn't really become a public menace until sanitation services were set up in heavily populated areas. Although these measures reduced the rates of cholera, typhoid, and a host of other infectious diseases, they also prevented middle- and upper-class infants from exposure to the polio virus. Then, when they were exposed at later ages, the disease took a heavier toll. For many years polio was considered a disease of the upper classes.

Second, as stated above, a polio infection usually resolves itself in a short bout of flu-like symptoms with diarrhea. It only infects the spinal cords of about 1% of the people who are exposed to it. That doesn't sound like a lot, but it means that if 10,000 children go swimming in a contaminated lake, 100 of them will experience some level of paralysis.

The paralysis caused by polio is motor only; sensation is still present. And because the motor nerves tend to overlap each other in the extremities, functioning muscle fibers still may be left even though a whole level of motor neurons may have been damaged. In other words, look at the dermatomes for the quadriceps. Even if all the impulses to the motor neurons in L_2 have been eliminated, other motor neurons to the same muscle group are provided by L_3. (See Figure 3.6.) Furthermore, anterior horn

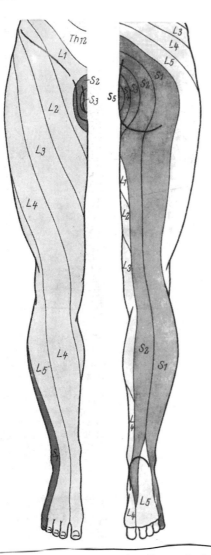

Figure 3.6. Dermatome patterns in the leg muscles allow multiple nerves to supply muscle groups. This way, if one nerve root is damaged, the muscle group is still useable.

cells that survive the initial attack can create new nerve connections to help reestablish motor control during recovery. Unfortunately, these cells can become overtaxed later in life, giving rise to *post polio syndrome* (this chapter, page 150).

The most serious form of this disease, *bulbar polio*, attacks not only the anterior horn cells, but the nuclei of some cranial nerves as well. Patients with this kind of damage risk death due to respiratory or heart failure. It was these patients, mostly children, who were confined to the "iron lungs" that were a big part of the American medical landscape in the 1930s and 1940s.

TREATMENT

Moist heat applications and massage have been used to treat polio survivors once the initial infection has subsided. Together, hydrotherapy and massage can help to limit contractures and keep functioning muscle fibers healthy and well-nourished.

PREVENTION

Polio is stunningly easy to prevent. There are two inexpensive, stable, easy-to-administer vaccines that are effective against this disease. The Salk vaccine injects inactivated polio virus into the bloodstream, causing the recipient to create a set of antibodies against it. This vaccine, although protecting the patient, does not eliminate the possibility of that person's transmitting the disease to someone else.

The Sabin vaccine, an oral medication, introduces weakened viruses into the digestive system, where they attract antibodies exactly where the virus first tends to reside. The advantages of the Sabin vaccine are that this approach prevents the patient from being a carrier of the disease, as well as creating an internal immune response, and because it is given orally rather than hypodermically, it can be administered by anyone. People who handle the diapers of infants who have received the oral vaccine need to be aware that live virus may be in the fecal matter. Immune-suppressed persons should avoid contact with infants who are undergoing this treatment.

State health departments vary in how they recommend polio vaccines be administered. Many of them now give both the oral and injected vaccines, giving the best of both worlds to their patients.

MASSAGE?

indicated!

Massage therapists in the United States are *extremely* unlikely to encounter an acute case of polio in their practice. Polio survivors will experience only a motor paralysis; sensation is still intact. So massage can be performed for these clients with good possibility of benefit and little risk of danger.

Post Polio Syndrome

DEFINITION: WHAT IS IT?

May not be on boards, Know Grey matter, white matter.

Now that *polio* (this chapter, page 148) is little more than a memory for most people (the last reported case in the Western Hemisphere was in 1991), an unexpected phenomenon is being found among its survivors. Some people who had polio as children, especially those who experienced significant loss of function, as they reach middle age find they have a sudden, and sometimes extreme, onset of fatigue, achiness, and weakness, not always in just the muscles originally affected. There may also be breathing difficulties, sleep disturbances, and trouble swallowing. These symptoms usually begin about 25 to 40 years after the original infection. This condition is called post polio syndrome, or PPS.

POST POLIO SYNDROME IN BRIEF

What is it?
Post polio syndrome is a group of signs and symptoms common to polio survivors, particularly those who experienced significant loss of function in the acute stage of the disease. *P.P.S.*

How is it recognized?
Symptoms of PPS include a sudden onset of fatigue, achiness, and weakness. There may also be breathing and sleeping difficulties. *Swelling*

Is massage indicated or contraindicated?
Massage under medical supervision is indicated for people with PPS.

DEMOGRAPHICS: WHO GETS IT?

There are 300,000 polio survivors in the United States. Of them, about 25% have some symptoms of PPS, although polio survivors are more than usually prone to arthritis, tendinitis, and other orthopedic problems that mimic PPS.

ETIOLOGY: WHAT HAPPENS?

PPS is *not* a resurgence of the original polio infection. Instead, it seems to be the result of normal aging combined with the loss of some percentage of anterior horn cells from the initial polio attack. The surviving cells, in spite of or because of whatever new synapses they were able to make in the recovery process, may be severely overtaxed. PPS may be the result of overstressed motor neurons.

TREATMENT

PPS does not result from a new infection. It is treated as a problem that may be ameliorated by reduced muscular and neurological stress: adjusted braces, a change in activity levels, exercise programs that encourage the use of muscles *not* supplied by the damaged nerves. People with PPS need to avoid excessive use of their affected muscles, since exercize of these damaged tissues can cause permanent damage to the working fibers.

MASSAGE?

Massage for persons with PPS is indicated: it will reduce muscle tone, improve local nutrition, and generally decrease strain on the nervous system.

Nervous System Injuries

Bell's Palsy

DEFINITION: WHAT IS IT?

It's important for massage therapists to be very familiar with this condition, because it's one of those things that a careless practitioner can actually induce, if the setting is right. This disorder is the result of damage to or impairment of cranial nerve VII, the Facial Nerve. This nerve is composed almost entirely of motor neurons, and is responsible for providing facial expression, blinking the eyes, and providing some taste sensation. (See Figure 3.7.) It exits the cranium through a small foramen just behind the earlobe. This spot is palpable by *gently* putting the index finger just behind the earlobe and slightly opening the mouth. *Sudden onset*

CAUSES

Causes of Bell's palsy vary widely. Rather than being a specific disease, it's a type of peripheral neuritis, that is, inflammation of a nerve, usually from some mechanical interference. Some possibilities include tumors, bone spurs at the foramen, upper cervical

---

BELL'S PALSY IN BRIEF

What is it?
Bell's palsy is a flaccid paralysis of one side of the face caused by inflammation or damage to cranial nerve VII.

How is it recognized?
Symptoms of Bell's palsy include drooping of the muscles on the affected side, difficulty with drinking and eating, and difficulty in closing the eye on one side. There may also be some pain, headaches, hypersensitivity to sound, and drooling.

Is massage indicated or contraindicated?
Massage is indicated for Bell's palsy, in the absence of contraindicated underlying causes.

BELL'S PALSY

Sir Charles Bell (1774–1842) was a Scottish surgeon, anatomist, and physiologist. He pioneered neurological research in several areas, including damage to the facial nerve and the structure of the spinal cord. (Bell's law states that the ventral horns of the spinal cord are for motor function while the dorsal horns are for sensory function.)

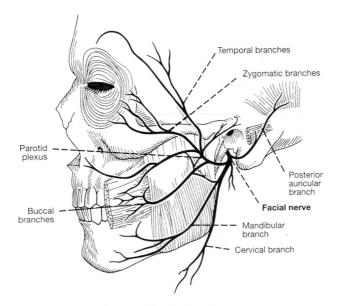

Temporal branches

Zygomatic branches

Parotid plexus

Posterior auricular branch

Facial nerve

Buccal branches

Mandibular branch

Cervical branch

Figure 3.7. The facial nerve.

BELL'S PALSY

Jim S.

No Dimple for a Year!

When I think about what may have precipitated my bout with Bell's palsy, I remember one of the most stressful years of my life. I had recently moved to the Pacific Northwest and had to go back to school to receive Washington State licensure as a massage practitioner. I was working three jobs and going to school. I had also spent some days plunging into the cold water of a tributary of the Breitenbush river. I was overcooked!

When the paralysis started, I thought it was a temporary effect of some bodywork I had received. I was told to take Advil and ice my neck. I was given massage to help with the pain. But nobody recognized the seriousness of the symptoms. Within a day I had full-on Bell's palsy, complete with hyperacusis (abnormal acuteness of hearing), full facial muscle paralysis, an eyelid that would not blink (with the inherent rolling of the eye up and out of danger when the lid would normally blink), and a distorted soapy beer taste on the affected side of my tongue.

It was clear in my subsequent research that these symptoms could not have been caused by a massage. With Bell's, the location of impediment on the facial nerve is proscribed by the symptoms. In other words, if I had only had facial paralysis, I would know that the nerve was impaired at a point above the jaw line. As you add symptoms (hyperacoustic sensitivity, taste impairment), you trace further up proximal to the geniculate ganglion, located inside the area near the ear.

Because I neglected to see a neurologist for over a week, my facial nerve degenerated and it took almost a year for nearly full function to resume. I couldn't use my dimple for a year! Now I'm adamant about people seeing a neurologist immediately when I hear of a case of Bell's palsy.

The whole experience was generally frustrating because there's a lot of poor information out there, but it was a great emotional process; when you've used your face for a calling card all your life and suddenly it's not available to you anymore, you have to really deal with what's underneath.

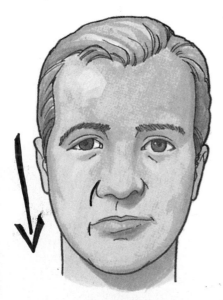

Figure 3.8. Bell's palsy: loss of motor function on one-half of the face

subluxation, and *TMJ disorder* (chapter 2, page 89), all of which can increase surrounding pressure on an already crowded area. Severe middle ear infections or a specific viral attack are rarer but also possible causes for Bell's palsy.

This condition is also associated with *diabetes* (see chapter 4, page 210), which is a frequent cause of peripheral neuritis. Lyme disease, Guillain-Barré syndrome, exposure to certain toxins, and facial infections are also seen hand-in-hand with Bell's palsy. Up to 75% of all recorded cases are preceded by an upper respiratory infection.

SIGNS AND SYMPTOMS

Symptoms of Bell's palsy are a result of the sudden loss of innervation to all the muscles on one side of the face: flaccid paralysis, drooping, and distortion of the affected side of the face. (See Figure 3.8.) It is difficult to eat, drink, and close the eye of the affected side. Sometimes the ear on that side becomes hypersensitive. Pain may be felt on the affected side, but not the sharp, electrical pain seen with *trigeminal neuralgia* (this chapter, page 164). This is a motor paralysis, not a sensory one (except for the Facial Nerve taste buds that may be affected) so sensation throughout the face will be intact.

COMPLICATIONS

Bell's palsy is usually a short-lived disorder that has few serious complications, but one of the most serious to consider is corneal ulcers. These can occur if the lubrication and cleaning of the eyeball provided by blinking is impaired.

TREATMENT

Treatment for Bell's palsy is usually conservative because most cases are self-limiting, that is, they take care of themselves without interference. More stubborn cases, however, may be treated with anti-inflammatories directed at the nerve itself, or even surgery to remove any physical obstacle that may be impeding nerve conduction.

PROGNOSIS

This condition almost always has a sudden onset (the textbook Bell's palsy patient will simply wake up with it one morning), and it also nearly always has a rapid recovery rate. Improvement is usually seen within two to three days, and complete restoration of function can be expected within weeks or months. Some cases take longer, however, and they will often see a less complete recovery because muscle tissue that is deprived of nerve flow atrophies and becomes fibrotic *much faster* than muscle tissue that is simply not used.

MASSAGE?

Bell's palsy is a flaccid paralysis with sensation left intact. If the underlying cause of the neuritis has been diagnosed as safe for massage (i.e., not a tumor, Lyme disease, infection, etc), then massage is a very appropriate treatment choice. Massage will keep the facial muscles elastic and the local circulation strong. This will set the stage for a more complete recovery when nerve supply is eventually restored.

Headaches

Headaches are one of the most common physical problems in the range of human experience. Up to 90% of adults in the United States will experience a headache each year; 45 million of them will see a doctor for relief. But although they can herald some serious underlying problems, most of the time headaches are self-contained, temporary problems, only peripherally related to other conditions in the body.

TYPES OF HEADACHES

In 1962 the National Institute of Neurological Diseases and Blindness divided headaches into three categories. Since then dozens more classifications have been created, but the three basic headings still stand as an organizing principle:

- Vascular headaches. These include classic and common migraines, cluster headaches, and possibly sinus headaches. They account for a total of about 6 to 8% of all headaches.
- Muscular contraction headaches. By far the most common type of headache people experience (90 to 92%), these are brought about by muscular tension,

---

HEADACHES IN BRIEF

What are they?

Headaches are pain caused by any number of sources. Muscular tension is the most common source of pain; congestive headaches are less common; and headaches due to serious underlying pathology are the rarest of all.

How are they recognized?

Tension headaches may be bilateral and generally painful. Vascular headaches are often unilateral and have a distinctive "throbbing" pain from blood flow into the head. Headaches brought about by central nervous system disease are extreme, severe, and prolonged. They can have a sudden or gradual onset.

Is massage indicated or contraindicated?

Massage is systemically contraindicated for headache due to infection or CNS disturbance. Massage is indicated for vascular headaches in the subacute stage. Massage is indicated for tension headaches.

bony misalignment, *TMJ disorders* (see chapter 2, page 89), *fibromyalgia* (chapter 2, page 50), or other muscular problems.

- Traction-inflammatory headaches. These account for 2% of the headaches people experience, and they are indicative of severe underlying pathology such as tumors, aneurysm, or infection in the central nervous system.

DANGER SIGNS

When are headaches really a harbinger of something much worse? Headaches in combination with extreme fever often have a bacterial or viral precipitator. They are usually short lived, subsiding when the fever passes the crisis point. The time to become concerned is when headaches are severe, repeating, and have a sudden onset, or when they have a gradual onset but no remission. In other words, if a severe headache doesn't go away in four to five days on its own, it may be a symptom of some serious underlying condition. This is particularly true if the headache is accompanied by slurred speech, numbness *anywhere* in the body, and difficulties with motor control. The first things to rule out in cases like this are a brain or meningeal infection, a tumor, or an aneurysm, i.e., a traction-inflammatory headache.

By far the largest number of headaches fall into the other two categories. They can be painful, even debilitating, but they seldom have serious long-term effects on general health.

Vascular Headaches

DEFINITION: WHAT ARE THEY?

These are headaches that have to do with blood flow to the brain. The pain they cause is from excess fluid pressing on the meninges, and they are characterized by a pain that "throbs" with the patient's pulse. These may also be called *congestive* headaches.

Migraines

These are considered by many to be the crème de la crème of headaches. Somehow people just don't take a headache seriously if it's not a migraine. Consequently, clients may report that they suffer migraines when what they really have are extremely severe tension headaches. This is significant because the treatment protocols for the two conditions are quite different. Only a doctor is qualified to make a conclusive diagnosis about what kind of headache is present; not a massage therapist, not even the client.

DEMOGRAPHICS: WHO GETS THEM?

About 23 million people in the United States suffer from diagnosed migraines. This malady is responsible for an overwhelming $50 billion in lost wages and medical expenses every year.

Women get migraines more often than men do. It is estimated that up to 18% of all women will have a migraine at some time in their lives, while about 6% of men will. Many migraines are genetically linked; 70 to 80% of migraine patients have other family members with the same malady.

ETIOLOGY: WHAT HAPPENS?

This is a fascinating and paradoxical phenomenon. Migraine headaches begin with extreme vasoconstriction in the affected hemisphere, which one would expect to be painful, but it's not. Instead the person often feels a sense of euphoria mixed with dread that the worst is yet to come. The vasoconstriction is then followed by a huge vasodilation: a veritable flood of blood into the affected part of the brain. It is all still contained within the vessels, of course, but all the excess pressure will press against the meninges, which causes excruciating pain. Migraine headaches are therefore *congestive* headaches.

CAUSES

No one has identified an exact reason for what sets up the process for migraines to take place. Some triggers have been identified, such as the consumption of certain kinds of foods, including red wine, cheese, chocolate, coffee, tea, and any kind of alcohol. Abnormal levels of stress can bring them on, as can hormonal shifts such as menstruation, pregnancy, and menopause. (These hormonal shifts can also make preexisting migraines disappear.) The good news about migraines is that they usually subside by middle age. It is not unheard of, but quite uncommon for mature people to suffer from migraines.

SIGNS AND SYMPTOMS

The word migraine comes from the French, hemi-craine, or "half-head." This is because migraine headaches have a very characteristic unilateral presentation. In classic migraines the pain will be preceded by blurred vision, the perception of flashing lights or auras, and even auditory hallucinations. Classic migraines comprise only about 15 to 20% of all migraines. Then, as with the common migraine, which does not include auras (the other 80 to 85% of migraines), the patient will experience extreme throbbing pain on one side of the head, which may cause the affected eye and side of the nose to water. Migraines will often be accompanied by hypersensitivity to light, nausea, and possibly vomiting. Symptoms can persist for anywhere from several hours to several days.

TREATMENT

Once a migraine has begun, little can be done except to wait for it to pass. Most treatment protocols focus on prevention: identifying particular triggers and avoiding them assiduously. Vasodilators, such as ergot, may be administered in the early stages of a headache, but the nausea that most people experience makes it difficult to take oral medication. A new approach, administering painkillers through a nasal spray, is getting good results.

For people who suffer from frequent, debilitating migraines, some medical options now are available to take on a prophylactic basis. That is, taken daily, these medicines will prevent the initial onset of a headache.

Another treatment for migraines is to give the patient a warm dark room and lots of privacy. Some doctors recommend using a cool cloth on the head to reduce blood flow; this works well in conjunction with a warm footbath for a derivative hydrotherapeutic effect.

Pain Killers, nasal Spray, dark room, cool Cloths

Cluster Headaches

These are a fairly rare, not well-understood variety of congestive or vascular headache. They are closely related to migraines, but unlike migraines, cluster headaches affect men more often than women. They come, one right after the other, for days or weeks at a time. Cluster headaches usually happen at night, with pain severe enough to wake a person out of a sound sleep. Similar to migraines, they will cause the eye and nostril of the affected side to water. They may also cause facial swelling and unilateral sweating. Cluster headache episodes may occur once or twice in a year, or just once in a lifetime.

Sinus Headaches

Sinus headaches are listed among the congestive headaches because they also have to do with congestion: of the sinuses rather than the cranium itself. When a person suffers from sinus-related allergies or sinusitis, their membranes can become irritated and inflamed. A further discussion of this problem can be found in the section titled *sinusitis,* chapter 6, page 255.

Muscular Contraction (Tension) Headaches

ETIOLOGY: WHAT HAPPENS?

The average head weighs about 18 to 20 pounds. The area of bone-to-bone contact where the occiput rests on the first cervical vertebra is about the same as two pairs of fingertips touching. The whole thing is kept in balance by tension exerted by muscles and ligaments around the neck and head. The muscles primarily responsible for the posture of the head form two inverted triangles just below the occiput. It is not surprising, then, that things can easily get a little out of balance, and the resulting pain will reverberate throughout the whole structure.

CAUSES

The causes are almost too numerous to list here, precisely because staying pain free involves such a delicate balance of muscle tension, bony alignment, and a myriad of other factors. Here are some of the major causes for tension headaches:

- Muscular, tendinous, or ligamentous injury to the head or neck structures (of these the ligaments are hurt most often; they are vulnerable to fraying and irritation with uncontrolled movement). (See *whiplash*, chapter 2, page 108.) Simple muscle tension in the suboccipital triangle or the jaw flexors can cause headaches. These muscles are especially vulnerable to the effects of emotional stress. When people are worried or angry, they tend to clench their jaws and tighten their necks.
- Subluxation or fixation of cervical vertebrae can irritate ligaments and/or cause muscle spasms, both of which lead to headaches.
- Structural problems in the alignment of the cranial bones (which are not completely immobile) or in the TMJ can cause headaches. (See *TMJ disorders*, chapter 2, page 89.)
- Trigger points in the muscles of the neck and head can refer pain all around the head. (See *fibromyalgia*, chapter 2, page 50.)
- Any kind of ongoing mental or physical stress can change postural and movement patterns, which will lead to muscle spasm, subluxation, fixation, and so on. Poor ergonomics, especially in repetitive work situations, is frequently the culprit behind chronic tension headaches.

MASSAGE?

The appropriateness of massage depends on what kind of headache the client has. If it is related to a serious underlying pathology, or even an ordinary bacterial or viral infection, any massage is obviously out of the picture. If it is a congestive headache, massage is best left for the subacute stage; clients in the throes of migraine or cluster headaches wouldn't be interested in massage in any case. But for the most common tension-related headaches, massage is resoundingly indicated.

Hyperesthesia

DEFINITION: WHAT IS IT?

Literally, this means, "too much feeling." Hyperesthesia is a symptom, not a disease. It is included as a topic here not because it's likely to appear as a diagnosis, but because massage therapists *must* respect this condition.

Hyperesthesia can accompany any nervous system disorder that involves irritated nerve endings; *herpes simplex* (chapter 1, page 10) and *herpes zoster* (this chapter, page 144) are perfect examples. Other possibilities include *herniated discs* (chapter 2, page 114), *carpal tunnel syndrome* (chapter 2, page 111), and any kind of *neuritis* (this chapter, page 157). Hyperesthesia also can be the by-product of stress or an emotional reaction to touch. Regardless of the cause, the first priorities of massage therapists are not to exacerbate pain and not to spread disease. Consequently, it's important to pinpoint why the client is experiencing such extreme sensitivity.

MASSAGE?

Once it is clear *why* the nerves are irritated or the skin is hypersensitive, massage therapists can make an informed decision about the appropriateness of their work. Knowing the cause of the pain will also indicate whether cautions are local or systemic. Someone with an inflamed carpal tunnel, for instance, is only locally contraindicated, while someone with an acute case of shingles is systemically off limits.

> ### HYPERESTHESIA IN BRIEF
>
> **What is it?**
> Hyperesthesia is extreme sensitivity in the skin, often because of stress or irritated nerves.
>
> **How is it recognized?**
> Hyperesthesiac clients are extremely sensitive and have very low pain thresholds.
>
> **Is massage indicated or contraindicated?**
> This depends entirely on the root cause of the problem.

Neuritis

DEFINITION: WHAT IS IT?

Neuritis means any inflammation of a peripheral nerve. This is a symptom rather than a disease; neuritis occurs *because* of some other problem, and the appropriateness of massage will depend on the precipitating factors. Inflammation of a single nerve, as seen in *trigeminal neuralgia* (this chapter, page 164), is referred to as mononeuropathy. If several nerves are involved, which occurs with *lupus* (chapter 5, page 241) for instance, it would be called polyneuropathy.

ETIOLOGY: WHAT HAPPENS?

Neuritis can be traced to several different problems. Here are some of the basic categories:

- Mechanical injuries. Nerve inflammation is often caused by some mechanical injury to the nerve. With a *herniated disc* (chapter 2, page 114) or *sciatica* (chapter 2, page 118), a hard object is pressing against the nerve root, irritating and inflaming it. Neuritis is also common with major body trauma such as bone *fractures* (chapter 2, page 60) because the nerves in the periosteum are inflamed, suffer bruises, or penetrating injuries.
- Other diseases. A host of other conditions include neuritis among their symptoms or complications: *herpes simplex* (chapter 1, page 10) and *zoster* (this chapter, page 144), *lupus* (chapter 5, page 241), and *peripheral neuropathy* (this chapter, page 142) all involve neuritis.
- Chemical exposure. Exposure to some chemicals can also cause neuritis: carbon monoxide and carbon tetrachloride can cause this disorder, as can exposure to heavy metals, some kinds of drugs, and alcohol. A deficiency in thiamin can also result in nerve inflammation.

> ### NEURITIS IN BRIEF
>
> **What is it?**
> Neuritis means inflammation of a nerve. It is usually a symptom or complication of some other problem.
>
> **How is it recognized?**
> Hyperesthesia is the primary symptom of this condition. Numbness, weakness, and parasthesia may also be present.
>
> **Is massage indicated or contraindicated?**
> Massage is at least locally contraindicated for any acute neuritis. Whether massage is systemically contraindicated will depend on the underlying pathology.

SIGNS AND SYMPTOMS

Hyperesthesia is the major symptom of neuritis: a lot of pain with very little (or no) stimulus. The pain may be localized, but more often it shoots down the dermatome with a characteristic electrical feel. Other symptoms include numbness or reduced sensation, weakness, and tingling or pins and needles.

One variety of neuritis is sometimes a precursor of another problem, a complication of another problem, or a disease unto itself. That is *optic neuritis*, which involves acute inflammation of the optic nerve. Symptoms include sudden loss of color vision or vision altogether and extreme pain on movement of the eye. Optic neuritis involves the swelling and destruction of the myelin sheath on the optic nerve, and is often linked to *multiple sclerosis* (this chapter, page 135). It may also arise as a complication of herpes zoster or lupus.

MASSAGE?

The appropriateness of massage will depend entirely on the cause of the nerve inflammation. Lupus has very different guidelines for massage than a broken bone. Obviously massage is at least locally contraindicated for any acutely inflamed nerve. Beyond that, it will be necessary to make a case-by-case judgment.

Spinal Cord Injury

DEFINITION: WHAT IS IT?

The definition of spinal cord injury is self evident: damage to some percentage of nerve tissue in the spinal canal. How that damage will be reflected in the body depends on where and how much of the tissue has been affected.

DEMOGRAPHICS: WHO GETS IT?

Frequency of spinal cord injuries in the United States is estimated at about 10,000 per year, excluding those persons who die at the scene of the accident. Of those who survive, 35% of injuries are due to motor vehicle accidents, 30.4% to violence, 19.5% to falls, 8.1% to sports injuries, and 6.9% to other accidents. Within sports injuries, 66% of spinal cord damage is caused by diving accidents, and almost *all* spinal cord injuries from sports cause quadriplegia, also called tetraplegia.

The neck is the most vulnerable part of the spine; about half of all injuries occur here. The levels most often injured, by order of frequency, are C_5, C_4, C_6, T_{12}, and L_1. Male patients outnumber females by about 4 to 1. Anywhere from 183,000 to 230,000 spinal cord injury patients are alive today.

ETIOLOGY: WHAT HAPPENS?

When the spinal cord is injured at a certain level, the damage will be reflected in all the muscles supplied at and below that level. The damage may be caused by a badly herniated disc that creates a permanent lesion on the spinal cord, a bone chip from a fractured vertebra, a bullet, or anything else. A "complete" injury means that all

---

SPINAL CORD INJURY IN BRIEF

What is it?
Spinal cord injury is a situation in which some or all of the fibers in the spinal cord have been damaged, usually by trauma but occasionally from other problems such as tumors or bony growths in the spinal canal.

How is it recognized?
Spinal cord injury will cause the loss of some muscle function, as well as sensory deprivation. The affected muscles, in the absence of nerve conduction, atrophy quickly.

Is massage indicated or contraindicated?
Mechanical types of massage are appropriate only if sensation is present and no underlying pathologies will be exacerbated by the work. Areas without sensation are contraindications for massage that intends to manipulate and influence the quality of muscle tissue.

supply inferior to the site of injury is interrupted. A "partial" or "incomplete" injury means that some supply remains below the site. Amazingly, up to 90% of all axons must be damaged before function is fully lost.

Nontraumatic damage to the spinal cord can also create paralysis. Sources of these problems include spinal cord tumors, damage from cancer-related radiation, thoracic aneurysm and subsequent surgery, and congenital spinal cord malformations like spina bifida or spinal canal stenosis.

SIGNS AND SYMPTOMS

Symptoms of spinal cord injury depend on what level has been damaged and what percentage of the spinal cord tissue has been affected. For specific information about different types of paralysis, see the accompanying sidebar.

COMPLICATIONS

Complications of spinal cord injuries depend on the extent of the damage. With any kind of sensory paralysis, a danger always exists of getting hurt without knowing it. Even minor abrasions can fester and become badly infected before they're noticed and treated. For patients who are bedridden or wheelchair-bound, *thrombophlebitis* (chapter 4, page 187) is a threat, especially in the first few weeks. *Urinary tract infections* (chapter 8, page 318) or other kidney problems are a constant danger because the bladder is never completely emptied. Likewise, a constant sitting or reclining posture makes it difficult to fight off respiratory infections; *pneumonia* (chapter 6, page 252) is the leading cause of death for persons with spinal cord injuries. Autonomic hyperreflexia is a situation in which patients with damage above T_6 have a sudden onset of hypertension, rapid heartbeat, sweating, and other sympathetic nervous system reactions. These can be extreme enough to culminate in seizure, stroke, and even death. Attacks of autonomic hyperreflexia are most often brought about by bladder obstruction, but can also be caused by bowel impaction, menstruation, and labor. It is also possible that deep abdominal work may precipitate an episode of autonomic hyperreflexia.

TREATMENT

In cases of traumatic spinal cord injury, surgical intervention to remove anything pressing on the spinal cord is critical. Since it has been found that only 10% of axons need to be intact to maintain function, preserving as many healthy fibers as possible from secondary injury has become a major priority in emergency spinal cord care. A steroidal medication called *methylprednisolone* (MP), in some cases reduces inflammation and acts as an antioxidant to the injury-generated oxygen-free radicals that can cause important secondary damage to spinal cord fibers. Drugs that improve the action potential of demyelinated fibers are also sometimes prescribed.

NERVE DAMAGE TERMINOLOGY

Nerve damage can manifest in several different ways. Familiarity with some of the vocabulary of nervous system damage can make it much easier to "talk shop" with clients and doctors dealing with these problems.

Paresthesia: a technical term for any abnormal sensation, particularly the tingling, burning, and prickling feelings associated with "pins and needles."

Hyperkinesia: excessive muscular activity.

Hypokinesia: a condition involving diminished or slowed movement.

Hypertonia: a general term for extreme tension, or tone in the muscles.

Hypotonia: the opposite of hypertonia; it means an abnormally low level of muscle tone, as seen with flaccid paralysis.

Spasticity: a type of hypertonia. It is a condition in which the stretch reflex is overactive. The flexors want to flex, but the extensors don't want to give way. Finally the extensors are stretched too far, and then they release altogether. This phenomenon is called the "clasp-knife effect."

Paralysis: comes from the Greek for "loosening." It means the loss of any function controlled by the nervous system.

Paresis: partial or incomplete paralysis.

Flaccid paralysis: typically a sign of *peripheral nerve* damage. It accompanies conditions like *Bell's palsy* (this chapter, page 151). Flaccid paralysis involves muscles in a state of *hypo*tonicity.

Spastic paralysis: indicates *central nervous system* damage. Spastic paralysis combines aspects of hypertonia, hypokinesia, and hyperreflexia. This situation is never resolved, which distinguishes it from mere *spasm* (chapter 2, page 57). (continued)

NERVE DAMAGE TERMINOLOGY, cont.

Types of spastic paralysis:

* *Hemiplegia* means one vertical half (or *hemi*sphere) of the body has been affected. This is the variation that most often accompanies *stroke* (this chapter, page 161).
* *Paraplegia* means the bottom half of the body, or some part of it, has been affected. These patients still have at least partial use of their arms and hands.
* *Diplegia* is a symmetrical paralysis of upper or lower extremities resulting from injuries to the cerebrum.
* *Quadra*plegia, or tetraplegia, means that the body has been affected from the neck down. Tetraplegics can eat, breathe, talk, and move their heads because these functions are controlled by the cranial nerves which are usually protected from injury.

Some other treatments for spinal cord injury include the implantation in muscles of electrodes, which are controlled from an external computer. These implants can provide pinching and gripping capabilities for people who otherwise would not have the use of their hands. Surgical transfer of healthy tendons can also be helpful. For some people, the triceps muscle may be paralyzed while the deltoid is not. Surgically extending the posterior deltoid tendon and attaching it to the olecranon can provide these people with the power it takes to use a wheelchair.

Until recently most cases of spinal cord injury were considered untreatable in terms of reversing any damage. Treatment for these patients has always been targeted at providing them with the skills to live as fully as possible, given their situation. Physical and occupational therapists may specialize in helping these patients gain the skills they need to function; mental/emotional therapists are also critical, especially for those who are adapting to their paralysis as a new way of life.

Although damage to central nervous system tissue has always been considered to be permanent, new research is finding that under certain circumstances it can be regenerated. This has important ramifications for the hundreds of thousands of people who live with spinal cord disability.

Research into the possibility of regenerating CNS fibers has achieved three major breakthroughs in the past decade:

* CNS axons will grow in a peripheral nervous system environment: peripheral nerves placed into a brain were invaded by CNS axons, which grew the length of the nerve.
* Certain proteins in the CNS stop nerve growth; these proteins can be inhibited to allow growth in laboratory settings.
* Growth factors in the CNS have been identified and isolated.

Other promising research involves the transplantation of PNS Schwann cells to replace the damaged myelin in the CNS.

MASSAGE?

Massage can be an important part of the life of people with spinal cord injuries, as long as four main cautions are kept in mind:

* Blood clots. Blood clots can form in the legs of any person who is bedridden or wheelchair-bound. This is true for spinal cord injury patients especially in the first few weeks of their condition, as the body is adjusting to a new way of life.
* No sensation. If a client cannot feel the hands of the massage therapist, then that therapist should *not* be trying to influence the texture or malleability of the client's tissues. Mechanical massage is appropriate for the parts of the body where sensation is intact; reserve the numb areas for energy work.
* Brittle fibers. Spastic fibers are not like regular, or even spasmed, fibers. They are brittle and easy to injure. This is another good reason to leave the paralyzed areas alone in terms of mechanically based massage.
* Hyperreflexia. Many people with spinal cord injuries have "gray areas" where sensation is partially intact. Massage can feel very good in these areas, but anything too stimulating can cause a hyperreflexive reaction; in other words, uncontrollable shaking or tremors that are not dangerous, but also are not pleasant to the client. Very

light stroking may also elicit a hyperreflexive response. It is important to treat each client individually, because each person will have different responses to massage.

Outside of these concerns, massage can be a wonderful part of a paralyzed client's life. These people are carrying a whole different load than uninjured persons, but they are prone to the same kinds of injuries as anyone else. Imagine being in a wheelchair and having shoulder tendinitis; wouldn't it be a relief to get rolling pain-free again? It takes a lot of courage to work with this population; fears include accidentally hurting the client, physically or emotionally, by saying or doing the wrong thing. But within this group is a very eager population of people waiting for massage.

Stroke

DEFINITION: WHAT IS IT?

Stroke, also called brain attack or cerebrovascular accident (CVA), is damage to the brain because of oxygen deprivation.

DEMOGRAPHICS: WHO GETS IT?

Stroke is the single most common type of central nervous system disorder there is. It is the third leading cause of death in the United States, coming in right behind heart disease and cancer. It is the leading cause of adult disability; three million Americans live with permanent impairments due to stroke.

This year, 550,000 Americans will have a stroke; that's one every minute. One-fourth of them will experience no lasting effects (until the next stroke); one-half of them will suffer some kind of permanent disability; and one-fourth of them will die. Of the people who survive a stroke this year, 10 to 18% will have another stroke within a year, and 33% of them will have another stroke within five years.

Cerebrovascular accidents cost approximately $30 billion per year in hospital, physician, and rehabilitation expenses.

ETIOLOGY: WHAT HAPPENS?

Oxygen deprivation in the brain can be caused by one of three things:

- Thrombosis, which is a clot of blood that forms inside the brain and becomes lodged in a brain vessel and starves off nerve cells. These strokes account for up to 88% of all CVAs.
- Embolism, which is much the same thing except that the clot has traveled to the brain from elsewhere in the body. Although this seems like a trivial distinction, it becomes significant when one considers diagnosis and treatment options. Emboli generally come from inefficient pumping of a heart with atrial fibrillations; incomplete and arrhythmic contractions allow blood in the left atrium to thicken and form clots before being forced out into the bloodstream. Emboli account for 8 to 14% of all CVAs.

  These two problems are called *ischemic strokes*, as they have to do with oxygen being cut off to affected tissues, and the subsequent death of those tissues. (See Figure 3.9.) Another type of stroke results from too much blood, although not within the proper blood vessels.

STROKE IN BRIEF

What is it?
A stroke is damage to brain tissue caused by either a clot lodged to block blood flow to brain tissue or an internal hemorrhage.

How is it recognized?
The symptoms of stroke are paralysis and/or numbness on one side, blurry or diminished vision, asymmetrically dilated pupils, dizziness, difficulty in speaking or understanding simple sentences, sudden extreme headache, and possibly loss of consciousness.

Is massage indicated or contraindicated?
Massage may be indicated during recovery from a stroke, but only with medical clearance, since this problem is usually associated with cardiovascular disease.

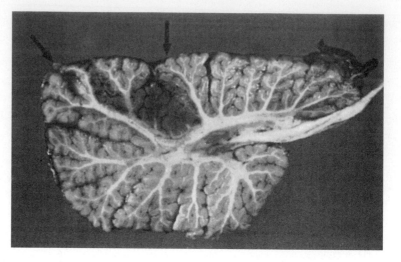

Figure 3.9. Stroke: damaged brain tissue is clearly visible.

- Hemorrhage, or the rupture of a blood vessel will also cause tissue death in the brain. Hemorrhages are often associated with *aneurysms* (see chapter 4, page 190), which may be a result of hypertension, bleeding disorders, or malformation of blood vessels. Hemorrhagic strokes are less age specific than ischemic strokes. They may occur in the subarachnoid space (7% of strokes) or in intracerebral area (10% of strokes).

Hemorrhagic and ischemic strokes are distinct from but highly associated with a related phenomenon: *transient ischemic attacks*, or TIAs. In a TIA, a very tiny blood clot creates a temporary blockage in the brain, but it quickly breaks apart and disperses before causing any lasting damage. Consequently, TIAs are associated with ischemic CVAs rather than hemorrhagic ones. Symptoms of TIAs are very similar to those of stroke, except that they last only a few minutes or hours. These are, however, like the muffled rumblings of an incipient eruption; about one-half of all people who experience a TIA will have a major stroke within five years.

RISK FACTORS

Although a person can have a genetic predisposition toward a CVA, many factors contribute to the likelihood of stroke that are well within the reach of personal control. Risk factors that can be controlled include:

- High blood pressure. Untreated hypertension is the biggest single contributing factor to the risk of stroke. See *hypertension*, chapter 4, page 199.
- Smoking. Nicotine constricts blood vessels and raises blood pressure.
- Atherosclerosis, high cholesterol. This situation also contributes to high blood pressure, as well as raising the risk of *emboli* (see chapter 4, page 182).
- Atrial fibrillation. Left untreated, this condition can help to form the emboli responsible for some ischemic embolic strokes.
- High alcohol consumption. This is generally considered to be more than two drinks per day.
- Obesity
- Sedentary lifestyle
- Diabetes. Untreated, this condition can contribute to high blood pressure and atherosclerosis (see chapter 4, page 193).
- High-estrogen birth control pills, especially when taken by a smoker. No similar risk has been found with postmenopausal estrogen replacement therapy.
- Overall stress

Risk factors that can't be controlled include:

- Age. Two-thirds of all stroke patients are over 65 years old. The risk of having a stroke doubles every year after 35.
- Gender. About 25% more men have strokes than women. However, women seem to have more severe strokes; 60% of all people who die from strokes are women.
- Race. African Americans have a higher incidence of hypertension than Caucasians. They are about twice as likely to have a stroke as Caucasians, and they are almost twice as likely to die from it.
- Family history. Having a family history of stroke and cardiovascular disease can be a predisposing factor. Congenitally weak blood vessels is an inherited disorder. However, in cases of ischemic strokes, the question needs to be asked: what is inherited, the status of the blood vessels, or the diet and exercise habits?
- Previous stroke. Having one stroke usually predisposes a person to having another. Predisposition is not predestination, however; by taking control of whatever factors are within reach, a person can take big steps toward reducing the chances that he or she will have another stroke.

SIGNS AND SYMPTOMS

It is important to be able to recognize the signs of stroke; the sooner treatment is administered, the less likely permanent damage will occur. Surprisingly, a huge proportion of Americans don't recognize the major symptoms of stroke, which are as follows:

- Unilateral weakness, numbness, or paralysis of the face, arm, leg, or any combination of the three.
- Suddenly blurred or decreased vision in one or both eyes; asymmetrical dilation of pupils.
- Difficulty in speaking or understanding simple sentences.
- Dizziness, clumsiness, vertigo.
- Sudden, very extreme headache.
- Possible loss of consciousness.

After a debilitating stroke, the extent of the damage will depend on what part and how much of the brain has been affected. Occasionally, a progressive degeneration may occur over one or two days, but usually a stroke is complete within a few hours.

Motor damage from strokes can result in partial or full paralysis of one side of the body; aphasia (loss of language); and memory loss and personality changes, which may be mild or severe. Sensory damage may result in permanent numbness and vision loss.

DIAGNOSIS

When a person suspects he may have had a stroke, he usually undergoes extensive testing to isolate the extent of the damage he may have sustained. This generally takes the form of CT scans, MRIs, EEGs, x-rays, and other tests. The goal is only partially to pinpoint the damage. More pertinent is to determine whether the stroke was hemorrhagic or ischemic. If it was ischemic, it is important to know if the clot was formed inside the brain (a thrombus) or elsewhere (an embolism). The answer to that question will yield different options to prevent further incidents.

TREATMENT

The treatment of choice for ischemic stroke survivors is anticoagulant medication to minimize the risk of more clotting. Severe brain damage may be averted if the anticoagulants are administered within a few hours of the stroke. If the CVA was caused by a hemorrhage, however, anticoagulant treatment could be dangerous, or even deadly.

Changing life habits that increase risk is also important: stopping smoking, improving diet and exercise habits, reducing stress. If necessary, surgery may be performed either on the blood vessels leading to the brain or inside it to widen the lumenae and reduce the possibility of more clots being caught or formed inside.

Interestingly, the prognosis for hemorrhagic strokes is often better than that for ischemic ones. Although the initial symptoms of a hemorrhagic stroke are often more severe because a larger mass of brain tissue is affected by the leakage of blood, once that leakage recedes, the oxygen supply to the brain is restored and some of the symptoms may abate. With ischemic strokes, a certain amount of tissue is starved for oxygen and there is no hope of spontaneous recovery.

Finally, and perhaps most important in terms of rehabilitation, physical and occupational therapy is recommended to help to "retrain" muscles that have suddenly lost their source of central nervous system information. Because the brain has a vast resource of backup wiring, this is often a very successful part of the recovery process. It needs to be started very soon after the CVA, though, in order to prevent the fibrosis and atrophy of muscle tissue that happen so quickly when nerve signals have been interrupted.

MASSAGE?

Massage can sometimes play a role in the recovery of a stroke survivor, but serious cautions should be considered. First and foremost is the client's general cardiovascular health. The vast majority of stroke patients have other circulatory problems. Therefore, it's *very important* to get medical clearance before proceeding with massage. Second, hemiplegia is a type of spastic paralysis, which carries specific cautions and guidelines for massage. See *nerve damage terminology* sidebar, this chapter, page 159.

Trigeminal Neuralgia

DEFINITION: WHAT IS IT?

Neur-algia means "nerve pain." This is another condition that is not a disease in itself, but a description or symptom of some other problem. Any nervous system disorder that causes pain along the length of sensory peripheral nerves can be said to have neuralgia among its symptoms. There are a few different types of specific neuralgias, but trigeminal neuralgia is by far the most common.

TRIGEMINAL NEURALGIA IN BRIEF

What is it?
Trigeminal neuralgia (TN) is pain along the trigeminal nerve, usually in the lower face and jaw.

How is it recognized?
The pain of trigeminal neuralgia is very sharp and severe. Patients report stabbing, electrical, or burning sensations. There may also be a muscular tic.

Is massage indicated or contraindicated?
Massage is locally contraindicated when a client is having an acute episode of TN. Otherwise, massage is appropriate. Work on the face and head of a client who has TN with their specific guidance.

ETIOLOGY: WHAT HAPPENS?

Several things can cause this condition because the trigeminal nerve is fairly vulnerable. Bone spurs at the foramina, tumors, TMJ imbalance, misalignment at the atlas, and certain drug reactions can all give rise to trigeminal neuralgia. It may be caused most often by a particular artery that wraps around the nerve and "strangles" it, which can damage the myelin sheath. Trigeminal neuralgia can also be an early sign of *multiple sclerosis* (this chapter, page 135).

Episodes of trigeminal nerve pain can be triggered by speaking, chewing, swallowing, sitting in a draft, a light touch to the wrong spot, and sometimes by no stimulus at all. Unlike *Bell's palsy* (this chapter, page 151), however, this is not necessarily a self-limiting condition. It is likely to continue, the attacks increasing in frequency, until the source of irritation is removed.

Trigeminal neuralgia is certainly the most common type of diagnosed neuralgia, but two other varieties of nerve pain deserve a mention too:

- Post herpetic neuralgia. This is a complication of *herpes zoster* (this chapter, page 144). It will occur wherever the shingles blisters appeared, but can outlast the visible lesions by several weeks or months.
- Atypical face pain. This is a condition similar to trigeminal neuralgia, and in some cases may be a predecessor to it. It is characterized by pain that is less severe than trigeminal neuralgia, but it tends to be continuous rather than intermittent. The pain may also go up over the back of the head and into the scalp, and it may involve the occipital as well as the trigeminal nerve.

Neuralgia outside of these classifications is rare, except as a symptom of nerve inflammation from *herniated discs* (chapter 2, page 114) or other mechanical pressures.

SIGNS AND SYMPTOMS

Tic douloureux, or trigeminal neuralgia, is a disorder involving Cranial Nerve V. The nerve, usually on only one side of the face, is irritated in some way to produce extremely painful sensations. Usually it's the lower two branches of the trigeminal nerve that are affected; this produces symptoms in the lower face and jaw. (See Figure 3.10.)

Some people call the pain of trigeminal neuralgia among the worst in the world. It's often described as sharp, electrical stabbing or burning sensations. The words "hot poker" appear in a lot of the literature associated with this condition. These episodes may last for 10 seconds to a minute, or several jabs may occur in rapid succession. A muscular tic sometimes develops along with the nerve pain. Patients are usually women between 50 and 70 years old, although anyone of any age can have this problem. Statistics vary, but it is estimated that trigeminal neuralgia affects less than 5 out of every 100,000 people in the United States.

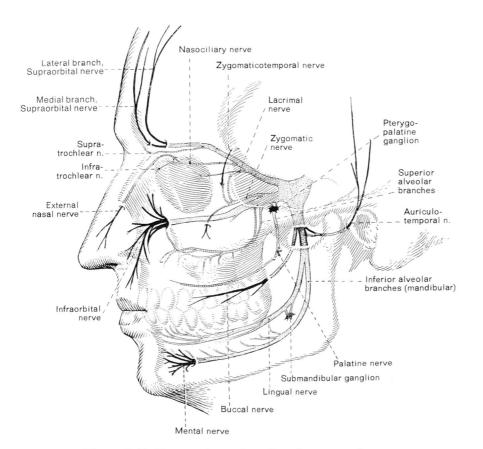

Figure 3.10. Trigeminal neuralgia affects the trigeminal nerve

TREATMENT

Obviously, treatment strategies for this problem depend on the source of the pain. Sinus and tooth infections can sometimes mimic trigeminal neuralgia, so an early step is to rule those out. Misalignment of cervical vertebrae or TMJ problems can be sorted out by the appropriate professionals. Acupuncture often works well for trigeminal neuralgia, as it does for many problems with nerve conduction.

The mainstream medical approach to TN starts with painkillers, then proceeds to anti-seizure drugs that inhibit nerve conduction. If a specific obstruction such as an artery or tumor has been identified, surgery may be successful in correcting the situation. In the worst-case scenarios, an injection of alcohol to deaden the nerve, or surgery to sever it may be suggested. The obvious disadvantage in these cases is that destroying the nerve also destroys sensation to half of the face; it will remain numb forever. This kind of intervention is to be avoided, if at all possible.

MASSAGE?

If a client is prone to trigeminal neuralgia attacks, massage is locally contraindicated during attacks, but is otherwise appropriate with a few cautions. The client will be able to indicate if it feels safe or comfortable to receive work on her face. Be especially careful around the facial foramina, because pressure where the nerve emerges can be extremely irritating.

Other Nervous System Disorders

Seizure Disorders

DEFINITION: WHAT ARE THEY?

Epilepsy, one type of seizure disorder, is one of the oldest conditions recorded in medical history. It was first described about 2000 years BC, but it was not studied as a specific problem—other than "demonic possession"—until the mid-nineteenth century. Epilepsy is not a disease itself, but rather an indication of an underlying neurological pathology that creates a tendency to have seizures. Seizure disorders are the second most common type of central nervous system problem in the country, so it is important to be familiar with them. (The most common neurological problem is *stroke*, this chapter, page 161.)

DEMOGRAPHICS: WHO GETS THEM?

World wide, it is estimated that approximately 1% of the population will experience a seizure at some point. In the United States, epilepsy affects about 2.5 million people, with around 100,000 new cases being reported each year. Men and women suffer from epilepsy equally.

Epilepsy usually begins in childhood. About two-thirds of all patients are diagnosed before their fouteenth birthday. Many children grow out of this condition with no lingering effects. A smaller percentage of people deal with some degree of seizure activity all their lives.

ETIOLOGY: WHAT HAPPENS?

When interconnecting neurons in the brain are stimulated in a certain kind of way, a tremendous burst of excess

---

SEIZURE DISORDERS IN BRIEF

What are they?
Seizure disorders are usually caused by neurological damage, although it may be impossible to delineate exactly what that damage is. Epilepsy is one type of seizure disorder.

How are they recognized?
Seizure disorders are diagnosed through CT scans and MRIs. Seizures may take very different forms for different people; they range from barely noticeable to life threatening.

Is massage indicated or contraindicated?
Massage is contraindicated during seizures, but is indicated at all other times.

electricity stimulates the neighboring neurons. The reaction is repeated and soon millions of neurons in the brain are giving off electrical discharge. This is the central nervous system "lightning storm" of the epileptic seizure, and it affects the rest of the body in a number of different ways.

For the most part, no one knows what starts the storm in the first place. Triggers will vary for different people. For some, sudden changes in light level, from dark to light or vice versa, will trigger a seizure. For others flashing or strobing lights, or the strobing effect created by ceiling fans, will be the trigger. For others certain sounds, or even particular notes of music, will cause a seizure. High anxiety or other sicknesses like cold or flu can also lead to seizures.

CAUSES

In some cases the cause of seizures can be definitively linked to a mechanical or chemical problem in the brain. Birth trauma, skull fractures, shaken baby syndrome, brain tumors, and penetrating wounds can all cause seizures, as can some types of metabolic disturbances, infections, exposure to some toxins, and extreme hypotension or hemorrhage. Rarely, epilepsy can be traced to a hereditary problem. But patients who can list a root cause for their problem comprise only one third of all cases. The other two out of three seizure patients have no identifiable cause for their disorder. In other words, seizures are, by and large, idiopathic.

SIGNS AND SYMPTOMS

Seizures take very different forms in each person they affect. From the original oversimplified categories of "petit mal" and "grand mal" seizures, over 30 different classes of seizures have been identified. These can range from the barely noticeable 5-to-10-second "absence seizures" to life-threatening, hours-long "static seizures" in which a new episode begins before the previous one has resolved. These seizures are estimated to cause 22,000 to 42,000 deaths per year in the United States.

The type of seizure that has been traditionally called "grand mal" is now referred to as a "tonic/clonic" seizure, and is characterized by a sudden stiffening with loss of consciousness followed by rhythmic shaking or contractions. They may last up to seven minutes, after which the patient is often disoriented and tired.

One aspect of seizure research focuses on where in the brain the electrical discharges are located. If they can be pinpointed to a specific lobe or side ("partial seizures"), they are less severe than the "general seizures" that involve abnormal electrical activity all over the brain.

Misfiring electricity in the brain can obviously trigger involuntary motor activity. Interestingly, sensory activity can be stimulated as well. Many patients report that before they experience a seizure they hear, see, smell, or even taste things that aren't there: hallucinations brought about by sensory neurons randomly firing in the higher centers of the brain. These "auras" may help to pinpoint exactly where in the brain the abnormal electrical discharges are happening.

DIAGNOSIS

Epilepsy is usually diagnosed by an EEG, a test which measures electrical activity in the brain. If an underlying mechanical cause is suspected, x-rays, CT scans, and/or MRIs may be used to look for identifiable lesions. Tests are conducted in part to delineate seizures from other conditions that produce seizure-like symptoms: fainting spells, heart arrhythmia, hypoglycemia, and reactions to some medications.

TREATMENT

Seizures are generally treated with anti-seizure medication which acts to make neurons in the brain harder to stimulate. Chemically, many of these drugs are very similar to valium.

As with most kinds of medication, there is a good side and a bad side to this picture. On the good side, they can be very effective at limiting seizures, making it possible for the patient to live a normal life. On the other hand, these drugs can have unpleasant side effects (drowsiness, nausea) and taking them is usually a life-long commitment. Furthermore, the stronger the medication, the more chance there is for dangerous reactions with alcohol or medicines taken for other reasons.

In some cases where the damaged tissue in the brain is easily isolated, surgery may be performed to remove the seizure-causing lesion.

Nonmedical interventions to reduce the severity and frequency of seizures include biofeedback and stress-reducing techniques. Although these have had some success with some patients, it is important that patients not change their anti-seizure medication without first consulting their physician.

MASSAGE?

It is inappropriate to try to massage someone who is in the midst of a seizure of any kind. In this situation, the practitioner's job is to make sure the client is safe, call 911 or the local emergency number, and then wait until the seizure has subsided. If a client has a history of seizures, it is perfectly fine to work with him at any other time, although if his seizures tend to come on fast with no warning, the therapist should be alert to the possibility of its happening during an appointment. Someone recovering from a severe seizure will probably find that he is sore and tender, as if he had been doing a lot of unaccustomed exercise, which in fact he has. It is also very possible to sustain serious injury when these seizures happen in unprotected surroundings. Sprains, bruises, even broken bones can happen during tonic/clonic seizures.

CHAPTER REVIEW QUESTIONS: NERVOUS SYSTEM CONDITIONS

1. What's the difference between spastic and flaccid paralysis? Where in the nervous system does each indicate damage?

2. How can a person who has experienced spinal cord damage at C_6 still have control of his head and neck?

3. Why is massage indicated for Bell's palsy, when it is contraindicated for most other types of paralysis?

4. Is post polio syndrome contagious? Why or why not?

5. Describe the safest course of action for a client who experiences an epileptic seizure during a massage.

6. A client who has multiple sclerosis comes for massage. The therapist performs a rigorous sports-massage type treatment and then recommends a soak in a hot tub. Is this a good idea? Why or why not?

7. Can a person who has had chicken pox catch herpes zoster from another person? Why or why not?

8. Name three conditions that can result in hyperesthesia.

9. What is neuritis? Name two conditions that can cause it.

10. A client is recovering from a major stroke. What are some of the key criteria on which to base a judgment about the appropriateness of Swedish massage?

BIBLIOGRAPHY, NERVOUS SYSTEM CONDITIONS

General References, Nervous System

1. Carmine D. Clemente, PhD. Anatomy: A regional atlas of the human body. 3rd ed. Baltimore: Urban & Schwarzenburg, 1987.
2. I. Damjanou. Pathology for the health-related professions. Philadelphia: Saunders, 1996.
3. Giovanni de Dominico, Elizabeth Wood. Beard's massage. Philadelphia: Saunders, 1997.
4. Deane Juhan. Job's body: A handbook for bodywork. Barrytown, NY: Station Hill Press, Inc., 1987.
5. Jeffrey R. M. Kunz, MD, Asher J. Finkel, MD, eds. The American Medical Association family medical guide. New York: Random House, Inc., 1987.
6. Elaine M. Marieb, RN, PhD. Human anatomy and physiology. Redwood City, CA: Benjamin/Cummings Publishing Co., Inc., 1989.
7. Ruth Lundeen Memmler, MD, Dina Lin Wood, RN, BS, PHN. The human body in health and disease. 5th ed. Philadelphia: JB Lippincott Co., 1983.
8. Mary Lou Mulvihill. Human diseases: A systemic approach. 2nd ed. Norwalk, CT: Appleton & Lange, A publishing division of Prentice-Hall, 1987.
9. Stedman's medical dictionary. 26th ed. Baltimore: Williams & Wilkins, 1995.
10. Taber's cyclopedic dictionary. 14th ed. Philadelphia: F.A. Davis Company, 1981.
11. Gerard J. Tortora, Nicholas P. Anagnostakos. Principles of anatomy and physiology. 6th ed. New York: Biological Sciences Textbook, Inc., A&P Textbooks, Inc., and Elia-Sparta, Inc. Harper & Row Publishers, Inc., 1990.
12. Janet Travell, MD, David G. Simons, MD. Myofascial pain and dysfunction: The trigger point manual. Baltimore: Williams & Wilkins, 1983.

Amyotrophic Lateral Sclerosis

1. ALS Brochure. American Academy of Neurology, 1997. URL: http://www.aan.com/public/bals.html. Accessed fall 1997.
2. Amyotrophic lateral sclerosis. Copyright 1998 ADAM Software, Inc., all rights reserved. Copyright 1998 CommuniHealth. URL: /www.healthanswers.com. Accessed winter 1998.
3. MedicineNet: Amyotrophic lateral sclerosis (ALS or "Lou Gehrig's Disease"). Information Network, Inc., 1995–1997. URL: http://www.medicinenet.com. Accessed fall 1997.

Chorea

1. Essential tremor. American Academy of Neurology, 1997. URL: http://www.aan.com/public/esse.html. Accessed fall 1997.
2. Huntington's disease. Copyright 1998 ADAM Software, Inc., all rights reserved. Copyright 1998 CommuniHealth. URL: /www.healthanswers.com. Accessed winter 1998.

Multiple Sclerosis

1. MS patient brochure. American Academy of Neurology, 1997. URL: http://www.aan.com/public/bmult.html. Accessed fall 1997.
2. Natural course of MS redefined. National Institute of Health, U.S. Department of Health and Human Services, October 28, 1997. URL: http://www.ninds.nih.gov/WHATSNEW/PRESSWHN/1990/10-16-90.HTM. Accessed fall 1997.
3. What is multiple sclerosis? The well-connected health reports. HealthGate Data Corporation. URL: http://www.healthgate.com/. Accessed fall 1997.

Parkinson's Disease

1. Dietrich Miesler. Parkinson's disease and massage therapy. Massage Therapy Journal 1996; 35(1):34–37.
2. Jan N. Mueller. Elderly parkinson's patient—Feeling good. Massage Therapy Journal 1996; 35(1):28–42.
3. Parkinson's disease. American Academy of Neurology, 1997. URL: http://www.aan.com/public/park.html. Accessed fall 1997.
4. Parkinson's update. Update Newsletter 1995; 54. Medical Publishing Company. URL: http://www.chronicillnet.org/news/PD_update.html. Accessed fall 1997.

Peripheral Neuropathy

1. Masatomi H. Ikusaka, MD. Peripheral neuropathy. In: University of Iowa Family Practice Handbook: Chapter 14: Neurology. The Author(s) and the University of Iowa, 1992–1997. URL: http://www.vh.org/Providers/ClinRef/FPHandbook/Chapter14/07-14.html. Accessed fall 1997.
2. Peripheral neuropathy. Copyright 1998 ADAM Software, Inc., all rights reserved. Copyright 1998 CommuniHealth. URL: /www.healthanswers.com. Accessed winter 1998.

Encephalitis

1. Encephalitis, arboviral. In: Center for Disease Control. Case definitions for public health surveillance. MMWR 1990;39 (No.RR-13):11–13. URL: http://www.cdc.gov/epo/mmwr/other/case_def/enceph1.html. Accessed fall 1997.

Herpes Zoster

1. Susan Fitzgerald. Chicken pox vaccine nears approval. Washington Post Health, August 24, 1993, p. 9.

Meningitis

1. Meningicoccal meningitis. New York State Department of Health Communicable Disease Fact Sheet, March 1996. URL: http://www.health.state.ny.us/nysdoh/consumer/menin.htm. Accessed fall 1997.
2. Meningitis. Copyright 1998 ADAM Software, Inc., all rights reserved. Copyright 1998 CommuniHealth. URL: /www.healthanswers.com. Accessed winter 1998.
3. World Health Organization. Emerging and other communicable diseases. Meningicoccal meningitis fact sheet. March 1996. URL://http:www.who.ch/programmes/emc/csmfacts.htm.

Polio, Post Polio Syndrome

1. A brief history of polio. Polio Virus Information Center Online, 1996–1997; Alan W. Dove. August 8, 1997. URL: http://128.59.173.136/PICO/Chapters/History.html. Accessed fall 1997.
2. Polio epidemiology. Polio Virus Information Center Online, 1996–1997; Alan W. Dove. August 8, 1997. URL: http://128.59.173.136/PICO/Chapters/Epidemiology.html. Accessed fall 1997.
3. Polio pathogenesis. Polio Virus Information Center Online, 1996–1997; Alan W. Dove. August 8, 1997. URL: http://128.59.173.136/PICO/Chapters/Pathogenesis.html. Accessed fall 1997.
4. Post polio syndrome: Public health education information sheet. March of Dimes Birth Defects Foundation, 1997. URL: http://www.modimes.org/pub/postpoli.htm. Accessed fall 1997.
5. World Health Organization.Global polio incidence declines by 82%. April 6, 1995. URL: http://www.who.ch/press/1995/pr95-25.html.

Bell's Palsy

1. Bell's palsy. Copyright 1998 ADAM Software, Inc., all rights reserved. Copyright 1998 CommuniHealth. URL: /www.healthanswers.com. Accessed winter 1998.
2. Bell's palsy. American Academy of Neurology, 1997. URL: http://www.aan.com/public/bell.html. Accessed fall 1997.
3. Doctor, what is bell's palsy? American Academy of Otolaryngology, Head and Neck Surgery, 1994. URL: http://www.netdoor.com/com/entinfo/facnvaao.html. Accessed fall 1997.

Headaches

1. Thomas V. Dibacco. Migraine's torment "the worst in the world." Washington Post Health, December 20–27, 1994, p. 14.
2. Headache. American Academy of Neurology, 1997. URL: http://www.aan.com/public/head.html. Accessed fall 1997.
3. MedicineNet: Migraine headache. What is a migraine headache? Information Network, Inc., 1995–1997. URL: http://www.medicinenet.com. Accessed fall 1997.
4. MedicineNet: Questions and answers about cluster headaches. Information Network, Inc., 1995–1997. URL: http://www.medicinenet.com. Accessed fall 1997.

Neuritis

1. Optic neuritis. American Academy of Neurology, 1997. URL: http://www.aan.com/public/bals.html. Accessed fall 1997.

Spinal Cord Injury

1. David Brown. Studies offer hope for fixing injured spinal cords. Washington Post Health, January 13, 1994, p. A10.
2. Current projects. Integrated Spinal Rehabilitation Foundation (INSPIRE). 9/21/97. URL: http://www.the-sett.demon.co.uk/inspire.htm#Projects. Accessed fall 1997.
3. Frequently asked questions. Cure Paralysis Now, 1997. URL: http://www.cureparalysis.org/faq/index.html. Accessed fall 1997.

Stroke

1. Sally Squires. Surgery to prevent strokes. Washington Post Health, October 4, 1994.
2. Stroke. American Academy of Neurology, 1997. URL: http://www.aan.com/public/stro.html. Accessed fall 1997.
3. Stroke. Copyright 1998 ADAM Software, Inc., all rights reserved. Copyright 1998 CommuniHealth. URL: http://healthanswers.com. Accessed winter 1998.
4. Stroke awareness. Stanford University Medical Center, June 18, 1997. URL:

http://www-med.stanford.edu/school/ stroke/part1.html. Accessed fall 1997.

5. Stroke (brain attack) statistics. American Heart Association, 1997. URL: http:// www.americanheart.org/heartg/strokes. html. Accessed fall 1997.

6. Stroke (brain attack) tests. American Heart Association, 1997. URL: http:// www.americanheart.org/heartg/strokete. html. Accessed fall 1997.

7. Stroke facts. National Stroke Association, March 9, 1997. URL: http://www.stroke. org. Accessed fall 1997.

8. Transient ischemic attack. American Academy of Neurology, 1997. URL: http://www.aan.com/public/tran.html. Accessed fall 1997.

Trigeminal Neuralgia

1. Leslie Carroll. Atypical face pain. Trigeminal Neuralgia Resources. URL: http:// neurosurgery.mgh.harvard.edu/TNR/. Accessed fall 1997.

2. Jakke Makela. TN—An introduction. Trigeminal Neuralgia Resources. URL: http://neurosurgery.mgh.harvard.edu/ TNR/. Accessed fall 1997.

3. MedicineNet: Questions and answers about trigeminal neuralgia. Information Network, Inc., 1995–1997. URL: http:// www.medicinenet.com. Accessed fall 1997.

4. Optic neuritis. Copyright 1998 ADAM Software, Inc., all rights reserved. Copyright 1998 CommuniHealth. URL: http:// healthanswers.com. Accessed winter 1998.

Seizure Disorders

1. Epilepsy. American Academy of Neurology, 1997. URL: http://www.aan.com/ public/epil.html. Accessed fall 1997.

2. Epilepsy FAQ. Epilepsy Foundation of America, August 1, 1997. URL: http://www.efa.org/FAQ/faq.htm. Accessed fall 1997.

3. Sally Squires. Warning on epilepsy drug poses dilemma: Risk of fatal blood disease must be balanced against felbamate's effectiveness against seizures. Washington Post Health, August 16, 1994, p. 7.

Circulatory System Conditions

4

OBJECTIVES

After reading this chapter, you should be able to tell . . .

- What the disorder is.
- How to recognize it.
- Whether massage is indicated or contraindicated for that condition.
- Whether a contraindication is local or systemic, or refers to a specific stage of development or healing.
- Why those choices for massage are correct.

In addition to this basic information, you should be able to . . .

- Describe the three tissue layers of most blood vessels.
- Describe the structural differences between veins and arteries.
- Name four ways in which the circulatory system works to maintain homeostasis.
- Name three varieties of anemia.
- Name two types of aortic aneurysm.
- Name four risk factors for developing atherosclerosis.
- Name three common symptoms of diabetes.
- Describe the difference between primary and secondary Raynaud's syndrome.
- Name the primary danger for complications of deep vein thrombosis.
- Name three causative factors for varicose veins.

INTRODUCTION

Most of the diseases that are contraindicated for massage are contraindicated because of the way the circulatory system works. This introduction gives a brief overview of how this system feeds, cleans, and protects the body, with a bit of emphasis on the aspects of the system that are relevant to the conditions listed in this chapter.

The body's cells are highly specialized and complex in their functioning and metabolism. The large majority of them are fixed, immobile, unable to move *toward* nutrition or *away* from toxic wastes. They depend on the circulatory system for the constant delivery of food and fuel, and the constant carrying away of garbage. Suppose a person needed someone to run to the grocery store for them *and* to flush their toilets *and* take out their trash. How long would she last if her service was interrupted? Massage can sometimes interrupt or interfere with circulatory service. If a massage therapist is going to make wise choices about to whom and when to give massage, he or she *must* have a strong understanding of how massage affects the cardiovascular system.

GENERAL FUNCTION: THE CIRCULATORY SYSTEM

The body depends on the process of *diffusion*, that random distribution of particles throughout an environment, for the exchange of nutrients and wastes. In order for diffusion to happen, a medium, an environment, must allow substances to move freely. What could be better than the combination of blood and lymph? The human body contains about six gallons of liquid. In every milliliter of this liquid, particles are flowing this way and that, chemicals are reacting, and *life* is happening.

The circulatory system, through the medium of the blood, works to *maintain homeostasis*, the tendency to maintain a stable internal environment. It does this in a number of different ways.

- Delivery of nutrients and oxygen. The blood carries nutrients and oxygen to every cell in the body. If for some reason the blood can't reach a specific area, cells in that area will starve and die. This is the situation with many disorders, including *stroke* (chapter 3, page 161), *myocardial infarction* (this chapter, page 206), and *decubitus ulcers* (chapter 1, page 36).
- Removal of waste products. While dropping off nutrients, the blood, along with lymph, simultaneously picks up the waste products generated by metabolism. These include carbon dioxide and other more noxious compounds that, left to stew in the tissues, can cause problems. Again, if blood and lymph supply to an area is limited, the affected cells can "drown" in their own waste products and be damaged or even die.
- Temperature. Superficial blood vessels dilate when it's hot, and they constrict when it's cold. Furthermore, blood prevents the hot places (the heart, the liver, working muscles) from getting too hot by flushing through and distributing the heated blood throughout the rest of the body. By keeping a steady temperature, the circulatory system maintains a *stable internal environment*.
- Clotting. This is an often overlooked but truly miraculous function of the circulatory system without which people would quickly die. Every time a rough place shows up in the endothelium of a blood vessel, a whole chain of chemical reactions result in the spinning of tiny fibers that catch cells to plug any possible gaps. Unfortunately, under certain circumstances, this reaction is sometimes more of a curse than a blessing.
- Protection from pathogens. Without white blood cells (WBCs), the body would have no defense against the hordes of microorganisms that are longing to gain access to it's precious (and precarious) internal environment. For a closer look at what actually happens to those would-be invaders, see the section in the introduction to Lymph and Immune System Conditions.
- Chemical balance. There is a very narrow margin of tolerance for variances in internal chemistry. A person can actually *die* if his or her blood gets even fifteen one-hundredths too alkaline or too acidic. Happily, blood components, including red blood cells (RBCs), are supplied with enzymes and other mechanisms specifically designed to keep pH balance within the safety zone.

Structure and Function: The Blood

ERYTHROCYTES

Almost all of the blood cells, red and white alike, are born in the red bone marrow. Red ones (erythrocytes) are created at the command of a hormone secreted by the kidneys called *erythropoietin*. RBCs are constantly being produced and dying, at a rate of about

2 million per second. They comprise 98% of all blood cells. Their life span is about four months, and during that time they do a single job: deliver oxygen to the cells and carbon dioxide to the lungs. They are so devoted to this task, they have given up their nuclei to make more room to carry their cargo. (One indicator of disease is the presence of nuclei in RBCs; this means RBCs are being released from the bone marrow prematurely.)

Red blood cells are tiny; 1 cubic milliliter of blood holds about 5 million of them. They are built around an iron-based molecule called *hemoglobin*. This molecule (250 million of them are in each RBC) is extremely efficient at carrying oxygen, slightly less so at carrying CO_2. Much of the carbon dioxide in blood is suspended in plasma, like a carbonated drink—which once prompted a student to ask why, when we jump up and down, don't we fizz up and explode. Another key quality to healthy RBCs is their shape: they are discs that are thinner in the middle than around the edges. They are very smooth, and should be flexible enough to bend and distort themselves to get through the tiniest capillaries. If for some reason they are not round, smooth, and flexible, big problems will occur.

LEUKOCYTES

Leukocytes, or white blood cells, aren't really white; they're more or less clear. Unlike RBCs, which are all identical, different classes of WBCs fight off different types of invaders in different stages of infection. Types of WBCs include neutrophils, basophils, eosinophils, monocytes, and lymphocytes. (See Figure 4.1.) More information about white blood cell function can be found in the Lymph and Immune System Conditions chapter.

PLATELETS OR THROMBOCYTES

These are not whole cells at all, but fragments of huge cells born in the red bone marrow. *Thrombo* means clot, and *cyte* means cell, so it's clear what thrombocytes do. As stated above, thrombocytes travel through the system looking for leaks or rough places in the

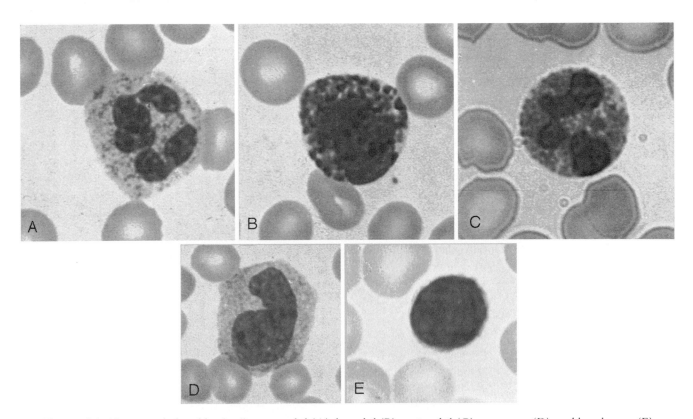

Figure 4.1. Varieties of white blood cells: neutrophil (A), basophil (B), eosinophil (C), monocyte (D), and lymphocyte (E)

blood vessels. If they should find one, a series of chemical reactions ensues that cause tiny threads of fibrin, a special protein, to be woven in the injured area. These act as a net to catch not only passing thrombocytes, but passing RBCs as well, forming a *crust* if it's on the skin, or a *clot* (*thrombus*) if it's internal. This is a good thing, it's very important, and it's usually not a problem because chemicals also circulate in the blood to *melt* clots; these are called *anticoagulants*. But under certain circumstances, this clotting mechanism has cause to overwork, which ultimately can become life threatening.

Structure and Function: The Heart

The heart is divided into left and right halves. The right half pumps blood to the lungs (the pulmonary circuit) while the left half pumps to the rest of the body (the systemic circuit). Each half of the heart is further divided into top and bottom. The small top chambers, where blood returning from the lungs and body enters, are called the atria (the singular form is *atrium* from the Latin for "entrance hall") and the larger bottom chambers are the ventricles (from the Latin for "belly"). The two-part "lub-dup" of the heartbeat is the coordinated contraction of first the atria and then the ventricles.

The cardiac muscle of the atria is much thinner and weaker than that of the ventricles. This is because the atrial contraction needs to push blood only a few centimeters downhill into the ventricles. The cardiac muscle of the ventricles, however, is much thicker and stronger than that found in the atria, because the ventricular contraction pushes blood out into the circulatory system—through the pulmonary circuit to the lungs from the right ventricle, and through the systemic circuit to the rest of the body from the left ventricle. The differences in how hard various parts of the heart have to work has great implications for the seriousness of myocardial infarctions; the location of the dead tissue determines how well the heart will function without it.

Structure and Function: Blood Vessels

The vessels *leaving* the heart are called *arteries* and *arterioles*; the vessels *going toward* the heart are called *venules* and *veins*; the vessels that connect them are called *capillaries*. Ideally this should be a closed system; that is, although WBCs are free to come and go through capillary walls, the RBCs should never be able to leave the 60,000 miles of continuous tubing that comprises the circulatory system. If they *do* leak out, it's because an injury is somewhere in the system, and a blood clot should be forming.

Arteries and veins share the same basic properties of most of the tubes in the body. They have an internal layer of epithelium (it's called *endo*thelium here, because it's on the inside); a middle layer of smooth muscle; and an external layer of tough, protective connective tissue. This combination of tissues makes these tubes strong, pliable, and stretchy.

Capillaries are delicate variations of basic tube construction. As the arteries divide into smaller arterioles, their outer layers become thinner and thinner. Finally all that is left is one layer of simple, squamous epithelium: the capillaries. This construction is ideal for the passage of substances back and forth, because most diffusion happens readily through single-cell layers. But because capillaries lack the tougher muscle and connective tissue layers of the larger tubes, they are much more vulnerable to injury.

Blood cells leave the heart through the thick-walled arteries, crowd into arterioles, and line up one by one to squeeze through the capillaries. Once they've dumped their cargo of oxygen and picked up their CO_2, they have more breathing room; now they're in the venules. Again the three-ply construction design is present, but with a difference. Much of the venous system operates against gravity. Blood flows upward in the legs, the arms, and the trunk partly by indirect pressure exerted by the heart on the arterial system, but also with the help of hydrostatic pressure and muscular contraction. To help the blood move along without backing up in the system, small epithelial flaps or *valves* line the veins. The smooth muscle layer is present here, but is thinner and weaker than in the arteries, which have to cope with much higher pressure coming directly from the heart. Veins become wider, bigger, and stronger as they approach the heart, but they are never as strong as arteries. Fortunately, the force with which blood moves through them is never as strong either.

When blood returns from the body to the heart (the systemic circuit), it then goes to the lungs to be reoxygenated (the pulmonary circuit). (See Figure 4.2.)

The chapter on cardiovascular conditions is the most self-referential portion of this book. Most of the conditions discussed here are caused by or are complications of (or both) other conditions in this chapter.

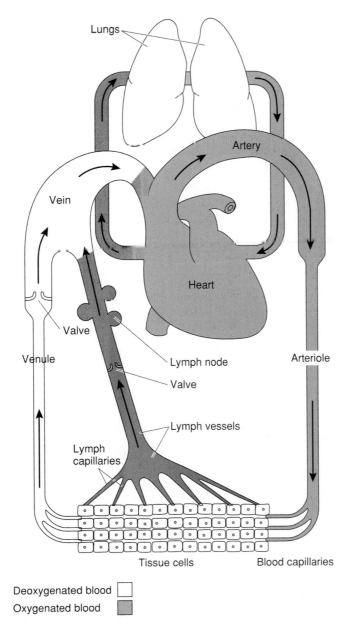

Figure 4.2. The right side of the heart pumps blood to the lungs in the pulmonary circuit. The left side of the heart pumps blood through the rest of the body in the systemic circuit.

CIRCULATORY SYSTEM CONDITIONS

Blood Disorders
  Anemia
  Embolism or Thrombus
  Hemophilia
  Hematoma
  Thrombophlebitis or Deep Vein
    Thrombosis

Vascular Disorders
  Aneurysm
  Atherosclerosis

Hypertension
Raynaud's Syndrome
Varicose Veins

Heart Conditions
  Heart Attack

Other Circulatory Conditions
  Diabetes Mellitus

Blood Disorders

Anemia

ANEMIA
Literally, "without blood." This is a bit of a misnomer because the blood volume for anemia patients may be perfectly normal. The ability of the blood to perform its function of delivering oxygen is compromised in some way.

DEFINITION: WHAT IS IT?

Anemia is the condition of having either an insufficient supply of RBCs, or an insufficient or somehow functionally impaired supply of hemoglobin within those cells, or both. In any case, "anemia" all by itself is not a diagnosis; it's a description. The diagnosis comes when one determines why there is a shortage of red blood cells or hemoglobin.

ETIOLOGY: WHAT HAPPENS?

Several different kinds of anemia exist, each with different guidelines for treatment and the appropriateness of massage. Some of the most common varieties will be examined here, with discussions of what is really happening in the body and how massage might positively or negatively affect it.

Idiopathic Anemias. These conditions, which have no well-understood cause, may be due to poor nutritional uptake because of how stress affects gastric juices, or to other more mysterious factors. But once other pathologies are ruled out, these anemias (which are usually comparatively mild) may respond well to massage.

Nutritional Anemias. These anemias occur because the body is missing something vital in its diet and no amount of massage—no matter how brilliantly administered—will replace it. However, most of these conditions will not be negatively affected by massage. The only exception to this rule is advanced cases of pernicious anemia.

- Iron deficiency anemia. Iron is the primary component of hemoglobin. An insufficiency of iron in the diet will lead to insufficiencies of hemoglobin, and then to "iron poor blood." Some controversy exists over how much iron is really necessary. Some recent research has established relationships between high iron levels and heart attacks. Evidently, excess iron

ANEMIA IN BRIEF

What is it?
Anemia is a symptom rather than a disease in itself. It indicates a shortage of red blood cells or hemoglobin or both.

How is it recognized?
Symptoms of anemia include pallor, shortness of breath, fatigue, and poor resistance to cold. Other symptoms may accompany specific varieties of anemia.

Is massage indicated or contraindicated?
Massage is indicated for idiopathic and nutritional deficiency anemias (except advanced pernicious anemia). Hemolytic, most aplastic, and secondary anemias contraindicate massage.

tends to produce oxygen-free radicals that can damage arterial walls, opening the door to *atherosclerosis* (this chapter, page 193). However, the FDA has maintained an 18 mg RDA on iron, and iron deficiency anemia is still considered the leading nutritional deficiency in the world.

- Folic acid deficiency anemia. Folic acid is a nutrient found in green leafy vegetables that is absolutely critical to the formation of red blood cells. If a person doesn't get enough, it's impossible to produce the two million cells per second needed to replace the cells that are dying. Folic acid is also water soluble. That means it can't be stored for later use; a steady fresh supply is necessary.

- B_{12} deficiency anemia. Vitamin B_{12}, or *cobalmine*, is another critical ingredient for the making of new RBCs. It is found only in animal food sources: meat and eggs. Total vegetarians must supplement their B_{12} supply or they could end up with the much more serious *pernicious anemia*.

- Pernicious anemia. Of all the nutritional anemias, this is the most serious because it can lead to irreversible damage to the central nervous system. The importance of B_{12} in the formation of red blood cells was just covered. Very few people in the United States suffer from a B_{12} deficiency, yet pernicious anemia does happen here. This is because in order to absorb B_{12}, a special chemical in gastric secretions called *intrinsic factor* is needed. Without it a person may take in all the B_{12} she requires, but her body has no access to it, and she will not produce enough erythrocytes to keep up with her needs.

  The causes behind reductions in intrinsic factor are not always understood. Sometimes it's a genetic tendency, or it may be autoimmune. Most often, though, it happens when some section of the stomach is surgically removed because of another condition. Whatever the reason, once it's gone, it's gone for good, and the affected person faces a lifetime commitment to supplementing B_{12} by injection.

  This pales in comparison to the alternative, however. B_{12} is also critical to the maintenance of the central nervous system. Left long enough without it, a person will experience the slow onset of paralysis and even brain damage. This is often irreversible, and it contraindicates massage, especially if any impairment in sensation is present.

- Other nutritional deficiencies. Anemia can be the result of shortages of several other substances, notably copper and protein. Massage will not improve this condition, and if it is very advanced (with extreme shortness of breath, fatigue, and low stamina), massage could possibly tax the already overworking heart in a dangerous way. Anemia this advanced is relatively rare, however.

Hemorrhagic Anemias. Hemorrhagic anemias are those brought about by blood loss. Usually it's from a slow leak, but occasionally it's from some trauma; this would be *acute hemorrhagic anemia*. The most common causes of hemorrhagic anemia are *ulcers* (chapter 7, page 278), heavy menstruation, and large wounds. Obviously, rigorous circulatory massage would be systemically contraindicated for bleeding ulcers and large wounds. Heavy menstruation wouldn't be badly influenced unless the therapist worked deeply in the abdomen during flow, but it is a sign that all is not right, and the client should be checked by a doctor to rule out some other disorder, such as *endometriosis* (chapter 9, page 328) or *fibroid tumors* (chapter 9, page 330).

SICKLE CELL ANEMIA AND MALARIA: A CLOSE CONNECTION

A person will have sickle cell anemia if he inherits a gene for it from *both* of his parents. If he inherits only one gene, he has the sickle cell *trait,* but not the disease. This is a crucial distinction because the sickle cell trait will usually *not* create any negative impact on the body, although some people experience a mild anemia. However, the presence of this one gene will limit the rupturing of erythrocytes during an attack of malaria!

Sickle cell genes are most often found in populations (and descendants of populations) from the Mediterranean, subtropical Africa, and Asia, otherwise called the *malarial belt*. Isn't it an amazing world?

Hemolytic Anemias.   This group of anemias involve the premature destruction of healthy red blood cells. In addition to the basic symptoms of anemia, other symptoms include *splenomegaly*—or abnormal growth of the spleen—as it works overtime to process all those dying RBCs, and the presence of reticulocytes in the blood. These are simply immature red blood cells that have not yet lost their nucleus, and therefore aren't equipped to carry the load of a normal mature cell. Reticulocytes are released from the bone marrow when the body senses that the supply of erythrocytes is becoming dangerously low.

In hemolytic anemias, the red blood cells may die for a variety of reasons, but they all leave their membrane, or "ghost," behind while their hemoglobin leaks into the blood instead of being processed in the liver as is normal. One consequence of this is the additional risk of blood clotting because of extra debris in the stream (see *embolism or thrombus*, this chapter, page 182). Furthermore, all that extra hemoglobin in the blood will break down into bilirubin, which may result in *jaundice*: a condition that can have a profound impact on the liver (see chapter 7, page 299).

Causes of hemolytic anemia range from genetics (sickle cell is an example of this) to allergic reactions to certain drugs to malaria.

- Sickle cell anemia. This is a special type of hemolytic anemia in which the hemoglobin molecules (remember, 250 million in each red blood cell) are not normal. They deteriorate after delivering their load of oxygen, which eventually leads to the collapse of the cell into the characteristic "sickle" shape. (See Figure 4.3.) Symptoms and complications of sickle cell anemia include blood that is viscous and prone to clotting; joint pain; *meningitis* (chapter 3, page 146); *seizures* (chapter 3, page 166); *stroke* (chapter 3, page 161); and several varieties of organ damage from blockages caused by blood clots. Trauma or infection can bring on extremely painful sickle cell "crises" when the body may suffer yet more damage from the sticky, lumpy blood flow. No cure exists for this condition; treatment is limited to addressing the symptoms alone. The average age of death for a man with sickle cell anemia is 42; for women, it's 46.

    Circulatory massage for any kind of hemolytic anemia is contraindicated.

Aplastic Anemia.   In aplastic anemia, bone marrow is sluggish or even completely inactive. The production of every kind of blood cell is suspended. When this moment's two million cells report to the spleen for destruction, no new RBCs replace them. Likewise, there are no new WBCs, so resistance to infection goes way down. And finally, the stream of thrombocytes has dried up too, making persons with aplastic anemia prone to uncontrolled bleeding.

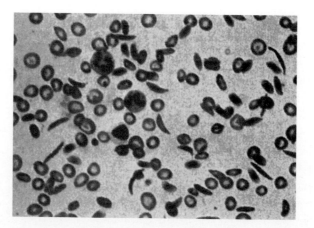

Figure 4.3. Sickle cell anemia

Aplastic anemia can be caused by bone marrow tumors, autoimmune disease, renal failure, folate deficiency, certain viral infections, exposure to some types of radiation, and some poisons. Bone marrow transplants have proven fairly successful at solving the problem if it's caught early.

Massage is probably contraindicated for aplastic anemia, especially if it includes a cancerous situation, but it's worth checking with the primary care physician. Someone with bone marrow inhibited by toxic exposure or radiation may be able to benefit from massage, but this client's immune system may be severely compromised. A massage therapist should work with this kind of client only after checking with the primary care physician, and only when feeling perfectly healthy herself.

Secondary Anemias.   Anemia is a frequent complication of other disorders. Sometimes a direct cause and effect relationship is apparent, and sometimes the association is a less obvious one, though still present. Here is a partial list of some of the conditions that anemia frequently accompanies.

- Ulcers. Gastric, duodenal, and colonic ulcers can all bleed internally. This might not be very obvious, but it results in a steady draining of red blood cells which can impair general oxygen uptake and energy levels. This is a description of the *hemorrhagic anemias* discussed above.
- Leukemia. There are two basic types of leukemia, with further subdivisions within them. One type involves the bone marrow that is supposed to be producing healthy *granulocytes*, a type of white blood cell. But what comes out instead are useless cells that have no immune function, that outlive normal WBCs, and that interfere with other body processes. Eventually the white-to-red blood cell ratio is disturbed. The bone marrow tumors can also grow to interfere with the cells that produce red blood cells and platelets. The appropriateness of massage for this and other cancerous conditions is controversial. See *cancer,* chapter 10, page 358.
- Kidney disease. The capillaries inside the kidneys have a tremendous workload. Not only are they filtering toxins and maintaining water balance, they are doing so under tremendous mechanical pressure from the renal arteries. Sometimes the kidney capillaries become damaged and leak red blood cells into the urine. Again, it's a leak not a gusher, but just as that dripping faucet will drive up a person's water bill, a leaking kidney will slowly but surely drain away viable red blood cells. Massage is systemically contraindicated for most kidney disorders (see chapter 8, page 314).
- Hepatitis. The liver contributes vital proteins to the blood, and it is responsible, along with the spleen, for breaking down and recycling the hemoglobin from dead erythrocytes. If liver function is disrupted for any reason, the quality and amount of hemoglobin available to new red blood cells may suffer. Massage is systemically contraindicated for acute hepatitis. (See *hepatitis,* chapter 7, page 296.)
- Acute infectious disease. For reasons that are not entirely clear, anemia seems to be a sign or indicator that the body is under attack. It is a frequent follower of pneumonia, tuberculosis, and rheumatoid arthritis. It's as if the body is so busy defending itself (even against itself), that new RBC production takes a back seat. Anemia in these cases usually clears up spontaneously once the primary condition has been resolved. Certainly massage is contraindicated until the primary condition has been resolved.

SIGNS AND SYMPTOMS

No matter what the cause of anemia is, some symptoms are dependable. These include . . .

- Pallor. Pallor is present because of either a reduced amount of RBCs or a reduced amount of hemoglobin to carry the oxygen, which gives the RBCs their color. Pallor is visible in the skin, and also in mucous membranes, gums, and nail beds. In dark skinned people, pallor shows as an ashy-gray appearance to the skin.

- Dyspnea. This is a fancy way of saying shortness of breath. Why is this a symptom of anemia? Because with less oxygen-carrying capacity, a person has to breathe harder and more often just to keep up. That's why another sign of anemia is a higher respiratory rate.
- Palpitations. This doesn't actually mean the heart is beating irregularly; it means it's probably beating faster and harder, and a person is more aware of it. Another term for this is *tachycardia*.
- Fatigue. Often this is the first noticeable symptom of anemia. The body simply has less oxygen to go around, so muscles wear out sooner and stamina is nonexistent. Unfortunately, a host of other conditions make a person feel worn out, so this is rarely enough for a whole diagnosis.
- Intolerance to cold. Oxygen is needed for muscle contraction and for heat production. Someone who is in short supply of oxygen will run out of steam in a hurry.

TREATMENT

Treatments, when applicable, are discussed within the descriptions of different types of anemia above.

MASSAGE?

The appropriateness of massage is addressed within the descriptions of different types of anemia above. Very advanced anemia of any kind is fairly rare. However, if the blood is especially low in hemoglobin or oxygen, the heart has to work extremely hard to pump the diminished supply through the body. For this reason, very advanced anemia of any kind contraindicates massage.

Embolism or Thrombus

EMBOLISM OR THROMBUS IN BRIEF

What are they?
Thrombi are stationary clots; emboli are clots that travel through the circulatory system. Emboli are usually composed of blood, but may also be fragments of plaque, fat globules, air bubbles, tumors, or bone chips.

How are they recognized?
Venous emboli land in the lungs, causing pulmonary embolism. Symptoms of PE include shortness of breath, chest pain, and coughing up sputum that is streaked with blood.

Arterial emboli can lodge in coronary arteries (heart attack), the brain (transient ischemic attack or stroke), kidneys, legs, or some other organ.

Is massage indicated or contraindicated?
Massage is systemically contraindicated in the presence of diagnosed thrombi or emboli, as it is for any disorder involving potential blood clots.

DEFINITION: WHAT ARE THEY?

An embolism is a traveling clot or collection of debris, and thrombus is a lodged clot. (See Figure 4.4.) Emboli and thrombi are part and parcel of the whole interrelated cardiovascular disease picture. They can cause heart trouble, and heart trouble can cause them.

ETIOLOGY: WHAT HAPPENS?

Blood leaves the left ventricle of the heart and goes to its destination in the body through smaller and smaller vessels: arteries, arterioles, capillaries. Nutrient-waste exchange happens at the capillary level, and then the vessels become larger as they zoom back toward the right atrium: venules, veins, and the vena cava. The same telescoping action happens in the pulmonary circuit: blood leaves the right ventricle through the huge pulmonary artery, and vessels going into the lungs become smaller and smaller. Oxygen and carbon dioxide are exchanged through capillaries in the lungs, and the freshly oxygenated blood goes back toward the heart through venules, veins, and finally the large pulmonary vein. (See Figure 4.2.)

Jagged-edged platelets constantly flow through the circulatory system looking for rough spots, which indicate injury. If they find something to stick to (i.e., a disruption in

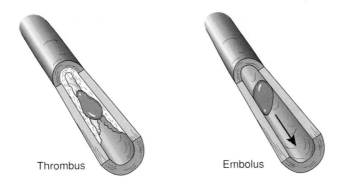

Thrombus   Embolus

Figure 4.4. A thrombus is a lodged clot and an embolism is a moving clot.

the walls of the blood vessels), they will. Then they start releasing the chemicals that cause blood proteins to weave fibers, making a net to catch other blood cells, and a clot is formed. Clots can also form in places where blood doesn't flow quickly; the clotting factors will accumulate enough to thicken the fluid even without platelets initiating the action. This is a danger in *aneurysms* (this chapter, page 190), and it's also a danger with atrial fibrillation, a condition in which the atria don't contract efficiently and blood tends to pool and thicken before moving into the ventricles.

The construction of the circulatory system is such that no passageway is large enough for a clot to move from the arterial side of the pulmonary circuit to the arterial side of the systemic circuit. Clots can form on the pulmonary side or the systemic side, and where they form will determine what kind of damage can happen.

Pulmonary Embolism

The lungs are the one and only destination for venous clots formed anywhere in the systemic circuit. When something, usually a sudden movement after prolonged immobility, knocks any clot in any vein loose, it will jet toward the heart in increasingly bigger tubes. It will make the rounds of the right atrium and ventricle, get into the pulmonary artery, and end up in the lungs. *Where* the embolism stops moving depends on how big it is. Size is also the deciding factor in how much damage is done. This can vary from a temporary loss of a tiny bit of lung function to total circulatory collapse when suddenly little or no blood returns to the heart from the lungs.

Every year about 5 out of every 10,000 people in the United States suffer a pulmonary embolism. Many of them resolve spontaneously. But 30% of those people whose embolisms are not diagnosed or treated will die. This condition is usually a complication of *thrombophlebitis or deep vein thrombosis* (this chapter, page 187).

RISK FACTORS

Risk factors for pulmonary embolism include other types of cardiovascular disease, extended bed rest, oral contraceptives, and any kind of surgery, although surgeries for femur and hip fractures have a particularly high embolism rate.

Women in advanced stages of *pregnancy* (chapter 9, page 347) are also at high risk for pulmonary embolism, as the weight of the uterus on the femoral vessels can cause blood to pool and thicken in the legs.

SIGNS AND SYMPTOMS

Classic symptoms of pulmonary embolism include difficulty breathing, chest pains, and coughing with bloody sputum. Other symptoms that may or may not be present are shortness of breath, lightheadedness, fainting, dizziness, rapid heart beat, and sweating.

TREATMENT

Treatment of non–life threatening pulmonary embolism situations is usually an aggressive course of anticoagulants and attention to the cause of the deep vein thrombosis. If it is a major embolism, surgery may be required to vacuum it out of the lung.

PREVENTION

Recent efforts have been made to identify especially high-risk patients in hospital settings, in order to take steps to prevent the formation of emboli in the first place. Preventative measures include low-dose anticoagulants starting shortly before surgery, tight stockings on the legs, elevation of the legs, external compression on the legs, and early ambulation following surgery.

Arterial Embolism

This is one of the many complications of *atherosclerosis* (this chapter, page 193). Emboli in the arteries can also be a complication of bacterial infection, atrial fibrillation, or rheumatic heart disease, which can create clots inside the heart. Emboli can be made of some foreign object in the bloodstream such as a bit of plaque, a bone chip, an air bubble, or a knot of cancer cells.

The main difference between arterial and venous emboli is the final resting place. If the clot is somewhere in the systemic arterial system, it could wind up virtually anywhere, *except* the lungs. Therefore the damage it will cause will be very different. The brain, the heart, the kidneys, and the legs are statistically the most common sites for arterial emboli to lodge.

SIGNS AND SYMPTOMS

Symptoms of emboli in organs may be nonexistent until significant loss of function is noticed in the affected tissue. This is particularly dangerous in the kidneys, where clots can come to rest somewhere in the renal arteries. If the legs are affected, however, the patient will quickly notice sharp, tingling pain, followed by numbness, weakness, coldness, and blueness. Left untreated, this tissue will develop gangrene (that is, it will start to die off) in a matter of hours; immediate medical attention is necessary.

If the embolism lodges in the brain, it is called a *transient ischemic attack* if the symptoms are short-lived, and a *stroke* (chapter 3, page 161) if they're more serious. And finally, if it lodges in a coronary artery, it's called a *heart attack* (this chapter, page 206).

TREATMENT

If a person has a tendency to form clots easily, anticoagulant medications may be prescribed in order to circumvent the complications of heart attack or stroke.

MASSAGE?

The tendency to form thrombi or emboli is a situation that systemically contraindicates rigorous circulatory massage. Lodged thrombi are a medical emergency. *If* a person knows an embolism is present in either the venous or arterial sides of the system, he should be under strict treatment. People who are taking blood thinners because of a tendency for clotting need medical clearance before receiving any massage that impacts the circulatory system.

Hemophilia

HEMOPHILIA
This word comes from the Greek *haima*, or "blood," and *philos* or "fond." Hemophiliacs were called, essentially, "blood lovers," probably because their blood had a tendency to seep away uncontrollably.

DEFINITION: WHAT IS IT?

This is a genetic disorder involving the absence of some plasma proteins that are crucial in the clot-forming process. Anyone who has studied Russian history has at least a vague idea about this disease; the last ruling family in Russia, the Romanovs, had it in their genes, and because it weakened the Royal Family, hemophilia influenced the course of world history.

Hemophilia is actually a collection of different types of genetic disorders, each one of them affecting a different clotting factor in the blood. Their presentations are all much the same, however, so the only people who need to know *which* type of hemophilia is present are the patients themselves, and the people who administer clotting factors after a bleeding episode.

DEMOGRAPHICS: WHO GETS IT?

In this country, hemophilia affects about 20,000 men. About 1 in every 4,000 live male babies will have hemophilia. The disease is carried on the X chromosome of female genes, but almost always affects males. One mild variety, called Von Willebrand's disease, affects women as well.

SIGNS AND SYMPTOMS

Hemophilia first appears in childhood. Extensive bruising and bleeding occurs with very mild irritation, and small scrapes and lesions tend to bleed for a long time. Hemophiliacs don't bleed *faster* than normal, but they do bleed *longer*. As the person matures, he will find that he is prone to subcutaneous bleeding (bruising), intramuscular hemorrhaging (see *hematoma*, this chapter, page 186), nosebleeds, blood in the urine (hematuria), and severe joint pain brought about by hemorrhaging in joint cavities. Bleeding episodes may follow minor trauma, or they may occur spontaneously.

Hemophilia is rated mild, moderate, or severe, depending on what percentage of normal levels of clotting factors the patient has. Severe hemophiliacs have less than 1% of normal levels.

COMPLICATIONS

Bleeding into joint cavities is the main problem for people with hemophilia today. Unless clotting factors are administered very soon after an episode, the blood inside the joint may collect and become very difficult for the body to reabsorb. This can lead to debilitating *arthritis* (chapter 2, page 80).

Infected blood products have been another major worry for people with hemophilia. At one time, contracting HIV was a significant risk for hemophiliacs. A specific variety of hepatitis virus has also posed a threat; it could result in chronic low-grade hepatitis, or flare to complete liver failure (see *hepatitis*, chapter 7, page 296). New screening and blood treatment techniques have eradicated those risks, and the blood supply available today is the safest in history.

TREATMENT

Treatment protocols for people with hemophilia have taken giant leaps forward in the past 30 years. Before 1965, the only treatment available was transfusions of whole blood: a time-consuming and inefficient means of replacing clotting factors for someone experiencing an internal hemorrhage. Consequently, most hemophiliacs were in wheelchairs by their teens, and their life expectancy was much shorter than the norm. In 1965, techniques were developed to isolate the specific missing clotting factors, allowing a much more efficient treatment. More recently, these clotting factors have been manufactured in

---

HEMOPHILIA IN BRIEF

What is it?
Hemophilia is a genetic disorder in which certain clotting factors in the blood are either inactive or missing altogether.

How is it recognized?
Hemophilia can cause superficial bleeding that persists for longer than normal, or internal bleeding into joint cavities or between muscle sheaths with little or no provocation.

Is massage indicated or contraindicated?
Massage is systemically contraindicated for most cases of hemophilia unless the case is very mild and the client gets medical clearance.

a form that can be self-administered, which radically increases a hemophiliac's independence and ability to work and travel.

All this comes at tremendous cost, however. It is estimated that the average annual bill for clotting factor replacement alone is $10,000. Further expenses for complications, hospitalizations, infections, and surgery can increase the cost of having hemophilia to $100,000 a year or more—and that's if the person doesn't have HIV or hepatitis. Furthermore, while hemophilia patients in industrialized countries may receive adequate care, it is estimated that 80% or more of the total world population with hemophilia doesn't have such access.

MASSAGE?

Mechanical, circulatory massage is contraindicated for people with moderate to severe hemophilia; people who have been diagnosed with a mild case should get medical clearance. Although the mechanisms that cause "spontaneous bleeds" in hemophiliacs are largely unknown, massage therapists should not put themselves in the position of being even indirectly responsible for tissue damage to a client. Energetic and noncirculatory techniques may be appropriate.

Hematoma

DEFINITION: WHAT IS IT?

This term refers to both extensive bleeding between muscle sheaths and to capillary seepage that causes deep and superficial bruising. Although the size and seriousness of these two conditions vary widely, their treatment guidelines are very much the same, so they will be considered together here.

HEMATOMA IN BRIEF

What is it?
A hematoma is a deep bruise (leakage of blood) between muscle sheaths.

How is it recognized?
Superficial hematomas are simple bruises. Deep bleeds may not be visible, but they will be painful, and if extensive bleeding is present, the affected tissue will have a characteristic "gel-like" feel.

Is massage indicated or contraindicated?
Massage is locally contraindicated for acute hematomas because of the possibility of blood clots and pain. In the subacute stage (at least two days later), when the surrounding blood vessels have been sealed shut and the body is in the process of breaking down and reabsorbing the debris, gentle massage within pain tolerance around the perimeter of the area and hydrotherapy can be helpful. Watch for signs of thrombophlebitis or deep vein thrombosis (this chapter, page 187), and if there is any doubt, consult a doctor.

SIGNS AND SYMPTOMS

Bruises are reddish or purplish (or black and blue) in the acute stage. They fade to yellowish green in the subacute stage, when the local macrophages have migrated in to clean up the debris. The processes for cleaning up capillary leaks deeper than the skin, for instance in a gastrocnemius that has been kicked, are invisible but otherwise identical.

Larger bleeds can involve quite a bit of inflammation along with discoloration. They can occur when an arteriole between deep muscle layers is injured. It will pour blood into an area until local pressure closes it off. A large acute hematoma feels like hot, half-congealed gelatin under the muscle layers, and it will be quite painful to the touch. They happen most often in large fleshy areas like the calf or buttocks.

A special variety of hematomas (subdural hematomas) happen in the brain; this is covered in *stroke* (chapter 3, page 161).

TREATMENT

Small bruises require no medical intervention, although they respond well to alternating hot and cold applications, which stimulate macrophages to come into the area and flush wastes from the tissue damage away. Larger bleeds, however, can be more complicated. If they're caught relatively early, they can be aspirated or drained, but if they're left too long they will have a tendency to congeal from the concentration of clotting factors in the blood. At that point, only time, hydrotherapy, and gentle movement will help to break up the pooled blood into a form that the body can reabsorb. An occasional complication of hematoma is *myositis ossificans* (see chapter 2, page 54).

MASSAGE?

Hematomas and bruises contraindicate local massage in the acute stage because of pain and the possibility of disturbing blood clots. In the subacute stages (at least two days after the injury occurs), the local blood vessels will be sealed off. Gentle massage may be appropriate around the edges of the lesions, always within the tolerance of the client. Watch for signs of *thrombophlebitis or deep vein thrombosis* (this chapter, page 187), which contraindicates massage.

Thrombophlebitis or Deep Vein Thrombosis

DEFINITION: WHAT ARE THEY?

Thrombophlebitis and deep vein thrombosis (DVT) refer to inflammation of a vein caused by clots. Usually thrombophlebitis is a term used for superficial veins, while deep vein thrombosis is much the same problem in a deeper vein. These clots can form anywhere in the venous system, but they are most often in the calves, thighs, and occasionally in the pelvis.

DEMOGRAPHICS: WHO GETS IT?

The clots of thrombophlebitis and DVT happen more commonly in women than in men, and they are especially associated with the elderly and the overweight. About 2 out of every 1000 people will experience thrombophlebitis at some point; it usually affects people over 60 years old.

ETIOLOGY: WHAT HAPPENS?

These conditions should be major concerns for well-trained massage practitioners. They involve thrombi—stationary clots—somewhere in the veinous system, where, if they break loose, nothing will stop them from traveling straight into the lungs, causing pulmonary embolism (see *embolism or thrombus*, this chapter, page 182).

CAUSES

The causes of thrombophlebitis and DVT can be many and varied. Any circumstance in which there is venous stasis (slowed movement of venous blood), increased coagulability, or blood vessel damage will increase the chances of developing this problem. Here are a few of the most common preciptitators of thrombophlebitis or DVT:

- Physical trauma. Being kicked or hit in the leg can damage the delicate venous tissue, which will then be prone to clot formation. Athletes are particularly vulnerable to this problem.
- Varicose veins (this chapter, page 204). These are another risk factor, since they, too, involve damaged tissue and the risk of clot formation.

> ## THROMBOPHLEBITIS OR DEEP VEIN THROMBOSIS IN BRIEF
>
> **What is it?**
> Thrombophlebitis and deep vein thrombosis (DVT) are inflammations of veins due to blood clots.
>
> **How is it recognized?**
> Symptoms for thrombophlebitis may or may not include pain, heat, redness, swelling, and local itchiness, and a hard cord-like feeling at the affected vein. Symptoms for DVT are often more extreme: possibly pitting edema distal to the site, often with discoloration, and intermittent or continuous pain that is exacerbated by activity or standing still for a long period of time.
>
> **Is massage indicated or contraindicated?**
> Massage is strictly systemically contraindicated for thrombophlebitis or deep vein thrombosis.

DEEP VEIN THROMBOSIS: CASE HISTORY

Anne, age 67

"It was just a broken knee!"

Anne is a retired schoolteacher who spends her winters in Arizona and summers in the mountains of Colorado. In May, one week after she had moved to her summer home, she took a bad fall over a curb and sustained a lateral plateau fracture to the tibia of her left leg: a leg with which she had a history of varicose veins and phlebitis.

Because her health maintenance organization was out of state (in Arizona), it was reluctant to cover any treatment for conditions not considered "life threatening." For that reason, Anne, a mildly overweight, moderate smoker, spent three weeks sitting in a chair all day at 10,000 feet of altitude (which thickens the blood because less oxygen is in the air). She was unable to move except with the use of a walker. Her broken knee was never set or seen by an orthopedist.

Eventually the swelling in the leg became so severely painful that she sought out a general practitioner in the Colorado town. He sent her to a local hospital for an ultrasound, which revealed a blood clot from her ankle to her groin. She immediately checked into the hospital and was put on anticoagulant medication.

Four days later she was sent home. Still basically immobile, but taking anticoagulants, she returned to sitting in her chair with her leg elevated for 12 to 14 hours a day. On her second night home, she woke in the night with severe chest pains and shortness of breath. The emergency medical team took her back to the hospital where it was revealed that she had thrown a large clot to the lung: a pulmonary embolism. At this point, her condition was too severe to be treated at a small rural hospital. After two days in the intensive care unit, she was transferred to a larger facility about 100 miles away where a filter was inserted into her vena cava to prevent any further clots from reaching her lungs.

When she checked out of the second hospital, she was prescribed supplemental oxygen to compensate for the loss of lung function and the high altitude. She used an oxygen tank for several weeks, and had to quit smoking in the process. Several months later, Anne has no severe pain in her knee, but it is constantly achy. She limps when she gets tired, which happens easily; her energy level never quite returned to what it used to be.

- Local infection. This can cause clots inside of veins.
- Reduced circulation. Physical restriction, such as too-tight socks or immobility, can cause the clotting factors in the blood to accumulate in amounts that will cause coagulation even without damage to a vessel wall.
- Pregnancy (chapter 9, page 347). In the advanced stages, pregnancy can increase risk when the weight of the fetus on femoral vessels slows blood return.
- Diseases. Diseases particularly disposed to complicate into thrombophlebitis or DVT are polycythemia and *sickle cell anemia* (this chapter, page 178). Both of these involve blood that is viscous, sticky, and not free-flowing.
- Surgery. This is another major risk for DVT. In fact, thrombosis and subsequent pulmonary embolism is the leading cause of death for orthopedic surgery, especially for knee and hip replacements. Heart and any kind of gynecological surgery also hold high risks for thrombosis.
- High-estrogen birth control pills. These can increase the risk of developing blood clots.

The majority of blood clots causing DVT or thrombophlebitis form in the lower legs, but the majority of clots that break off and go to the lungs originate in the thigh or pelvis. Sudden movement or change in position is often the factor that will cause part of a clot to detach and become a pulmonary embolism. Another alarming fact is that a patient who is immobile because of some leg injury is almost as likely to throw a clot from the *uninjured* leg as she is from the injured side. This is because lack of ambulation can thicken the blood systemically, even where no damage to blood vessels exists.

SIGNS AND SYMPTOMS

Thrombophlebitis can show the major signs of inflammation: pain, heat, redness, swelling. Along with those, sometimes it is accompanied by itchiness, a hard cord where the vein is affected, and edema with discoloration distal to the area. (See Figure 4.5.) If it is caused by a local infection, a general fever and illness will be present as well. The trick is that although thrombophlebitis *may* show these signs, it may *not* as well. A client may complain of an ache deep in her calf that she really wants "worked out." This is a reasonable request except the massage therapist may "work out" a blood clot that will land the client in the hospital with the other 650,000 pulmonary embolism cases this year.

Deep vein thrombosis is considered the most dangerous of these two conditions, because the clots in deeper veins can be big enough to do more serious damage in the lungs. It usually shows much greater swelling and edema than thrombophlebitis, because the clot will inhibit blood flow back to the heart. The backup will force extra fluid out of the capillaries and into the interstitial spaces, thus adding general edema to any localized swelling

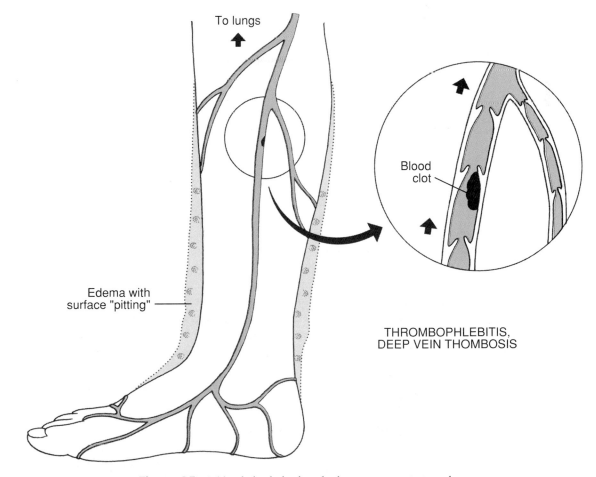

To lungs

Blood clot

Edema with
surface "pitting"

THROMBOPHLEBITIS,
DEEP VEIN THOMBOSIS

Figure 4.5. A blood clot lodged in the leg can cause pitting edema.

of the vein. Often the capillary exchange will become so sluggish that the edema will "pit," or leave a little dimple wherever it's touched. Pitting edema is a huge red flag for massage therapists. It is an indication that this person's circulation is absolutely not capable of dealing with the internal changes brought about by massage.

Occasionally deep vein thrombosis will develop in the pelvis. In this case, no obvious symptoms may be present until a piece of the clot detaches and travels to the lung.

DIAGNOSIS

Thrombophlebitis and DVT can be diagnosed in a couple of ways, each with inherent benefits and disadvantages. Ultrasound is a fast and noninvasive technique, but it tends to yield a lot of "false positives," leading to unneccesary prescriptions of anticoagulants that can lead to risks of uncontrolled bleeding. Venography—injecting the blood vessel with dye and watching how it moves through the system—can be more accurate, but it is slow and the injection itself can damage delicate tissue.

TREATMENT

The treatment for both of these conditions is anticoagulants. The risk is that these chemicals will make a person very prone to heavy bleeding: another caution for massage. If the patient is bedridden, a pneumatic compression may be used: a machine will mimic the pumping action of exercise by inflating and deflating a tubular balloon around the affected leg. Support hose to prevent the accumulation of postoperative edema are sometimes recommended.

For high-risk patients who have clotting disorders that make anticoagulants prohibitive, a special filter may be implanted in the vena cava to prevent clots from reaching the lungs.

Thrombosis that occurs as a surgical complication is undergoing close scrutiny now. Doctors hope to be able to prevent the clots from forming, and therefore to eradicate the risk of pulmonary embolism. Prophylactic preoperative doses of anticoagulants are being investigated as one prevention measure. Interestingly, the stress of dealing with postoperative pain contributes to the formation of clots (increased clotting factors in the blood is part of the sympathetic reaction) so increased and more efficient methods of pain control are being found to reduce the rates of postoperative DVT.

MASSAGE?

Massage is systemically contraindicated for thrombophlebitis and DVT. Unfortunately, it's a common enough problem that most massage therapists probably *will* run across it someday.

It is not possible to absolutely rule out phlebitis when a client complains of deep calf pain, but one sign that may help is this: passive dorsiflexion of the foot will cause pain with DVT; this is called "Homan's sign." Passive dorsiflexion may also cause pain with a muscular injury, but *so will resisted plantarflexion*, although it may take a good deal of resistance to get a positive sign, since the calf muscles are so strong. Resisted dorsiflexion should not cause pain with a DVT.

Vascular Disorders

Aneurysm

DEFINITION: WHAT IS IT?

An aneurysm is a permanent bulge in the wall of an artery brought about by any combination of genetically weak smooth muscle tissue, high blood pressure, atherosclerosis, and compromised connective tissue. Aneurysms are potentially quite serious and worth knowing about because some types of massage on an aneurysm patient could put that person at great risk.

ETIOLOGY: WHAT HAPPENS?

The three-ply construction of the arteries has already been discussed: the endothelial inside layer, the smooth muscle middle layer, and the tough connective tissue outer layer. The blood pressure in the aorta, the largest artery, is very high. If those muscle and connective tissue layers are somehow impaired, they can bulge wide with blood. This bulge is an aneurysm. Nothing short of surgery will ever make it recede. As the aneurysm swells, the walls will stretch and become weaker, increasing the risk of rupture and subsequent death.

Aneurysms happen most often (75%) in the abdominal aorta and at the base of the brain. Thoracic aneurysms are usually associated with specific diseases such as Marfan's syndrome, which frequently exhibits a congenital weakness of the aorta. Occasionally aneurysms will appear in more distal vessels, but those cases are generally much less serious because the blood pressure pushing on the vessels further away from the heart is much lower.

> ## ANEURYSM IN BRIEF
>
> ### What is it?
> An aneurysm is a delicate dilation or outpouching in an artery, usually part of the aorta or at the base of the brain.
>
> ### How is it recognized?
> Symptoms of aneurysms are hard to pin down. Thoracic aneurysms may cause chronic hoarseness; abdominal aneurysms may cause local discomfort, reduced urine output, or severe backache. Cerebral aneurysms may be silent, or may cause extreme headache when they are at very high risk for rupture.
>
> ### Is massage indicated or contraindicated?
> Massage is systemically contraindicated for diagnosed aneurysms, and is strongly cautioned for clients who fit the profile for aneurysms, but have not been diagnosed.

CAUSES

Several different factors can contribute to the chances of developing an aneurysm:

* Compromised smooth muscle. Atherosclerotic plaques will invade and weaken aortal muscle (see *atherosclerosis*, this chapter, page 193). Aortic aneurysms are a serious complication of atherosclerosis and *hypertension* (this chapter, page 199).
* Congenitally weak arterial wall muscle. Sometimes the tissue simply isn't strong enough to put up with normal blood pressure, and with no warning an aneurysm can rupture. This happens most often in the arteries at the base of the brain. When a high school basketball player drops dead on the court, this is usually the kind of situation that causes it. (See *stroke*, chapter 3, page 161.)
* Inflammation. A few diseases, such as polyarteritis nodosa or bacterial endocarditis, can cause inflammation of the aortal tissue. These will weaken the tissue to the extent that aneurysms may occur. Fortunately, these conditions are relatively rare; it is unlikely that someone with them will come looking for massage.
* Trauma. Mechanical injury to a vessel may sometimes damage the outer layers while leaving the inner one intact. This will result in the characteristic bulging and stretching of the most delicate arterial tissue.

TYPES OF ANEURYSMS

Aneurysms come in a variety of shapes and sizes, some of which are particular to where the lesion occurs. (See Figure 4.6.)

* Saccular. These are usually the case with thoracic or abdominal aortic aneurysms. The aortal wall bulges like a small (or large) rounded sack that throbs and pushes against neighboring organs and other structures.
* Fusiform. This is also common for aortic aneurysms; in this case, the bulge is less round and more tubular, as if the aorta were widened like a sausage for a few inches.

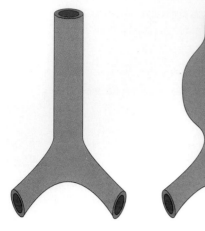

Normal artery   Artery with aneurysm

Common types of aneurysms

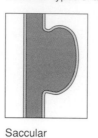
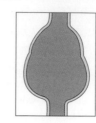
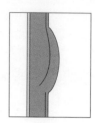

Saccular   Fusiform   Dissecting

Figure 4.6. There are several different types of aneurysms.

- Berry. This is a term for several small aneurysms clustered together in the brain.
- Dissecting. This is the least common and most painful type of aneurysm. Again affecting the aorta, in this situation the blood pressure actually *splits* the layers of the blood vessel. It can happen between the tunica intima (innermost layer) and the tunica media (muscular layer), or between the tunica media and the adventitia (outer layer). In some cases, this type of aneurysm can seal itself off when the blood trapped inside the split coagulates and solidifies.

SIGNS AND SYMPTOMS

Aneurysms can be difficult to identify by symptoms because they often aren't painful until they are actually a medical emergency. This is certainly true of cerebral aneurysms. The swelling of aortic aneurysms may create some warning signals, usually when the bulge is pressing on something else or interfering with another organ's functioning. Thoracic aneurysms will sometimes create difficulty with swallowing (*dysphagia*), chest pain, hoarseness, and coughing that is not relieved with medication, because the protrusion is pressing on and irritating the larynx. Abdominal aneurysms will sometimes show as a throbbing lump, loss of appetite, weight loss, reduced urine output, and, if it's pushing against the spine, severe backache.

This should be extremely alarming to massage therapists! How is a person supposed to tell if a client's backache is from a muscle spasm or an abdominal aneurysm? That's why it's vital to take a complete history before a first massage session. People with aneurysms will generally have a history of heart disease, atherosclerosis, and/or high blood pressure. If a client fits the profile for an aneurysm, explain to him that, for his own benefit, he needs medical clearance before receiving massage.

DIAGNOSIS

Thoracic and abdominal aneurysms are sometimes diagnosed by accident, when a patient undergoes ultrasound testing for some other reason, and the test shows abnormal widening of the aorta. Otherwise they are diagnosed by angiograms: dye is injected into the blood, and its progress through the vessels is tracked on screen.

COMPLICATIONS

For those rare aneurysms that are not in the aorta or the brain, no serious complications may accompany them unless they become large enough to impede blood flow, which can lead to gangrene. The more typical aneurysm will at the very least press against its neighbors, which can be uncomfortable or even interfere with function; for example, aneurysms in the ascending aorta pressing against the larynx. The good news is that this may be the first sign of trouble. If the bulge is stable and blood pools in it for any length of time, it can help to form clots as the stagnant blood congeals and then finds its way back into the stream again. (See *embolism or thrombus*, this chapter, page 182.) And of course, *a rupture could always occur*, which would lead to hemorrhaging in the best case and shock followed by collapse of the circulatory system in the worst case. Of all people whose aneurysms rupture, 75 to 80% will die as a result.

TREATMENT

Surgery is generally the treatment for aneurysms. They don't spontaneously retreat, because the pressure that caused them never really lets up, especially if extensive tissue damage results. Surgery involves clamping off the artery above and below the lesion, and attaching either a replacement graft or a dacron substitute to the two ends. This is usually successful, but it has to be done *before* a rupture occurs. Some thoracic aortic aneurysms are simply inoperable.

Controversy surrounds the question of when surgery for aneurysm should be performed. Normal aortic size is about 2 cm; a dangerously distended aneurysm is about 5 to 6 cm. Many doctors recommend checking aneurysm size by ultrasound every 6 months until it is big enough to pose a serious threat.

A new technique being developed will insert a replacement tube at the site of an aneurysm without major surgery, in much the same way angioplasties are performed. At this point, this procedure is useful only for the small percentage of aneurysm patients whose bulges are the right size and in the right place, but it may well be developed to apply to more people.

MASSAGE?

If a massage therapist works on a client who subsequently experiences a ruptured aneurysm and dies, the therapist could be held responsible. Even if the aneurysm might have eventually ruptured regardless of massage, it is important to avoid raising even the *possibility* that massage might be responsible for a client's death.

Any condition involving damaged blood vessels requires extreme caution for massage. *Massage changes the internal environment.* It dilates some blood vessels and constricts others. It reroutes circulation mechanically through compression and friction on the skin, via the parasympathetic nervous system, and by changing hormonal balance (reducing adrenalin), which shifts blood from the skeletal muscles (a sympathetic state) to the internal organs (a parasympathetic state). If a client can't tolerate the radical shift of his internal environment in terms of blood vessel dilation, chemical distribution, and autonomic state, he isn't a good candidate for massage.

Atherosclerosis

DEFINITION: WHAT IS IT?

Atherosclerosis is a condition in which lipid deposits infiltrate and weaken layers of large blood vessels, particularly the aorta. It is compounded by the fact that damage to the aorta can cause it to spasm, while blood clots will form at the site of these deposits. These features contribute to the restriction of the diameter, or *lumen* of the blood vessel, as well as to the risk of creating and loosening blood clots in the system.

DEMOGRAPHICS: WHO GETS IT?

Random samplings of arteries taken from autopsies of people who died from something other than heart disease reveal that the incidence of atherosclerosis is very high in the

ATHEROSCLEROSIS IN BRIEF

What is it?

Atherosclerosis is a condition in which the arteries become partially or completely occluded due to atherosclerotic plaques.

How is it recognized?

Atherosclerosis has no symptoms until it is very advanced. However, it is connected to several other types of circulatory problems, including hypertension, arrhythmia, coronary artery disease, cerebrovascular disease, and peripheral vascular disease.

Is massage indicated or contraindicated?

Circulatory massage is systemically contraindicated for advanced atherosclerosis.

A BRIEF DISCOURSE ON CHOLESTEROL

Cholesterol is a fatty substance available in any animal product. Dietary saturated fat is also easily converted into cholesterol in the liver. It is used by many cells as an important part of metabolism.

Cholesterol by itself has no access to the body's cells. Just as glucose must be escorted by insulin, cholesterol must be escorted by *lipoproteins,* other chemicals also produced by the liver. When a cholesterol measurement is taken, it is actually the lipoproteins that are being counted.

The three varieties of lipoproteins are LDLs, HDLs, and triglycerides. The LDLs ("bad cholesterol") are only bad when the body's cells have no more need for their cargo. At that point the LDLs will deposit the cholesterol in artery walls. The HDLs ("good cholesterol") are involved in a process called "reverse cholesterol transport." In this process, LDL cholesterol is moved out of the arteries and back to the liver for metabolic processing. The third type, triglycerides, are a type of fatty acid independent of the other two. Studies have shown that elevated triglyceride levels will contribute to plaque formation. So in a cholesterol reading, it's useful for a person to know not just what his or her overall levels are, but in what ratios the fat types occur. A good ratio to aim for is 3.5 to 4 parts HDL to every 1 part LDL or triglyceride.

United States, although it doesn't always become symptomatic. In some cultures, this disease is completely unknown; they are generally found in third world countries where dietary diseases are related to famine rather than to excess. The good news is that people have some control over how much atherosclerosis will affect them. The leading risk factors for developing pathological atherosclerosis are largely controllable.

ETIOLOGY: WHAT HAPPENS?

The process of developing atherosclerosis is a complex one that is not yet completely understood. Several theories have been formed, but as research reveals more secrets about this condition, the reality may turn out to be quite different from what people have always believed.

One theory for the development of atherosclerosis maps out various steps beginning with damage to the endothelial layer of the aorta. Deviations in the disease process will occur in different people, but the basics follow:

1. Endothelial damage. The inside layer of arteries is sometimes called the tunica intima. It is made of delicate epithelial tissue and is subject to a lot of abuse. A variety of things may hurl the first insult at the tunica intima: constant *hypertension* (this chapter, page 199) in the aorta and arteries surrounding the heart; carbon monoxide from cigarette smoke; even a high level of iron in the blood may produce oxygen free radicals that begin the process of endothelial erosion (see *anemia,* this chapter, page 178).

2. Monocytes arrive. These small white blood cells are attracted to any site of damage in the body. The monocytes infiltrate the epithelial layer and turn into macrophages—big eaters.

3. Macrophages take up LDL. The reasons for this are unclear. LDLs are the low density lipoproteins that are the "bad guys" of the cholesterol world. Actually, they have an important job, which is to escort usable cholesterol to all the cells in the body. But when those cells don't need any more cholesterol, they stop accepting it. This leaves extra LDLs with nowhere to go. They are consumed by the white blood cells in the tunica intima, which are then called "foam cells." This is the beginning of the development of fatty streaks that characterize atherosclerosis.

4. Foam cells infiltrate the next layer. Foam cells secrete growth factors; this causes the smooth muscle cells in the arterial wall to proliferate all around them. The grayish-white lumps of plaque found inside dissected arteries are made of these extra muscle cells and cholesterol-filled macrophages. Furthermore, these foam cells can release enzymes that damage arterial walls and cause bleeding and clot formation.

ATHEROSCLEROSIS: CASE HISTORY

Mary, age 55

"There's chest pain, and then there's chest pain."

I have a history of bursitis in my left shoulder. Six years ago I started having pain in my left shoulder again, so I went to my family practitioner. He gave me some pain medicine, but he said if it wasn't better by the end of the weekend to call him back. Well, on Monday it was still bad, so I went back to see him.

The doctor I saw was someone I had never visited before, so he didn't know me or my history at all. He said, "I don't know why, but I know you *have* to be in the hospital." He put me in a wheelchair and checked me into intensive care.

The internist there looked me over and said, "I don't think there's anything wrong with you. Why not check yourself out and go home?" But my doctor said I couldn't go until all the tests were run. Nothing on the tests showed up until they did a stress test on a treadmill. I wasn't on it for two minutes when they took me off and put me in an ambulance to a nearby hospital with a cardiac unit.

They did a catheterization, which is a scope that goes up blood vessels from the legs into the heart to look around. (*This describes a test that visualizes blood flow through the vessels surrounding the heart.*) They found out that there was a serious blockage, *and* I have a congenital defect in my coronary arteries—there's a missing section, which increases the risk for heart attack. Then they did two angioplasties, but it didn't solve the problem. They finally did open heart surgery: a single bypass operation where they used a section of my mammary artery to go around the blockage and the place where the artery wasn't complete. They said it was a miracle I hadn't had a heart attack and because of where the blockage was, if I had had one, it probably would have been fatal.

Things were pretty good after that. I got into a cardiac rehabilitation unit and was exercising regularly, until I started developing tumors on my foot bones. They weren't cancerous, but the doctors said they could get to be. I had to have surgery to remove a part of the bone, which ended the exercise for about six months.

After I recovered from that, I developed a neuroma on the bottom of my foot. As a complication of that surgery, I developed hammer-toes, and then the neuroma came back. Then one day I was going to another doctor appointment and I tripped on the sidewalk. My right wrist swelled way up. It wasn't broken, but it didn't go down for about six months. They said it was reflex sympathetic dystrophy.

Five years later, a little more than a year ago, I went shopping for some shirts for my husband. While I was standing in the store, the chest pains hit me. There's chest pain and then there's chest pain. There's no way to describe what it feels like; if you've ever had it, you'll know what I'm talking about.

I let the pain pass, bought the shirts, and they hit me again. I barely made it to my car. I just sat there and cried. I thought, "This couldn't be happening *again!*" The traffic to my house was awful, so I ended up just going to the doctor's office instead. They did an EKG, but it was negative; they never show anything unless the heart muscle has been damaged. I checked back into the hospital and they did two catheterizations but they didn't clear the blockage; it was in an awkward spot, sort of around a bend in the artery, and the probe couldn't get in.

We wanted to try to insert a stent which would keep it open, but it turned out that my arteries are too small. We finally decided it was necessary to do another open-heart surgery. This time they took an artery from my forearm. And so far, so good. It's just a miracle that I've never had a heart attack. (continued)

ATHEROSCLEROSIS: CASE HISTORY, cont.

Mary works as a special education teacher at an elementary school. She was diagnosed with Non-Insulin Dependant Diabetes (NIDDM) about nine years ago. She had controlled the diabetes with drugs and diet until her first surgery, when she went on insulin. Between surgeries she was able to get off the insulin, but went back on after her second operation. Today she is gradually moving toward controlling her diabetes and atherosclerosis with diet, exercise, and medication. She also takes one child's aspirin per day, a mild diuretic, and a cholesterol lowering medicine. Her cholesterol count is in the normal range for someone with no history of heart problems, but her doctors feel it's important to lower it further. Mary's blood pressure is normal (112/72 at the last reading) and she has no edema or kidney problems.

5. Platelets arrive. Attracted by the changing texture of the arterial wall, platelets arrive and release their chemicals, which do three unpleasant things:
   • Growth factors are secreted, which reinforces the proliferation of new smooth muscle cells.
   • Clots form.
   • Vascular spasm occurs because the chemical that inhibits it can't get through all the plaque.

When vascular spasm and clots combine, partial or total occlusion of the artery can occur. Symptoms of this will depend on the location of the blockage and the amount of tissue that is affected.

Another explanation of the development of atherosclerosis begins with the depostion of LDL cholesterol in the subendothelial spaces of the arteries, where it undergoes chemical changes (oxidation) that make it impossible to leave the artery wall. Circulating monocytes are attracted to the LDL deposits. They infiltrate the arterial wall and literally gorge themselves on the embedded cholesterol, becoming foam cells.

The monocytes can consume so much that they rupture, releasing their contents in the area. Among the chemicals released are growth factors that stimulate smooth muscle cell proliferation in the arterial wall. These sites become raised lesions or *plaques*. Calcium is eventually deposited there. The rough texture they create attracts passing thrombocytes, which then contribute to clot formation and the subsequent dangers discussed above.

RISK FACTORS

Risk factors for atherosclerosis can be divided into situations that can be modified and others over which a person has little or no control.

Modifiable Risk Factors

• Smoking. Carbon monoxide from cigarette smoke is extremely damaging to endothelium. Furthermore, nicotine causes the release of epinephrine and norepinephrine, leading to vasoconstriction and high blood pressure.
• High cholesterol levels. A predictable statistical link has been established between high cholesterol levels and the development of pathological atherosclerosis. Over 52% of Americans have cholesterol readings above the recommended maximum of 200 mg/dl. Over 20% have readings over 240 mg/dl.
• High blood pressure. Chronic high blood pressure will contribute to aortic damage, which opens the door to the formation of plaques.
• Sedentary lifestyle. Regular, moderate cardiovascular exercise, perhaps more than any other factor, can reduce the risk of atherosclerosis.

Nonmodifiable Risk Factors

- Family history of cardiovascular disease. This factor no one can control. But a family history is not a death sentence; controlling other factors will significantly reduce the chance of developing problems.
- Kidney disorders. Atherosclerosis can sometimes lead to kidney problems. But if the kidney problems predate the circulatory ones, high blood pressure brought about by kidney failure can be a precipitating cause of atherosclerosis.
- Diabetes. People with uncontrolled diabetes are especially susceptible to atherosclerosis because of the way their bodies metabolize food. However, if the diabetes is controlled, the risk of atherosclerosis is much lower.

SIGNS AND SYMPTOMS

What are the symptoms of atherosclerosis? Until the damage has progressed to dangerous levels, *there are none!* An artery has to be *75 to 80% occluded* before the person has any awareness of a problem. This is largely because the body doesn't depend on any single artery to do a job. Most parts of the body have two or three alternate vessels that can be pressed into service if one of them becomes clogged.

COMPLICATIONS

The complications of atherosclerosis are sometimes the first symptoms of the disease. They include, but are not limited to . . .

- High blood pressure. Hypertension is both a cause and a result of this disease; it will contribute to the original damage to the tunica intima, and it will arise when the arterial walls are too brittle to adjust to the constant changes in blood volume flowing through them.
- Aneurysm. When the wall of an artery is rendered inelastic and defective, it can bulge, become thin and weak, and become susceptible to rupture. (See this chapter, page 190.)
- Thrombus or embolism. A thrombus is a stationary clot; an embolism is a traveling clot. No matter where it goes, it will probably do damage when it lands. Thrombi are the link between atherosclerosis and stroke, and between atherosclerosis and pulmonary embolism. (See *embolism or thrombus*, this chapter, page 182.)
- Coronary artery disease (CAD). This is a result of having coronary arteries so impaired that the cardiac muscle receives an inadequate supply of oxygen. The results can range from chest pain (*angina pectoris*) to *heart attack* (this chapter, page 206) to cardiac arrest and death. CAD can be brought about by atherosclerosis alone, or in combination with some of its partners in crime: thrombi caught in the coronary artery or vascular spasm. (See Figure 4.7.)
- Transient ischemic attack (TIA). This happens when an embolism (a traveling clot) temporarily blocks some blood supply to the brain. The symptoms are similar to those of a mild stroke, but the clot is small enough to break up or move out of the way without causing permanent damage. TIA, however, is considered a warning sign of the possibility of a cerebrovascular accident (stroke).
- Arrhythmia. Advanced atherosclerosis can contribute to the development of irregular or uncoordinated beating of the cardiac muscle, as blood supply through the coronary arteries is periodically interrupted. Arrhythmia can cause clots to form in the atria when the chamber is not completely emptied. These clots can travel to the lung (pulmonary embolism) or the brain (stroke).
- Peripheral circulatory damage. The coronary arteries are not the only ones that become hard and brittle. The carotid artery is vulnerable, as are renal arteries and the arteries of the extremities, especially the legs. Some types of peripheral circulatory

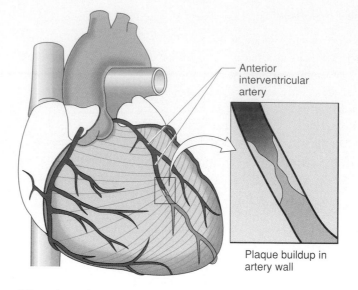

Anterior
interventricular
artery

Plaque buildup in
artery wall

Figure 4.7. Atherosclerotic plaque can deprive the heart muscle of blood supply.

problems that accompany advanced atherosclerosis are stasis dermatitis, gangrene, and skin ulcers. (See *diabetes*, this chapter, page 210.)

DIAGNOSIS

The traditional way to check for *stenosis*, or narrowing of arteries, is to inject them with dye and take a series of x-rays to watch the movement of fluid through the tubes; this procedure is called an *angiogram*. Computer technology, though, has produced a new, faster, less intrusive test called an *Ultrafast CT Scanner*, which takes very fast, clear pictures of the insides of arteries with about one chest x-ray's worth of radiation. It is not yet as complete a test as an angiogram, but it can be used to screen out high-risk patients who have no symptoms but who want to find out at what stage their disease exists.

TREATMENT

Treatment for advanced atherosclerosis starts simply. If the situation has been caught before it gets out of hand, it can often be dealt with by changing eating and exercise habits. Radically reducing the fat calories in the diet from 45% (the American average) to closer to 5% or 10%, along with mild exercise and stress reduction techniques, can yield success in reversing even advanced cases of atherosclerosis nonsurgically. The goal is to reduce serum LDL levels to under 100 mg/dl in order to reverse the disease.

Some drugs and other substances, notably niacin and chromium, have been found to increase HDL levels, which will in turn reduce LDL levels in the blood. Lipid lowering agents can be successful, but they often have side effects. Unfortunately, plaques that have been long in place are only about 15% soluble fats; the rest are composed of cellular debris, connective tissue, foam cells, and smooth muscle cells.

More advanced cases, and more standardized medical approaches, will often involve drugs and/or surgery. The drugs are generally smooth muscle relaxants that will cause the blood vessels to dilate. Aspirin can be useful, but it causes stomach irritation for many people. Specially coated tablets have been designed to avoid this problem in the treatment for the prevention of CAD.

Surgical intervention for atherosclerosis used to mean automatic bypass surgery. Surgeons would remove the damaged piece of coronary artery and replace it with something else, often a graft from the internal mammary artery or a piece of femoral vein. A single, double, triple, or however-many bypass refers to how many sections of artery are being replaced.

Recently good results have been found with a much less intrusive option: *angioplasty*. In this procedure, the artery may first be treated with a laser to vaporize plaques (laser angioplasty); then a small balloon is inflated to widen the artery (balloon angioplasty). Unfortunately, the scarring that occurs when the balloon is removed ("restenosis") can be a difficult, even dangerous complication of this procedure; such rapid proliferation of new cells occurs where the endothelium was scraped, the patient may be worse off after the procedure than before. The latest techniques to deal with this problem include altering the genes of a small stretch of affected artery in a way to make them receptive to drugs designed to inhibit new growth; the insertion of a small coil, called a *stent*, to keep the artery widened; and in some procedures, the "welding," with a laser, of the inside of the artery into a permanently smooth shape.

In yet another type of procedure called *catheter atherectomy*, a tiny rotating drill is inserted into clogged arteries to shave off plaque. The shavings are then trapped and removed.

With the exception of bypass surgery, all of these procedures can be done by inserting special tubes into arteries in the arms or legs and guiding the equipment to where it needs to go. Obviously the amount of shock to the system is less and the recovery process is much easier than it used to be. But new emphasis is being put on *maintaining* the structural changes brought about by surgery; if the patient reverts to former eating and exercise habits, his or her arteries can reach the same sorry state in just a few years.

MASSAGE?

It is impossible to tell if a person has a subclinical buildup of plaque. The deciding factor is whether the client can adjust to the change in internal environment that massage will bring about. In other words, he is not a good candidate for massage if his ability to maintain homeostasis will be completely overcome during a session.

If a client is taking *any* kind of medication for circulatory problems, it is vital to receive medical clearance before proceeding; this is one of the most important questions on a medical history form.

Hypertension

DEFINITION: WHAT IS IT?

Hypertension is a technical term for *high blood pressure*; the terms are interchangeable in this book. The definition is blood pressure persistently elevated above 140 mg Hg systolic and/or 90 mg diastolic.

DEMOGRAPHICS: WHO GETS IT?

Hypertension is a virtual epidemic in this country. Statistics vary, but they indicate that anywhere from 45 to 75 million people in the United States have high blood pressure. It strikes men about twice as often as women, until women reach the age of 60. Then it evens out and affects both genders equally. African Americans are about twice as likely to have hypertension as anyone else. Other predisposing factors include obesity, smoking, atherosclerosis, and water retention. Some evidence exists for a genetic tendency for high blood pressure, but sometimes it's hard to know what's been inherited: high blood pressure genes or high blood pressure habits.

HYPERTENSION IN BRIEF

What is it?
Hypertension is the technical term for high blood pressure.

How is it recognized?
High blood pressure has no dependable symptoms. The only way to identify it is by taking several blood pressure measurements over time.

Is massage indicated or contraindicated?
For borderline or mild high blood pressure, massage may be useful as a tool to control stress and increase general health, but other pathologies related to kidney or cardiovascular disease must be ruled out. High blood pressure that requires medication usually contraindicates circulatory massage, but under some circumstances, massage may be appropriate with a doctor's approval.

ETIOLOGY: WHAT HAPPENS?

With hypertension, the blood vessels are stressed by internal or external forces. In order to understand how these forces cause damage, it is necessary to take a brief look at exactly what blood pressure is.

A *sphygmomanometer* is an instrument that measures the pressure blood exerts against arterial walls at two different moments: ventricular contraction (systole) and ventricular relaxation (diastole). As a measure of the general health and resiliency of the cardiovascular system, the *diastolic* pressure, taken at the moment of relaxation, clearly gives more information than the *systolic* pressure, which is taken at the moment of contraction.

The variables involved in measuring blood pressure are fourfold: total blood volume; pressure from *inside* the vessel (which would increase with any buildup of material inside); pressure from the *outside* of the vessel (which would increase from excess fluid pressing all around); and blood vessel diameter. If any of these factors is out of balance, it will influence total body blood pressure, which will in turn influence the health and longevity of blood vessels.

The two types of high blood pressure are: *essential*, which means "not due to some other pathology," and *secondary*, which is a temporary complication of some other condition such as pregnancy, kidney problems, adrenal tumors, or hormonal disorders. Secondary high blood pressure will clear up as soon as the precipitating cause is dealt with. About 95% of all hypertension is essential. For both essential and secondary high blood pressure, another variable is *malignant hypertension*. In this condition, the diastolic pressure rises very quickly, over a matter of weeks or months. It is extremely damaging to the circulatory system, a high risk for ischemic or hemorrhagic *stroke* (chapter 3, page 161), and left untreated, is often fatal. Malignant high blood pressure is a medical emergency.

Here are some basic guidelines for grading the severity of hypertension in adults, based on the averages of more than two readings taken at each of more than two visits after an initial screening.[1] The blood pressure cuff translates the pressure into millimeters of mercury (mm Hg).

Category	Systolic BP (mm Hg)	Diastolic BP (mg Hg)
Normal	<130	<85
High Normal	130–139	85–89
Hypertension		
Stage 1 (mild)	140–159	90–99
Stage 2 (moderate)	160–179	100–109
Stage 3 (severe)	180–209	110–119
Stage 4 (very severe)	≥210	≥120

Massage therapists are not generally required to take blood pressure measurements; these numbers are just an indicator of possible trouble. Also be aware that blood pressure can change significantly from hour to hour. It's not uncommon to see it shoot up, from anxiety, in a doctor's office; this is known as "white coat hypertension."

SIGNS AND SYMPTOMS

This disease, often called "the silent killer," has few recognizable symptoms. A few subtle signs are occasionally observed, however, so they are included here: shortness of breath after mild exercise; headaches or dizziness; swelling of the ankles, especially during the daytime; excessive sweating or anxiety. Any combination of these symptoms indicates that a visit to the doctor would be a good idea.

---

[1] Joint National Committee (1993). The fifth report of the Joint National Committee on detection, evaluation and treatment of high blood pressure. Archives of Internal Medicine 153:154–183.

COMPLICATIONS

This is a very important list. Having hypertension can shorten a person's life span. Here's how:

- Edema. High blood pressure will force extra fluid out of the capillaries at the nutrient/ waste exchange sites. This adds to overall levels of interstitial fluid, causing edema. In a typically vicious circle, edema will further raise the blood pressure by putting external force on blood vessels. See more in *edema*, chapter 5, page 224.
- Atherosclerosis. Having blood pushing against arteries in an unceasing torrent will simply wear out the walls, especially when the arteries have naturally lost some of their resiliency from age. The moment the slightest damage occurs for a platelet to cling to, the atherosclerotic process will begin. This will reinforce high blood pressure by narrowing arterial diameters. See more in *atherosclerosis*, this chapter, page 193.
- Stroke. Someone with hypertension is four times more likely to suffer a stroke than someone who does not have hypertension. The stroke may be from an embolism or it may be from ruptured arteries in the brain. See more in *stroke*, chapter 3, page 161.
- Enlarged heart, heart failure. Making the heart push against narrowed arteries will cause the left ventricle to grow considerably, but the coronary arteries will not grow with it to handle the extra load. The muscle fibers also lose elasticity. Therefore, the contractions are actually weaker, because the muscle is not well supplied with blood, and it can't contract fully. This can also cause angina. When the ventricles of the heart are so overtaxed that they simply cannot keep up with the workload, the patient risks heart failure. This condition is six times more likely to happen to someone who is hypertensive than someone who is not. See more in *heart attack*, this chapter, page 206.
- Aneurysms. This is the result of high blood pressure causing a bulge in the arteries. See more in *aneurysm*, this chapter, page 190.
- Kidney disease. In a way, this is the most interesting complication of high blood pressure, because a circular relationship exists between hypertension and kidney dysfunction. Problems can start in either place—the kidneys or the circulatory system. If it starts with the circulatory system, here is one process: hypertension can cause atherosclerotic plaques to form in the renal arteries, which are subject to *tremendous* blood pressure. This will cause reduced blood flow into the kidney, which will impair kidney function, leading to kidney damage and systemic edema, which will exert even more pressure on the outsides of blood vessel walls. Hypertension can also cause kidney dysfunction through direct pressure on the delicate kidney tissues. Injury to the nephrons will decrease kidney function. This will result in systemic fluid retention, which increases blood pressure and puts even more stress on the kidneys.

     If the problem starts in the kidneys, a decrease of kidney function is seen (see more under *renal failure*, chapter 8, page 314). This will often be accompanied by extra release of *renin*, the kidney-based hormone that regulates some electrolyte balance. Excess renin results in vasoconstriction, water and salt retention, increased edema and blood volume, and high blood pressure.

TREATMENT

Hypertension is a highly treatable disease, but because it has virtually no symptoms until it has progressed to very dangerous levels, it is frequently untreated or incompletely treated (i.e., someone not taking his medication because he feels fine).

     Diet is the first way to approach this condition. Reducing salt and fat intake, while increasing calcium, magnesium, and potassium, has been an effective beginning to controlling hypertension. Restricting salt alone can lower diastolic pressure by as much as 5 points for half the people who try it. Exercise is crucial for the development of healthy new blood vessels, as well as weight control. Medication, if it's called for, includes diuretics to cope with edema and general fluid volume, vasodilators, and sometimes beta blockers, which decrease the force of ventricular contraction. Once beginning on medication, however, the patient is making a lifetime commitment. Even though he may feel fine, stopping the medication will put him back at risk for all the complications of high blood pressure.

Medicating high blood pressure is a bit problematic. Because the disease itself has no strong symptoms, and because the medicines often have mild but unpleasant side effects, there has been great difficulty in educating hypertension patients to be consistent with their medications. Recent statistics indicate that in the United States only 65% of the people who have hypertension are aware of it, less than half of those people who are diagnosed treat it at all, and only 21% of those who treat it, treat it successfully.

MASSAGE?

If a client knows that he has high blood pressure but he is not required to take medication for it, conservative massage is probably fine. It can help to lower the general blood pressure and levels of stress that contribute to it. It's important, however, to rule out kidney and other advanced cardiovascular problems before beginning. Watch especially for signs that massage is overchallenging the body: clamminess, bogginess, and possible edema in the days after the treatment.

If a client *is* taking medication for high blood pressure, circulatory modalities are usually strongly cautioned. Some cases of high blood pressure are relatively simple to treat and may not put a client at risk, but consulting a well-informed doctor is the only way to make a responsible judgment regarding massage. Techniques that don't strongly influence fluid flow may be appropriate, but rigorous, fast-paced work may be too much of a challenge for an impaired ability to maintain homeostasis.

Regardless of whether the client is on blood pressure medication, *deep abdominal work is contraindicated for high blood pressure*. It is possible to accidentally trip the vaso-vagus reaction. Unintentionally overstimulating the vagus nerve can result in amplified parasympathetic reactions, leading to systemic vasodilation and faintness from lack of blood to the brain. Another possibility is that the body could experience a sympathetic rebound effect. Ordinarily a vaso-vagus reaction is unpleasant but not dangerous—*unless* the blood vessels are not equipped to handle a rapid demand to dilate and constrict. Once again, a client's health is determined by his ability to maintain a stable internal environment during massage.

Raynaud's Syndrome

DEFINITION: WHAT IS IT?

This is a condition involving the status of the smallest blood vessels in the hands and feet, although it can also affect the nose, ears, lips, and even the tongue.

ETIOLOGY: WHAT HAPPENS?

In Raynaud's syndrome, the blood vessels in the extremities experience a spasm of smooth muscle tissue. It occurs in temporary episodes at first, but the vasoconstriction can become a permanent situation.

PRIMARY CAUSES

Raynaud's syndrome can be a primary problem or a secondary one, which appears as a symptom of another disease. When it's a primary problem, unconnected to underlying pathology, it is called *Raynaud's disease*. It may be caused by emotional stress (the autonomic nervous system will route blood away from the skin during emergencies), cold, or because of a mechanical irritation, such as operating machinery that influences blood vessel dilation. Pianists and typists are particularly vulnerable. Raynaud's disease generally has a very slow onset, and the attacks are less severe than when the symptoms occur as a secondary problem.

SECONDARY CAUSES

Occasionally, extreme vasoconstriction is a complication of some other disorder. In this case the condition is called *Raynaud's phenomenon*. It will generally have a much faster on-

---

RAYNAUD'S SYNDROME

This condition is named for Dr. Maurice Raynaud, a French physician who lived from 1834–1881. He was the first doctor to document this chronic vasoconstrictive disorder.

set than Raynaud's disease, and it can get quite a lot worse before it will respond to treatment. Some conditions associated with Raynaud's phenomenon are . . .

- *Arterial diseases* that involve occlusions, such as *diabetes* (chapter 4, page 210), *atherosclerosis* (this chapter page 193), and Buerger's disease (a rare condition involving inflammation and blood clots in the arteries).
- *Connective tissue diseases* such as scleroderma (a rare connective tissue disease similar to lupus), *lupus* (chapter 5, page 241), and *rheumatoid arthritis* (chapter 2, page 80).
- *Drug sensitivity* to certain drugs including beta-blockers and ergot compounds.
- *Neurovascular compression* in situations such as *carpal tunnel syndrome* (chapter 2, page 111) or *thoracic outlet syndrome* (chapter 2, page 120).

RAYNAUD'S SYNDROME IN BRIEF

What is it?
Raynaud's syndrome is defined by episodes of vasospasm of the arterioles, usually in fingers and toes, but occasionally in the nose, ears, lips, and tongue.

How is it recognized?
Affected areas will often go through marked color changes of white, or ashy gray for dark-skinned people, to blue to red. Attacks can last for less than a minute or several hours. Numbness and/or tingling may accompany attacks and recovery.

Is massage indicated or contraindicated?
Massage is indicated for Raynaud's syndrome that is not associated with underlying pathology. Otherwise, follow the guidelines for the precipitating condition.

SIGNS AND SYMPTOMS

Raynaud's syndrome is usually bilateral and affects many more women than it does men. During an attack, the skin will undergo a characteristic cycle of colors: white, as the blood is shunted away from the area (on dark-skinned people, the skin looks ashy-gray); blue, as the cells are starved for oxygen; and red, as the attack subsides, the arterioles reopen, and the blood returns to the affected area. (See Figure 4.8, Color Plate 29.)

Attacks of Raynaud's phenomenon can last anywhere from less than a minute to several hours. In very advanced cases, a wasting of flesh and ulcerations on the starved skin

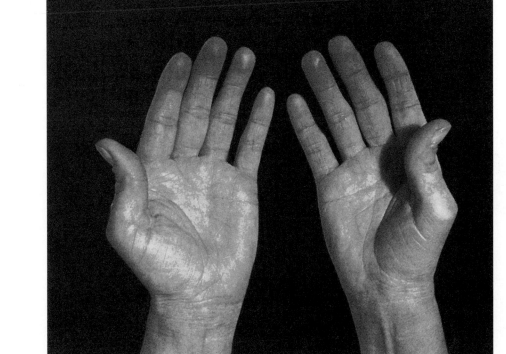

Figure 4.8. Raynaud's syndrome

may appear. The fingers may taper and the skin can become smooth and shiny. Gangrene is a rare but possible complication for these extreme cases. More often, ongoing weakness and loss of sensation may occur.

TREATMENT

Treatment obviously depends on whether the patient has a primary or secondary case of Raynaud's. Generally a noninvasive approach is taken first, at least for primary Raynaud's disease. Hydrotherapy, dressing appropriately for the weather, protecting the hands when working with cold or frozen foods, making sure that shoes aren't too tight, even moving to a warmer climate are all suggested before more intervention is sought.

If results are unsatisfactory, the next step is medication to dilate the blood vessels. Other drugs work to counteract norepinephrine, the stress-related hormone that initates vasoconstriction. A *sympathectomy*, or surgical severing of the nerves that control vasodilation, may be attempted, but this is rarely successful in the long run, as the nerves may grow back after surgery.

MASSAGE?

The good news about Raynaud's is that though the primary version of the syndrome is fairly common (some surveys estimate that 5 to 10% of the population is affected), the secondary version is rather rare. It tends to accompany serious diseases, patients of which are unlikely to seek out massage. As long as any dangerous underlying causes for the vasoconstriction have been ruled out, Raynaud's syndrome is indicated for massage. In fact, massage can work with the parasympathetic nervous system to stimulate reflexive vasodilation and help to restore normal circulation.

Varicose Veins

DEFINITION: WHAT ARE THEY?

Varicose veins are distended, often twisted or "ropey" superficial veins. They are caused by damage to the internal valves, which make sure that blood only goes one way: toward the heart. When blood backs up along the system, the affected vein is stretched, distorted, and generally weakened. (See Figure 4.9.) Varicose veins can happen at the anus (hemorrhoids), at the esophagus (esophageal varices), or at the scrotum (varicoles). Most often they occur in the legs, which will be the focus of the rest of this discussion.

DEMOGRAPHICS: WHO GETS THEM?

Women get varicose veins more often than men, largely due to the way a fetus can obstruct fluid return through the femoral vein, which can set the stage for later problems (see *pregnancy*, chapter 9, page 347). It is estimated that about 1 in 10 people will have varicosities at some point, mostly after 50 years of age.

ETIOLOGY: WHAT HAPPENS?

The veins in the legs have a fascinating construction that assists the heart in getting the blood from the toes all the way back to the chest. Small veins pick up the blood from the internal muscle capillaries. These veins tend to run on

---

VARICOSE VEINS IN BRIEF

What are they?
Varicose veins are distended veins, usually in the legs, caused by valvular incompetence and a backup of blood returning to the heart.

How are they recognized?
Varicose veins are ropey, slightly bluish, elevated veins that twist and turn out of their usual course. They happen most frequently on the medial side of the calf, although they are also found on the posterior aspects of the calf and thigh.

Is massage indicated or contraindicated?
Massage is locally contraindicated for extreme varicose veins and anywhere distal to them. Mild varicose veins contraindicate deep, specific work, but are otherwise safe for massage.

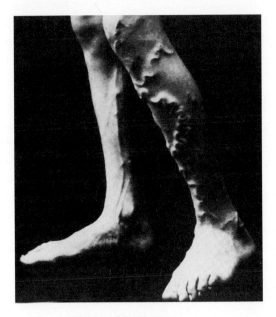

Figure 4.9. Varicose veins

the superficial aspect of muscles. They feed into larger veins that perforate the muscle bellies, and then into the very big, deep veins that run under the muscles, close to the bones. When the leg muscles contract, the perforating veins are squeezed, sending their contents to the deep veins. When the leg muscles relax the perforating veins draw in new blood from the smaller veins. The contraction and relaxation of the leg muscles (especially the soleus—"sump pump of the leg") is crucial to blood return. The valves inside the perforating veins and the deep veins ensure that blood will not collect in the smaller, weaker superficial veins.

CAUSES

What can damage the valves in the veins? It could be simple wear and tear: being on one's feet for many hours a day, especially if the legs muscles are not allowed to fully contract and relax during that time, will weaken the veins. It could also be a mechanical obstruction to returning blood: knee socks that are too tight, for instance, or a fetus pressing on the femoral vein. Systemic congestion from kidney problems or liver backups has caused problems, too. Finally, it simply could be congenitally weak veins. Once a valve is damaged, anywhere in the system, blood will back up and put pressure on the next valve down. Valvular incompetence will ultimately cause the weakest superfical veins to become distorted, dilated, and twisted off their regular pathway. The biggest, deepest veins are seldom affected by this weakening process because their walls are thicker and the leg muscles act as built-in support hose.

SIGNS AND SYMPTOMS

Varicose veins look like lumpy bluish wandering lines on the surface of the skin. They are often visible on the back of the calf, but more often they affect the great saphenous vein and show up anywhere from the ankle to the groin on the medial side. They may only be visible when the patient is standing. When they are especially bad, they may be achy or slightly itchy, and the sluggish movement of fluid through the circulatory system will force an excess accumulation of interstitial fluid: distal edema.

COMPLICATIONS

Although varicosities are seldom anything more than annoying, occasionally they create some unpleasant side effects. Chronically impaired circulation may result in varicose ulcers, which won't heal until circulation is restored. Skin irritation from poor circulation will occasionally lead to a type of *eczema* (chapter 1, page 21) that again won't resolve until the varicosity is relieved. Also, stagnant blood in a distended vein may coagulate, raising the strong possibility of *thrombophlebitis* (this chapter, page 187).

TREATMENT

Mild varicose veins are usually treated with good sense. Support hose or elastic bandages can give extra help to damaged veins, and avoiding long periods of being erect without full contraction and relaxation of the muscles is often recommended. Reclining with the feet slightly elevated will also reduce symptoms. Whether or not the veins can actually *heal* is somewhat controversial. If the damage has not progressed too far, relieving the mechanical stresses while strengthening the smooth muscle tissue (with hydrotherapy, for instance) can yield good results.

Surgery for mild varicose veins is not generally recommended, except as a cosmetic intervention. However, varicose veins are a progressive condition; they don't usually spontaneously reverse, and left untreated, their complications can be serious. Therefore, a certain number of patients will eventually seek treatment for health, rather than cosmetic concerns.

The two traditional approaches for treating varicosities that threaten to become more serious are surgery to remove the affected vein ("stripping") and injections of sclerosing chemicals into the vein, which will cause it to completely close down. Sclerosing procedures recently have been seen to have high recurrence rates, and stripping can be very traumatic, involving a hospital stay and several weeks of postoperative edema. A new alternative, called *ambulatory phlebectomy*, is becoming the standard surgical intervention. In this procedure, only small lengths of the affected veins are taken, through very tiny incisions. It can be done as an outpatient procedure with little risk of complications. In all of these treatments, the body's remarkable ability to generate new blood vessels will quickly accommodate the closure or removal of the affected vein.

MASSAGE?

Massage is locally contraindicated for varicose veins, particularly for veins that are elevated from the skin and that have visibly been distorted from their original pathway. Heavy massage distal to these veins is cautioned also.

If the vein is only slightly darkened and not elevated or causing any pain, it is still wise to avoid local heavy pressure, but otherwise massage is safe. The tiny reddened "spider veins" are slightly dilated venules, and are safe for massage.

Heart Conditions

Heart Attack

DEFINITION: WHAT IS IT?

A heart attack is damage to some portion of the cardiac muscle as a result of ischemia, which starves and kills some of the muscle cells. The ischemia is usually caused by coronary artery disease (CAD), or *atherosclerosis* (this chapter, page 193), of the coronary arteries, which supply the cardiac muscle with oxygen and nutrition. If these arteries are completely occluded by plaque, thrombi, or any combination of the two, some piece of the muscle will die. (See Figure 4.10.) The muscle tissue will not grow back; it is replaced by inelastic, noncontractile scar tissue. The damaged area is referred to as an *infarct*. Another term for heart attack is *myocardial infarction* (MI).

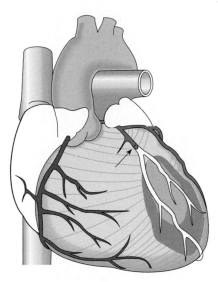

Figure 4.10. Heart attack

HEART ATTACK IN BRIEF

What is it?
A heart attack, or myocardial infarction (MI), is damage to the myocardium caused by a clot or plaque fragment getting lodged somewhere in a coronary artery, or atherosclerosis so complete that it deprives the cardiac muscle of oxygen.

How is it recognized?
Symptoms of heart attacks include angina, shortness of breath, a feeling of great pressure on the chest, and pain around the left shoulder and arm, jaw, and back.

Is massage indicated or contraindicated?
Massage is contraindicated for patients recovering from heart attacks. After complete recovery, heart attack patients may be good candidates for massage but not without medical clearance.

DEMOGRAPHICS: WHO GETS THEM?

More than 60 million people in this county have been diagnosed with some form of cardiovascular disease; over 42% of all deaths in this country are linked to these conditions. Coronary artery disease (CAD) is the leading cause of death in the United States, claiming close to half a million lives every year. Approximately one and a half million heart attacks occur per year in this country; two out of three people survive, while the other third die within 2 hours. Close to 14 million Americans alive today are survivors of one or more heart attacks.

Most people are familiar with the high-risk profile for heart attack victims: sedentary lifestyle, *hypertension* (this chapter, page 199), high cholesterol levels, smoking. Other contributing factors include *diabetes* (this chapter, page 210), obesity, and stress. Males, people with a family history of cardiovascular disease, and women over 35 who take birth control pills also have an increased chance of suffering a heart attack. Also, people who make less than $5,000 per year, regardless of race or gender, are about twice as likely to die of some sort of heart disease than people who make more than $50,000 per year. This label of "low socioeconomic standing" is adjusted for level of education, job skills, and whether or not the person is married or has a life partner.

ETIOLOGY: WHAT HAPPENS?

When a portion of the cardiac muscle is killed off by ischemic attack, the ability to contract with coordination and efficiency is badly damaged. Atrial fibrillations (rapid, incomplete, and weak attempts at contraction) may occur, especially if any part of the sinoatrial node, the heart's electrical "pacemaker," has been damaged. Incomplete contractions allow blood to pool and thicken in the chambers of the heart, and may contribute to the risk of *stroke* (chapter 3, page 161) or simple brain damage by oxygen de-

OTHER HEART CONDITIONS

Heart Failure

Heart failure is the term for what happens when the heart is not strong enough to keep up with its work load. Heart failure comes in three varieties.

- Left heart failure. This is also called *congestive heart failure*. In this case the left side of the heart is badly impaired in its function. A backup of congestion in the pulmonary circuit leads to the seepage of fluid back into the alveoli. This condition, if it becomes severe and is not corrected, will result in pulmonary edema. Symptoms of left heart failure include severe shortness of breath and stubborn coughing, perhaps with bloody sputum. One serious complication of this condition is the risk of *pneumonia* (chapter 6, page 252) in the functionally impaired lungs.   *(continued)*

OTHER HEART CONDITIONS, cont.

- Right heart failure. In the absence of left heart failure, this is also called *cor pulmonale*. It commonly results from pulmonary disease and high vascular resistance in the lungs. In other words, it becomes difficult to pump blood through the pulmonary circuit. The backup is felt through the rest of the body. Symptoms include severe *edema* (chapter 5, page 224), especially in the legs. Someone with this type of heart failure will have ankles that look like they're spilling over the sides of his shoes. If the patient is bedridden, the edema may occur in the abdomen or low back—wherever gravity is pulling most. The most common cause of right heart failure is left heart failure.

- Biventricular heart failure. This is left and right side failure simultaneously. Symptoms incorporate both left and right side signs. If this condition shows no improvement with conventional therapies (drugs or surgery), a heart transplant may be considered. Otherwise, a different surgical innovation might be applied: *cardiomyoplasty*. In this surgery the distal end of the latissimus dorsi is freed from the humerus and wrapped around the weakened heart. A special pacemaker that coordinates the fast-twitch fibers of the latissimus with the heart's slow-twitch fibers is implanted between them. Two million people in the United States have biventricular heart failure, and an estimated 400,000 more are diagnosed every year. About one-half of these people will die within five years of being diagnosed.

Heart Murmurs

The heart can make dozens of types of noises during its contractions. These are referred to as *murmurs*. They often, but not always, point to some type of valvular dysfunction within the heart. A client with a persistant heart murmur needs to be cleared for massage by a primary care physician.

Angina Pectoris

Literally "chest pain," this is a description of the symptoms that can occur when the heart muscle doesn't receive adequate oxygen. Angina pectoris is frequently a consequence of coronary arteries that are severely occluded, but other possible causes of chest pain include severe anemia or hyperthyroidism. This condition may involve severe pain or a feeling of heavy pressure around the chest, left shoulder and arm, and into the jaw and back.   (continued)

privation. Ventricular fibrillations, because they interfere with blood flow to the entire body, will result in death if they are not treated quickly. Intervention with CPR mimics the healthy pumping of the ventricles, decreasing the risk of brain damage until help arrives.

The seriousness of a heart attack is determined by the size and location of the blockage. If it is relatively small and blood flow is impaired to an area that doesn't have to work especially hard, the heart attack is not a serious one. But if the infarct, or area of damaged tissue, is large enough to weaken the heart's ability to contract, or if the damaged tissue contains the electrical conduction system for the heart, major intervention will be necessary to aid in recovery. Because the right side of the heart pumps blood only to the lungs and back, while the left side pumps blood all over the body, left-sided infarctions are generally considered to be more serious than right-sided ones.

SIGNS AND SYMPTOMS

One of the first (and often only) warning signs of a heart attack is angina, or chest pain, which often happens during physical activity when the cardiac muscle demands more oxygen than it can get. The impaired coronary arteries spasm, or suffer temporary interruptions in blood flow, or simply can't deliver adequate amounts of blood, which causes the cardiac muscle pain. The difference between angina and a true heart attack, however, is that angina will cease when the unusual exercise or tax on the circulatory system stops or after the administration of nitroglycerin, a coronary vessel dilator. Heart attack pain will continue.

Other symptoms of heart attack include a feeling of heavy pressure in the chest. Sometimes pain that begins in the center of the chest can also be felt in the face, jaw, stomach, and left shoulder and arm. Other possible signs include dizziness, dyspnea (shortness of breath), sweating, chills, nausea, and fainting.

COMPLICATIONS

Several of these conditions are expounded upon elsewhere in this chapter; diseases of the cardiovascular system are highly interrelated. Furthermore, with heart disease it's hard to say what comes first: the infarct or the thrombus. In other words, a circular chronology to the events may occur, rather than a straight line.

- Embolism. A heart attack can actually cause blood clots to form in the heart itself, which then exit through the aorta and travel to wherever the bloodstream takes them. These are arterial emboli, and they can land in the brain, causing a stroke, or the renal arteries, where they can contribute to *renal failure* (chapter 8, page 314). Prolonged bed rest can also promote *deep vein thrombosis* (this chapter, page 187), which then carries a risk for pulmonary embolism (see *embolism or thrombus*, this chapter, page 182).

- Aneurysm. Weakened cardiac tissue can create a bulge in the heart muscle itself similar to *aneurysms* (this chapter, page 190).

- Heart failure. Contrary to what it sounds like, this is not the same as cardiac arrest. Heart failure means that the muscle is no longer strong enough to do its work, and the body pays the price. See the box on *Other Heart Conditions* for more information.

- Shock. With shock, the circulatory system swings reactively from sympathetic to parasympathetic, opening all the arteries to a maximum diameter in the process. The main danger with shock is loss of blood to the brain from radically decreased blood pressure.

TREATMENT

The first priority with heart attack patients is to identify where the blockage is, and to get rid of it as quickly as possible. This is done with clot-dissolving drugs, which can take effect in 90 minutes or less, and with immediate balloon angioplasty, which can open up most clogged arteries in about an hour. The technical term for this procedure is *percutaneous transluminal coronary angioplasty*, or PTCA. Other immediate care options include the administration of oxygen and pain management with nitroglycerin and/or morphine.

Later care usually includes more clot dissolvers and nitroglycerin, which works to relax the smooth muscle tissue in the arteries. After the emergency has passed, the main treatment for heart attacks is observation. A barrage of tests is conducted to determine the location and extent of damage to the cardiac muscle. These tests will then indicate one of three future courses of action: 1) if the infarct was minor, it requires no further medical intervention; 2) prescriptive anticoagulants are indicated; or 3) a serious and permanent narrowing of a coronary artery requires surgery to open and repair. This surgery may be a more complete version of the angioplasty, or it may be coronary bypass surgery in which damaged sections of the coronary artery are replaced with grafts of healthy vessels from elsewhere in the body.

Treatment in heart attack and heart surgery recovery must also embrace the lifestyle changes that will support a healthier future: eating sensibly, exercising regularly, controlling high blood pressure, and quitting smoking are the most important factors.

Some studies have indicated that taking aspirin regularly can decrease the chance of a repeat heart attack for people with a history of heart disease. Specially coated tablets have been designed to minimize gastrointestinal

OTHER HEART CONDITIONS, cont.

Angina is typically brought on by periods of extreme stress or exertion, and is relieved by rest and drugs, among them nitroglycerin (to dilate coronary vessels) and beta-blockers (to reduce heart rate).

Angina itself does not imply that a heart attack is happening; however, it does suggest cardiovascular problems that may put a person at risk for myocardial infarction. Any client who has episodes of angina pectoris should be cleared by a primary care physician before receiving massage.

Hypertrophy of the Heart

This condition, which is seen most dramatically in the left ventricle, is brought about by chronically high systemic pressure in the blood vessels. If the heart has to fight against constricted arteries to push blood through the body, it will hypertrophy, or grow larger. It may increase in strength as well, for a while, but as the need for oxygen outgrows the supply from the coronary arteries, the tissue will eventually experience ischemia, possible myocardial infarction, and eventually congestive heart failure.

Congenital Heart Problems

A person may be born with any of approximately 35 different structural problems, most of them focusing around valve function. Approximately 32,000 people a year are born with these problems, although new surgical techniques with infants (and even babies still in utero) are making it more rare to see adults with debilitating congenital heart defects.

Rheumatic Fever

Rheumatic fever is an autoimmune complication of exposure to streptococcus in which antibodies attack the heart valves, especially the mitral valve. It affects about 1.3 million Americans, and is responsible for close to 6,000 deaths per year. Mitral valve damage will affect the way the heart can pump blood through the body. It can lead to arterial emboli or congestive heart failure.

Infectious Diseases of the Heart

A couple of varieties of streptococcus prey on endocardium. If they find a way in (which can happen from something as innocuous as an abscessed tooth, but is more often a complication of open heart surgery) they will also cause clots that are then released into the arterial system.

(continued)

OTHER HEART CONDITIONS, cont.

Massage? For most of these conditions, massage is systemically contraindicated. Work that mechanically pushes fluid through the system will hinder, rather than help, these damaged structures.

problems, but this intervention carries a slight possibility of an increased chance of subdural hemorrhage, so patients must consider carefully all the implications of taking aspirin on a daily basis.

MASSAGE?

The appropriateness of massage absolutely depends on the individual, the extent of the damage they survived, and how long ago it occurred. Some heart attack survivors make themselves healthier than they ever were before, while others will re-accumulate high levels of plaque on their arteries within just a few years of surgery. The safety of massage will depend on how easily the client can withstand those changes in internal environment that this work will bring about. If in doubt, always check with a doctor.

Other Circulatory Conditions

Diabetes Mellitus

DIABETES
This word comes from the Greek for "a siphon" or "to pass through," referring to the tendency for diabetics to urinate very frequently.

DEFINITION: WHAT IS IT?

Diabetes is not a single disease, but rather a group of related disorders that all result in hyperglycemia, or elevated levels of sugar in the bloodstream, which is then shed in the urine.

Diabetes is not strictly speaking a circulatory system condition. It more properly belongs under the heading of endocrine disorders, but since it has such a profound impact on the circulatory system, this discussion fits best here.

DEMOGRAPHICS: WHO GETS IT?

Diabetes is the seventh leading cause of death in the United States, and the sixth leading cause of death by disease. About 625,000 new cases are diagnosed every year. An estimated 16 million Americans have it, but about half of them don't know it.

Diabetes, a largely treatable and even preventable disease, costs approximately $92 billion a year in direct medical costs and indirect costs of disability, lost wages, and premature mortality.

DIABETES MELLITIS IN BRIEF

What is it?
Diabetes is a group of metabolic disorders characterized by glucose intolerance or deficiency and disturbances in carbohydrate, fat, and protein metabolism.

How is it recognized?
Early symptoms of diabetes include frequent urination, thirstiness, and increased appetite along with weight loss, nausea, and vomiting.

Is massage indicated or contraindicated?
Massage is indicated for people with diabetes as long as their tissue is healthy and they receive medical clearance.

ETIOLOGY: WHAT HAPPENS?

In diabetes, glucose builds up in the blood because of decreased or completely nonexistent levels of insulin output from the pancreas, or sometimes from malfunctioning insulin receptors on target cells. Insulin is required to escort glucose molecules into cells where it can be consumed to produce energy. In the absence of insulin, the body cannot burn this remarkably clean fuel source, and must resort first to fat reserves, and then finally to proteins. Eventually, in the absence of any other fuel source, the body will burn its own muscle tissue. The problem is that these fuel sources don't burn cleanly. They leave behind a lot of toxic debris, which is largely responsible for the complications associated with diabetes.

Several types of diabetes mellitis exist; the two most common varieties will be considered here.

Type I. *Insulin dependent diabetes mellitus* (IDDM) is an autoimmune disorder. It can be brought about by a number of different factors, including exposure to certain drugs and chemicals, or as a complication of some kinds of infections. It has been linked to a specific protein in the mumps and coxsackie virus (a fairly common virus that gives flu-like symptoms) that is almost identical to a protein in the insulin-making cells of the pancreas. This protein is called GAD, and the killer T cells of people with IDDM attack it, destroying the rest of the islet cell along with it. The destruction of the islet cells leads to a deficiency in insulin. The most exciting aspect of this research is the promise of being able to modify the body's response to GAD, either by injecting it into the thymus before exposure to the coxsackie virus (this would ensure tolerance of this particular protein) or even by eating GAD, which seems to stimulate suppresser cells.

IDDM usually shows up in teens, almost always before age twenty. It is the rarer, and more serious, of the two basic types of diabetes. About 300,000 people in the United States have IDDM, and about 30,000 new cases are diagnosed each year. It accounts for 5 to 10% of all diabetes in this country. Because IDDM requires self-administered doses of insulin instead of the constant steady production provided by a healthy pancreas, Type I diabetics can experience very extreme cycles of blood sugar levels— from very, very high, which can cause acidosis and diabetic coma, to dangerously low, which can lead to insulin shock.

Type II. This variety is also called *non-insulin dependent diabetes mellitis* (NIDDM). It is more common for women than men. Approximately 80% of people with NIDDM are overweight. NIDDM is especially prevalent in African American, Hispanic, and Native American populations. In fact, in some Native American tribes, almost 50% of the adults have NIDDM. Type II diabetes is usually controllable with diet, exercise, and possibly some anti-diabetes drugs, depending on how advanced it is when treatment begins.

The exact cause of adult-onset diabetes is uncertain, and is probably different for different people. For some it seems clear that a lifelong habit of a high carbohydrate diet simply wears out the pancreas, and makes the insulin-producing cells less efficient. In others the insulin production may be at normal levels, but the incoming flood of sugar is too much to deal with. And for still others, insulin production may be normal or even above normal, but for some reason the target cells have fewer receptor sites to receive the insulin. In any case, the results are the same: frequent urination, excessive thirst, and excessive hunger, along with the possibility of dangerous accumulations of atherosclerosis.

Other types of this disorder include *gestational diabetes*, in which a woman develops a transient case while pregnant. Left untreated, it can cause birth defects in the child. Women who have gestational diabetes also have a 50% chance of developing NIDDM later in life. *Secondary diabetes* may develop with damage or trauma to the pancreas, or as a symptom of some other endocrine disorder such as acromegaly (too much growth hormone) or Cushing syndrome (hyperactive adrenal glands).

SIGNS AND SYMPTOMS

Identifying diabetes early is a great challenge. Very often the first symptoms are too subtle or nonspecific to cause a serious problem, and by the time it's diagnosed, the progression of the disease already may have caused permanent damage.

The three defining "polys" that all types of diabetes have in common include: *Polyuria*, or frequent urination, resulting from elevated blood sugar, which acts as a diuretic. It pulls water from the cells in the body, then pulls excess water into the kidneys and urine. *Polydipsia* means excessive thirst, which accompanies the loss of water with polyuria. *Polyphagia* refers to increased appetite, since diabetics must obtain all their energy from fats and proteins instead of carbohydrates, which are the most efficient kind of fuel. Other symptoms of diabetes include fatigue, weight loss, nausea, and vomiting.

DANGER SIGNS

People with diabetes may experience two medical emergencies, both of which can be fatal if not treated promptly.

Ketoacidosis.   This involves a critical *shortage* of insulin and lack of glucose in the cells. In this situation, the body will partially metabolize fats for fuel, and the acidic by-product of that metabolism dangerously changes the pH balance of the blood. Ketoacidosis is identifiable by a characteristic sweet or fruity odor to the breath. It can be brought on by stress, infection, or trauma, and can lead to shock, coma, and death.

Insulin Shock.   This emergency is at the other end of the scale. In this case, *too much* insulin is circulating, either because too much has been administered or because insufficient calorie intake, sudden exertion, stress, infection, or trauma has resulted in the consumption of available blood sugar. The consequence of having too much available insulin is a dangerously low blood sugar level. Symptoms of diabetic shock include dizziness, confusion, weakness, and tremors. It, too, can lead to coma and death if not treated (with the intake of juice, candy, or non-diet soda) quickly.

COMPLICATIONS

Complications of diabetes are many and serious.

*   Cardiovascular disease. Diabetics are especially prone to these problems because residue left from the metabolism of fats and proteins contributes to high rates of *atherosclerosis* (this chapter, page 193). And, unlike many atherosclerosis patients, diabetics don't accumulate plaque only on coronary arterial walls, but systemically throughout the body. Diabetes also increases the risk of *stroke* (chapter 3, page 161), *hypertension* (this chapter, page 199), and *aneurysm* (this chapter, page 190).

    Some degree of cardiovascular disease is present in 75% of all diabetes-related deaths. About 65% of people with diabetes have high blood pressure.
*   Edema. This condition develops in the extremities because of sluggish blood return. This can also give rise to stasis dermatitis.
*   Ulcers, gangrene, amputations. Imagine what would happen if *all* the body's blood vessels were caked with plaque. Absence of blood flow carrying nutrients and white blood cells would make it difficult or impossible to heal from even minor skin lesions. Ingrown toenails can become life threatening for diabetics; instead of healing, they become gangrenous. The tissue either dies from starvation or is infected with pathogens that are impossible to fight, forming characteristic diabetic ulcers, usually on the feet. (See Figure 4.11, Color Plate 30.) Diabetes accounts for more than half of all amputations (about 57,000) performed in the United States every year.
*   Kidney disease. Renal vessels become clogged with plaques very readily, since they're one of the first diversions from the descending aorta. The kidneys also have a hard time functioning with excess blood sugar, which acts as a powerful diuretic. Not surprisingly, then, diabetes is the top cause of renal failure (see *renal failure*, chapter 8, page 314).

    Renal failure is the leading cause of death for people with diabetes. Recent research indicates that *very* frequent monitoring and adjustments of blood sugar levels (meaning 4 to 6 times per day, as opposed to the more usual 1 to 2 times) can significantly reduce the amount of glomerular buildup in diabetic kidneys, thus reducing the risk of secondary hypertension by about 50%.
*   Impaired vision. The capillaries of the eyes of diabetic persons can become abnormally thickened, depriving eye cells of nutrition. Diseased capillaries will leak blood and proteins into the retina. Microaneurysms may form, cutting off circulation. All of these contribute to diabetic *retinopathy*. Excess glucose also binds with special pro-

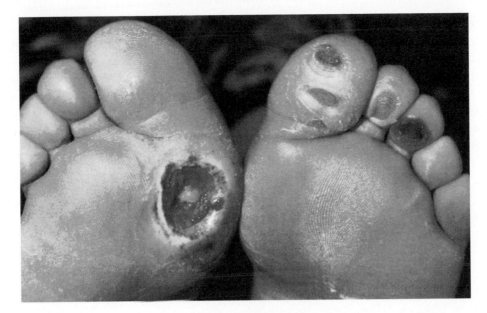

Figure 4.11. Diabetic ulcers

teins in the lens causing first cataracts, then blindness. This disease is the leading cause for new blindness in the United States: up to 24,000 cases per year.

About one-half of all diabetes patients will experience some level of visual impairment within 10 years of being diagnosed. Close to 80% will have some vision loss within 15 years.

- Peripheral neuropathy. Lack of capillary circulation and excess sugar in the blood both contribute to nerve damage. Symptoms of diabetic neuropathy include tingling or pain, and eventual numbness. It often affects the spinal nerves, but can damage autonomic cranial nerves as well. If this is the case, the patient can experience low blood pressure, diarrhea, constipation, or sexual impotency.

    Peripheral neuropathy generally appears about 10 to 20 years after diabetes is diagnosed. It is estimated that up to 25% of all diabetes patients will experience some degree of neuropathy.

- Others. Diabetes affects just about every body system in some way. It is linked to *urinary tract infections* (chapter 8, page 318), candida, birth defects, and higher than normal rates of gum disease and tooth loss.

TREATMENT

Before the development of insulin in 1921, the diagnosis of diabetes was a death knell. Most people lived only a few years after the disease was identified. Nowadays the goal of insulin treatment is to keep blood sugar levels as stable as possible. IDDM is treated primarily with insulin supplementation from bovine or porcine sources, although an artificial form of human insulin is now being found to reduce allergic reactions. Techniques to administer insulin more regularly have been developed to minimize the dangerous roller coaster ride of too much to too little blood sugar.

NIDDM is first approached with changes in diet and exercise. It has recently been found that exercise will improve insulin uptake in resistant target cells, and a sedentary lifestyle may be more responsible for the rising statistics in NIDDM in the United States and all developed nations than diets high in saturated fats and simple carbohydrates. About 35% of NIDDM patients are treated with insulin supplementation. Hypoglycemic agents may also be prescribed.

MASSAGE?

Massage may be appropriate for people with diabetes, under the right circumstances. The main condition is that the client must have healthy, responsive tissue with good blood supply, *and* clearance from her doctor. For clients with advanced diabetes and atherosclerosis, circulatory massage is probably out of the question, but energetic techniques are certainly appropriate. Be aware that diabetic neuropathy can involve lack of sensation. Someone with adult-onset diabetes may be completely unaware of her condition until someone points out her ulcers, which often occur on the feet.

CHAPTER REVIEW QUESTIONS: CIRCULATORY SYSTEM CONDITIONS

1. Describe the process of the development of atherosclerosis.

2. What indication of diabetes might a massage therapist be the first person to notice?

3. Where will all venous emboli go? Why?

4. Name three places arterial emboli can go to cause significant damage.

5. Heart attacks involve blockages where: in the heart itself or in the coronary arteries?

6. Which chamber of the heart is the worst place to experience a myocardial infarct? Why?

7. Why is hypertension called the "Silent Killer"?

8. Describe the relationship between high blood pressure and kidney dysfunction.

9. Describe how a person may experience any three of the following conditions at the same time: high blood pressure, chronic renal failure, edema, atherosclerosis, diabetes, aortic aneurysm, stroke.

10. A client has ropey, distended varicose veins on the medial aspect of the right knee. Distal to the knee, the tissue is clammy and slightly edematous. Pressing at the ankle leaves a dimple that takes several minutes to disappear. What cautions must be exercised with this client? Why?

BIBLIOGRAPHY, CIRCULATORY SYSTEM CONDITIONS

General References, Circulatory System

1. Carmine D. Clemente. Anatomy: A regional atlas of the human body. 3rd ed. Baltimore: Urban & Schwarzenburg, 1987.

2. I. Damjanou. Pathology for the health-related professions. Philadelphia: Saunders, 1996.

3. Giovanni de Dominico, Elizabeth Wood. Beard's massage Philadelphia: Saunders, 1997.

4. Deane Juhan. Job's body: A handbook for bodywork. Barrytown, NY: Station Hill Press, Inc., 1987.

5. Jeffrey R. M. Kunz, Asher J. Finkel, eds. The American Medical Association family medical guide. New York: Random House, Inc., 1987.

6. Elaine M. Marieb. Human anatomy and physiology. Redwood City, CA: Benjamin/Cummings Publishing Co., Inc., 1989.

7. Ruth Lundeen Memmler, Dina Lin Wood. The human body in health and disease. 5th ed. Philadelphia: JB Lippincott Co., 1983.

8. Mary Lou Mulvihill. Human diseases: A systemic approach. 2nd ed. East Norwalk, CT: Appleton & Lange, A publishing division of Prentice-Hall, 1987.

9. Stedman's medical dictionary. 26th ed. Baltimore: Williams & Wilkins, 1995.

10. Taber's cyclopedic dictionary. 14th ed. Philadelphia: F.A. Davis Company, 1981.

11. Gerard J. Tortora, Nicholas P. Anagnostakos. Principles of anatomy and physiology. 6th ed. New York: Biological Sciences Textbook, Inc., A&P Textbooks, Inc., and Elia-Sparta, Inc.; Harper & Row Publishers, Inc., 1990.

12. Janet Travell, David G. Simons. Myofascial pain and dysfunction: The trigger point manual. Baltimore: Williams & Wilkins, 1983.

Anemia

1. Aplastic anemia answer book. University of Texas Houston Medical School, 1997. URL: http://medic.med.uth. Accessed fall 1997.

2. PV (Polycythemia Vera) FAQ. MPD Research Center, Inc., 1996. URL: http:// www.acor.org/diseases/hematology/MPD/ PVFAQ.html. Accessed fall 1997.

3. John Schwartz. Drug prevents sickle cell anemia attacks. Washington Post, January 31, 1995:A1.

4. Kristy Woods. Sickle cell disease: Beyond the pain: A comprehensive approach to care. University of Chicago Primary Care Group Topics, 1994. URL: http://uhs.bsd. uchicago.edu/uhs/topics/sickle.cell.html. Accessed fall 1997.

Embolism or Thrombus

1. Arterial embolism. Copyright 1998 ADAM Software, Inc., all rights reserved. Copyright 1998 CommuniHealth. URL: http://www.healthanswers.com. Accessed winter 1998.

2. Blood clots. Copyright 1998 ADAM Software, Inc., all rights reserved. Copyright 1998 CommuniHealth. URL: http://www.healthanswers.com. Accessed winter 1998.

3. National Institutes of Health consensus development conference statement: Prevention of venous thrombosis and pulmonary embolism. Originally published: Prevention of venous thrombosis and pulmonary embolism. NIH Consensus Statement, 1986; 6(2):1–8. URL: http://text. nlm.nih.gov/nih/cdc/www/54txt.html. Accessed fall 1997.

4. Pulmonary embolus. Copyright 1998 ADAM Software, Inc., all rights reserved. Copyright 1998 CommuniHealth. URL:

http://www.healthanswers.com. Accessed winter 1998.

Hemophilia

1. Bleeding disorder treatments. National Hemophilia Foundation. URL: http:// www.infohforg/bleeding_info/hemophilia/ symptoms_hemo.html. Accessed fall 1997.

2. Complications in hemophilia and its treatment. National Hemophilia Foundation. URL: http://www.infohforg/bleeding_ info/hemophilia/comp_hemo.html. Accessed fall 1997.

3. How is hemophilia treated? World Federation of Hemophilia. URL: http://www.wfh. org/hemotret.html. Accessed fall 1997.

4. What you should know about bleeding disorders. National Hemophilia Foundation, Greene Street, Suite 303, New York, NY 10012. URL: http://www.hemophilia. org. Accessed winter 1998.

5. What is hemophilia? National Hemophilia Foundation. URL: http://www. infohforg/bleeding_info/hemophilia/ hemo.html. Accessed fall 1997.

Thrombophlebitis or Deep Vein Thrombosis

1. Doug Alexander. Deep vein thrombosis and massage. Massage Therapy Journal 1993; 32(2): 56–63.

2. Deep vein thrombosis. Cleveland Clinic Foundation. URL: http://www.anes.cof. org:8080/pilot/orhto/dvt.htm. Accessed fall 1997.

3. Deep venous thrombosis. Boston University Medical Center. Community Outreach Health Information System, 1995–1996. URL: http://web.bu.edu:80/COHIS/ cardvasc/vessel/vein/dvt.htm. Accessed fall 1997.

4. Deep venous thrombosis. Copyright 1998 ADAM Software, Inc., all rights reserved. Copyright 1998 CommuniHealth. URL: http://www.healthanswers.com. Accessed winter 1998.

5. MedicineNet: Questions and answers about phlebitis. Information Network, Inc., 1995–1997. URL: http://www. medicinenet.com. Accessed fall 1997.

6. Phlebitis. Boston University Medical Center: Community Outreach Health Information System, 1995–1996. URL: http://web.bu.edu:80/COHIS/cardvasc/ vessel/vein/phlebtis.htm. Accessed fall 1997.

7. Thrombophlebitis. Copyright 1998 ADAM Software, Inc., all rights reserved. Copyright 1998 CommuniHealth. URL: http://www.healthanswers.com. Accessed winter 1998.

Aneurysm

1. Aneurysms. Texas Heart Institute, 1997. URL: http://www.tinc.edu/thi/aneurysm.html#Aneurysms. Accessed fall 1997.
2. Aortic aneurysm. American Heart Association, 1997. URL: http://www.americanheart.org/heartg/aneurysm.html. Accessed fall 1997.
3. M. David Tilson. Answers to FAQs about abdominal aortic aneurysms. URL: http://www.columbia.edu/~mdt1/faqs.html. Accessed fall 1997.

Atherosclerosis

1. Peter M. Abel. Is coronary artery disease reversible? Cardiovascular Institute of the South, 1996. URL: http://www.cardio.com/articles/reversal.htm. Accessed fall 1997.
2. Atherosclerosis. American Heart Association,1997. URL: http://www.americanheart.org/heartg/athero.html. Accessed fall 1997.
3. Cardiovascular disease statistics. American Heart Association, 1997. URL: http://www.americanheart.org/heartg/cvds.html. Accessed fall 1997.
4. The gallery of the pathogenesis of atherosclerosis. Bristol-Myers Squibb Co., 1991. ER Squibb & Sons, Inc. 541-417 4/91.
5. Gina Kolata. Genetic approach to preventing regrowth of arterial plaque. NY Times Medical Science, August 9, 1994:B6.
6. William R. Ladd. Angioplasty and bypass surgery: Are they really "alternatives"? Cardiovascular Institute of the South, 1996. URL: http://www.cardio.com/articles/altrntiv.htm. Accessed fall 1997.
7. William R. Ladd. Atherosclerosis isn't a universal malady. Cardiovascular Institute of the South, 1996. URL: http://www.cardio.com/articles/atherosc.htm. Accessed fall 1997.
8. Sally Squires. Cardiac images show blockage in arteries. Washington Post Health, August 30, 1994:Z07.
9. What is ultrafast CT scanning? Center for Cardiovascular Education, Inc., 1996–1997. URL: http://www.heartinfo.org/ctscan/html. Accessed fall 1997.

Hypertension

1. Blood pressure. American Heart Association, 1997. URL: http://www.americanheart.org/heartg/bp.html. Accessed fall 1997.
2. Factors that contribute to high blood pressure. American Heart Association, 1997. URL: http://www.americanheart.org/heartg/hbpf.html. Accessed fall 1997.
3. High blood pressure causes. American Heart Association, 1997. URL: http://www.americanheart.org/heartg/hbpc.html. Accessed fall 1997.
4. High blood pressure. American Heart Association, 1997. URL: http://www.americanheart.org/heartg/hbp.html. Accessed fall 1997.
5. MedicineNet: Power points about high blood pressure. Information Network, Inc., 1995–1997. URL: http://www.medicinenet.com. Accessed fall 1997.

Raynaud's Syndrome

1. Questions and answers about raynaud's phenomenon. National Institute of Arthritis and Musculoskeletal and Skin Diseases, January 1997. URL: http://www.nih.gov/niams/healthinfo/ar125fs.htm. Accessed fall 1997.
2. Raynaud's phenomenon. Boston University Medical Center: Community Outreach Health Information System, 1995–1996. URL: http://web.bu.edu:80/COHIS/cardvasc/vessel/vein/raynaud.htm. Accessed fall 1997.

Varicose Veins

1. MedicineNet: Power points about varicose and spider veins. Information Network, Inc., 1995–1997. URL: http://www.medicinenet.com. Accessed fall 1997.
2. New technique for difficult varicose veins. Modern Medicine 1996: 64; 2. URL: http://www.modernmedicine.com/modern/fyi91.htm. Accessed fall 1997.
3. Varicose veins. Boston University Medical Center: Community Outreach Health Information System, 1995–1996. URL: http://web.bu.edu:80/COHIS/cardvasc/vessel/vein/varicose.htm. Accessed fall 1997.
4. Varicose veins. Copyright 1998 ADAM Software, Inc., all rights reserved. Copyright 1998 CommuniHealth. URL: http://www.healthanswers.com. Accessed winter 1998.

Heart Attack

1. Congenital heart disease statistics. American Heart Association, 1997. URL: http://www.americanheart.org/heartg/conghds.html. Accessed fall 1997.
2. Heart attack and angina statistics. American Heart Association, 1997. URL: http://www.americanheart.org/heartg/has.html. Accessed fall 1997.
3. MedicineNet: Power points about heart attack. Information Network,

Inc., 1995–1997. URL: http://www.medicinenet.com. Accessed fall 1997.

4. MedicineNet: Power points about palpitations. Information Network, Inc., 1995–1997. URL: http://www.medicinenet.com. Accessed fall 1997.

5. Peter W. Pendergrass, Carolyn diGuiseppi. Aspirin prophylaxis for the primary prevention of myocardial infarction. US Preventive Services Task Force. URL: http://text.nlm.nih.gov.cps/www/cps.75.html. Accessed fall 1997.

6. Rheumatic heart disease statistics. American Heart Association, 1997. URL: http://www.americanheart.org/heartg/rhds.html. Accessed fall 1997.

7. Rheumatic heart disease/rheumatic fever. American Heart Association, 1997. URL: http://www.americanheart.org/heartg/rhd.html. Accessed fall 1997.

8. Risk factors and coronary heart disease. American Heart Association, 1997. URL: http://www.americanheart.org/heartg/riskfact.html. Accessed fall 1997.

9. Jay Siwek. Guidelines on treating congestive heart failure. Washington Post Health (Consultation), November 22, 1994:Z15.

Diabetes Mellitus

1. Diabetes: A serious public health problem. Centers for Disease Control, 1996. URL: http://www.cdc.gov/nccdphp/ddt/glance.htm. Accessed fall 1997.

2. Diabetic neuropathy. Copyright 1998 ADAM Software, Inc., all rights reserved. Copyright 1998 CommuniHealth. URL: http://www.healthanswers.com. Accessed winter 1998.

3. Diabetic neuropathy: The nerve damage of diabetes. National Institute of Diabetes Digestive and Kidney Diseases: NIH Publication No. 95-3185, July 1995. E-text updated: 27 November 1996. URL: http://www.niddk.nih.gov/DiabeticNeuropathy/DiabNeur.htm. Accessed fall 1997.

4. Exercise hailed as "best drug" for insulin resistance syndrome. American Diabetes Association, June 8, 1996. URL: http://www.diabetes.org/ada/amsat1.html. Accessed fall 1997.

5. Keith Jenkins. Many who have diabetes don't know it. Washington Post Health, January 31, 1995:Z5.

6. MedicineNet: Power points about diabetes mellitus. Information Network, Inc., 1995–1997. URL: http://www.medicinenet.com. Accessed fall 1997.

7. National diabetes information clearinghouse: Diabetes overview. National Institute of Diabetes Digestive and Kidney Diseases. URL: http://www.niddk.nig.gov/overview.overview.html. Accessed fall 1997.

8. Boyce Rensberger. Scientists cite breakthrough on diabetes. Washington Post, October 4, 1993:A1.

Lymph and Immune System Conditions

OBJECTIVES

After reading this chapter, you should be able to tell . . .

- What the disorder is.
- How to recognize it.
- Whether massage is indicated or contraindicated for that condition.
- Whether a contraindication is local or systemic, or refers to a specific stage of development or healing.
- Why those choices for massage are correct.

In addition to this basic information, you should be able to . . .

- Name five ways that lymph can be moved through the body.
- Name the type of immunity supplied by T cells and by B cells.
- Name three places in the body where macrophages are concentrated for immune system defenses.
- Name two "indicator diseases" for AIDS.
- Name three criteria, besides fatigue, necessary for a positive diagnosis of chronic fatigue syndrome.
- Name two examples of edema that contraindicate circulatory massage, and one example of edema that indicates massage.
- Name three good reasons to let a mild fever run its course without interference.
- Name the four cardinal signs of inflammation. What is a fifth possible sign?
- Name what lupus can do to the musculoskeletal system organs.
- Name the most dangerous complication of lymphangitis.

I ♡ You

LYMPH SYSTEM INTRODUCTION

The lymphatic system is a critically important system for massage practitioners to understand. It's a bit peculiar; its components are not even vaguely symmetrical, and it functions as a sort of subsystem to both the circulatory and immune systems. The conditions listed under this heading may be influenced by either of these other two systems. A brief reminder of how the lymphatic system works follows.

LYMPH SYSTEM STRUCTURE

As blood travels away from the heart, it travels through progressively smaller tubes—the aorta branches into the arteries, which branch into arterioles, which finally divide into the very tiny and delicate capillaries. The pressure and speed with which blood travels decreases as it gets further away from the heart. Still, everything should keep moving at a good pace; a blood cell can complete its circuit through the body about every 60 seconds.

The walls of the capillaries are made of one-cell-thick squamous epithelium, designed for maximum efficiency of diffusion. The diameter, or luminae, of capillaries is so tiny that the red blood cells must line up one by one to pass through. This is the moment for the transfer of nutrients and wastes in the tissue cells. Also, having dropped off oxygen and picked up carbon dioxide, the vessels turn from arterial capillaries into venous capillaries. Finally, fluid from the arterial blood is squeezed out of the capillaries by external pressure. In other words, *this* is the origin of interstitial fluid.

Interstitial fluid is absolutely vital! All the body's nutrients and wastes travel via this medium. But it needs to keep moving; if it stagnates, toxins can accumulate and cause problems. Interstitial fluid keeps moving through the system by flowing into a different type of capillary: a lymphatic capillary. Lymphatic capillaries are similar to circulatory capillaries in construction, with one major difference: they are part of an *open* system. That is, interstitial fluid and even small particles can flow into lymphatic capillaries at almost any point along the length of that capillary. (Circulatory capillaries are *closed* to the extent that red blood cells are *not* able to come and go unless the vessel has been damaged.) (See Figure 5.1.)

When interstitial fluid has moved into a lymphatic capillary, it is officially called *lymph*. Lymph is composed mainly of plasma that has been pressed out of the bloodstream, loads of metabolic wastes that have been exuded by hardworking cells, and some chunks of particulate waste as well.

Interstitial fluid in the lymph system is drawn to a series of cleaning stations called *nodes* where the wastes are neutralized and any small particles are filtered out. The nodes are also home to most of the body's specific immune response cells, so if any pathogens have been picked up and marked by macrophages in the lymph, this is where the immune response really begins. Eventually the cleaned-up fluid is deposited back into the circulatory system; this happens just above the right atrium of the heart where the right and left thoracic ducts empty into the right and left thoracic veins, respectively.

LYMPH SYSTEM FUNCTION

Lymph flows through the lymphatic capillaries into ever bigger vessels, usually against the pull of gravity and without the aid of the heart's direct pumping action. What moves it along? Several things:

- Gravity. Gravity will help move lymph if the limb is elevated.
- Muscle contraction. When muscle fibers squeeze down around lymphatic vessels, they push fluid through just like a hand squeezes around a tube of toothpaste.
- Alternating hot and cold. Hydrotherapy applications can cause contractions in the smooth muscle tissue of lymphatic vessels to move fluid along.
- Breathing. Deep breathing draws lymph up the thoracic duct like an expanding bellows during inhalation and squeezes it muscularly during exhalation.
- Massage. Big mechanical manipulative strokes such as petrissage and deep effleurage can increase lymph flow, but even small, extremely superficial reflexive strokes can cause stagnant fluid to be drawn into lymphatic capillaries.

If everything is working well, fluid levels in the tissues should be constant, but not stagnant. The amount of fluid being squeezed *out* of circulatory capillaries should be almost

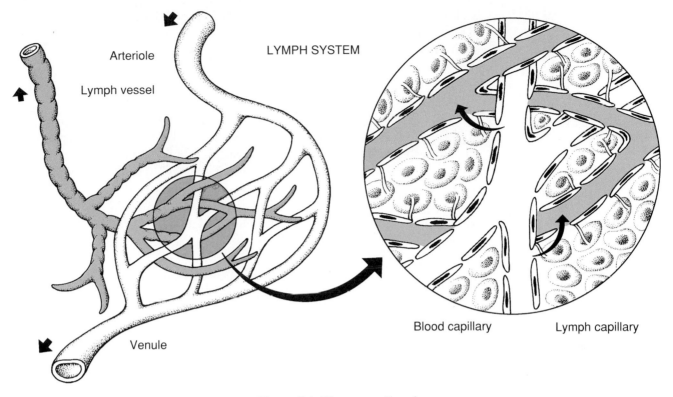

Figure 5.1. The origin of lymph

equal to the amount being drawn *into* lymphatic capillaries; this is called Starling's Equilibrium. But a backup anywhere in the system could result in major changes in fluid balance. If lymph vessels or nodes are blocked, for instance, the body won't stop producing interstitial fluid. This fluid will accumulate between tissue cells. It will cause swelling and quickly become a hindrance to diffusion and other chemical reactions, rather than the transfer medium it is designed to be. This is the problem with many of the diseases of the lymph system, and this is a serious situation for massage practitioners, who generally should *not* be trying to push fluid through an already overtaxed system.

IMMUNE SYSTEM INTRODUCTION

The immune system is unique; it is not comprised of a collection of organs each performing a task for a coordinated total effort, like the cardiovascular, muscular, nervous, or other systems in the body. Instead, it is a nebulous, incredibly complex collection of cells and chemicals stationed all over the body whose coordinated function is not to turn food into energy or to distribute oxygen, but to do something even more fundamental to keep the whole organism alive. Because the immune system is composed of specialized cells rather than organs, this discussion will focus on the function rather than the structure of the system.

IMMUNE SYSTEM FUNCTION

The primary function of the immune system is to distinguish what is "self" from what is "non-self" and to eradicate anything that is "non-self" as quickly as possible. Immune system devices range from being very general to highly specific in identifying exactly which pathogens to attack. Some white cells will simply ignore a pathogen if it's not their particular target. Most of the nonspecific immune devices, such as intact skin and the acidity of the gastric juices, won't be discussed here, but it is worthwhile to look at some of the *specific* immune machinery because when it's working well it's positively miraculous, and when it's *not* working well, or when it makes mistakes, things can go terribly wrong.

T cells and B cells

The two interlocking branches of the specific immune responses are cellular immunity (T cells) and humoral immunity (B cells). Neither of these extremely complicated systems is worth a penny if the pathogen it's trying to fight hasn't been tagged. Specific immune system cells cannot recognize a pathogen unless it is displayed by a macrophage. So *that* is the first step in fighting off an infection: a macrophage must find, eat, and display a piece of the microorganism in question. Fortunately, macrophages are distributed generously all through the blood and interstitial fluid, and they are concentrated in such places as the superficial fascia, lymph nodes, lungs, and liver, where the chance of meeting pathogens is especially high.

Consider what happens when someone touches a contaminated doorknob and then wipes his eye: rhinovirus 14 has just been introduced into the body. A passing macrophage eats the pathogen, and it is drawn through lymphatic capillaries into a nearby lymph node. A T cell is waiting there. It just happens to be especially designed to recognize the flag of rhinovirus 14. The T cell becomes very busy, replicating itself into several different forms that travel into the bloodstream in search of more virus to attack. In the process, the original T cell stimulates its B cell partner. This B cell clones, and the new cells start producing rhinovirus 14–specific antibodies at a mind-boggling pace: 2000 antibodies per second! Antibodies are *not* alive. They are Y-shaped chemicals forged especially to lock onto their target pathogen and "retire" it. This happens in many different ways, depending on the pathogen and the antibodies involved.

Back when the T cells and B cells first became active, they each made a few copies of themselves that would outlive the infection, and circulate through the body on the lookout for future attempts by the same pathogen to invade. These are *memory cells*, and thanks to them, people very seldom get sick with the same pathogen twice. If rhinovirus 14 gains access to the body again, an immune attack against it will occur so quickly, a person will never know he is in danger.

The way in which T and B cells somehow recognize their own special pathogens and launch just the right attack against them makes the immune system seem miraculous. It's even been shown that B cells will produce antibodies that can disable *manmade* pathogens that don't occur in nature. *That's* being prepared! But the immune system occasionally makes mistakes. Sometimes it will launch a full-scale attack—complete with an inflammatory response, antibody production, and all the rest—against an antigen that's not really dangerous: cat dander or pollen, for instance. The immune system may also mistake a part of the body for a dangerous pathogen; that is, it fails to distinguish self from nonself. Conditions involving this type of mistake are called *autoimmune disorders*.

Hypersensitivity Reactions

Autoimmune disorders and allergies are *hypersensitivity reactions*, and they refer to immune system function that goes beyond the call of duty. Four types of hypersensitivity reactions occur, and because two of them can involve the skin and the other two can involve systemic disorders, it's useful for massage therapists to be familiar with them.

Type I
A Type I hypersensitivity reaction is an immediate reaction to an antigen, or particle of "non-self." In this situation, IgE, a specific type of antibody, quickly sensitizes nearby mast

cells to the presence of an "enemy"—which could be a fragment of pollen, the proteins from peanuts or shellfish, or a droplet of bee venom. The alerted mast cells then release histamine and other chemicals, which create dramatic changes in vascular permeability and attract other white blood cells to the area. This inflammatory response creates the symptoms associated with typical allergic reactions: redness, swelling, itching, weepy eyes, and runny nose with hay fever; nausea, vomiting, and diarrhea with certain food allergies. If the irritated mast cells are in the respiratory tract, the hypersensitivity reaction will occur as a bout of bronchial *asthma* (see chapter 6, page 259).

One of the distinguishing features of a Type I reaction is that the IgE antibodies stay local in the affected tissues. The histamine and other chemicals that are released, however, may be carried through the bloodstream to other parts of the body. If enough of these chemicals are present, and if the body's reaction is severe enough, the result may be *anaphylactic shock*. This type of shock causes the vascular dilation stimulated by histamine and other inflammatory substances to become so extreme and far reaching that a person may be at risk of death from a combination of low blood pressure, pulmonary edema, and circulatory collapse.

Examples of Type I hypersensitivity reactions include hay fever, atopic dermatitis (also known as *eczema*, chapter 1, page 21), *hives* (chapter 1, page 24), and bronchial asthma.

HYPERSENSITIVITY REACTIONS AND MASSAGE OIL

Type I hypersensitivity reactions typically occur within several seconds to a few minutes of exposure to an irritating substance. However, a late-phase Type I reaction will sustain allergic symptoms long after the irritation has been removed. *Arachidonic acid* is a substance associated with late-phase Type I reactions, especially in the form of bronchial asthma. The significance of this for massage therapists is that some types of massage oils can break down into arachidonic acid on the skin. A client who is sensitive to this type of reaction may have no immediate skin symptoms, but may wonder several hours later why he is coughing, wheezing, and feeling short of breath.

Oils particularly prone to breaking down into arachidonic acid are composed mostly of Omega-6 sized molecules. These include safflower, soy, almond, sunflower, and corn oils. Although they can be pleasant and convenient to use for massage, they are the most likely to cause skin irritation and allergic reactions. Therefore, when it is recommended to avoid potentially irritating oils for certain conditions, these are the ones to eliminate first.

Type II

Type II hypersensitivity reactions are far less common than Type I. They involve inflammatory cytotoxic ("cell killing") reactions against a specific substance that may or may not belong to the body.

Examples of Type II reactions include myasthenia gravis, hemolytic *anemia* (chapter 4, page 178), and reactions to the transfusion of mismatched blood.

Type III

In Type III reactions, antibodies bind with antigens, but the particles they form are too small to be phagocytized. These tiny conglomerates eventually become caught in the body's most delicate fluid filters: in the kidneys, the eyes, the brain, and the serous membranes surrounding the heart, lungs, and abdominal cavity. They stimulate immune system activity, which results in inflammation and damage to these very delicate structures.

Examples of Type III reactions include *systemic lupus erythematosis* (see chapter 5, page 241), a specific type of *glomerulonephritis* (see chapter 8, page 309), and possibly *rheumatoid arthritis* (see chapter 2, page 80).

Type IV

Type IV, or "delayed" reactions, are cell mediated; they rely on T cells to stimulate an immune response to an irritant. In some cases, large clumps called *granulomas* are formed of immune system cells. In other cases, an immune system overreaction occurs without the formation of granulomas.

Contact *dermatitis* (see chapter 1, page 21) is an example of a Type IV hypersensitivity reaction. In this case, an inflammatory reaction on the skin occurs after exposure to an irritating substance such as plant toxins (e.g., poison ivy), certain dyes, soaps, metals, or latex. This typically delayed reaction may occur 24 to 48 hours after exposure.

That's a very brief summary of specific immunity, and it's a lot more than was known just 20 years ago. Another aspect to this system that scientists are just beginning to investigate is the fact that immune system cells actually *talk* to each other, discussing in a language made of chemicals called cytokines what their strategies are for fighting off infection. These chemical messages are beginning to be deciphered, and some of them say things like "act like me," "come over here," and "eat this."

Furthermore, it turns out that immune system cells don't just talk to each other. Some of the chemical messages they're sending out are picked up and acted on by other systems in the body, especially the nervous and endocrine systems. Receptor sites exist on white blood cells for brain chemicals; in other words, the nervous system can "talk" directly to the immune system. Some of the lymphokines secreted by white blood cells are similar, maybe even identical, to the neurotransmitters previously assumed to exist only in the central nervous system. Other lymphokines, specifically interleukin-1, are secreted by macrophages, but relay information to the hypothalamus. This creates some major implications about how health and resistance to disease are related to mental and emotional state. Intuitively this makes a lot of sense, and for the first time, it is possible to back up these theories with empirical evidence. A branch of science called *psychoneuroimmunology* has developed specifically to explore these relationships. Bit by bit, that imaginary division between "mind" and "body" is disappearing.

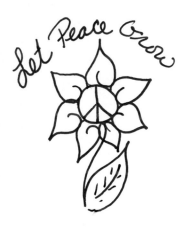

LYMPH AND IMMUNE SYSTEM CONDITIONS

Lymph System Conditions
- Edema
- Hodgkin's Disease
- Lymphangitis

Immune System Conditions
- Chronic Fatigue Syndrome
- Fever
- HIV/AIDS
- Inflammation
- Lupus

Lymph System Conditions

Edema
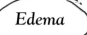

DEFINITION: WHAT IS IT?

Edema is the accumulation of fluid between cells. It may be associated with inflammation or poor circulation. In either case, the stagnant fluid needs to be pulled into lymphatic capillaries and processed by the lymph system.

ETIOLOGY: WHAT HAPPENS?

The Starling Equilibrium states that the forces that cause fluid to leave blood capillaries should *almost* equal the forces that cause fluid to be reabsorbed by blood capillaries, and that anything left over (which should be about 10%) should be taken in and processed by the lymph system. Lymph capillaries are perfectly designed to pick up excess interstitial fluid: each squamous cell is anchored to surrounding tissue by a collagen filament. When excess fluid accumulates in any area, these anchoring filaments pull back on the squamous cells, thus increasing the lymph capillary's ability to take in fluid. Sometimes, though, more fluid builds up in the tissues than the circulatory and lymph systems combined can accommodate, and this is called edema. This occurs in conditions where blood return is somehow impaired, which pushes excess fluid out of the vessels around the capillaries. Edema isn't generally noticeable until interstitial fluid volume is about 30% above normal.

CAUSES

Edema can have several causes; most of them are a combination of mechanical and chemical factors. Mechanical factors may involve a weakened heart or an obstruction of some kind; chemical causes of edema usually have to do with the accumulation of proteins in the interstitial fluid, which causes the area to retain water.

MASSAGE?

Most types of systemic edema, and *every* instance of pitting edema, contraindicate massage because of the impact massage has on fluid flow.

Contraindicated Edemas.

- If the heart is overtaxed (i.e., *congestive heart failure*, chapter 4, page 206) and is not pumping the volumes it should be, fluid will accumulate in the tissues. Vigorous massage will not improve this situation, and could quite possibly make it worse by putting an even greater load on the system.
- If the kidneys are not filtering blood fast enough or completely enough because of chemical imbalance or mechanical obstruction, edema will develop and massage could make the situation much worse. (See *renal failure*, chapter 8, page 314.)
- If the liver is congested, the puffiness and bogginess of typical edema may be less visibly apparent, but the same rules apply: pushing blood through a system that is chemically or mechanically impaired will do only damage. (See *enlarged liver*, chapter 7, page 300.)
- If edema is due to local infection, massage is contraindicated because of the risk of pushing bacteria into the lymphatic and circulatory systems before the body has had a chance to tag it and marshal appropriate defenses. (See *inflammation*, this chapter, page 237.)
- If a chance exists of mechanical blockage anywhere in the circulatory system, massage is contraindicated because it can damage delicate structures in the circulatory system or, even worse, it could break loose an embolism or thrombus. Some examples of mechanical blockages include edema associated with pregnancy, blood clots, or emboli and elephantiasis. (See *embolism or thrombus*, chapter 4, page 182.)

Indicated Edemas.
All this is not to say that every type of edema absolutely contraindicates massage under every kind of circumstance. Edema is a red flag for massage therapists, and it calls for caution before proceeding. But if a client has fluid retention related to a subacute musculoskeletal injury, skilled massage is *very* indicated, and in fact could be vital to the healing process (see *sprains*, chapter 2, page 87). Likewise, if a client is temporarily confined to bed or is even partially immobilized for some reason that does *not* contraindicate massage, massage can be valuable to the health of his or her injured tissues as long as the risk of blood clotting has been ruled out.

Hodgkin's Disease

DEFINITION: WHAT IS IT?

Hodgkin's disease is a type of slow-growing lymphoma, or cancer of the lymph nodes. It involves the mutation of macrophages into large, malignant multinucleate cells called

---

EDEMA IN BRIEF

What is it?
Edema is the retention of interstitial fluid either because of electrolyte or protein imbalances or because of mechanical obstruction in the circulatory or lymphatic systems.

How is it recognized?
Edematous tissue is puffy or boggy. It may be hot, if associated with local infection, or quite cool, if it is cut off from local circulation.

Is massage indicated or contraindicated?
Massage is contraindicated for most edemas, particularly pitting edema, where the tissue does not immediately spring back from a touch. Indicated edemas include those due to subacute soft tissue injury or temporary immobilization caused by some factor that does *not* contraindicate massage.

HODGKIN'S DISEASE

Thomas Hodgkin (1798–1866) was a British physician who documented this disorder.

HODGKIN'S DISEASE IN BRIEF

What is it?

Hodgkin's disease is a slow-growing lymphoma that typically begins in the lymph nodes of the neck, axilla, or inguinal areas, but may spread to attack internal organs.

How is it recognized?

Painless swelling of lymph nodes is the cardinal sign of this disease, along with the possibility of fatigue, low-grade fever, night sweats, itchiness, and loss of appetite.

Is massage indicated or contraindicated?

Rigorous circulatory massage is generally not recommended for a person who is fighting cancer, although this may be a case-by-case decision. For someone who has been cancer-free for 5 years or more, massage is appropriate. Noncirculatory types of massage may be appropriate for Hodgkin's patients, with medical clearance.

Reed-Sternberg cells. It is seen most often in the submandibular nodes, but can also occur at the axillary and inguinal nodes. Eventually the growths will spread to organ tissues, particularly the liver, or bone marrow.

CAUSES

The cause of Hodgkin's is unknown. Possible reasons include genetic predisposition, disturbance of immune system function, or susceptibility to the Epstein-Barr virus, which has been linked to several other cancers as well. But for the most part, no specific cause or list of risk factors have been identified.

SIGNS AND SYMPTOMS

The primary symptom of Hodgkin's disease is painless, non-tender swelling of lymph nodes in the axilla, around the neck, or around the inguinal area. (See Figure 5.2.) Other symptoms include fatigue, weight loss, night sweats, itching, and loss of appetite. Late stage Hodgkin's disease involves decreased immunity and susceptibility to secondary infection.

TREATMENT

Hodgkin's disease is a very treatable form of cancer, but early detection is vital. The first step in treating this condition after the Reed-Sternberg cells have been identified is to stage its progress; this is accomplished through MRIs or CT scans of the abdomen, lymphangiograms, physical exams, and examinations of blood chemistry. Stage I Hodgkin's disease means that only one lymph node is affected. Stage II means that two or more sites of growth have been found, but they are on the same side of the diaphragm. In Stage III, growths may be found above and below the diaphragm, while in Stage IV, growths are present at lymph nodes all over the body and the liver and bone marrow are also affected.

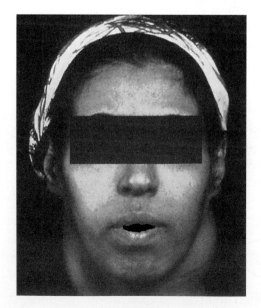

Figure 5.2. Hodgkin's disease

Treatment begun in Stage I or II may be restricted to radiation to kill off the cancer cells. If the disease is caught in Stage III or IV, radiation may be combined with chemotherapy. For cases particularly resistant to treatment, very extreme radiation followed by a bone marrow transplant to replace the damaged cells may be recommended. In this procedure, samples of the patient's own marrow are taken and stored before treatment begins, thus insuring a good tissue match.

PROGNOSIS

Of patients who begin treatment in Stage I or II of Hodgkin's disease, 70 to 80% will live 10 years or longer. Of those who begin treatment in Stage III or IV, up to half of them live 5 years or more. A person who has a history of Hodgkin's disease needs to be conscientious about keeping track of his condition, though, because this cancer does recur on some occasions. Also, people who have had Hodgkin's have a higher risk of developing some other kind of cancer, especially leukemia, later in life.

MASSAGE?

The general rule for Swedish massage and cancer of any kind has been that a 5-year period with no evidence of new growth should pass before a client receives rigorous circulatory massage. Massage that improves immune response with minimal circulatory impact (e.g., reflexology, trigger points along the spine, energy work, etc.) *may* be indicated earlier than 5 years, although only with medical clearance.

Rules for massage and cancer are undergoing close scrutiny as many cancer patients, even those with recent tumor removal or who are undergoing chemotherapy, are experiencing great benefits from massage. See more under *cancer*, chapter 6, page 358.

Lymphangitis

DEFINITION: WHAT IS IT?

Lymphangitis is an infection with inflammation in the *lymphangions*: lymphatic capillaries.

DEMOGRAPHICS: WHO GETS IT?

People with depressed immunity and/or poor circulation are especially susceptible to lymphangitis and lymphadenitis (inflammation of the lymph nodes), because their macrophage activity is likely to be sluggish, while their colonies of bacteria are more than happy to take advantage of the opportunity to set up shop.

Massage practitioners have a much greater chance of developing lymphangitis than most clients do. This condition is an occupational hazard for bodywork professionals because repeated immersions of the hands in soapy water may lead to hangnail formation and drying and cracking of nail beds, which in turn increases the chance of infection.

ETIOLOGY: WHAT HAPPENS?

In lymphangitis, the lymph capillaries become infected, usually with some of the colonies of streptococcus bacteria that congregate on the skin. This condition can be a complication of cellulitis or from a viral or *fungal infection* (see chapter 1, page 7). If the pathogens are successful, they can

---

LYMPHANGITIS IN BRIEF

What is it?

Lymphangitis is an infection of lymph capillaries. If it proceeds to the nodes, it is called *lymphadenitis*. If it travels past the lymphatic system, it is called blood poisoning (*septicemia*), and it can be life threatening.

How is it recognized?

Lymphangitis includes all the signs of local infection: pain, heat, redness, swelling. It also often shows red streaks from the site of infection running toward the nearest lymph nodes.

Is massage indicated or contraindicated?

Massage is systemically contraindicated for lymphangitis until the infection has been completely eradicated.

LYMPHANGITIS: CASE HISTORY

Rebecca, age 24

"It was the most miserable night of my life."

One winter I was working four jobs at once. I was a tutor for a massage school, I was setting up a small practice of my own, I was a nanny during the afternoons, and I was also working in a theatre company, doing anything that needed doing, which was usually a lot.

I remember it was the week before Christmas, which was a really busy time for the theatre company—we went on tour doing shows for young children. I had also done several massage treatments that week, which was unusual for me. I was working in the light booth at the theatre one morning when I noticed that a hangnail on my right index finger suddenly seemed swollen, hot, and tender. I could do nothing about it. I remember sitting there for about an hour watching it get bigger, redder, and more painful.

That afternoon I had to leave town to be with my family over the holidays. The airport had been socked in with fog for three days, which delayed all the flights, so I missed my connection and had to spend the night on the floor of O'Hare Airport in Chicago. It was one of the most miserable times I can remember. I was feverish and shaking, and my hand hurt like hell.

By the time I finally reached D.C., all I wanted to do was go to bed. I spent practically the entire holiday flat on my back. The swelling of my finger finally subsided, but not before I broke out in intensely painful fever blisters all over my mouth. My doctor back home told me they were probably just an opportunistic outbreak while my defenses were low. All I know is they made it impossible to eat and I missed all my favorite Christmas foods.

I found out much later that I had probably had lymphangitis, and that I was very lucky it didn't develop into blood poisoning, especially since I didn't see a doctor until the whole thing was over. If I had it to do over again, I'd make sure I *never* let myself get so run-down, and I'd be sure to cover any noticeable hangnails before doing massage. I wouldn't wish an experience like that on my worst enemy.

set up an infection in the lymph vessel before macrophages or other white blood cells can stop them. Infections that infiltrate the lymph nodes themselves are called *lymphadenitis*.

SIGNS AND SYMPTOMS

Symptoms of lymphangitis include signs of local infection: pain, heat, redness, swelling. The infected lymph vessel will often light up with a visible scarlet track running proximally from the portal of entry, which is usually some lesion in the skin such as a hangnail, a knife cut, or an insect bite. If the infection remains unchecked by white blood cells, it will quickly move further into the lymph system, leading to swollen nodes, fever, and a general feeling of misery. This can happen very quickly; lymphangitis can become a systemic infection in a matter of hours.

COMPLICATIONS

Lymphangitis is an infection of the *lymph* system, not the circulatory system. However, if even a few bacteria move past the filtering action of the lymph nodes, the infection *will* enter the bloodstream at the right or left subclavian veins. Then the situation changes to a much more serious one: septicemia, or blood poisoning, which is life-threatening. This is why, if lymphangitis is a possibility, medical intervention is advisable at the earliest possible opportunity.

TREATMENT

Lymphangitis is usually treated successfully with antibiotic therapy. Treatment must begin soon after the infection has been identified, however, or the infection may complicate into blood poisoning or cellulitis.

MASSAGE?

Lymphangitis sufferers feel so sick so fast that it's highly unlikely that an infected client would try to keep an appointment. While a client who has lymphangitis should not *receive* massage, a practitioner who has it likewise should not *give* massage. Therefore, massage therapists must keep their hands clean and own a good pair of cuticle scissors. They must *not* allow hangnails and other lesions to remain uncovered or untrimmed, and perhaps most important, they must *not* allow their health to degenerate to the point that they are vulnerable to this kind of infection.

If a massage therapist has an open hangnail or other wound on a finger, the threat of lymphangitis is an excellent reason to cover it with a "finger cot" during massage appointments.

Immune System Conditions

Chronic Fatigue Syndrome

DEFINITION: WHAT IS IT?

Chronic fatigue syndrome (CFS) is a recently recognized, distinct collection of signs and symptoms that varies in severity from being mildly limiting to completely debilitating.

This condition was officially named in 1988 by scientists at the Centers for Disease Control. They purposefully kept the name vague because this disease affects different people in very different ways, and they feared any more specificity about causes or symptoms would exclude some people who are badly affected by this condition. Nonetheless, some people feel this title trivializes their condition, and CFS is therefore also called CFIDS (*chronic fatigue immune dysfunction syndrome*). In Europe this same condition is called *myalgic encephalomyelitis*, or ME.

CFS probably has been around since at least the nineteenth century. Florence Nightingale suffered from debilitating fatigue for decades; it is suspected that she had CFS. This condition may also be behind other vague diagnostic labels such as "neurasthenia," "iron poor blood," and, more recently, "yuppie flu."

DEMOGRAPHICS: WHO GETS IT?

This is an interesting question. Many medical professionals still don't recognize this emerging disease, making it hard to say accurately what part of the population is affected

---

CHRONIC FATIGUE SYNDROME IN BRIEF

What is it?
Chronic fatigue syndrome (CFS) is a collection of signs and symptoms that indicate an ongoing immune response. The original stimulus of the response may be an identifiable pathogen, or it may simply be a dysfunction of the immune system.

How is it recognized?
The central symptom to CFS is debilitating fatigue. It may be accompanied by swollen nodes, slight fever, muscular and joint aches, headaches, excessive pain after mild exercise, and nonrestorative sleep.

Is massage indicated or contraindicated?
Massage is indicated for CFS except during fever, and can be a very helpful part of a treatment plan.

most. To date, this disease is reported mainly by white middle and upper class women from 25 to 45 years old; this is the origin of the term "yuppie flu." In fact, it's been found that this slice of the population is simply most likely to seek medical help; they are not the only people affected. CFS affects all segments of the population and is probably not gender specific. Current estimates suggest that anywhere from 200,000 to 500,000 adults in the United States may be affected to some extent. Although it is known that CFS can also affect young children and teens, statistics on childhood incidence are not available.

ETIOLOGY: WHAT HAPPENS?

Blood studies show that someone with CFS is trying hard to fight off an infection. Antibody, T-cell, and interleukin levels are much higher in his blood than in a healthy person's. It seems as though the CFS patient was at one time infected with some pathogen that initiated a normal immune response. For many people, the original infection may have been Epstein Barr (the virus associated with mononucleosis); for others, it may have been herpes, a bad cold, or anything else. But long after that infectious agent is cast out of the body, the immune system still tries to fight it. Some people may not have had an original infection, but an emotionally or physically stressful event may trigger the onset of CFS. This condition is very similar to an ongoing allergic reaction: the body is trying desperately to fight something off, *even though there is no danger*. What's becoming clear is that the symptoms of CFS are *not* caused by the original infectious agent, but by immune system hyperactivity.

The process of fighting a disease, especially a disease that isn't really there, is literally exhausting: to the adrenal glands (which are pumping out both adrenaline and cortisol to fight a nonexistent infection); to energy levels because the adrenal glands become so depleted; and to one's emotional equilibrium. Who can cope with feeling sick and weak and nonfunctional *all the time* without becoming depressed? And depression adds a whole different list of chemical reactions to the equation.

Some of the latest research in CFS points to a dysfunction in the pituitary-adrenal axis: the vital link between the nervous and endocrine systems that helps to cope with stress and changes in the immediate environment. Several phenomena support this theory. For one thing, CFS is strongly linked with a neurological disorder called *neurally mediated hypotension*, in which messages from the brain to the circulatory system keep the blood vessels from contracting enough to maintain a normal blood pressure. This condition is connected to an inappropriate response to adrenaline. People with CFS typically have extremely low levels of cortisol in the blood, which indicates adrenal exhaustion as a part of the picture. And finally, many people with CFS report moderate to severe allergies: a further example of inappropriate immune response and adrenal depletion.

CAUSES

A lot of research in CFS has focused on trying to identify a specific pathogen that dependably initiates this ongoing immune response. Some of the viruses under investigation have included human herpesvirus-6, Epstein Barr, some retroviruses including HIV, enteroviruses, and other factors such as toxic exposure or genetic predisposition. So far, no single pathogen or environmental factor has been identified as a cause for CFS. It's not even clear whether it's contagious. In rare circumstances, it appears in clusters: whole households or a high percentage of a workplace may be affected. But for the most part, CFS appears randomly across a wide spectrum of the population.

SIGNS AND SYMPTOMS

Fatigue that is unending and not restored by sleep or rest is the central symptom of CFS. Other symptoms vary, but may include general muscular or joint pain, low-grade fever, swollen lymph nodes, headaches, and sore throat.

CFS usually has a fairly specific onset: it is possible to identify when symptoms began and to differentiate new patterns in headaches or general muscle pain. Occasionally, though, CFS has a less obvious point of onset and only gradually becomes debilitating.

Typically, people who experience a sudden onset of the disease will eventually also experience sudden relief; it simply stops, although it may be many years before that relief occurs. People who have a gradual onset are more likely to live with this disease as a lifelong condition.

DIAGNOSIS

No special marker exists for CFS, contributing to the difficulty many medical professionals have to accepting CFS as a real disease. This condition is diagnosed first by ruling out other diseases with a similar profile. Once that has been accomplished, CFS is diagnosed based on the following criteria:

- Presence of clinically evaluable fatigue with a specific onset not traced to physical labor. The fatigue is not relieved by rest, and it forces a reduction in all normal activities. This is present for a minimum of 6 months.
- At least four of the following additional symptoms must be present. They must not predate the onset of fatigue, and they must be a consistent problem for 6 months or more:
  - short-term memory loss
  - tender lymph nodes
  - pain that lasts longer than 24 hours after mild exercise
  - confusion
  - muscle pain
  - nonrestorative sleep
  - sore throat
  - joint pain without signs of inflammation
  - headaches of a new type or pattern since the onset of symptoms

DIFFERENTIAL DIAGNOSES

Several conditions present similarly to CFS, although they may seem quite different from each other. These conditions must by ruled out as a primary cause for the fatigue of CFS, although some of them may be secondary complications of the disease, or they may occur simultaneously with CFS:

- fibromyalgia
- post polio syndrome
- hepatitis
- cancer
- Gulf War syndrome
- Lyme disease
- diabetes
- anorexia
- lupus
- allergies or chemical sensitivities
- clinical depression
- other mental conditions that can cause similar symptoms

TREATMENT

The primary treatment for CFS is making lifestyle choices that support the body as fully as possible. This means avoiding stress as much as possible (here, "stress" means anything—emotional or physical—that requires the body to adapt to a change); modifying diet to minimize stimulants (caffeine, sugar) and depressants (alcohol) as much as possible; and exercising very gently, within tolerance so as not to exacerbate symptoms.

Chemical intervention can be helpful, but it is sometimes difficult to find exactly the right combination of drugs. Many CFS patients are extremely hypersensitive to chemicals; often one-quarter of the regular dosage is adequate. A powerful combination for many people is immune-suppressant drugs combined with low-dose tricyclic antidepressants.

MASSAGE?

Massage can be a wonderful part of a treatment plan for someone with CFS. It stimulates a parasympathetic response; it cleanses tissues and stimulates circulation when exercise may be too much to handle; it can relieve muscle and joint pain; and it can improve sleep. Because CFS doesn't appear to be contagious or a condition that spreads through the circulatory system, gentle massage is a safe and appropriate choice for CFS patients.

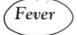

Fever

DEFINITION: WHAT IS IT?

Fever is an abnormally high body temperature usually brought about by bacterial or viral infection, but is sometimes stimulated by other types of tissue damage.

ETIOLOGY: WHAT HAPPENS?

Several steps lead to actually having a fever.

1. A person is infected with some microorganism: bacteria, for instance.
2. Macrophages find and eat those invaders.
3. Some pieces of the bacterial cell membranes are displayed by the macrophages. They stimulate white blood cells to secrete a lymphokine called interleukin-1. Other lymphokines and substances that are secreted include interleukin-6 and tumor necrosis factor (TNF).
4. Interleukin-1 circulates through the system, finding its way to the brain. A series of chemical reactions involving prostaglandins tell the hypothalamus to reset the body's thermostat to a higher level. In this situation, interleukin-1 is acting as a *pyrogen*: a *fever-starter*.
5. Orders from the hypothalamus ripple downward through the body, setting up the muscular and glandular reflexes that will raise the core temperature. These reflexes include shivering, constriction of superficial capillaries, and increased metabolism.

The characteristic shivering and "chills" that accompany a rising fever are part of the mechanism to increase the core temperature. Once that goal has been met, the shivering will stop but the body processes will keep working to maintain the increased temperature until the stress and stimulating chemicals have been removed. Reaching this peak is called the *crisis* of the fever. When the crisis has passed, the body's cooling mechanisms take over: sweating and capillary dilation. These are signs that the worst is over and the fever has broken.

This culture has a strange and somewhat troubling discomfort with discomfort. In general, people would rather *hide* a symptom than *feel* it and figure out what it's trying

---

FEVER IN BRIEF

What is it?
Fever is an increased core temperature brought about by immune system reactions, usually to invasion by some pathogens.

How is it recognized?
Fever is identifiable by thermometer.

Is massage indicated or contraindicated?
Massage is systemically contraindicated for fever, which indicates that the body is fighting infection. This condition can be recognized at a glance (or touch). Massage therapists are not, by the way, usually required to keep thermometers in their offices.

to tell them. This is particularly true with fever, which can be disagreeable and inconvenient. In rare cases, fevers can become high enough to do some serious damage. But for the vast majority of the time, fever is a sign that the body is working in the most efficient way possible to rid the body of invading pathogens. Here's how:

- The presence of interleukin-1 and other cytokines will not only help to reset the body's thermostat, but will stimulate T-cell production. Increased T-cell production will then stimulate B cells and antibodies.
- In the presence of fever, *interferon,* a powerful antiviral agent, is much more active.
- Increased temperature limits iron secretion from the liver and spleen, starving off and slowing bacterial and viral activity.
- Increased temperature will raise the heart rate (10 beats per minute per degree), which in turn increases the distribution of white blood cells throughout the body.
- Increased temperature increases cell wall permeability and speeds chemical reactions. This promotes faster recovery for damaged tissues.

Sometimes people even use a sauna to induce an "artificial fever" in an attempt to stimulate immune system activity. Infection *not* accompanied by fever is considered to be much more serious than the fever itself. Aspirin, ibuprofen, and acetaminophen all work to inhibit fever by interrupting the chemical processes in the hypothalamus that reset the thermostat.

COMPLICATIONS

Fever occasionally complicates into a dangerous situation, particularly when they measure over 104°F. The most common complications are *dehydration* (from prolonged sweating), *acidosis* (the blood becomes too acidic), and once in a great while, brain damage. Death from fever will occur somewhere around 112° to 114°F for adults. If a fever comes down too fast, it can quickly dilate blood vessels. This situation can turn into *shock,* which can be dangerous, especially to older patients.

MASSAGE?

Massage is systemically contraindicated in the presence of fever. Energetic techniques that don't impact blood flow may be helpful for someone having a hard time getting past the crisis point.

HIV/AIDS

DEFINITION: WHAT IS IT?

The human immunodeficiency virus attacks various agents of the immune system with disastrous results. Infection with the virus will eventually develop into AIDS. AIDS was first recognized as a specific disease in the United States in 1981, but research since then indicates it has been present since 1979, and in Africa and the Caribbean long before that.

DEMOGRAPHICS: WHO GETS IT?

Accurate statistics on HIV and AIDS are difficult to collect because of the lack of consistent reporting.

Worldwide. The World Health Organization estimates that 29.4 million people around the world are HIV positive. About 8.4 million of them have AIDS. Women, formerly thought to be less at risk for the disease, now comprise 42% of the people infected, and that number is climbing. Projections suggest that by the year 2000, 40 million people will be infected with the disease.

HIV/AIDS IN BRIEF

What is it?

Acquired Immune Deficiency Syndrome (AIDS) is a disease caused by the Human Immunodeficiency Virus (HIV), which attacks and disables the immune system, leaving a person vulnerable to a host of diseases that are not a threat to uninfected people.

How is it recognized?

Most people with HIV will experience a week or two of flu-like symptoms within a few weeks of being infected. Then an interval passes with no symptoms. When the virus has successfully inactivated the immune system, infections will occur by opportunistic conditions such as cytomegalovirus or pneumocystis carinii. At this point, the HIV infection becomes AIDS.

Is massage indicated or contraindicated?

Massage is indicated for all stages of HIV infection as long as the practitioner is healthy and doesn't pose any risk to the client, and the client is able to keep up with the changes that massage brings about in the body.

About 3.1 million new HIV infections were reported in 1996 alone. That amounts to 8500 each day: 7500 adults plus 1000 infants who were infected prenatally or through breast feeding. About 70% of new infections around the world occur from heterosexual intercourse. People in developing countries account for 90% of new infections.

In 1996, 1.5 million people worldwide died of AIDS; 350,000 of them were children. Cumulative deaths to date amount to 5 million adults and 1.4 million children.

United States. In the United States, approximately 1 million people reportedly are HIV positive, with about 50,000 new cases reported every year. Current cases of AIDS equal about 58,000. Cumulative deaths from this disease add up to over 340,000. Infections and deaths from AIDS are disproportionately high in African Americans and Hispanics. AIDS is the leading cause of death for men from 25 to 44 years old.

ETIOLOGY: WHAT HAPPENS?

Viruses consist of a protein coat of variable complexity wrapped around a core of DNA or RNA. Outside of a host cell, viruses have no metabolic functions and cannot replicate. Inside a host cell, the virus shoots its core into the nucleolus, and reprograms the functions of that cell to reproduce the virus. In other words, the host cell becomes a virus factory. When the factory is full of inventory, it will literally burst at the seams, releasing hordes of new viruses in search of other hosts. Enormous amounts of damage occur with any viral infection, not only to the cells attacked by the virus, but also to the cells the body will sacrifice in order to fight back.

The primary targets of the HIV are helper T cells and some other nonspecific white blood cells. The virus' portals of entry to these cells has been a subject of intensive research. One identified entryway is a specific protein in membranes of target cells, called CD4. This molecule is found in the membranes of helper T cells, as well as some monocytes and macrophages. Because of this particular protein in the cell membrane, helper T cells are sometimes called CD4 cells.

These viral targets are significant for a couple of reasons. First, if the virus pools in macrophages before moving up in the immune system hierarchy, its presence would not immediately trigger the production of antibodies, which makes it difficult to identify in a blood test. Second, consider the consequences of a virus that targets, as its ultimate goal, the helper T cells. Helper T cells are the vital link between humoral and cell-mediated immunity. They tell the B cells when to produce plasma cells and antibodies; they govern the activities of macrophages and monocytes through the secretion of lymphokines; and they also stimulate killer T cells and natural killer cells. Without helper T cells, the entire immune system collapses and leaves the body vulnerable to a wide array of opportunistic diseases.

The core of the HIV virus is RNA, rather than DNA, which holds the blueprints for our own cells. This retrovirus uses an enzyme called *transciptase* to convert its RNA to DNA. In the process, the virus is sometimes minutely altered, just enough to make it resistant to treatment. Drug treatments for AIDS currently focus on interrupting the complex processes of viral transcription and replication inside the host cells.

PROGRESSION

Each stage of this disease is associated with decreasing numbers of active helper T cells and increased viral titres (counts of virus). The typical pattern looks like this:

- Phase 1. A person is infected with HIV. The virus is present in the body, but may be pooling in white blood cells rather than eliciting an immune response. Consequently, tests are negative and no symptoms are present, but the person is very contagious because the "viral load," that is, the level of virus in the blood, is very high. This incubation phase can last a year or more, although the average is three weeks to six months in sexually transmitted cases.
- Phase 2. In the acute primary HIV infection, antibodies will become detectable in blood tests. About 70% of people will experience fatigue, swollen glands, fever, weight loss, headaches, drowsiness, and confusion within several weeks of exposure. These symptoms will usually last about two weeks, and are often mistaken for the flu or mononucleosis.
- Phase 3. This is the inactive period of infection. Usually no symptoms are present, and no opportunistic diseases occur. Although the virus is continuing to replicate while decimating immune system cells, the body is able to keep up with the process. During this phase, medical intervention will limit viral growth and prolong life expectancy. The length of the inactive phase varies widely, depending on the initial health of the person, what kind of treatment is given, and several other factors. It can last anywhere from 1 to 15 years, with a median average of 10 years.
- Phases 4 and 5. During this time, symptoms of opportunistic diseases or AIDS-related cancers become apparent and eventually debilitating. A normal helper T cell count is 800 to 1000 cells per cubic milliliter of blood. AIDS is diagnosed when these levels drop to 200 cells/ml or below.

[handwritten margin notes: — HIV infection — Flu like Symptoms — ↓ immune cells — other disease become present]

SIGNS AND SYMPTOMS

Signs and symptoms of HIV depend on the stage of infection. Specific guidelines are given in the discussion of phases of the disease above.

COMPLICATIONS

When AIDS has virtually disabled normal immune function, the body is incapable of fending off attacks from pathogens with which healthy people have no problems. A list of formerly obscure diseases are now so closely associated with AIDS; they are called "indicator diseases." Here are some of the most common and serious ones:

[handwritten margin note: Related Diseases]

- Pneumocystis carinii pneumonia (PCP): This is a protozoal infection of the lungs.
- Cytomegalovirus (CMV): This can cause retinitis and blindness, colitis, pneumonia, and infection of the adrenal glands.
- Kaposi's sarcoma (KS): This is a type of skin cancer. (See Figure 5.3.)
- B-cell lymphomas: HIV has recently been found to specifically initiate the cancer cell replication with a variety of lymphomas, as well as KS.

Other opportunistic diseases associated with AIDS include *toxoplasmosis*, which can cause encephalitis or pneumonia; *candida*, a yeast infection that can cause thrush or esophagitis; and *cryptococcus neoformans*, a fungal infection that can cause meningitis and pneumonia. In addition to these "indicator diseases," people with AIDS are highly susceptible to gastrointestinal disturbances, herpes simplex, shingles, a specific type of tuberculosis, meningitis, cervical cancer, and many other conditions.

DIAGNOSIS

Infection with HIV is determined by the presence of antibodies in the blood. This is a bit problematic since the peculiar nature of this pathogen prevents the body from tagging it

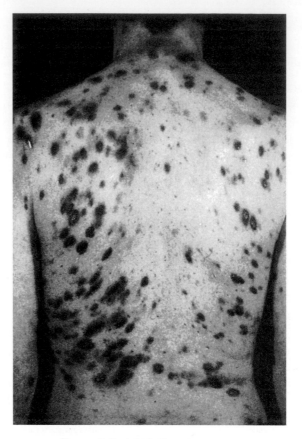

Figure 5.3. AIDS: Kaposi's sarcoma

and initiating antibody production until the virus is widespread. In order to get a truly dependable diagnosis, AIDS tests must be conducted for up to 6 months after the last incidence of high risk behavior: sharing IV drug needles, unprotected sex with a potentially infected partner, or the use of blood or blood products.

Typically the first blood test given is an ELISA (enzyme-linked immunosorbent assay) test. Because this extremely sensitive test sometimes yields false positives, a positive reading is followed by a second ELISA test and/or a Western Blot test. If both tests are negative and the person is clearly in a high-risk population and shows signs of being sick, tests may be conducted to look for signs of the virus itself in the blood, rather than antibodies to the virus.

TREATMENT

One of the things that makes finding a cure for AIDS so difficult is that in the process of converting its core from RNA to DNA, the virus can minutely change, just enough to make it resistant to drugs. The answer to that problem has been to combine various drugs in order to anticipate the mutations of the virus. This has been highly successful in laboratory settings, but these drug combinations are often prohibitively toxic to the actual patients.

The most successful AIDS treatments so far have involved interrupting viral replication at two stages. AZT and AZT-like drugs interfere with the initial stages of conversion from RNA to DNA. They don't eradicate the virus altogether, but they are successful at slowing down the rate of replication, and thus increasing the life expectancy of the patient. A more recent addition to the battle against AIDS has been a group of drugs called *protease inhibitors*. These work to interrupt the later maturing phase as the viruses linger in the T cells and macrophages before they're released. Combining

AZT-type drugs with protease inhibitors has been the most promising combination of drug therapies yet developed.

The future of drug treatment for AIDS looks bright, as new breakthroughs promise better treatments. One of the most recent discoveries includes finding out exactly how the virus gains access to target cells. The CD4 protein in the membranes of helper T cells, monocytes, and macrophages is one important attachment site for the virus. But that molecule alone was not sufficient to admit the virus into the cell; another entry had to exist. A recent discovery has revealed other docking sites for the virus. A class of chemicals called *cytokines* are involved with the inflammatory process. It has been found that HIV will attach at certain cytokine receptors on target cells. But, if the receptors are blocked with the cytokines themselves, the virus has no access. Further, if the receptor sites are somehow damaged or altered, the virus cannot attach. This may account for the rare phenomenon of some people who are actually not susceptible to AIDS at all.

Translating this breakthrough into a treatment strategy may mean trying to genetically alter target cells so their cytokine receptors are resistant to HIV, or developing artificial cytokines that can block the receptors from the virus.

As people with AIDS are contemplating a longer life expectancy than ever before, their needs will be changing. Already a shift has moved away from providing terminal care to providing people with housing, jobs, and protection from discrimination.

The picture for people with AIDS in the United States is rosier than it's been since the disease was identified in 1981. Although treatment can cost $50,000 a year or more, many people with AIDS in the United States at least have access to that treatment. This is not the case in developing countries where AIDS statistics are growing the fastest. Some 90% of the world's AIDS patients have little or no access to treatment.

MASSAGE?

AIDS is spread through the exchange of bodily fluids: semen, breast milk, blood, and vaginal secretions. Research has not shown that it can be transmitted through sweat or casual contact. Therefore, the person most at risk for getting sick when an AIDS patient receives massage is not the therapist but the client. The practitioner must take care not to carry active pathogens that may put the AIDS client at risk.

Massage for HIV-positive clients who are asymptomatic is absolutely indicated. Although in advanced stages of AIDS, opportunistic diseases can make circulatory massage problematic, other types of work may reduce stress, which in turn strengthens the immune system. It can be a very appropriate treatment option, and an important source of support and comfort for people who are often rejected, ignored, or actively persecuted by our society.

Inflammation

DEFINITION: WHAT IS IT?

Inflammation is a protective device in response to injury or infection. It involves localized swelling and chemical reactions to isolate the area and to resolve the damage through immune response.

ETIOLOGY: WHAT HAPPENS?

When a person sustains tissue damage, cells are injured, ripped open, destroyed. The damage may occur from mechanical or thermal stress (a sprain, a laceration, or a burn, for instance); it may be due to pathogenic invasion; or tissue may be injured by toxic chemicals. When cells are injured, they release certain proteins that start a chain of events

INFLAMMATION IN BRIEF

What is it?

Inflammation is a protective device in response to injury or infection. It involves localized swelling and chemical reactions to isolate the area and to resolve the damage through immune response.

How is it recognized?

The signs of inflammation are redness, pain, swelling, heat, and loss of function.

Is massage indicated or contraindicated?

Massage is contraindicated for acute inflammation, but may be appropriate for subacute situations, depending on the causative factors.

designed to minimize total damage. This chain of events is called inflammation: a reaction of injured tissue to defend and protect the body from invasion. The different aspects of this reaction are specifically designed to achieve three basic goals: to dispose of pathogens and cellular debris; to prevent the spread of pathogens in the body; and to prepare the injured area for healing.

Three basic components contribute to all stages of inflammation. The *chemical* components include inflammation mediators, such as histamine and cytokines, released from nearby cells to participate in cell-to-cell communication. The *vascular* components of inflammation involve vasodilation, vasoconstriction, and changes in the permeability of vessel walls to allow the migration of certain blood cells. The *cellular* component of inflammation includes white blood cell movement to the area of infection or injury, and phagocytosis as those WBCs consume pathogens and/or debris.

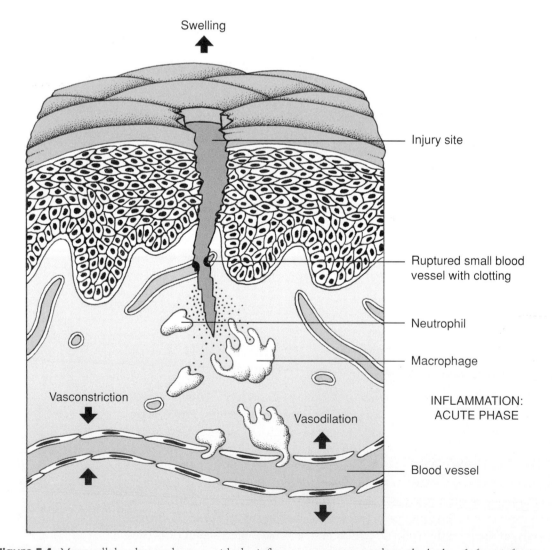

Figure 5.4. Many cellular changes happen with the inflammatory response to keep the body safe from infection.

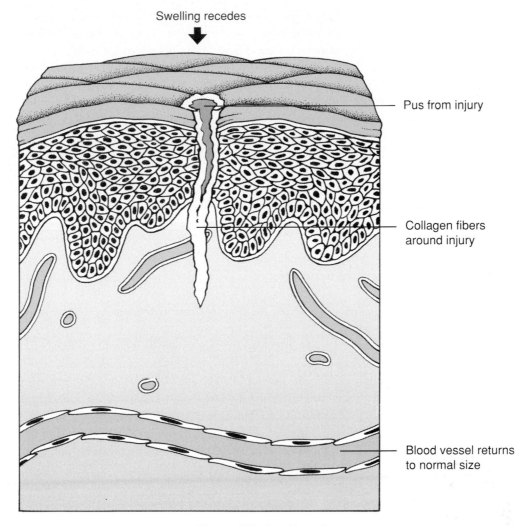

Swelling recedes

Pus from injury

Collagen fibers
around injury

Blood vessel returns
to normal size

Figure 5.4. *(continued)*

PROGRESSION

Step 1: The injury—acute vascular response. For the sake of simplicity, consider a basic laceration or puncture wound as a model, although the same principles will hold true for any kind of local injury. (See Figure 5.4.) In the *very first moments*, especially if it was a very serious injury, vasoconstriction will occur. This is a protective mechanism against excessive bleeding. The vasoconstrictive stage is over within a few seconds for a minor injury, and several minutes for a more serious one.

Following vasoconstriction is a period of arteriolar vasodilation, which is the most important step in the whole inflammatory process. Injured cells, especially mast cells stationed in superficial fascia and epithelial membranes all over the body, release a host of chemicals that all cause increased permeability of blood vessel walls and capillary dilation. When those two features occur together, substances can quickly get *out* of the bloodstream and *into* the damaged area. Specifically, neutrophils are usually the first white blood cells to arrive, but they are accompanied by antibodies and clotting factors equally crucial in the inflammatory process. In addition to bringing new material in, this increased fluid flow also tends to flush wastes out, including dead cells and pathogenic toxins.

Step 2: Fibrin formation. A complicated chain of events causes certain blood proteins to precipitate out and form fibrous nets. These nets serve a double purpose of making a clot to close off any broken blood vessels, and to catch loose pathogens before they enter the bloodstream. Blood clots help to isolate infection from the rest of the body.

Step 3: White blood cells arrive.   One of the chemicals released early by damaged cells goes to bone marrow and stimulates it to produce extra *neutrophils*, the cannon fodder of the immune system. These little cells arrive within a few minutes to a few hours of the inflammatory signals, sacrificing themselves to eat or at least slow down any pathogens they can find. Later in the cycle of the infection, the macrophages show up. They are bigger than the neutrophils; they have bigger appetites and can disable more than one pathogen, while the neutrophils can only serve once. Macrophages eat pathogens as well as the body's own dead and damaged cells.

Step 4: Inflammatory exudate formation.   Exudates are any fluids expressed from tissues that are in the process of healing. One example of exudate is pus. Pus is comprised of dead and living white blood cells, along with whatever pathogens they've managed to kill. Pus is usually walled in by the thickened connective tissues surrounding the infection site. It can be expressed through the surface of the skin, aspirated, or, if left alone long enough, it will usually be reabsorbed by the body (macrophages will eventually clean it up).

Step 5: Tissue healing.   Fibroblasts, like white blood cells, migrate to an injured area. Early in the inflammatory process, nearby fibroblasts are stimulated to start spinning new collagen fibers. They produce loads of collagen to be used to knit together torn fibers or to thicken and toughen the nearby connective tissue membrane walls: another isolation mechanism.

Steps 1 through 4 happen in what would be considered the acute phase of infection: they begin within moments of the injury, and remain the primary activity for up to 3 days, depending on the severity of the damage.

The rebuilding of damaged tissue usually begins 3 to 4 days after the injury and continues for 2 weeks or more. The maturation phase, when the scar tissue molds and changes according to the stresses put upon it, can last up to two years, depending on the severity of the injury, the general health of the person, and other variables.

SIGNS AND SYMPTOMS

Every massage therapist should know this litany: the symptoms of inflammation are pain, heat, redness, swelling, and sometimes loss of function. In some cases, itching, clotting, and pus formation could be added to the list.

It's easy to see how each of these symptoms comes about. Vasodilation brings about the redness, heat, and swelling by drawing extra blood to a small area. Pain and itching can be the result of several factors: edemic pressure, damaged nerve endings, irritating pathogenic toxins, even irritating chemicals released by other cells. If the inflammation limits joint movement, the patient experiences loss of function. Clotting and pus formation have already been discussed. Not all of these symptoms will be present in all cases of inflammation.

With long-lasting infectious inflammations, the types of white blood cells present will vary, and it may take days or weeks to completely eradicate all traces of the pathogens. (Some pathogens are never completely eradicated, but simply become dormant: see *herpes zoster*, chapter 3, page 144.) Also some traces of pathogens will cause a system-wide reaction accompanied by *fever* (this chapter, page 232). Musculoskeletal injuries will also include subacute and chronic stages. For more information on what can be done in those situations, see *sprains*, *strains*, and *tendinitis*, chapter 2, pages 87, 59, and 103, respectively.

TREATMENT

The typical treatment for inflammation is no surprise: anti-inflammatories. These can be steroidal, e.g., cortisone, or nonsteroidal, e.g., aspirin. Regardless of their chemical impact on the body, anti-inflammatories may have significant impact on massage: they may hide the results of overtreatment, thus raising the risk that massage could cause injury. If a client is taking anti-inflammatories for a condition that does not contraindicate massage, suggest that she make her appointment just as her dose is wearing off. That way it will be possible to get much more accurate information about what massage is actually doing to her body.

MASSAGE?

Acute localized infections and inflammation at the very least locally contraindicate massage. Thickened fascial walls will isolate the infection to a certain extent, but working distally to a badly infected knee may be asking for trouble. Work proximally only. For a view of a worst case scenario, see *lymphangitis*, this chapter, page 227. If the infection is systemic, as in *influenza* (chapter 6, page 251), it is also a systemic contraindication, at least in the acute stage.

In the postacute stages of infection and inflammation, massage can be very helpful in flushing out debris and improving circulation that may have been sluggish and congested for a while.

Inflammation does not always imply the presence of infection. Sprains and *dermatitis* (chapter 1, page 21) are two examples among many conditions in which an inflammatory process may exist without invading pathogens. When inflammation is present without infection, the general rule for massage is to wait for the subacute stage, during which bringing more fluid to the area is not likely to make matters worse. For more specific guidelines, check the appropriate sections.

Lupus

DEFINITON: WHAT IS IT?

Lupus is an autoimmune disease in which the connective tissues are attacked by the body's own antibodies. Although it only rarely becomes life threatening, lupus has the potential to be devastating. The human body is composed of more connective tissue than anything else, and lupus antibodies interpret all that connective tissue as the enemy. Lupus tries to destroy the very tissues that holds the body together.

DEMOGRAPHICS: WHO GETS IT?

Statistics on this disease vary greatly. Population surveys estimate that the incidence of lupus in the United States is between 1.4 and 2 million people. African Americans and Asians have higher rates than Caucasians, and Caribbean blacks have the highest rates of all.

Lupus affects people at any age, but it is most common in people between 10 and 50 years of age. It affects women far more than men; depending on the age group studied, women with lupus outnumber men by as much as 9 to 1.

ETIOLOGY: WHAT HAPPENS?

Three varieties of lupus have been identified: drug-induced lupus erythematosis, discoid lupus erythematosis (DLE), and systemic lupus erythematosis (SLE).

- Drug-induced lupus. This is a situation in which some rarely prescribed medications for high blood pressure, heart arrhythmia, and epilepsy can create lupus symptoms. These symptoms will disappear when the medications are discontinued.
- Discoid lupus erythematosis. This is a chronic skin disease. It can involve small scaly red patches with

LUPUS

From the Latin word for "wolf," several possibilities exist for the origin of this name. It could refer to the characteristic "butterfly mask" on the face that looks like the facial markings of a wolf, or it could refer to the lesions that may appear on the face or elsewhere on the body that were thought to resemble wolf bites.

LUPUS IN BRIEF

What is it?
Lupus is an autoimmune disease in which antibodies attack various types of connective tissue throughout the body. Three varieties have been identified, of which *systemic lupus erythematosis* is the most serious.

How is it recognized?
Eleven specific criteria are used to identify lupus. They include, among other things, arthritis in two or more joints, pleurisy, pericarditis, and kidney and nervous system dysfunction.

Is massage indicated or contraindicated?
Massage is systemically contraindicated for acute flares of lupus. It *may* be indicated in the subacute stage, depending on the health of the tissues.

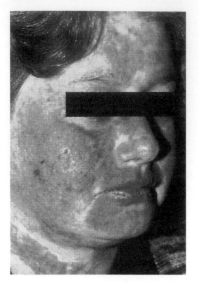

Figure 5.5. Lupus

sharp margins that don't itch, or it can create the characteristic "butterfly rash" of redness over the nose and cheeks. (See Figure 5.5, Color Plate 31.) The skin can become very thin and delicate. If the lesions scar, permanent hair loss may follow. About 10% of people with DLE will go on to develop systemic lupus erythematosis.

- Systemic lupus erythematosis. This is a situation in which antibody attack are launched against a variety of connective tissues throughout the body. This can result in *arthritis* (chapter 2, page 80), *renal failure* (chapter 8, page 314), bleeding disorders, psychosis, seizures, inflammation of the heart, and pleurisy. This very serious disorder can usually be controlled but, at this time, cannot be cured. SLE sometimes begins as DLE, but not always.

CAUSES

The precise cause or causes of lupus are unknown. A genetic link has been found, but a child of a parent with lupus has only a 5% chance of developing the disease. Environmental factors may include exposure to certain viruses, ultraviolet light, certain medications, and high levels of estrogen. Women with lupus often report a change in symptoms with their menstrual cycle, and recent research shows that estrogen replacement therapy employed to reduce the risk of *osteoporosis* (chapter 2, page 62) can increase the risk of lupus for some women.

SIGNS AND SYMPTOMS

The rest of this discussion will focus on SLE, which creates the most far-reaching and long-lasting symptoms of the three varieties of lupus.

Lupus can affect virtually every system in the body. Although no two patients will ever share the same symptoms, a brief overview of some of its most common manifestations is helpful:

- Musculoskeletal System. Of all people with lupus, 80 to 90% will eventually develop arthritis. Some will even experience necrosis (tissue death) of bone and joint tissue, especially in the hips and shoulders. Nonspecific muscle pain is another common symptom, and often some overlap exists between lupus and *fibromyalgia* (chapter 2, page 50).
- Integumentary System. The characteristic butterfly rash seen with lupus has already been mentioned. These rashes, which can appear anywhere on the body, are badly exacerbated by sunlight in a condition called *photosensitivity*. Lupus can also cause ulcers in the mucus membranes, particularly in the nose, throat, and mouth.
- Nervous System. Twenty-five percent of people with lupus will have some nervous system dysfunction. This can range from migraine headaches to psychosis to *seizures* (chapter 3, page 166). Lupus is occasionally misdiagnosed as epilepsy.
- Cardiovascular System. Lupus is associated with a specific clotting disorder that involves slow clot formation and slow clot dissolving. This problem affects 30 to 50% of lupus patients, and can lead to *stroke* (chapter 3, page 161) or *pulmonary embolism* (chapter 4, page 183). The serous membranes of the heart can be affected too, which results in inflammation, arrhythmia, and severe chest pain. *Anemia* (chapter 4, page 178) and *Raynaud's syndrome* (chapter 4, page 202) are other circulatory system complications of lupus.
- Respiratory System. A common complication of lupus is pleurisy: inflammation and fluid accumulation in the serous membranes that line the lungs.
- Urinary System. Tissue damage in the kidneys creates *glomerulonephritis* (chapter 8, page 309), a condition seen in 50% of people with lupus. Kidney damage can accumulate without symptoms until the kidneys are on the brink of *renal failure* (chapter 8, page 314).

- Reproductive System. The specific clotting disorder associated with lupus can make it difficult to carry a child to term. Repeated spontaneous miscarriages are sometimes the first sign of the disease that will lead to a diagnosis.

DIAGNOSIS

It is clear from this long and varied list of symptoms that lupus can look like a lot of different diseases. Fortunately, it leaves some specific clues in the blood that can help to identify the disease. Unfortunately, those clues are sometimes present in people *without* lupus so they can't be used as a definitive diagnosis.

A collection of eleven signs and symptoms are common for lupus patients. If any four of these criteria are present at any time, a positive diagnosis of lupus can be made. The four signs do *not* need to be present simultaneously.

- malar (butterfly) rash
- discoid skin rash (can cause permanent scarring)
- photosensitivity
- mucus membrane ulcers, particularly in the mouth, nose, or throat
- arthritis in more than two joints
- pleurisy and/or pericarditis
- kidney problems: blood or protein in the urine
- brain irritation: seizures or psychosis
- blood count abnormalities: low RBCs, WBCs, or platelets
- immunologic disorders: special lupus cells are present in the blood
- lupus antibodies (ANA) present in the blood

This condition, like other autoimmune conditions, is exacerbated by certain kinds of stimuli. Exposure to certain drugs, including penicillin, sulfa, and tetracyclene, will initiate an attack. So will excess exposure to sunlight, emotional stress, injury, infection, or trauma. Someone who has lupus must identify those stimuli that are particularly potent for her and avoid them carefully.

TREATMENT

Treatment for lupus begins with trying to minimize the kinds of events that tend to trigger attacks. Drug therapy will start with nonsteroidal and then steroidal anti-inflammatories. Immunosuppressive drugs are sometimes used to quell the needless attacks on the connective tissues.

PROGNOSIS

In the 1950s, one-half of all people diagnosed with lupus died within 5 years. Today, 80 to 90% of new lupus patients live 10 years, and after they reach the 10-year mark, their life span is essentially the same as the general population. These remarkable advances are due to earlier detection of the disease and better drug therapies that keep system-wide inflammation under control. Although no cure currently exists for lupus, the length and quality of life these patients can expect are better than they've ever been.

MASSAGE?

Active flares of lupus mark periods of inflammation that can damage the heart, the lungs, the kidneys, and the joints. Massage during these acute episodes is systemically contraindicated. Subacute periods *may* be appropriate for massage, especially as a treatment strategy against the stress that can trigger attacks, but care must be taken to ensure that the circulatory system is capable of handling the changes in internal environment brought about by massage.

CHAPTER REVIEW QUESTIONS:
LYMPH AND IMMUNE SYSTEM CONDITIONS

1. What is an allergy?

2. What is an autoimmune disease? Give two examples.

3. What are lymphokines, and what do they do?

4. What type of cell is the primary target for HIV?

5. Who is most at risk for getting sick when a massage therapist works with an AIDS patient? Why?

6. What is the link between chronic fatigue syndrome and the immune system?

7. Describe how the inflammatory process causes pain, heat, redness, and swelling.

8. What are the dangers of working with a client who is taking anti-inflammatories?

9. How is lupus generally treated medically? Why?

10. Why are massage therapists particularly at risk for lymphangitis?

BIBLIOGRAPHY, LYMPH AND IMMUNE SYSTEM CONDITIONS

General References, Lymph and Immune Systems

1. Carmine D. Clemente. Anatomy: A regional atlas of the human body. 3rd ed. Baltimore: Urban & Schwarzenburg, 1987.

2. I. Damjanou. Pathology for the health-related professions. Philadelphia: Saunders, 1996.

3. Giovanni de Dominico, Elizabeth Wood. Beard's massage. Philadelphia: Saunders, 1997.

4. Deane Juhan. Job's body: A handbook for bodywork. Barrytown, NY: Station Hill Press, Inc., 1987.

5. Jeffrey R. M. Kunz, Asher J. Finkel, eds. The American Medical Association family medical guide. New York: Random House, Inc., 1987.

6. Elaine M. Marieb. Human anatomy and physiology. Redwood City, CA: Benjamin/Cummings Publishing Co., Inc., 1989.

7. Ruth Lundeen Memmler, Dina Lin Wood. The human body in health and disease. 5th ed. Philadelphia: JB Lippincott Co., 1983.

8. Mary Lou Mulvihill. Human diseases: A systemic approach. 2nd ed. East Norwalk, CT: Appleton & Lange, A publishing division of Prentice-Hall, 1987.

9. Stedman's medical dictionary. 26th ed. Baltimore: Williams & Wilkins, 1995.

10. Taber's cyclopedic dictionary. 14th ed. Philadelphia: F.A. Davis Company, 1981.

11. Gerard J. Tortora, Nicholas P. Anagnostakos. Principles of anatomy and physiology. 6th ed. New York: Biological Sciences Textbook, Inc.; A&P Textbooks, Inc.; and Elia-Sparta, Inc., Harper & Row Publishers, Inc., 1990.

12. Janet Travell, David G. Simons. Myofascial pain and dysfunction: The trigger point manual. Baltimore: Williams & Wilkins, 1983.

Hodgkin's Disease

1. Adult hodgkin's disease. National Cancer Institute/PDQ Patient Statement, October 1997. URL: http://rex.nci.nih.gov/INTRFCE_GIFS/INFO_PATS_INTR_DOC.htm. Accessed fall 1997.

2. Hodgkin's disease. Copyright 1998 ADAM Software, Inc., all rights reserved. Copyright 1998 CommuniHealth. URL: http://www.healthanswers.com. Accessed winter 1998.

3. MedicineNet: Power points about hodgkin's disease, adult. Information Network, Inc., 1995–1997. URL: http://www.medicinenet.com. Accessed fall 1997.

Lymphangitis

1. Lymphadenitis and lymphangitis. Copyright 1998 ADAM Software, Inc., all rights reserved. Copyright 1998 CommuniHealth. URL: http://www.

healthanswers.com. Accessed winter 1998.

Chronic Fatigue Syndrome

1. The CFS FAQ, Version: 1.32 (last revised March 19, 1997). Roger Burns on behalf of the CFS Internet Group, 1997. URL: http://www.cais.net/cfs-news/faq.htm; *or* http://www.jmas.co.jp/FAQs/medicine/ chronic-fatigue-syndrome/cfs-faq. Accessed fall 1997.
2. Chronic fatigue syndrome. National Institute of Allergy and Infectious Diseases, March 1995. URL: http://www.niaid.nih. gov/factsheets/cfs.htm. Accessed fall 1997.
3. Clinical aspects and demographics for CFS. Center for Disease Control, June 10, 1997. URL: http://www.cdc.gov/ncidod/ diseases/cfs/facts2.htm. Accessed fall 1997.
4. Overview of the NIAID chronic fatigue syndrome research program. National Institute of Allergy and Infectious Diseases, April 1997. URL: http://www.niaid.nih. gov/factsheets/cfsoverview.htm. Accessed fall 1997.
5. Understanding CFIDS. The CFIDS Association of America, Inc., 1996. URL: http://www.cfids.org/cfids.html. Accessed fall 1997.

Fever

1. Peter Slavkovsky. Fever and inflammation. Academic Electronic Press, 1995. URL: http://www.savba.sk/logos/books/ scientific/Inffever.html. Accessed fall 1997.

HIV/AIDS

1. The evidence that HIV causes AIDS. National Institute of Allergy and Infectious Diseases, July 1995. URL: http://www. niaid.nih.gov/factsheets/evidhiv.htm. Accessed fall 1997.
2. HIV infection and AIDS. National Institute of Allergy and Infectious Diseases, May 1997. URL: http://www.niaid.nih. gov/factsheets/hivinf.htm. Accessed fall 1997.
3. HIV/AIDS statistics worldwide. National Institute of Allergy and Infectious Diseases, September 1997. URL: http://www. niaid.nih.gov/factsheets/aidsstat.htm. Accessed fall 1997.
4. How HIV causes AIDS. National Institute of Allergy and Infectious Diseases, August 1996. URL: http://www.niaid. nih.gov/factsheets/howhiv.htm. Accessed fall 1997.
5. MedicineNet: Power points about AIDS. Information Network, Inc., 1995–1997. URL: http://www.medicinenet.com. Accessed fall 1997.
6. Presidential Advisory Council on HIV/ AIDS, July 8, 1996: Executive Summary Progress Report. CDC National AIDS Clearinghouse. URL: http://hivinsite.ucsf. edu/ads/9607/96071511.html. Accessed fall 1997.

Lupus

1. Estrogen and lupus. Arthritis Today, Scientific Frontiers 1995(Nov/Dec). URL: http://www.arthritis.org/at/archive/1995/ 11_12/ossf.shtml. Accessed fall 1997.
2. Robert G. Lahita. Symptoms of lupus. July 30, 1996. URL: http://www.hamline. edu.lupus.articles.symptoms_of_lupus. html. Accessed fall 1997.
3. Lupus anticoagulant. Copyright 1998 ADAM Software, Inc., all rights reserved. Copyright 1998 CommuniHealth. URL: http://www.healthanswers.com. Accessed winter 1998.
4. Lupus—Improved prognosis, but still difficult to diagnose. Mayo Foundation for Medical Education and Research. Mayo Health O@asis: May 1996. URL: http://www.mayo.ivi.com/mayo/9605/htm/ lupus.htm. Accessed fall 1997.
5. MedicineNet: Power points about systemic lupus erythematosis. Information Network, Inc., 1995–1997. URL: http:// www.medicinenet.com. Accessed fall 1997.
6. Systemic lupus erythematosis. Copyright 1998 ADAM Software, Inc., all rights reserved. Copyright 1998 CommuniHealth. URL: http://www.healthanswers.com. Accessed winter 1998.
7. Systemic lupus erythematosis. National Jewish Medical and Research Center, 1996. URL: http://www.njc.org/PRhtml/ !k_Lupus.htm. Accessed fall 1997.

Respiratory System Conditions

6

OBJECTIVES

After reading this chapter, you should be able to tell . . .

- What the disorder is.
- How to recognize it.
- Whether massage is indicated or contraindicated for that condition.
- Whether a contraindication is local or systemic, or refers to a specific stage of development or healing.
- Why those choices for massage are correct.

In addition to this basic information, you should be able to . . .

- Describe the basic mechanics of breathing, listing the main muscles involved.
- Describe where in the lungs gaseous exchange occurs and what structures are involved.
- Name two possible factors behind the recent rise in asthma statistics.
- Name two differences between influenza and the common cold.
- Know how Type A flu viruses can reinfect the same person.
- Name three risk factors for the development of emphysema.
- Briefly describe stages 0 through IV of lung cancer.
- Tell which is more common, primary or secondary pneumonia, and why.
- Name three possible causes for sinusitis.
- Know the prevalence of tuberculosis worldwide.

INTRODUCTION

STRUCTURE

The easiest way to discuss the structure of the respiratory system is to follow a particle of air through it. (See Figure 6.1.) Take a deep breath: air drawn in through the nose encounters mucous membranes. Mucous membranes line any cavity in the body that communicates with the outside world: the respiratory system, the digestive system, the reproductive system, and the urinary system. In the respiratory system, the mucous membranes start inside the nose and mouth and line the sinuses and throat, all the way down into the smaller tubes in the lungs. The wet, sticky mucous membranes in the respiratory system are responsible for warming, moistening, and filtering all the air that passes by.

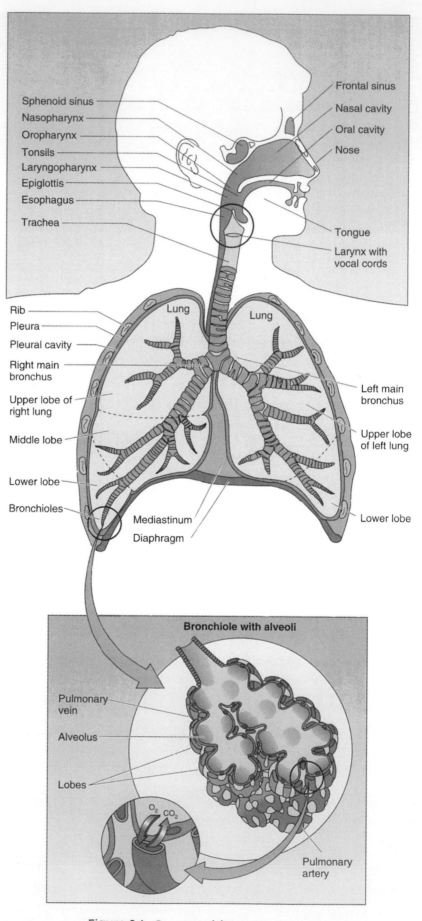

Figure 6.1. Overview of the respiratory system

Once past the nose and mouth, air enters first the pharynx, then the larynx, then the bronchi. The bronchi are asymmetrical: the right bronchus is bigger, wider, and straighter, leading into the three right lobes of the lungs. The left bronchus, on the other hand, is smaller in diameter, and it curves off to the side in order to reach the two lobes of the left lung. This is significant, because if any object should ever be inhaled into the lungs, it almost always follows the path of least resistance to the right side. The next section of tubing is the bronchioles, which subdivide 23 times until finally ending in microscopic alveoli. These little grape-shaped clusters of epithelium are like tiny balloons surrounded by blood capillaries. Gaseous exchange occurs through the alveoli. If for any reason they are impaired or not functioning correctly, the body won't be able to trade its carbon dioxide for oxygen.

The structure of the lungs themselves is well suited for fighting off infection. Within each lung are two or three lobes, and within each of those lobes are smaller segments. This isolation of different areas makes it difficult for pathogens to infect the whole structure. The whole respiratory tract is lined with mucous membrane, which traps pathogens and other particles. This "mucous blanket" slowly creeps toward the mouth and nose for expulsion. Smooth muscle tissue helps to support all the tubes down to the smallest bronchi; once an irritant has gotten into these tubes, a healthy cough reflex will quickly move it out of the body.

FUNCTION

Air cycles through the lungs anywhere from 12 to 20 times per minute. The lungs themselves do not have any muscle tissue to make them fill up or empty; they are simply two limp-walled sacs that inflate or deflate according to the air pressure inside and outside of them. Changes in air pressure are brought about by changing the shape of the thoracic cavity. If the cavity is made larger, the air pressure inside will be low until air rushes in to equalize it. In other words, the act of inhaling is simply filling a vacuum. When the pressure inside and outside the lungs has been equalized, air eases out again: exhalation. Exhalation is usually a passive process; it doesn't involve muscular activity unless a person specifically tries to remove air from his lungs.

Most of the conditions examined in this chapter deal with the vulnerability of the respiratory system to infection. Fortunately, thanks to the sticky mucous membranes and lungs that have carefully isolated segments, those infections seldom get a strong enough grip to do lasting damage.

RESPIRATORY SYSTEM CONDITIONS

Infectious Respiratory Disorders
    Common Cold
    Influenza
    Pneumonia
    Sinusitis
    Tuberculosis

Inflammatory Respiratory Disorders
    Asthma
    COPD/Emphysema

Other Respiratory Disorders
    Lung Cancer

Infectious Respiratory Disorders

Common Cold

DEFINITION: WHAT IS IT?

This condition is brought about by any of about 200 different viruses. Over the course of a lifetime, people are exposed to multitudes of viruses. They get sick, they establish

COMMON COLD IN BRIEF

What is it?

The common cold (or upper respiratory tract infection—URTI) is a viral infection from any of about 200 different types of viruses.

How is it recognized?

The symptoms of colds are nasal discharge, sore throat, mild fever, dry coughing, and headache.

Is massage indicated or contraindicated?

Massage is indicated for colds in the subacute stage only.

immunity to that particular pathogen, and they move on to the next infection. Much of this happens in childhood; by adulthood, people have encountered the majority of what they're likely to see, and the frequency of infections generally subsides. But no single infectious agent is responsible for the so-called common cold, and the viruses themselves keep mutating and changing. This is why an effective cure may never exist for this condition.

DEMOGRAPHICS: WHO GETS IT?

It is difficult to project just how common the common cold really is. One estimate suggests that about 1 billion colds occur in the United States in an average year. Children can have an average of six to eight colds a year, and adults generally have two to four per year. Colds are a major cause of school and work absenteeism, and cost untold millions of dollars in health care and lost productivity.

SIGNS AND SYMPTOMS

The symptoms of a cold are probably familiar to everyone: runny nose, sneezing, sore throat, dry coughing, headache, and perhaps a mild fever. They are typically limited to infections of the respiratory tract, which is why colds are sometimes called URTIs, for *upper respiratory tract infections*. Symptoms generally last less than 2 weeks, although the virus may be present in the body for a day or two before symptoms begin. This incubation period is also a contagious period, which can make the spread of infection hard to control.

COMPLICATIONS

Colds are seldom dangerous, except when they complicate into other disorders. The compromised integrity of the membranes and the accumulations of mucus, a perfect growth medium, leaves the body vulnerable to a bacterial onslaught that can include ear infections, bronchitis, laryngitis, *sinusitis* (this chapter, page 255), and *pneumonia* (this chapter, page 252).

PREVENTION

Cold viruses can live for up to 3 hours outside the body. The viruses are airborne after an infected person coughs or sneezes, but they are much more easily spread when they attach to someone's hand or face and find access into the body through a portal of entry: the mouth, the nose, or the eye. The disease spreads efficiently when someone picks up a virus on the hands or from a face pad, a doorknob or a piece of money, and then rubs the nose or eye.

The best way to prevent the spread of colds and other infectious diseases is by frequently washing the hands, focusing on the cuticles and nails, using soap or detergent, and scrubbing for 15 seconds or more before rinsing.

TREATMENT

Because these are viral infections, antibiotics are useless for treating colds. Getting extra rest, drinking lots of fluids, and isolating oneself away from family, classmates, and coworkers who could become infected, are all high priorities. A humidifier may relieve some of the irritation to mucous membranes, although it's important to be aware that some types of humidifiers can actually breed bacteria, and it's important to keep them scrupulously clean. Over-the-counter drugs can relieve the symptoms of a cold, but they will not reduce recovery time. In fact, by inhibiting the ways a body fights off infection (reducing fever, drying up the sinuses), over-the-counter drugs may actually increase the amount of time the infection is present in the body. Some research shows that aspirin can also increase the concentration of virus shed in nasal secretions, thus increasing the possibility of spreading the disease.[1]

Concern has recently been expressed over the prescription of "just in case" antibiotics. Only about 20% of colds will develop into bacterial infections, and the frequent administration of needless antibiotics doesn't improve recovery time, but can contribute to the creation of new and more drug-resistant strains of bacteria.

Alternative healthcare strategies for dealing with colds include plenty of vitamin C, echinacea, lysine (an amino acid with antiviral properties), zinc lozenges (also antiviral), and perhaps licorice root as an expectorant. Hydrotherapy options include artificial fevers to boost immune function (see *fever*, chapter 5, page 232), and cold double-compresses or packs.

MASSAGE?

Massage is appropriate for colds only in the subacute phase. If someone receives massage in the acute stage of a cold, it can be spread through the body much more effectively than would happen naturally, and that is *not* a benefit. On the other hand, if someone is on the postacute side of an infection, massage can help it to process through the body much faster. It's important to ask permission though, because this will sometimes make the person feel like he's having a relapse. It means, after all, squeezing three days of recovery into one day of feeling crummy again.

Influenza

DEFINITION: WHAT IS IT?

Like colds, influenza is a viral infection. However, while the primary mode of transmission for the cold virus is via the hands (see *common cold*, this chapter, page 249), flu viruses can also be spread through the air.

ETIOLOGY: WHAT HAPPENS?

Flu viruses have been classified into three different types. The type A viruses are the most virulent and are responsible for the major epidemics that claimed millions of lives in the early part of this century. The Spanish Flu epidemic of 1918–1919 was from a type A virus. It killed half a million people in the United States and 20 million others around the world. Type A viruses mutate quickly, therefore causing repeated infections in the same person. Type B flu viruses can also cause epidemics, and they mutate into different forms, but not nearly on the same scale as the type A's. Type C flu viruses are not associated with epidemics, and they are relatively stable. They also create much less severe symptoms than the other types.

SIGNS AND SYMPTOMS: FLU VERSUS COLD

Frankly, it doesn't really matter whether a person has a cold or the flu in terms of treatment. Since both are viral infections, they are treated the same way: rest, isolation, lots of fluids, and good nutrition. But to be technical, flu is a lot worse than a cold. It involves a fever up to 104°, and instead of being limited to the upper respiratory tract like a cold, flu can also cause swollen lymph nodes, and joint

INFLUENZA

This word comes from Italian for *influence*, specifically of the planets or stars. The original source was the Latin, *in-fluo*, to flow in. A synonym for flu is grippe, from the French *gripper*, to seize.

INFLUENZA IN BRIEF

What is it?
Influenza ("flu") is a viral infection of the respiratory tract.

How is it recognized?
The symptoms of flu include high fever, and muscle and joint achiness that may last for up to 3 days, followed by a runny nose, coughing, sneezing, and general malaise.

Is massage indicated or contraindicated?
Massage is indicated for the flu in the subacute stage only.

[1] Fact sheet: The common cold. National Institute of Allergy and Infectious Diseases; June 1996. URL: http://www.niaid.nih.gov/factsheets/cold.htm. Accessed fall 1997.

and muscle pain. A flu generally takes about 4 days to incubate, and then symptoms can last anywhere from 1 to 2 weeks. The fever alone may take 3 days to resolve, and it is often followed by upper respiratory symptoms very similar to those of a cold: a runny nose, sneezing, and coughing.

A chief characteristic of flu outbreaks is very high incidence rates. When a true flu virus is active, up to 50% of a local population may be affected; family members, colleagues, and classmates are all likely candidates. Cold viruses, although contagious, are not as virulent as flu viruses.

Influenza rarely causes intestinal inflammation with nausea, vomiting, and diarrhea. Although these symptoms are sometimes called a "stomach flu," they are almost always the result of a different kind of infection: salmonella, for instance. (See *gastroenteritis*, chapter 7, page 276.)

COMPLICATIONS

The real danger with flu is the possibility of an opportunistic bacterial infection in the shape of *pneumonia* (this chapter, page 252) or bronchitis. This is a particular danger for the very young, the very old, heavy smokers, diabetics, or people with other chronic lung problems, such as *emphysema* (this chapter, page 262).

The chances of dying from the flu these days are much lower than they used to be, thanks to antibiotics that deal with secondary infection. However, in the United States, flu still kills about 20,000 people, mostly the very young or very old, every year.

TREATMENT

Just as with colds, rest, liquids, alternative regimens, and chicken soup are the best therapies for a flu sufferer. Over-the-counter drugs may abate the symptoms, but will not speed healing. They can be useful, however, if the symptoms are preventing a person from getting the sleep needed to heal. One antiviral medication called *rimantadine* can reduce the duration of symptoms of flu if they are caused by a type A virus. Rimantadine is ineffective, however, for type B or C viruses.

Every year the Food and Drug Administration distributes a vaccine to fight a combination of type A and type B viruses. Unfortunately, these vaccines are composed several months before "flu season" (late fall to early spring) really hits. Consequently the vaccine may or may not be effective against the viruses circulating when it's administered. Furthermore, because viruses mutate so quickly, flu vaccines need to be updated every year. Nonetheless, flu vaccines are highly recommended for high-risk populations: the elderly, people with chronic lung problems or reduced immunity, and people working in healthcare settings.

MASSAGE?

Just as with colds, massage is indicated for influenza only in the subacute stage. And again, it is important to get a client's permission to temporarily exacerbate the symptoms, so the body can detoxify, flush out residual wastes, and recover more efficiently.

Pneumonia

DEFINITION: WHAT IS IT?

Pneumonia is also known as *pneumonitis*, a name which is more descriptive of the disease. It is not a single malady but any kind of inflammation of the lungs.

DEMOGRAPHICS: WHO GETS IT?

Pneumonia is the most common infectious cause of death in the United States, largely because it takes advantage when a patient's defenses are down due to other disorders. Every

PNEUMONIA
The Greek root of this word is *pneumon*, which means lung. The suffix *-ia* indicates "condition."

year about 3 million people in the United States contract pneumonia; half a million of them receive hospital care. Severity of the infection ranges from being not much worse than a bad cold, to being a cause of death within 24 hours.

ETIOLOGY: WHAT HAPPENS?

The alveoli are the most vulnerable structures in the lungs. They are the tiny air balloons with walls made of squamous epithelium. The capillaries of the pulmonary circuit surround the alveoli for the exchange of oxygen and carbon dioxide in the bloodstream. When an infection strikes in the lungs, these tiny air balloons may begin to fill up; dead white blood cells, mucus, and fluid backed up from the capillaries will pour into the alveoli until the diffusion of gases is impossible. If the capillaries are damaged, red blood cells will find their way in as well. Abscesses may also form.

In *lobar pneumonia*, fibrin, a blood protein responsible for clotting, will begin to thicken the fluid in the alveoli until it becomes a gelid mass. This is known as *consolidation*. Consolidation doesn't happen in all forms of pneumonia; in most cases, the alveolar exudate remains liquid, but is still a hindrance to diffusion. Edema is not always limited to the alveoli. In extreme cases, fluid may be found between the visceral and parietal layer of the pleurae. This can lead to pleurisy: scarring and limitation of movement between the pleurae during breathing.

CAUSES

Several infectious agents cause pneumonia. Each one of them has a different treatment protocol in terms of medicine, although not in terms of massage. It is also possible for more than one type of pathogen to be present at a time, a fact that makes diagnosis of this condition a special problem.

- Viruses. Viral infections account for about one-half of all pneumonia cases. Influenza A and B and syncytial virus are the most common culprits. Other viruses include cytomegalovirus, herpes simplex, and adenovirus. The incubation period (time between exposure to the pathogen and exhibiting symptoms) of viral pneumonia is 1 to 3 days.
- Bacteria. Bacterial pneumonia can be caused by staphylococcus, streptococcus, or a specific pathogen called pneumococcus. The toxins released by the bacteria initiate an inflammatory response. This inflammation leads to changes in the lungs, including the deposition of fibrin, and consolidation. The inflammation and resulting edema cause the terminal bronchioles to fill with exudate and other debris. One distinguishing feature of bacterial pneumonia is the production of greenish or yellowish sputum. This kind of infection usually responds well to antibiotics.
- Mycoplasma. Mycoplasma are infectious agents that are neither bacteria nor viruses. Mycoplasma pneumonia is extremely contagious and often affects whole families. The incubation period is quite lengthy (1 to 4 weeks), and because it tends to be not as severe as bacterial or viral types of infection, it is sometimes called "walking pneumonia." Fortunately, like bacterial pneumonia, mycoplasma pneumonia responds well to antibiotics.
- Pneumocystis carinii. Pneumocystis carinii is a protozoan infection almost exclusively associated with immunosuppressed patients such as those with AIDS and those receiving cancer chemotherapy or immunosuppressive drugs to prevent the rejection of organ transplants.

PNEUMONIA IN BRIEF

What is it?
Pneumonia is an infection in the lungs brought about by bacteria, viruses, or other pathogens.

How is it recognized?
The symptoms of pneumonia include coughing, occasional fever, pain on breathing, and shortness of breath.

Is massage indicated or contraindicated?
Massage is indicated for pneumonia in the subacute stage, under medical supervision.

- Others. Other pathogens that can cause pneumonia include chlamydia, rickettsia, and tuberculosis bacilli.

Pneumonia appears in several forms. Each one may present with different cautions attached to it, so it's worthwhile to be familiar with the most common types.

- *Primary pneumonia* is relatively rare. In this case, no predisposing factor exists; it is simply a bacterial attack directly on the lungs.
- *Secondary pneumonia* is by the far the most common situation. A viral or bacterial assault on lung tissue occurs because the body's immune system is weakened by another disease. Even if the primary disease is viral, the accumulation of mucus is a perfect growth medium for bacteria, leaving the patient vulnerable to this kind of infection.

Within the headings of primary or secondary, pneumonia may also be classified by the location of the infection.

- Bronchopneumonia. This type starts as a bronchial inflammation (bronchitis) and spreads into the lungs. It appears in a patchy pattern all over the lungs, not segregated to a specific area.
- Lobar pneumonia. This type is restricted to one lobe of the lungs. A particular thickening of the liquid in the alveoli called consolidation occurs there and gradually the whole lobe may be affected.
- Double pneumonia. This affects both lungs. It can be bacterial or viral.

A final classification for pneumonia determines the source of the infectious agent.

- *Community acquired pneumonia* is the most common form, and is usually a bacterial infection of streptococcus pneumoniae or haemophilus influenzae.
- *Nosocomial*, or *hospital-acquired pneumonia*, is an infection in a person who has been a hospital inpatient for at least 72 hours or an inpatient within the previous 1 to 3 weeks.

SIGNS AND SYMPTOMS

Signs and symptoms of pneumonia vary widely, depending on the causative factor and how much of the lung is affected. Some of the possible symptoms of pneumonia include coughing, very high fever, chills, sweating, delirium, chest pains, cyanosis, thickened green or yellow phlegm, blood-streaked phlegm, shortness of breath, muscle aches and pains, and pleurisy.

Pneumonia can have a sudden or gradual onset. Very often it follows the same course as a cold, but instead of getting better, the respiratory symptoms rapidly worsen and a fever of up to 104° will present.

TREATMENT

Treatment depends entirely on what type of pneumonia is present. Bacterial pneumonias generally respond well to antibiotics, and a vaccine for the pneumococcus bacterium is especially recommended for people who are immune-suppressed for any reason.

Viral pneumonias are untreatable with antibiotics. Symptomatic relief and supportive therapy involve breathing humidified air, drinking ample fluids, and supplementing oxygen if necessary. Pneumonia due to influenza viruses may be prevented through vaccination, if the vaccine is designed for the flu viruses circulating at the time.

PROGNOSIS

Considering the delicacy of the epithelium in the lungs, it is amazing that if a pneumonia infection is short lived, it is completely reversible. The body can reliquify and absorb the consolidated matter in affected alveoli, as it can reabsorb the fluid from any inflamed part of the lung. If a patient is generally healthy, he or she can expect to recover within 2 weeks.

In long-standing cases where fibrosis and scar tissue accumulate, the elasticity of the epithelial tissue, or the freedom with which the lungs move in the pleural cavity, may sustain permanent damage. This raises the risk for future infections.

For people who develop this condition as a complication of a more serious underlying disorder, pneumonia can be life threatening. Secondary pneumonia is an opportunistic disease. It kills more people every year than any other kind of infection, because it takes advantage of low defenses. It is often the final complication of other serious diseases, even noninfectious ones. People with stroke, heart failure, alcoholism, and cancer die of pneumonia more often than any other disease. People who are bedridden or paralyzed are susceptible, too, because their cough reflex is often impaired; they cannot expel mucus easily. Preexisting chest problems, such as flu, bronchitis, emphysema, or asthma, are open invitations. And finally, being immune-suppressed because of tissue transplants, AIDS, steroids, leukemia, or cytotoxic drugs will make a person particularly vulnerable to pneumonia.

MASSAGE?

Pneumonia patients can receive massage in the subacute stage under medical supervision. This serious and complicated condition frequently accompanies other serious conditions. Under the right circumstances, pneumonia can respond very well to the mechanical impact of percussive massage, which can help to move mucus from the alveoli into the bronchial tubes where muscle action can take over to expel it from the body.

Sinusitis

DEFINITION: WHAT IS IT?

Sinusitis, as the name implies, is a condition in which the mucous membranes that line the sinuses become inflamed and swollen.

ETIOLOGY: WHAT HAPPENS?

Sinuses are hollow areas located lateral to, above, and behind the nose. (See Figure 6.2.) They provide extra surface area for sticky mucous membranes to trap pathogens on their

SINUS
From the Latin for channel, hollow place, or tunnel.

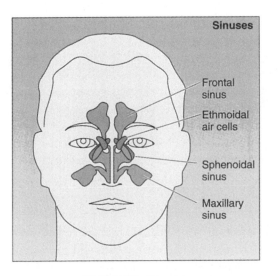

Figure 6.2. Sinusitis

SINUSITIS IN BRIEF

What is it?
Sinusitis is inflammation of the paranasal sinuses from infection, obstruction, or allergies.

How is it recognized?
Symptoms include headaches, localized tenderness over the affected area, runny or congested nose, facial or tooth pain, fatigue, and, if it's related to an infection, thick opaque mucus, fever, and chills.

Is massage indicated or contraindicated?
Massage is contraindicated for acute infections, but for chronic or noninfectious situations, it can be appropriate.

way in; they provide resonance for the voice; and they lighten the weight of the head considerably. But when the mucous membrane that lines the sinuses becomes red and inflamed, and the hollow area becomes filled with mucus that for one reason or another cannot drain, the sinuses can become a tremendous source of pain and discomfort.

CAUSES

Sinusitis can be caused by several different things. It's important to remember that inflammation is not necessarily infection, and some types of sinusitis do not involve pathogens at all.

- Viruses. The most serious types of sinusitis begin as viral infections. Then, when defenses are low, the bacteria that normally colonize the skin and mucous membranes take advantage of the situation and begin to multiply. This is nearly always a complication of a preexistent viral infection such as cold or flu. Dental work very occasionally causes sinusitis, if the contents of an abscessed tooth are somehow released into the nasal cavity. Any kind of infectious sinusitis is a serious condition. The client should not be massaged without a doctor's approval.
- Allergic rhinitis. Hay fever will also cause inflammation of the sinus membranes, but no underlying infection is present, and consequently, no danger of infectious complications exists. Hay fever is often distinguished from infectious sinusitis by the lack of congestion and the quality of the nasal discharge: it tends to be thin and runny, rather than thick and sticky.
- Structural problems. A deviated septum or the growth of nasal polyps can obstruct the flow of mucus out of the sinuses. This is not an infectious situation to begin with; but since mucus held back from normal flow is a perfect growth medium for bacteria, what begins as a structural anomaly can become a true infection.
- Fungal infections. Persons who are immune-suppressed are at particular danger for this type of sinusitis. Fungi such as Aspergillus or Curvularia are not threats to most people, but can be sources of sinus infection to AIDS patients or others whose immune systems are compromised.
- Medicine intolerance. Occasionally a reaction to aspirin or ibuprofen can produce inflammation in the mucous membranes of the sinuses.

SIGNS AND SYMPTOMS

Symptoms of sinusitis vary according to the cause of the inflammation. Symptoms may be short term and severe (acute sinusitis), or long term and less severe (chronic sinusitis), or they may vacillate between the two.

Severe headache is a key feature, especially upon waking. Bending over will make it much worse, because that position increases pressure on already stressed membranes. The affected area may be extremely painful to the touch, and some visible swelling or puffiness may be noticeable. With an acute bacterial infection, symptoms will be accompanied by fever and chills. Sore throat, coughing (caused by postnasal drip), and congestion or runny nose may appear with any type of sinus irritation, and regardless of whether it's an infectious or allergic situation, people with chronic sinusitis are likely to experience fatigue and general malaise because the body is fighting hard to cast off an invader.

COMPLICATIONS

It is rare but not unheard of for sinus infections to spread and become very serious situations. The infection can infiltrate facial bones, causing osteomyelitis and permanent bone damage, or it can gain access to the central nervous system and cause *meningitis* (chapter 3, page 146).

TREATMENT

Treatment for sinusitis begins with self-help measures: staying in humid air or breathing steam to help moisturize and liquefy the clogged mucus is an important step. Using air filters to remove irritating particles from the air can also help.

Drugs prescribed for this disorder begin with antibiotics, if the infection is bacterial. Decongestants are sometimes recommended to shrink the mucous membranes, but these are only appropriate for short-term use because they can create a terrible "rebound effect" when usage is stopped. Corticosteroids in nasal spray form can reduce swelling without many of the dangers inherent in other steroid drugs. Allergies may be treated with antihistamines to limit the inappropriate immune response that causes inflammation. In very extreme cases, surgery is recommended to go through one of the nasal bones into the nasal sinus and flush it out with sterile water, or to remove or repair any structural obstructions such as a deviated septum or nasal polyps.

MASSAGE?

For allergic rhinitis, massage is fine because no bacterial or viral infection is present to be spread, caught, or to complicate into a more serious condition. But for infectious acute sinusitis, if pus appears in the mucus, or if fever and general achiness is present, massage is contraindicated. If it's unclear what stage the client is in, obtain medical clearance before proceeding.

Tuberculosis

DEFINITION: WHAT IS IT?

Tuberculosis is a disease involving pus and bacteria-filled *tubers*, or bumps. These usually occur in the lungs, but sometimes appear in other places too.

DEMOGRAPHICS: WHO GETS IT?

The World Health Organization reports that tuberculosis affects one-third of the world's population. Eight million people become sick with it every year, and three million people die; that's more than the deaths from AIDS, malaria, and all tropical diseases combined. It was considered virtually conquered in the United States, because in the 1950s, a series of antibiotics was developed that finally managed to kill it. It steadily declined until 1986, when suddenly it began to rise again. It is up 16% since 1986 to infect 10 million Americans. Of those, about 10%, or one million people, will go on to develop the disease.

Why these vast increases? A few reasons are possible. The 1980s saw vast cuts in health and social services and vast increases in a population particularly vulnerable to this kind of infection: AIDS patients. Also, a great influx of immigrants were no longer tested as they entered the United States. At the same time, several new types of the tuberculosis bacteria developed, probably as a result of patients not finishing their prescriptions. This is a problem because some of the newer varieties of bacteria are extremely drug-resistant. It is estimated that up to 9% of the TB cases in the United States are of this new, possibly untreatable variety.

TUBERCULOSIS
From the Latin *tuber*, a swelling or bump, plus *osis*, condition. The word *tubercle*, which is a common anatomical term denoting a bump or protrusion, has the same root.

TUBERCULOSIS IN BRIEF

What is it?
Tuberculosis is a bacterial infection that usually begins in the lungs, but may spread to bones, kidneys, lymph nodes, or elsewhere in the body. It is a highly contagious airborne disease.

How is it recognized?
Infection with the tuberculosis bacterium may produce no symptoms. If the infection turns into the actual disease, symptoms may include coughing, bloody sputum, fatigue, weight loss, and night sweats.

Is massage indicated or contraindicated?
Massage is contraindicated for active tuberculosis disease, unless the client has been on consistent medication for several weeks and has medical clearance. Massage for clients with tuberculosis infection but no disease is fine, but these people should be under medical supervision as well.

ETIOLOGY: WHAT HAPPENS?

Tuberculosis is an airborne disease, although it requires prolonged contact to be spread from person to person. It is caused by the mycobacterium tuberculosis, a microorganism with a peculiar waxy coat that gives it many advantages over regular bacteria. This pathogen exists quite happily outside of the body. The saliva or mucus that might initially surround it will eventually dry up, but the bacteria will wait on, often suspended in the air, until a rich growth medium comes its way again. Ordinary antiseptics and disinfectants won't touch it. Even boiling it isn't dependable. The only thing that will always kill mycobacterium tuberculosis is direct sunlight.

PROGRESSION

Tuberculosis moves in the body in two phases.

- Primary phase. A bacterial infection sets up the usual inflammatory reaction in the lungs. But instead of engulfing the invader, tagging it, and launching a successful attack against it, the body builds a protective fibrous wall around the site of infection: a tubercle. These are usually found in the lungs, but if some of the bacteria seep out into the bloodstream, they will set up the same process elsewhere in the body. Kidneys and bones are the most common other sites.

  This is where it all stops for most people. This is tuberculosis infection, but not the active disease. Antibodies are produced that will react to another contact with the bacillus, as in the "scratch test" that looks for past exposure. The inhaled bacteria will remain stuck inside this tidy little fibrous package until something happens to set them free, usually a future depression in immune system function.

- Secondary phase. In about 10% of the people exposed to tuberculosis, the infection will become an active disease later in life. The bacteria will grow and spread into other areas in the lungs, or wherever else in the body they may be stationed. They will still be surrounded by bigger and bigger fibrous capsules, which can cause permanent scarring. Pleurisy, the scarring and sticking of the pleurae, is nearly always a complication of tuberculosis. Inside the capsules, the bacteria destroy cells; the tissue is necrotic, or dead. (See Figure 6.3.)

  New tubercles will eventually take up enough room in the lungs to impede function. A cough will begin and will gradually produce bloody sputum. This phlegm actually contains detached pieces of the bacteria-infested tubercles, which is why tuberculosis is so very contagious. If several of the tubercles join together, their necrotic centers can cause a cavity in the lung. Surrounding blood vessels will have a tendency to hemorrhage into the cavity, which leads to coughing up blood. Similar cavities can develop in the kidneys, if the tubercles form there. Tubercular infections in the bones tend to destroy articular cartilage.

RISK FACTORS

HIV (see chapter 5, page 233) puts people very much at risk for active tuberculosis. In an otherwise healthy person, the bacterium would enter the body and be largely controlled by the immune system. Only 1 in 10 people without HIV who are exposed to tuberculosis go on to develop the disease. But a person who is HIV positive who is exposed to TB has a chance of developing the disease that increases 7 to 10% *per year of being infected.* TB infection turns into TB disease in one out of every two or three people who are HIV positive, and these people can then, in turn, infect others. In fact, TB is the only airborne sickness that AIDS patients can transmit to healthy people.

SIGNS AND SYMPTOMS

The primary phase of tuberculosis is so benign a person may never know she's been exposed; the symptoms, if any show at all, are the same as for a mild flu. But the active dis-

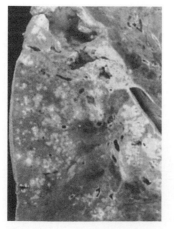

Figure 6.3. Post-primary tuberculosis

ease shows much more severe symptoms. They include fever, sweating, weight loss, and exhaustion. Chest pain and shortness of breath may also be present. A stubborn cough that starts dry and becomes productive of bloody or pus-filled phlegm is a cardinal sign. Other symptoms will arise if other organs have been infected as well.

TREATMENT

In the old days, tuberculosis patients were sent to sanitaria where it was hoped that sunlight, rest, and good food would enable them to outlive their infection. That's still a good approach, but it's even better when it's combined with the right antibiotics. Up to 90% of all tuberculosis patients have full recovery if their treatment is completed.

The important point is that *these antibiotics need to be taken with unfailing consistency.* In addition, several different types of antibiotics may be prescribed, in order to circumvent the bacteria's resistance to any single variety. This can mean up to 13 pills a day, for many months. Not surprisingly, studies indicate that approximately one-third of all patients do not take their medication as directed. This is not only irresponsible, it is downright dangerous, because this bacterium may mutate into a form drugs can't affect, and whoever is infected with this new strain will be likewise untreatable. It is estimated that a person with untreated TB disease infects about 14 people per year. A person with regular mycobacteria tuberculosis costs about $2000 to treat. A person with multi-drug resistant tuberculosis costs about $250,000 to treat.

In a study done of "directly observed therapy" (that is, when social workers directly observed their clients taking their medication for each and every dose), the rate of acquired drug resistance sank to 2.1%, down from 14%. Directly observed therapy, short term ("DOTS") is now considered the gold standard for TB treatment. The World Health Organization estimates that if 12 key countries instituted this treatment plan, the incidence of TB worldwide would drop by some 70%.

People who have a tuberculosis infection without the disease can prevent the development of the disease with a course of antibiotics that lasts about 6 months. People who have the regular TB disease without the drug-resistant strain can expect a similar treatment, although the antibiotics may be different. And people with drug-resistant strains of the disease may have to take multiple medications for 18 months or more.

Assuming a complete cure is successful, significant scarring and tissue damage from the fibrous capsules may result. Surgery may be necessary to restore function to affected tissues.

MASSAGE?

Tuberculosis can travel in the blood. If a client has the active disease, massage can spread it through the body and help to set up tubercles where they would not otherwise have occurred. Tuberculosis is also contagious; therapists won't do their clients much good if their own careers are cut short by this condition. However, if a client has been exposed to the bacterium and is taking medication, or if a client has had the active disease but has been under medication for several weeks, massage may be appropriate, with medical clearance.

Inflammatory Respiratory Disorders

Asthma

DEFINITION: WHAT IS IT?

Asthma may be brought about by external factors, such as allergens, but it is also directly linked to internal factors, such as emotional stress.

ASTHMA: CASE HISTORY

Richard L., age 52

I didn't contract asthma until I was 22, after I got back from Viet Nam. I was living in Los Angeles, and I got a very bad case of bronchitis. I was diagnosed then with just a common smog problem.

Then I moved to Corvallis, Oregon, and ran into the Willamette Valley Crud: they have pollination 10 months out of the year there. I saw an allergist who gave me skin tests, and I came up positive to 95% of the things he tested me for. Then I realized it wasn't just the smog; I had a lung problem.

At that time I started taking desensitization shots. I did that for about five years, but it didn't really help. I ended up quitting, and just medicating myself with aspirin, Sudafed, and over-the-counter inhalants. I didn't have any really bad episodes that I couldn't handle, but I was working in construction, and I knew that I couldn't be sawing or working in a closed room because I would stop breathing; my lungs would just shut down.

Then I moved to Bellingham, Washington, and went into a roofing business. I was working with hot tar, and this stuff called "torch down" that lets off a lot of fumes. A couple of times I ended up in the emergency room with breathing problems. They gave me a prescription inhalant and prednisone.

When I moved to Seattle, I wound up with an asthma specialist who's been really good for me. I've had a few bouts down here; one time, a cold put me in the hospital for about a week. I work in a shipyard now. I can stay away from the worst of the fumes, but about once a year I get a bad attack and go on prednisone until it clears up.

I've been doing massage since the 1960s but just recently went to school and became licensed. I'm really sensitive to perfumes, and massage schools are 90% female, so I'd always choose where to sit, to be away from anyone wearing perfume. But I never thought about massage oils until we got into it. I knew to stay away from oils and lotions that are scented at all. When I got a massage with almond oil, I noticed my skin would turn really red, but it wasn't until someone worked on my chest and back that I noticed about an hour later my breathing was affected. Since then I only use unscented lotion.

Asthma affects my life in all kinds of ways. My lung capacity is only about 65% of normal. I like to go listen to music, but the venues where the good bands play are always too smoky. I have to stay away from flower shops. It used to be almost impossible to go into a mall because you have to walk past the perfume counter to get through the big department stores, but that seems to be less of a problem now. Asthma really limits my social life, too. When someone asks us over to dinner, our first question has to be, "Do you have any pets?"

As my massage clientele builds, I'm able to cut back at the shipyard. Eventually I'll be able to do massage full time. My focus now is on controlling my environment—keeping out the things I know will trigger an attack and trying to stay as healthy as possible.

DEMOGRAPHICS: WHO GETS IT?

Asthma is on a distinct rise in this country; between 1990 and 1994, the number of people who reported having asthma increased from 10.4 million to 14.6 million. Deaths from asthma doubled between 1980 and 1993. Some theories about this increase include higher levels of air pollution and more airtight houses and office buildings where dust, dander, and other allergens can concentrate in the air.

Children are more often affected by asthma than adults. They often seem to grow out of the condition, but they are at high risk for having it reappear later in adulthood. Low-income children are the highest risk group of all; asthma is highly associated with cockroach-related allergens, incompletely vented heating sources, stoves, and secondhand smoke.

African-American children are about four times more likely to be hospitalized with asthma than Caucasian children. Recent genetic research shows that African Americans may be at increased risk for asthma because of a prevalence of certain immune system molecules in their bodies. This finding is a significant step toward being able to treat asthma more effectively.

ETIOLOGY: WHAT HAPPENS?

All bronchioles are sensitive to foreign debris, but the bronchioles of an asthmatic are extremely hair-trigger. Someone with asthma is exposed to a stimulus that causes a sympathetic reaction, which is then followed by a parasympathetic reaction. If the appropriate allergen (dust mites or pollen, for instance) comes along, the bronchioles first dilate (a sympathetic reaction), and then the body overcompensates by sending them into spasm. The irritated membranes lining these tubes swell up and secrete extra mucus. (See Figure 6.4.) People with asthma find it very difficult to breathe, especially to exhale, during an attack.

Three common types of asthma have been identified, along with a few others that occur more rarely.

- Extrinsic asthma. This is a typical example of a type 1 hypersensitivity reaction. In this situation, the mast cells located in the mucous membrane secrete a lot of histamine. Histamine causes vasodilation, increases cell permeability, and in the respiratory system, initiates excess mucus production. What counteracts histamine? Cortisol is the best chemical neutralizer available, but asthmatics, along with many allergy sufferers, seem to be short on this important adrenal hormone.
- Intrinsic asthma. This situation is more common in adults than in children. It involves attacks that may have no known origin, or which may be related to exercise,

ASTHMA IN BRIEF

What is it?
Asthma is the result of spasmodic constriction of bronchial smooth muscle tubes in combination with excess mucus production and mucosal edema.

How is it recognized?
Asthma attacks are sporadic and involve coughing, wheezing, and difficulty with breathing, especially exhaling.

Is massage indicated or contraindicated?
Massage is indicated for asthma as long as the individual is not in the throes of an attack. Between episodes, massage can be useful to reduce stress and deal with some of the muscular problems that accompany difficulty with breathing.

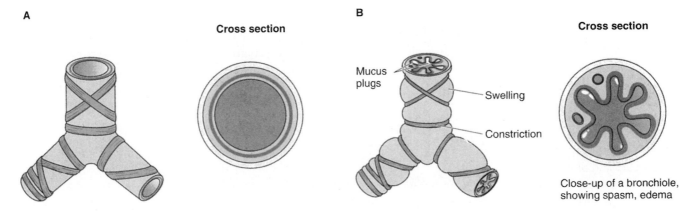

A   Cross section

B   Cross section

Mucus plugs — Swelling — Constriction

Close-up of a bronchiole, showing spasm, edema

Figure 6.4. Normal bronchiole (A) and bronchiole under asthma attack (B)

upper respiratory tract infection (see *common cold*, this chapter, page 249), or emotional stress.

- Mixed asthma. This combination of extrinsic and intrinsic factors is probably the most common situation.
- Others. A few other types of asthma are less common. They include occupational asthma, which is a reaction to work-related substances such as detergents, plastics, resins, and fumes, and cardiac asthma, which is related to *congestive heart failure* (see chapter 4, page 206), and the resulting excess fluid in the lungs.

SIGNS AND SYMPTOMS

Symptoms of asthma include dyspnea (shortness of breath), wheezing (the sound of air moving through tightened and clogged up bronchioles), and coughing, which may or may not be productive. It feels especially difficult to expel air; the alveoli may not be emptying sufficiently with each breath.

Asthma can show symptoms in several different ways. Bronchial asthma involves tight bronchioles with excess mucus production and wheezing; exercise-induced asthma occurs with physical exertion; silent asthma shows no symptoms leading up to an episode, when the patient suddenly finds himself dangerously short of breath; cough-variant asthma shows coughing alone as its primary symptom.

If symptoms are extreme and prolonged, the asthmatic person may start to feel panicky, adding sweating, increased heart rate, and anxiety to the list of symptoms. In emergency situations, the lips and face may take on a bluish cast (cyanosis) when access to oxygen is severely restricted.

Asthma attacks are sporadic, lasting anywhere from a few minutes to a few days. Between attacks, the lungs are generally normal. Someone who has had asthma for a long time may be at risk for other respiratory disorders, particularly bronchitis and *emphysema* (this chapter, this page).

TREATMENT

Medical treatment for extrinsic asthma begins with trying to identify and avoid the stimuli that cause the attacks. If someone is very familiar with her problem and is capable of predicting when her attacks will occur, prophylactic drugs may be taken on a short-term basis. These generally start with bronchodilators: variations on adrenaline that dilate the bronchioles without the other sympathetic nervous system effects. If bronchodilators are insufficient, steroids may be administered for their anti-inflammatory action. These can have serious side effects, however, and cannot be used successfully for very long. In emergency situations, adrenaline may be injected. This restimulates the sympathetic nervous system and redilates the bronchi, but can also cause panic-like symptoms.

MASSAGE?

Massage is absolutely indicated for asthma in the postacute stage. No one who is fighting for breath during an acute attack will be comfortable on a massage table. But massage can help with the number of different muscular reflections of asthma that someone who struggles with this problem will probably have. Watch for hypertonic intercostals, scalenes, serratus posterior inferior, and diaphragm. These muscles of inspiration will be chronically tight for someone who doesn't breathe easily, and the tightness will further interfere with her breathing.

EMPHYSEMA
This comes from the Greek words *en* (in) and *physa* (bellows). Emphysema means blown up, as in inflated, not exploded.

COPD/*Emphysema*

DEFINITION: WHAT IS IT?

Emphysema, along with chronic bronchial asthma and bronchitis, is one of a group of diseases called chronic obstructive pulmonary disease, or COPD.

DEMOGRAPHICS: WHO GETS IT?

It is estimated that 15 million Americans have some form of COPD, and about 500,000 new cases are reported every year. Most emphysema patients are between 65 and 75 years old. More than 80% of emphysema cases can be traced to cigarette smoking. Others may be due to occupational hazards: working with grain dust, in coal mines, or quarries can increase risk. A small percentage of emphysema patients have a genetic lack of the alpha-1 antitrypsin protein that protects alveolar walls. These people will generally develop the disease before they are 50 years old.

ETIOLOGY: WHAT HAPPENS?

When the delicate epithelium that lines the respiratory tract is constantly irritated (cigarette smoke and air pollution are the two biggest culprits), the cilia that are supposed to trap pathogens and particles will eventually disintegrate. Then the bronchioles produce excess mucus in an effort to fight off environmental irritations; this is the chronic bronchitis that usually accompanies emphysema.

Each lung has 300 million alveoli to provide sites for oxygen–carbon dioxide exchange. They should all be supplied with a specific substance called alpha-1 antitrypsin (AAT). This protein protects the delicate tissue from damage by environmental forces. Long-term exposure to cigarette smoke or other pollutants overcome the protective abilities of AAT, resulting in the destruction of the alveolar elastin fibers. The alveoli become less elastic and fill up with mucus, which interferes with their ability to exchange oxygen and carbon dioxide. Instead of emptying and filling with every breath, they only partially empty, or stay altogether full. This usually begins in a small area, but if the irritation continues, it will spread throughout the lung. The alveolar walls eventually break down and merge with each other, forming larger sacs, called bullae. These sacs have less volume and less surface area for gaseous exchange than the uninjured alveoli did. (See Figure 6.5.)

As the alveoli fuse and surface area for gaseous exchange is lost, the emphysema patient has to work much harder to move air in and out of the lungs. A person with healthy lungs expends about 5% of his energy in the effort of breathing. A person with advanced emphysema puts closer to 50% of his energy into this job, and he must do it all the time, 24 hours a day.

Less gaseous exchange means reduced oxygen levels in the blood, or *hypoxia*. This situation is toxic to brain cells. It also causes the epithelial walls of the alveoli to thicken into tough, fibrous connective tissue, which allows even less diffusion. As breathing becomes more difficult (the emphysema patient must consciously exhale—it no longer happens spontaneously), the respiration rate slows. This leads to even higher concentrations of carbon dioxide in the blood. The blood vessels supplying the damaged alveoli also sustain damage; it becomes harder to pump blood through the pulmonary artery. Hypoxia also leads to spasm of pulmonary blood vessels. All of these factors may contribute to pulmonary hypertension and right-sided heart failure, or *cor pulmonale*. Eventually the untreated emphysema patient experiences respiratory and circulatory collapse.

SIGNS AND SYMPTOMS

It can take many years for emphysema to advance to a stage where a person seeks medical help. Because it usually affects people over 65 years of age, early symptoms are often

---

COPD/EMPHYSEMA IN BRIEF

What is it?
Emphysema is a condition in which the alveoli of the lungs become fibrous and inelastic. They merge with each other, decreasing surface area, and limiting oxygen-carbon dioxide exchange. It is one of a group of diseases called *chronic obstructive pulmonary disease*, or COPD.

How is it recognized?
Symptoms of emphysema include shortness of breath with mild or no exertion, rales, cyanosis, and susceptibility to secondary respiratory infection.

Is massage indicated or contraindicated?
Massage is indicated for emphysema under medical supervision.

WHAT DOES "LUNG CAPACITY" MEAN?

In a normal, healthy person at rest, the act of breathing consumes approximately 5% of the body's energy. This percentage rises if the respiratory system has structural or functional problems; the act of breathing, of providing the tissues with oxygen, can become an exhausting labor.

Massage can do little to change the structure of the lungs, but it *can* affect the efficiency of the muscles of inspiration. Work with the diaphragm, the scalenes, and the intercostal muscles can make the act of breathing easier and less effortful, which in turn can make a person feel generally more energetic.

The size of a person's lungs depends largely on his height and general build. An average male can hold up to six liters of air, but only a small portion of that total is exchanged with each breath.

- *Tidal volume* is the amount of air moved in and out of the lungs during normal resting breathing. It involves about 500 ml of air.
- *Inspiratory reserve volume* is the amount of air that can be consciously inhaled beyond tidal volume inhalation. It averages about 3100 ml.
- *Expiratory reserve volume* is the amount of air that can be consciously exhaled beyond tidal volume exhalation. It averages about 1200 ml.
- *Vital capacity of the lungs* is all the air that it is possible to consciously inhale and exhale. That is, vital capacity is tidal volume, plus inspiratory reserve volume, plus expiratory reserve volume. Vital capacity accounts for a total of about 4800 ml.
- *Residual volume* is the amount of air left in the lungs after a maximum exhalation. This volume is necessary to prevent the alveoli from collapsing. Residual volume is about 1200 ml in a healthy adult.

Therefore, total lung capacity is the vital capacity plus the residual volume, about 6000 ml, or 6 liters for an average adult male in good health.

Highly trained athletes work to increase the accessibility of oxygen to their tissues. They look for a balance between breathing deeper and faster to bring more air in, and expending a minimum of energy on the act of breathing. Massage therapists can influence this balance by working with the muscles of respiration to reduce resistance and increase efficiency.

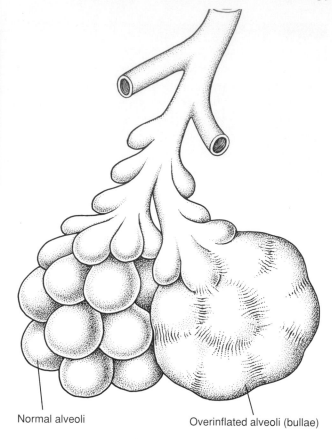

Normal alveoli

Overinflated alveoli (bullae)

Figure 6.5. COPD/Emphysema

assumed to be normal signs of aging. Symptoms of emphysema include pain with breathing, shortness of breath, coughing, and wheezing. Weight loss may occur as a person who must exert so much energy in breathing has little interest in eating. Listening to a patient breathe reveals decreased breath sounds. "Rales," a characteristic bubbling, rasping sound of air moving through a narrowed passage, may occur with some cases. Difficulty in exhaling will also be reflected in a test that measures expiration volume; decreased volume is a cardinal sign of emphysema. Exhalation takes longer, and the patient may develop a habit of pushing air out through pursed lips. This is an attempt to push against increasing back pressure in the lungs. Because the lungs no longer deflate normally with each breath, the diaphragm becomes permanently flattened. The emphysema patient often develops "barrel chest"; that is, the intercostals lock into a position that holds the rib cage out as wide as possible.

COMPLICATIONS

Emphysema patients are extremely vulnerable to *influenza* (this chapter, page 251) and *pneumonia* (this chapter,

EMPHYSEMA: CASE HISTORY

Roberta F., age 68

Roberta is 5'2" and weighs 100 pounds. She started smoking in 1947 and quit in 1984. She first experienced pulmonary symptoms in the mid 1980s. These included frequent shortness of breath, low energy, and consistent headaches on rising each morning. She was unable to walk far or fast. In an effort to catch her breath, she hyperventilated easily, which only made matters worse. Stress and frustration accompanied the fact that breathing was so difficult and that she could no longer accomplish the things she wanted to do.

Roberta's original doctor diagnosed her with chronic obstructive pulmonary disease (COPD) and chronic bronchitis. A pulmonary specialist then diagnosed her with emphysema. This finding was based on a number of tests, including a chest x-ray, spirometry (a measurement of respiratory gases), an analysis of arterial blood gases, and a measurement of the air volume she was able to expel.

Emphysema makes it hard for Roberta to do anything. The activities of daily living are difficult, and all daily routines have to be altered to accommodate the disease. Stairs and hills are especially difficult. Emphysema dulls the thinking by depriving the brain of oxygen. It reduces her appetite, and the lack of oxygen reduces the benefit from what food she does eat. It also strains her heart because it has to work harder to push more blood, which contains less oxygen, through the body.

Roberta's x-ray for emphysema also revealed that she has some degree of osteoporosis. This condition, in combination with her breathing difficulties, has significantly altered her posture. Her shoulders rise to her ears in her body's attempt to get more air. Also, her shoulders tend to roll forward. Because of the increased tension Roberta experiences while trying to breathe, some muscle stiffness and pain was occasionally a problem.

Another aspect of Roberta's experience with emphysema is how it has seriously affected her resistance to disease. Some medicines Roberta takes to help her breathe weaken her immune system, so it is harder for her to ward off respiratory ailments. In March 1997, she had a crisis that hospitalized her for 10 days. At that time, she began supplementing oxygen by nose. She was in a rehabilitation facility for 2 weeks, working with physical and occupational therapists who taught her ways to accomplish more with less energy.

In June 1997, Roberta suffered from a bad cold, which put her in the hospital for 4 days. In January 1998, Roberta contracted pneumonia, which was confirmed by chest x-ray. She was in the hospital for 5 days. The pneumonia cleared up with antibiotics, and she returned home.

Roberta is now feeling better. She still supplements oxygen, and her daily activities have become a little easier. She tries to keep up with her exercises, eat properly, and reduce stress. She also attends Better Breathing Club meetings sponsored by the American Lung Association to keep up with new information about techniques to deal with her disease, and she sees her pulmonary specialist regularly.

page 252) because they've lost much of the ability to resist secondary infection. Another complication occurs if the bullae should rupture. This allows air into the pleural space (which is supposed to be a vacuum), and ends in total lung collapse. The stress to the circulatory system if the lungs sustain this kind of damage is very great. The right ventricle, trying to pump blood through the partially collapsed pulmonary circuit, will enlarge and may eventually end in *heart failure* (chapter 4, page 206). The risk of blood clots forming somewhere in the circuit is also high, which results in *pulmonary embolism* (chapter 4, page 183).

TREATMENT

Emphysema is basically an irreversible disease. If it is found and treated early, further damage can be avoided. But once the alveoli have begun to break down, they cannot be replaced. The first course of action, of course, is to remove the irritating stimulus; usually this is cigarettes. Drugs may be administered to dilate the bronchi and take pressure off the alveoli, to remove mucus and edema from the lungs, and to ward off potential lung infections. Oxygen supplementation may be recommended during sleep or following exercise. A new surgery called "lung shaving" removes only damaged portions of the lung. This increases thoracic capacity for the diaphragm to work and improves circulation. Statistics on how it affects longevity, however, are not yet available. In rare cases, a heart and lung transplant may be necessary.

MASSAGE?

If a client is in the early stages of this disease, and limits his exposure to the irritating stimulus, and his tissues are healthy and responsive (that is, his skin shows signs of normal blood flow by appropriate temperature and color changes with massage), and he has medical clearance, massage for the emphysema client may be appropriate. Back, neck, and chest massage may be especially helpful. Advanced cases, in which a is experiencing difficulty breathing and shortness of breath, may not be appropriate for rapid, vigorous Swedish strokes, but calming reflexive work may be excellent for dealing with anxiety and the stress of quitting smoking, as well as the inevitable fatigue these individuals experience. Massage can also address the muscular contribution to "barrel chest." Emphysema clients often cannot tolerate laying completely prone or supine; they may be more comfortable receiving work in a reclining chair or on a massage chair.

Other Respiratory Disorders

Lung Cancer

DEFINITION: WHAT IS IT?

Lung cancer is the growth of malignant tumors in the lungs. (See Figure 6.6.) The epithelium in the lungs is particularly susceptible to damage from inhaled substances, and the propensity to grow tumors may be related to this tissue's tendency to regenerate quickly.

DEMOGRAPHICS: WHO GETS IT?

Lung cancer kills over 150,000 Americans a year and approximately one million people worldwide. It used to be primarily a men's disease, but after WWII it became more socially acceptable for women to smoke. Consequently, today's lung cancer rate for women is rising rapidly while it is declining slightly for men, but men with lung cancer still outnumber women significantly. Lung cancer is the third leading cause of death in the United States, coming in just behind heart disease and stroke, both of which are conditions that can also be linked to smoking. Close to 180,000 new cases of lung cancer are diagnosed every year.

LUNG CANCER IN BRIEF

What is it?
Lung cancer is the development in the lungs of malignant tumors that quickly spread to the lymph system and other organs in the body.

How is it recognized?
The early symptoms of lung cancer are a chronic cough, blood-stained sputum, and recurrent bronchitis or pneumonia.

Is massage indicated or contraindicated?
Massage is systemically contraindicated for lung cancer.

TYPES OF LUNG CANCER

Many different types of lung cancer have been identified, but they have been broken into two main groups: small cell carcinoma and non–small cell carcinoma.

- Small cell carcinoma. This is also called "oat cell" carcinoma. It is responsible for 15 to 20% of all lung cancers. Small cell lung cancer is fast growing, highly invasive, and usually inoperable.
- Non–small cell carcinoma. This includes several different types of cancers, depending on which cells they affect first. Non–small cell carcinomas account for 80 to 85% of all lung cancers. They include squamous cell carcinoma, adenocarcinoma, large cell carcinoma, and several others. Most of these grow more slowly than small cell carcinoma, but the symptoms they create are so subtle that diagnosis doesn't usually occur until long after the cancer has spread beyond its original area.

RISK FACTORS

The most obvious risk factor for lung cancer is smoking. About 80% of all lung cancer patients are smokers. It *is* possible to contract lung cancer without being a smoker, however. It is an occupational risk for people working with asbestos insulation, coal miners, and people who work with other toxic chemicals. Exposure to radon, excessive radiation, or a history of tuberculosis also increases risk. Living or working with a smoker increases the chances for developing lung cancer, as well as other respiratory disorders. An estimated 3000 Americans die every year from lung cancer connected to secondhand smoke; that's more deaths than from all other air pollutants combined.

The link between smoking and lung cancer is clear. Cigarette smoke contains over 40 known carcinogens, and the tar in cigarettes holds the damaging chemicals close to the delicate linings of the lungs. Light smokers are about 10 times more likely to get this disease than nonsmokers; heavy smokers are 25 times more susceptible. But if the person stops smoking, the chances of remaining healthy rise quickly. Precancerous changes in the lung have been seen to reverse after a person quits smoking. After 10 years of nonsmoking, the chances of developing lung cancer will be about the same as those for a lifetime nonsmoker.

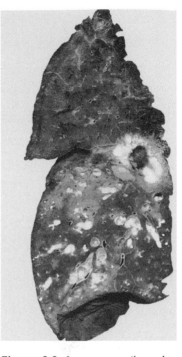

Figure 6.6. Lung cancer (bronchiolar carcinoma)

SIGNS AND SYMPTOMS

The primary symptom of lung cancer is a persistent cough, which is often confused with a regular smoker's cough. Some bloodstained phlegm and some shortness of breath may also be present. If tumors develop in the outer layers of the lung, chest pains develop, which become sharper with deep inhales. People with lung cancer are susceptible to recurrent bronchitis and pneumonia. If the cancer has spread to other parts of the body, it may create other symptoms such as bone pain, abdominal pain, or neurological signs such as headaches or numbness.

DIAGNOSIS

Lung cancer isn't hard to diagnose; the hard part is identifying the early symptoms in time to catch the tumors while they're still isolated. Only 15% of all lung cancers are found this early. Diagnostic tests include examinations of sputum that can show cancer cells, fiberoptic exams of bronchial tubes, needle aspirations of lung tissue for biopsy, and x-rays, CT scans, and MRIs to locate growths.

Once the presence of cancerous cells has been established, the next job is to identify what stage the disease is in, which determines the best treatment options. The TNM classification system is often used for lung cancer. This stages the progression of the disease by T: tumor size; N: nodal involvement; and M: extent of metastasis. In addition to this classification, staging for small cell and non–small cell carcinomas follow the same basic pattern: from Stage 0 to Stage I, the cancer is localized. In Stage II, it has invaded nearby lymph nodes in the mediastinum. Stage III tumors may have invaded the chest wall, the diaphragm, and lymph nodes in the neck. Stage IV lung cancer is systemic through the body; it can affect the brain and spinal cord, the bones, and abdominal organs, particularly the liver and pancreas.

TREATMENT

Most lung cancer patients don't seek medical help until the disease has progressed beyond the point when surgery can excise all the growth. Over 50% of newly diagnosed patients have cancer that has metastasized to elsewhere in the body. The three basic treatment options are radiation, chemotherapy, and surgery, which can range from a wedged resection (removal of a very small portion of damaged tissue), to a lobectomy (removal of a lobe), to a complete pneumonectomy (removal of a whole lung).

Small cell carcinoma grows so fast and spreads so quickly, it is generally treated with radiation and chemotherapy alone; surgery usually has no chance of containing the extent of the growth.

The prognosis for someone with lung cancer is usually very poor. Only 10% of all cases are permanently cured. About one-half of all people diagnosed with inoperable lung cancer die within a year. Only 13% of all people diagnosed with lung cancer live five years or more, but the life expectancy of people who are diagnosed in early stages is much higher than for those who are not.

MASSAGE?

Circulatory massage is contraindicated in any stage of lung cancer unless the client is dying and has decided to include massage as a comfort measure. In this case, it is often best to teach family members some techniques they can do themselves. If the client has had a "clean bill of health" for 5 years or more, massage may be appropriate. In any case, medical supervision is vital. For more information on massage and cancer, see *cancer*, chapter 10, page 358.

CHAPTER REVIEW QUESTIONS:
RESPIRATORY SYSTEM CONDITIONS

1. What is the purpose of mucous membranes? Where are they found?

2. How does the structure of the lungs work to limit the spread of infection?

3. Explain the sympathetic/parasympathetic swing that occurs with asthma.

4. What is the best defense against catching or spreading the cold virus?

5. What is the danger associated with taking broad spectrum antibiotics for a cold, "just in case"?

6. What are the repercussions of having alveoli fuse together, as happens with emphysema?

7. Why is the prognosis for lung cancer generally so poor?

8. What feature of the tuberculosis bacterium distinguishes it from most other pathogens?

9. What happens when prescriptions of antibiotics for tuberculosis (or other bacterial infections) are not completed as directed? Why is this a particular danger for TB?

10. A client has sinusitis. Her mucous is thick, opaque, and sticky. She has had a headache and a mild fever for several days. Is she a good candidate for massage? Why or why not?

BIBLIOGRAPHY, RESPIRATORY SYSTEM CONDITIONS

General References, Respiratory System

1. Carmine D. Clemente. Anatomy: A regional atlas of the human body. 3rd ed. Baltimore: Urban & Schwarzenburg, 1987.
2. I. Damjanou. Pathology for the health-related professions. Philadelphia: Saunders, 1996.
3. Giovanni de Dominico, Elizabeth Wood. Beard's massage. Saunders: Philadelphia, 1997.
4. Jeffrey R. M. Kunz, Asher J. Finkel, eds. The American Medical Association family medical guide. New York: Random House, Inc., 1987.
5. Elaine M. Marieb. Human anatomy and physiology. Redwood City, CA: Benjamin/Cummings Publishing Co., Inc., 1989.
6. Ruth Lundeen Memmler, Dina Lin Wood. The human body in health and disease. 5th ed. Philadelphia: JB Lippincott Co., 1983.
7. Mary Lou Mulvihill. Human diseases: A systemic approach. 2nd ed. East Norwalk, CT: Appleton &Lange, A publishing division of Prentice-Hall, 1987.
8. Stedman's medical dictionary. 26th ed. Baltimore: Williams & Wilkins, 1995.
9. Taber's cyclopedic dictionary. 14th ed. Philadelphia: F.A. Davis Company, 1981.
10. Gerard J. Tortora, Nicholas P. Anagnostakos. Principles of anatomy and physiology. 6th ed. New York: Biological Sciences Textbook, Inc., A&P Textbooks, Inc. and Elia-Sparta, Inc.; Harper & Row Publishers, Inc., 1990.
11. Janet Travell, David G. Simons. Myofascial pain and dysfunction: The trigger point manual. Baltimore: Williams & Wilkins, 1983.

Common Cold

1. Cold, flu or pneumonia? Do you have the one you think you do? Mayo Foundation for Medical Education and Research. Mayo Health O@sis: 1996. URL: http://www.mayo.ivi.com/mayo/9311/htm/coldflu.htm. Accessed fall 1997.
2. Fact sheet: The common cold. National Institute of Allergy and Infectious Diseases; June 1996. URL: http://www.niaid.nih.gov/factsheets/cold.htm. Accessed fall 1997.
3. Handwashing: Here's a habit that helps keep you healthy. Mayo Foundation for Medical Education and Research. Mayo Health O@sis: 1997. URL: http://www.mayo.ivi.com/mayo/9306/htm/handwash.htm. Accessed fall 1997.
4. Lessons from the literature: Antibiotics and the common cold. Centers for Disease Control. URL: http://www.niv.ac.za/lessons/current/les8_3.htm#cold. Accessed fall 1997.

Influenza

1. Cold, flu or pneumonia? Do you have the one you think you do? Mayo Foundation for Medical Education and Research. Mayo Health O@sis: 1996. URL: http://www.mayo.ivi.com/mayo/9311/htm/coldflu.htm. Accessed fall 1997.
2. Fact sheet: Flu. National Institute of Allergy and Infectious Diseases, April 1995. URL: http://www.niaid.nih.gov/factsheets/flu.htm. Accessed fall 1997.
3. Influenza. Copyright 1998 ADAM Software, Inc., all rights reserved. Copyright 1998 CommuniHealth. URL: www.healthanswers.com. Accessed winter 1998.
4. Influenza. New York State Department of Health, Communicable Disease Fact Sheet, March 1996. URL: http://www.health.state.ny.us/nysdoh/consumer/influ.htm. Accessed fall 1997.
5. Influenza prevention and control. Centers for Disease Control and Prevention. Last revised May 27, 1997. URL: http://www.cdc.gov/ncidod/diseases/flu/fluvirus.htm. Accessed fall 1997.

Pneumonia

1. Atypical pneumonia. Copyright 1998 ADAM Software, Inc., all rights reserved. Copyright 1998 CommuniHealth. URL: www.healthanswers.com. Accessed winter 1998.
2. MedicineNet: Power points about pneumonia. Information Network, Inc., 1995–1997. URL: http://www.medicinenet.com. Accessed fall, 1997.
3. Pneumonia. American Lung Association, 1997. URL: http://www.lungusa.org/homepage.html. Accessed fall 1997.
4. Viral pneumonia. Copyright 1998 ADAM Software, Inc., all rights reserved. Copyright 1998 CommuniHealth. URL: www.healthanswers.com. Accessed winter 1998.
5. Walking pneumonia. Copyright 1998 ADAM Software, Inc., all rights reserved. Copyright 1998 CommuniHealth. URL: www.healthanswers.com. Accessed winter 1998.

Sinusitis

6. Fact sheet: Sinusitis. National Institute of Allergy and Infectious Diseases, August 1996. URL: http://www.niaid.nih.gov/factsheets/sinusitis.htm. Accessed fall 1997.
7. MedicineNet: Sinusitis. Information Network, Inc., 1995–1997. URL: http://www.medicinenet.com. Accessed fall 1997.
8. Sinusitis. National Jewish Medical and Research Center, 1993. URL: http://www.njc.org/MFhtml/SIN_MF.html. Accessed fall 1997.

Tuberculosis

1. Brief history of tuberculosis. New Jersey Medical School, National Tuberculosis Center, 1996. Revised July 23, 1996. URL: http://www.umdnj.edu/~ntbcweb/history.htm. Accessed fall 1997.
2. 'Directly observed' therapy effective against TB. Washington Post, April 28, 1994, A10.
3. Epidemiology of tuberculosis. New Jersey Medical School, National Tuberculosis Center, 1996. Revised April 26, 1996. URL: http://www.umdnj.edu/~ntbcweb/tidepi.htm. Accessed fall 1997.
4. Fact sheet: Tuberculosis. National Institute of Allergy and Infectious Diseases, March 1997. URL: http://www.niaid.nih.gov/factsheets/tb.htm. Accessed fall 1997.
5. Anita Manning. Tuberculosis makes a menacing comeback. USA Today, November 17, 1992, p. 4D.
6. Tuberculosis fact sheet. Global Tuberculosis Programme, World Health Organization. URL: http://www.who.ch/gtb/publications/factsheet/index.htm. Accessed winter 1998.
7. Tuberculosis. American Lung Association, 1997. URL: http://www.lungusa.org/homepage.html. Accessed fall 1997.
8. Tuberculosis. New York State Department of Health Communicable Disease Fact Sheet, March 1996. URL: http://www.health.state.ny.us/nysdoh/consumer/tb.htm. Accessed fall 1997.

Asthma

1. Asthma: A concern for minority populations. National Institute of Allergy and Infectious Diseases, August 1996. URL: http://www.niaid.nih.gov/factsheets/minorasthma.htm. Accessed fall 1997.
2. Asthma and allergy statistics. National Institute of Allergy and Infectious Diseases, June 1996. URL: http://www.niaid.nih.gov/factsheets/allergystat.htm. Accessed fall 1997.
3. Asthma update: Report from Mayo Clinic grand rounds, December 6, 1995. Mayo Health O@sis, 1996. URL: http://www.mayo.ivi.com/mayo/9512/htm/asthma.htm. Accessed fall 1997.
4. Bronchial asthma. Copyright 1998 ADAM Software, Inc., all rights reserved. Copyright 1998 CommuniHealth. URL: www.healthanswers.com. Accessed winter 1998.
5. MedicineNet: Power points about asthma. Information Network, Inc., 1995–1997. URL: http://www.medicinenet.com. Accessed fall 1997.

COPD/Emphysema

1. Emphysema. Copyright 1998 ADAM Software, Inc., all rights reserved. Copyright 1998 CommuniHealth. URL: www.healthanswers.com. Accessed winter 1998.
2. Emphysema: Advances can help you breathe more easily. Originally published in Mayo Clinic Health Letter, April 1995. Mayo Foundation for Medical Education and Research, 1996. URL: http://www.mayo.ivi.com/mayo/9504/htm/emphysem.htm. Accessed fall 1997.
3. Emphysema: When you can't catch your breath. Healthbeat, May 23, 1995. University of Washington Health Sciences Center. URL: http://healthlinks.washington.edu/your_health/hbeat/hb950523.html. Accessed fall 1997.
4. Emphysema. American Lung Association, 1997. URL: http://www.lungusa.org/homepage.html. Accessed fall 1997.
5. Pamela Klimowitch. Massage for sufferers of respiratory disease. Massage Therapy Journal, Spring 1993, Vol. 32, No. 2, pp. 42–43.
6. Vince Mak. Chronic obstructive pulmonary disease (COPD), the UK perspective. Last updated June 9, 1997. Priory Lodge Education, Limited, 1996, 1997. URL: http://www.u-net.com/priory/cmol/copd.htm. Accessed fall 1997.

Lung Cancer

1. Jeffrey Kern. Ten questions about lung cancer. University of Iowa, 1992–1997. URL: http://www.vh.org/Providers/Lectures/KernLecture/KernContents.html. Accessed fall 1997.
2. Lung cancer: You may have a role in your risk for this disease. Originally published in Mayo Clinic Health Letter, June 1996. Mayo Foundation for Medical Education and Research, 1996. URL: http://www.mayo.ivi.com/mayo/9606/htm/lung.htm. Accessed fall 1997.

3. MedicineNet: Power points about lung cancer. Information Network, Inc., 1995–1997. URL: http://www.medicinenet. com. Accessed fall 1997.

4. Non-small cell lung cancer. National Cancer Institute/PDQ: Patient Statement. Last modified September 1997. URL: http://rex. nci.nih.gov/INTRFCE_GIFS/INFO_ PATS_INTR_DOC.htm. Accessed fall 1997.

5. Quitters do win. Originally published in Mayo Clinic Health Letter, June 1996. Mayo Foundation for Medical Education and Research, 1996. URL: http://www. mayo.ivi.com/mayo/9606/htm/lung_sb. htm. Accessed fall 1997.

6. Secondhand smoke: Clearing the air of a cloudy debate. August 11, 1997. Mayo Foundation for Medical Education and Research, 1997. URL: http://www.mayo. ivi.com/mayo/9708/htm/2nd_hand.htm. Accessed fall 1997.

7. Small cell lung cancer. National Cancer Institute/PDQ: Patient Statement. Last modified October 1997. URL: http://rex. nci.nih.gov/INTRFCE_GIFS/INFO_ PATS_INTR_DOC.htm. Accessed fall 1997.

Digestive System Conditions

7

After reading this chapter, you should be able to tell . . .

- What the disorder is.
- How to recognize it.
- Whether massage is indicated or contraindicated for that condition.
- Whether a contraindication is local or systemic, or refers to a specific stage of development or healing.
- Why those choices for massage are correct.

In addition to this basic information, you should be able to . . .

- Name three functions of the liver.
- Name three conditions that mimic symptoms of appendicitis.
- Name five complications of cirrhosis.
- Know why anemia is part of the profile for ulcerative colitis.
- List the recommendations for colon cancer screenings for people over 40 years old.
- Identify the difference between diverticulosis and diverticulitis.
- Name two complications gallstones can cause.
- Name three possible causes of gastroenteritis.
- Name which variety of hepatitis is the most communicable.
- Name three ways in which bacteria can gain entry to the peritoneal space.

INTRODUCTION

THE DIGESTIVE TRACT: STRUCTURE AND FUNCTION

The best way to discuss how the digestive tract works is to follow a piece of food through the system. (See Figure 7.1.)

When the teeth pulverize a bite of food, it is broken into small pieces so the digestive enzymes in the saliva and the rest of the gastrointestinal (GI) tract have more access to the nutrients. The food moves from the mouth, down the esophagus, and into a wide place within that tube: the stomach. Here it is further pulverized by powerful muscular contractions of the stomach, while being exposed to more chemicals (the secretion of which is largely dependent on emotional state). Accessory organs make their chemical contributions as the former food, now referred to as chyme, moves into the small

273

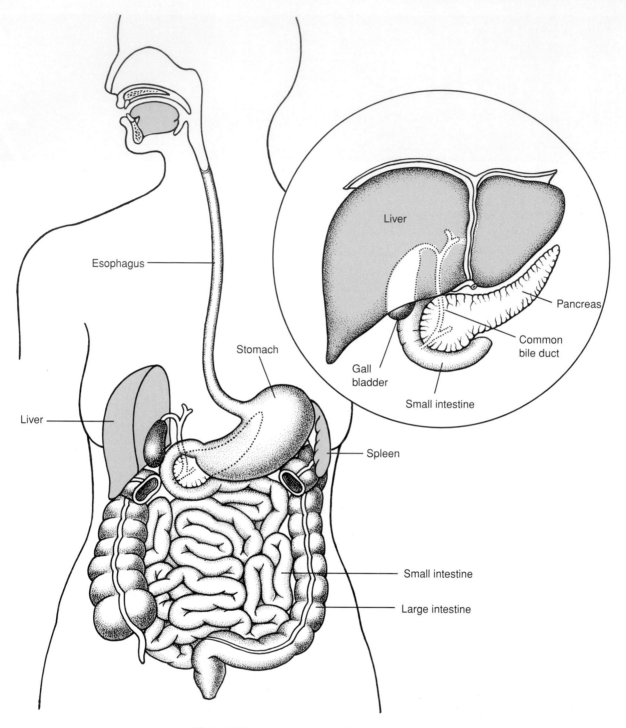

Figure 7.1. Overview of the digestive system

intestine. By now the barrage of digestive enzymes has reduced the meal into its most primitive building blocks: sugars, fats, and proteins.

The small intestine loops and twirls around the abdomen, secured by sheets of connective tissue membrane called the mesentery, a part of the peritoneum. It is lubricated on the outside by other layers of the peritoneum, which allow it to move freely as a person twists, squirms, and changes positions. The inside of a healthy small intestine looks like velvet or velour, with millions of tiny villi, each one supplied with blood and lymph capillaries for the absorption of nutrients and fats. From the villi, the nutrients enter the bloodstream while fats are drawn into the lymph system. Rhythmic waves of smooth muscle contraction should gently ease the food along the tube until, at the distal end of the small intestine, it passes through the ileocecal valve: the entryway to the colon.

The colon is a much shorter and wider section of tubing than the small intestine, and it differs also in the absence of villi and the presence of anchoring pieces of connective tissue that bind the colon down at the four flexures, or corners, of the abdomen. A healthy colon has segments called haustra. In this part of the tube, water is squeezed out of the bolus and resorbed back into the body; this is also the site of vitamin K synthesis. The colon is a kind of trash compactor; everything left of a meal that makes it this far is condensed and excreted.

THE ACCESSORY ORGANS: STRUCTURE AND FUNCTION

The continuous tube that winds from mouth to anus is only one part of the digestive system. The accessory organs also contribute to the process of turning food into energy or building blocks. These organs include the liver, gall bladder, and pancreas, each of which produces or releases chemicals into the digestive tract. Here is a brief review of each of these organs.

The Liver

This is an organ of immense complexity, with literally hundreds of functions. One of the things that makes the liver unique is its powers of regeneration; it is made mostly of epithelial tissue, the fastest tissue type to heal. The liver also holds twice the blood supply of most other organs. With the hepatic artery delivering oxygen, and the portal vein delivering fresh products of digestion from the small intestine, it's no wonder that this organ is hot and dark red, and that its internal blood pressure is very high.

The liver is the largest of the glands in the body. It is the destination of the portal system detour, receiving all the vitamins, amino acids, and glucose that are not immediately needed in the body. By storing glucose as glycogen until it is called for, the liver also acts as a sugar buffer. This prevents some of the radical swings in blood glucose levels that would occur if no intermediate stop for sugar existed. The liver is also the site for much of the most vital protein synthesis in the body. Many of the enzymes that sponsor cellular activity are born here; this is also the origin of blood proteins that regulate intracellular fluid and blood clotting.

Detoxification functions of the liver are well known. The liver alters many drugs into a form suitable for excretion. A functioning liver prevents many substances, including alcohol, from reaching toxic levels in the body. It also processes the poisonous wastes generated by protein digestion, changing them to uric acid to be excreted by the kidneys. In addition to these functions, specialized leukocytes in the liver, called Kupffer cells, are constantly watching for any pathogens they can eradicate. Finally, the liver helps to recycle dead red blood cells, producing bile, a substance that is vital for the digestion of fats. The liver produces up to three cups of bile each day. Bile leaves the liver via the cystic duct and enters the gall bladder.

The Gall Bladder

The gall bladder is a small bright green sack that hangs off the liver about halfway along the costal angle on the right side of the body. Its function is fairly simple: it receives bile from the liver, stores it, and concentrates it. The gall bladder can hold up to one cup of bile at a time. On neural or hormonal command, it releases the bile into the duodenum via the common bile duct. There the bile helps to emulsify fats: the fats are held in tiny globlets to make them easier to digest. The gall bladder and its ducts are susceptible to dysfunction, which can have serious repercussions.

The Pancreas

This is a fascinating gland that holds the distinction of being both an exocrine gland, releasing digestive juices into the intestine via the pancreatic duct, and an endocrine gland, releasing hormones directly into the bloodstream. Its exocrine secretions are so alkaline, they can be corrosive. Any blockage in the pancreatic duct can lead to very serious tissue damage, as the pancreas is quite capable of digesting itself.

GASTROINTESTINAL PROBLEMS AND MASSAGE

Most of the GI tract problems that respond well to massage are related to autonomic imbalance; when a person is under stress, digestion becomes a low priority. If this state continues for a long time, problems will develop. The most common disorders of this type are spastic or flaccid constipation, indigestion, and gas.

The first concern, however, is to eliminate the possibility of more serious conditions that would contraindicate circulatory massage. Massage practitioners are sometimes put in the position of deciding whether their work is going to help someone overcome her stress-related stomachache, or put her in the hospital. Symptoms that are a red light for something very serious include severe localized pain, bloody stools, anemia, bloating, and fever. Follow the general rule of thumb: if symptoms have persisted for 3 weeks or more, it's time to visit the doctor.

Problems in the GI tract are impossible to pin down without diagnostic tests, and fortunately, this is not within the scope of practice of massage therapy. Massage should not be performed when the client has any unexplained or undiagnosed pain. Any relief that a massage provides may delay the client from getting medical assistance for a serious and acute illness. The symptoms of colon cancer, for example, can look a lot like spastic constipation. One may indicate massage; the other definitely does not.

DIGESTIVE SYSTEM CONDITIONS

**Disorders of the Stomach
and Small Intestine**

Gastroenteritis

Ulcers

Disorders of the Large Intestine

Appendicitis

Colon Cancer

Diverticulosis/Diverticulitis

Irritable Bowel Syndrome

Ulcerative Colitis

Disorders of the Accessory Organs

Cirrhosis

Gallstones

Hepatitis

Jaundice

Liver, Enlarged

Other Digestive System Conditions

Peritonitis

Disorders of the Stomach and Small Intestine

Gastroenteritis

DEFINITION: WHAT IS IT?

Gastroenteritis is inflammation of the gastrointestinal (GI) tract, specifically the small intestine.

ETIOLOGY: WHAT HAPPENS?

Gastroenteritis has several causes. Although each pathogen may create slightly different symptoms, the basics (nausea, vomiting, diarrhea) are consistent.

- Viruses. The most common cause of GI inflammation is an infection with rotavirus or Norwalk virus. Any of the hepatitis viruses can also cause it, as can the enterovirus. Viral gastroenteritis is highly contagious, and can reach epidemic levels in environments such as day care centers, because most infants have not yet developed antibodies against infection, and the chance of fecal-oral contamination is very high.
- Bacteria. Bacterial gastroenteritis may be at fault when people complain of "stomach flu." (In reality, no flu virus attacks the GI tract.) Common bacterial pathogens include Salmonella, Shigella, and staphylococcus. Bacterial gastroenteritis usually spreads through improperly stored or prepared food, or contaminated water. "Travelers' diarrhea" is almost always from the E. Coli bacterium.
- Others. Other causes of gastroenteritis include parasites (i.e., Giardia), fungal infections (i.e., candida), toxins (i.e., poisonous mushrooms), dietary problems (i.e., food allergies), medications (i.e., antibiotics or magnesium-containing laxatives or antacids), or other conditions such as *appendicitis* (this chapter, page 280), *ulcerative colitis* (this chapter, page 290), or *diverticulitis* (this chapter, page 285).

COMPLICATIONS

The most serious complication of gastroenteritis is dehydration resulting from the massive fluid and mineral loss caused by diarrhea. This can lead to the loss of critical electrolytes, and can actually send someone into shock. The people most at risk for this extreme reaction are infants and the elderly since their systems are less able to cope with this extreme change in internal environment.

TREATMENT

Gastroenteritis is seldom a serious condition and is generally not treated with anything more sophisticated than rest and fluid replacement. Viruses do not respond to antibiotics, and antibiotics for bacterial infections tend to make intestinal inflammation worse. The use of anti-diarrhea medications is often discouraged, because the body is shedding pathogens: interfering with that process may prolong the infection. If supplementing fluids by mouth only serves to aggravate vomiting, it may be necessary to use intravenous fluid replacement in a hospital setting.

PROGNOSIS

Most cases of gastroenteritis are self-limiting and will resolve within 2 to 3 days without medical intervention. If

---

GASTROENTERITIS IN BRIEF

What is it?

Gastroenteritis is a form of gastrointestinal inflammation, which may be caused by a viral or bacterial infection, a parasite, fungus, toxic exposure, or other factors.

How is it recognized?

Symptoms of gastroenteritis include nausea, vomiting, and diarrhea.

Is massage indicated or contraindicated?

Massage is at least locally contraindicated for anyone with acute gastrointestinal inflammation, and systemically contraindicated for people with acute intestinal infections.

HIATAL HERNIA

Hiatal hernia is actually a muscular problem addressed briefly in chapter 2. However, because its symptoms primarily affect the gastrointestinal tract, it deserves a special mention here.

Occasionally the esophageal hiatus, the hole in the diaphragm through which the esophagus passes on its way to the stomach, becomes stretched and loose. The stomach itself may push up or *herniate* through this hole in the diaphragm muscle. The problem with this situation is that the stomach contents, including hydrochloric acid and digestive enzymes, can then splash up into the unprotected esophagus. This is especially likely to happen if the esophageal sphincter, a circular muscle designed to prevent the movement of materials back up into the esophagus, is weak or overstressed.

This situation is called *gastroesophageal reflux disease*. Symptoms include heartburn, chest pain that mimics heart attacks, difficulty in swallowing, and in advanced cases, tooth damage from exposure to corrosive acids. Changes in the lining of the esophagus may also occur. These tissue changes sometimes lead to esophageal cancer. Not all people with hiatal hernias experience gastroesophageal reflux disease, although close to 80% of all people with gastroesophageal reflux disease have hiatal hernias.   *(continued)*

HIATAL HERNIA, cont.

Treatment for gastroesophageal reflux disease and hiatal hernias includes changes in eating habits to avoid filling the stomach to capacity, medication to limit the output of stomach acid, and if necessary, surgery to repair the hernia and insert a mechanical valve to help or replace the ineffective esophageal sphincter.

symptoms persist longer than 2 to 3 weeks, it is no longer considered an acute infection, but a chronic condition. This would lead medical professionals to look for an underlying condition such as *irritable bowel syndrome* (this chapter, page 288), *diverticulitis*, *ulcerative colitis*, or *AIDS* (chapter 5, page 233).

MASSAGE?

Massage is contraindicated for someone with gastroenteritis because of the presence of infection and the possibility of spreading it.

Ulcers

DEFINITION: WHAT ARE THEY?

Ulcers of the stomach and duodenum will be discussed in this section, but an ulcer is an ulcer, whether it's in the GI tract or on the skin. An ulcer is the result of tissue damage that never gets better because it is subject to constant irritation and the healing process may be somehow impeded. Cells die, are sloughed off, and a crater develops but doesn't crust over. An ulcer is a perpetually open sore, an invitation to infection. (See Figure 7.2.) For more information on skin ulcers, see *decubitus ulcers*, chapter 1, page 36.

DEMOGRAPHICS: WHO GETS THEM?

Ulcers are common in the United States; about four million new ulcers are diagnosed each year. Men are more prone than women to develop ulcers in the duodenum, and they generally appear between the ages of 30 and 50 years. Women get more stomach ulcers than men, and they appear a bit later: usually after 60 years of age.

Ulcers lead to approximately 40,000 surgeries each year. Complications from ulcers are responsible for 6,000 deaths each year.

ETIOLOGY: WHAT HAPPENS?

Ulcers in the digestive system are called peptic ulcers, named for the protein-digesting enzyme pepsin that contributes to their development. The general understanding of how ulcers come about has undergone some radical changes in the last several years.

ULCERS IN BRIEF

What are they?

Ulcers are sores that, for various reasons, don't experience a normal healing process, but instead, remain open and vulnerable to infection.

How are they recognized?

The symptoms of gastric and peptic ulcers include general burning or gnawing abdominal pain between meals that is relieved by taking antacids or eating.

Is massage indicated or contraindicated?

Massage is locally contraindicated for someone with ulcers; specific work on the abdomen may exacerbate symptoms.

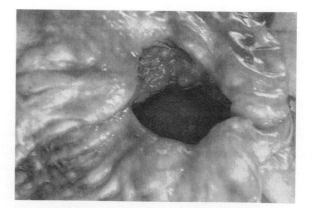

Figure 7.2. Perforating gastric ulcer

The relationship between emotional state and gastrointestinal health has long been established. During a sympathetic reaction, blood flow to the stomach is reduced. This limits the amount of protective mucus the stomach can produce, allowing digestive acids and pepsin to damage the stomach wall. Ulcers were traditionally treated with antacids, medicines that limit mucus production, and the avoidance of alcohol, cigarettes, and foods that tend to aggravate the stomach. Unfortunately, although symptoms were sometimes relieved, ulcers often recurred and became a life-long affliction.

In 1982, the discovery of a particular bacterium, *Helicobacter pylori*, in nearly all samples of ulcer tissue led to the conclusion that this pathogen is part of their cause. This theory was confirmed when it was found that treating ulcers with antibiotics, as well as antacids and mucus-stimulating medicines, almost always leads to a permanent solution of the problem. Helicobacter pylori is found in most, but not all, ulcer tissue samples. About 20 to 30% of ulcers have nothing to do with bacteria; they are brought about by the use of aspirin and other nonsteroidal anti-inflammatory drugs (NSAIDs) for other aches and pains, or to avoid the risks of heart attack or stroke.

SIGNS AND SYMPTOMS

The primary symptom of peptic ulcers is burning pain in the chest or abdomen that lasts anywhere from 30 minutes to 3 hours. The pain's occurrence in relation to eating varies greatly from one person to the next (it can depend on the location of the ulcer), but it is generally relieved by antacids or eating more food.

COMPLICATIONS

The possible short-term complications of ulcers are quite serious. They include bleeding, either slowly and constantly which leads to *anemia* (chapter 4, page 178), or hemorrhaging, which can occur when tissue damage invades artery walls. This can lead quickly to shock and death, if left untreated. Ulcers can also perforate or eat all the way through the organ wall, releasing bacteria and partially digested food into the peritoneal space (see *peritonitis*, this chapter, page 301). Perforation happens about 20 times more often with duodenal than stomach ulcers. (See Figure 7.2.) Finally, ulcers can create a combination of scar tissue and inflammation that can throw the pyloric valve into spasm, thus completely obstructing the digestive tract. If this situation is not quickly resolved, surgery may be required to reopen the digestive tract.

DIAGNOSIS

Blood tests for Helicobacter are a useful tool, but they can reveal false-positive findings. For that reason, a series of x-rays of the gastrointestinal tract typically are taken after the patient drinks a barium preparation. This will reveal not only the presence, but the precise location of the ulcers. Endoscopy, running a flexible tube down the throat with a camera attached, can also give precise information about ulcers, although it's a more complex and expensive process than x-rays. Once the presence of an ulcer has been determined, looking for Helicobacter will determine whether a bacterial infection is part of the picture.

It is important to go through the steps of diagnosis for peptic ulcers because the symptoms can sometimes mimic stomach cancer, and it's important to rule out this disease as quickly as possible.

TREATMENT

Up until recently, ulcers were healed fairly easily if the irritating influences were ceased, but they also recurred very easily, especially with smokers. Long-term effects of living with ulcers include increasingly poor nutrition, weight loss, depressed immunity, and in some cases, an increased chance of stomach cancer.

These days, treatment for most ulcers includes antibiotics for the Helicobacter pylori, bismuth to protect the delicate stomach lining, and medicines that limit acid production. Patients treated this way have up to a 90% chance of permanent recovery.

Ulcers caused by the use of nonsteroidal anti-inflammatory drugs will not respond to antibiotic therapy. The only way to limit them is to suspend the use of the medications that are damaging the stomach lining.

Occasionally a patient won't respond to medical therapy, or an ulcer is so far advanced that surgery becomes an important option. Surgeries for ulcers take one of three forms. A *vagotomy* severs the vagus nerve (the branch of the parasympathetic nervous system that stimulates gastric secretion). Recent advances in neurosurgery mean that just the part of the vagus nerve that controls gastric secretions can be cut. With an *antrectomy*, the lower part of the stomach (the antrum) is removed. A *pyloroplasty* is surgery that enlarges the pyloric valve to allow a better flow from the stomach into the duodenum. Antrectomies and pyloroplasties are generally performed in conjunction with vagotomies.

MASSAGE?

Massage is unlikely to make an ulcer any worse, unless the therapist is mechanically manipulating the stomach or intestines. Consider the abdomen a local contraindication for deep specific work. Otherwise, massage can be very helpful in reestablishing the autonomic balance that will promote permanent healing.

Disorders of the Large Intestine

APPENDIX
The Latin root of appendix is *appendo*, which means, "hang something on." This refers to the appendix's location, hanging off the cecum of the large intestine.

APPENDICITIS IN BRIEF

What is it?
Appendicitis is inflammation of the vermiform appendix, often due to infection, but sometimes related to physical obstruction, as well as pathogens.

How is it recognized?
The symptoms of appendicitis are widely variable, but include general abdominal pain that gradually settles in the lower right quadrant. Fever, nausea, vomiting, food aversion, and diarrhea may also be present.

Is massage indicated or contraindicated?
Massage is systemically contraindicated for acute appendicitis. Postoperative massage may be appropriate (see chapter 10, page 367.)

Appendicitis

DEFINITION: WHAT IS IT?

Appendicitis describes the inflammation of the vermiform appendix, a structure that dangles off the cecum. In some animals, the appendix performs a vital role in digestion and immunity. In people, however, its function is not completely understood. In fact, for a while it was standard procedure to remove the appendix during any abdominal surgery, just in case it should someday cause a problem. It is now recognized that the lymphatic follicles lining the appendix may help to produce some types of immunoglobulins, so the appendix is only taken out when leaving it in poses significant danger.

ETIOLOGY: WHAT HAPPENS?

Appendicitis is generally precipitated by an obstruction of the opening into the cecum; the cause could be a tumor, a foreign body (an old wives' tale suggests that swallowing watermelon seeds or bubble gum can cause appendicitis), fecal matter, or even a simple kink in the organ. Sometimes abdominal inflammation elsewhere will cause the appendix to be obstructed. As infection develops, usually thanks to Escherichia coli, the appendix will become inflamed, and may even develop abscesses or gangrene.

SIGNS AND SYMPTOMS

Symptoms of appendicitis often start with central abdominal pain, which eventually settles into the lower right quadrant. Nausea, vomiting, and anorexia, or food aversion, are often present as well. Pain is dull at first, and then becomes quite severe. It is aggravated by coughing, sneezing, or abdominal movement. If the appendix ruptures, the pain will often temporarily subside, since the pressure has been relieved, and it may take the infection a few hours to completely overtake the system.

Appendicitis is notorious for presenting itself differently in different people. Pregnant women and the elderly, in particular, tend to have a very different pattern of symptoms, leading to misdiagnosis and severe complications. In fact, although people over 60 years of age account for only 5 to 10% of appendicitis cases, they account for up to 50% of deaths from this infection.

COMPLICATIONS

In a worst-case scenario, the appendix may completely rupture, leaking its colonies of bacteria into the peritoneal cavity, almost certainly causing peritonitis. Occasionally, the greater omentum may be positioned to smother a perforated appendix, which can temporarily localize the infection. But this generally leads to internal adhesions and abscesses that, without medical intervention, would probably rupture as well.

In some situations the appendix itself may develop abscesses: small, painful, localized infections. In this case, the risk of infection being released by surgery is high, so the abscesses must be resolved with antibiotic therapy before the appendix is removed.

DIAGNOSIS

Although the ability to identify intestinal disorders has taken quantum leaps forward with CT scans, ultrasounds, and laparoscopies, appendicitis remains extremely difficult to diagnose. It resembles several other serious conditions, including *gastroenteritis* (this chapter, page 276), *kidney stones* (chapter 8, page 310), *urinary tract infection* (chapter 8, page 318), Crohn's disease, *pelvic inflammatory disease* (chapter 9, page 346), and *ovarian cysts* (chapter 9, page 341).

Ultimately, appendicitis is usually diagnosed through the patient history and a physical exam. One fairly dependable sign is "rebound pain": when the doctor pushes on the lower right side of the abdomen, and then lets go suddenly, the pain is worse on the release than with the initial pressure.

Laparoscopies (inserting a tiny camera into the abdomen to look around) can successfully diagnose appendicitis, but they must be done under anesthesia, which carries its own set of risks. Fortunately, if the appendix is infected, the surgery to remove it can be done at the same time.

TREATMENT

Once infection in the appendix has been identified, surgery is performed to remove it. This has traditionally been done through a small incision close to the site of the appendix, but recent advances have made laparoscopies a viable option. This technique has the advantages of creating a smaller wound and requiring a much shorter recovery time than traditional abdominal surgery.

It is best to perform this simple surgery in the early stages of inflammation before gangrene, rupture, or abscesses create further complications.

MASSAGE?

Someone with appendicitis needs immediate care, not massage. Even a chronic low-grade infection can flare up quickly, and the risk of rupture and peritonitis is very high. For guidelines about working with someone recovering from an appendectomy, see *postoperative situations*, chapter 10, page 367.

COLON CANCER IN BRIEF

What is it?

Colon cancer is the development of malignant tumors in the colon or rectum. Growths can block the bowel and/or metastasize to other organs, particularly the liver.

How is it recognized?

Colon cancer has different symptoms, depending on what part of the colon is affected. The most dangerous symptoms are extreme changes in bowel habits—diarrhea or constipation—that last more than 10 days. Other symptoms include blood in the stool, iron-deficiency anemia, and weight loss.

Is massage indicated or contraindicated?

Circulatory massage is contraindicated for active cases of colon cancer, as it is for most cases of cancer, although decisions must be made on a case-by-case basis. For more information about massage and cancer in general, see *cancer*, chapter 10, page 358.

Colon Cancer

DEFINITION: WHAT IS IT?

Colon cancer is the development of tumors anywhere in the large intestine from the ascending right side to the rectum. Although the two conditions are linked, malignant colon cancer is not the same thing as the presence of *adenomas*, or colon polyps.

DEMOGRAPHICS: WHO GETS IT?

The overall incidence of colon cancer in the United States is about 2 people per 1000. Men and women are affected equally. About 160,000 Americans are diagnosed, and about 60,000 people die from this disease every year.

Colon cancer is often symptomless. Some find it unpleasant to screen for, and it metastasizes easily. It is also statistically linked to diets high in fats, while low in fiber. All of these factors make colon cancer, which if caught early has a very high survival rate, the second leading cause of death by cancer in the United States: only lung cancer has a higher death rate.

Familial adenomatous polyposis and *hereditary nonpolyposis colorectal cancer syndrome* are two genetic conditions that predispose some people to the development of colon cancer. Although these people have a much greater than average chance of developing the disease, the vast majority of colon cancer cases are found in people who are *not* part of these high-risk groups.

ETIOLOGY: WHAT HAPPENS?

The colon, or bowel, is the last and widest section of the digestive tract. In this 6-foot long piece of tubing, the remnants of food are compacted, needed water is reabsorbed into the body, and feces are stored in the rectum until they are expelled. The inner lining of the colon is composed of epithelium which, as has been seen in other discussions of cancer, is particularly susceptible to uncontrolled growth.

The majority of colon cancers begin with the development of adenomas: small polyps in the bowel. Minor chromosome damage is believed to cause the formation of these polyps: the cells in the mucosa of the colon simply multiply without any reason and create these small pileups of excess tissue. (See Figure 7.3.) But if the polyps are present for a long period of time, the chromosome damage may accumulate and cause these benign growths to become malignant. They can invade the deeper layers of the bowel's muscular tube, they can obstruct the movement of fecal matter, and they can metastasize through the lymph system to other places in the body: notably, the brain, liver, and lungs. This is the transition from polyps to colon cancer, and it generally happens without warning.

CAUSES

No one knows what prompts common colon polyps, which occur in 30 to 40% of older Americans, to become malignant. Large polyps and ones that have been present for long periods of time are the most likely to become cancerous, but what actually causes the shift is still a mystery. One theory is that high-fat foods linger in the colon longer than others, and some of their by-products are carcinogenic, or cancer-causing. The presence of these chemicals may contribute to chromosome damage in the polyps, causing them to repro-

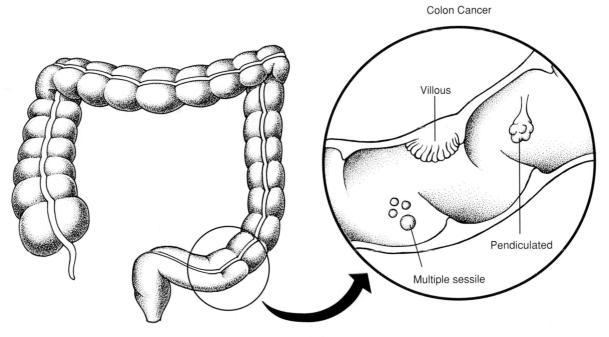

Figure 7.3. Colon cancer

duce at even more abnormal rates. This theory also suggests that diets high in fiber cause matter to move through the colon faster and more completely, "scrubbing" the bowel walls of damaging or irritating materials.

These theories make some sense, and they are statistically demonstrable in population studies that show colon cancer rates are much higher in cultures that follow a western diet (North America, Australia, and Europe) than in cultures that don't (South America, Africa, and Asia). Furthermore, colon cancer rates are increasing in countries currently moving toward a westernized diet standard. However, when discussing individual cases, no specific study proves that any particular diet will prevent, or even decrease, the chances of developing this disease. This is not to say that no connection exists between diet and colon cancer; it's just to point out that no one has yet defined exactly what the connection is.

RISK FACTORS

As stated above, some specific genetic conditions can predispose some people to the development of colon cancer, but the largest portion of people who have this disease do not come from this population group. Some of the other factors that can increase the chances of developing colon cancer include . . .

- Obesity. People who are obese have a statistically higher chance of developing colon cancer.
- Family history. Outside of the two genetic anomalies that can lead to colon cancer, a person who has a close relative with colon cancer has a slightly higher than normal chance of developing the disease herself.
- Ulcerative colitis. This condition is very highly connected with colon cancer. The younger a person is when diagnosed with ulcerative colitis, the greater her chances will be of eventually developing colon cancer. The risk is so high that for some people, preventive surgery to remove the whole colon is suggested before the cancer has a chance to develop. (See *ulcerative colitis*, this chapter, page 290.)
- Age. The chances of having colon cancer rise with age. This disease is the leading cause of death by cancer for people over 75 years old.

SIGNS AND SYMPTOMS

Like so many other types of cancer, colon cancer often doesn't show distinctive symptoms until it has progressed to dangerous levels. Symptoms will also vary according to where tumors are growing. Cancer in the spacious ascending colon is often first manifested as unexplained anemia: tumors can bleed continuously into the colon, making less iron, and therefore less oxygen, available to body cells. Growths in the more constricted descending colon, however, will be experienced as extreme constipation or narrowed stools. Other signs of colon cancer that a person may or may not be aware of are blood in the stools (sometimes it is obvious and bright red; sometimes it occurs in invisible, microscopic amounts), lower abdominal pain, and weight loss.

DIAGNOSIS

Colon cancer isn't difficult to diagnose; what's difficult is getting people to agree to be tested. Interestingly, a survey of oncologists revealed that even they don't follow the approved guidelines for regular colon cancer screening.

Basic screening for colon cancer begins with a digital rectal exam. This procedure, which is the same as that for prostate cancer, will reveal masses in the rectum. Fecal occult blood tests—special examinations of stool samples that indicate the presence of microscopic amounts of blood in the stool—are another early screening technique. Although several conditions exist that can cause blood in the stool, this is a serious sign that must be investigated.

If stool samples are positive for abnormal levels of blood, the next step is usually a barium enema, which will reveal through x-rays any particular masses in the colon, or a sigmoidoscopy, an exploration of the colon via a small tube with a camera attached. This scope looks for polyps that may have become malignant. The sigmoidoscopy is limited to the sigmoid colon; a full colonoscopy can be performed if tumors are suspected higher up in the structure.

If a test reveals the presence of suspicious polyps, tissue samples must be obtained to examine them for cancerous cells. The advantage of sigmoidoscopies and colonoscopies is that tissue biopsies can be performed at the same time as the initial exam. Although barium enemas are cheaper and easier to perform, a positive test will always require surgery to extract a tissue sample.

The ultra-fast CT scanner that has been in development for the screening of high-risk atherosclerosis patients can also be applied to colon screenings. This test is much shorter and more comfortable than other screening techniques, but, as with barium enemas, any indication of abnormal tissues always requires further intervention.

All these screening techniques sound to many people almost worse than having the disease itself. However, statistics that compare survival rates for people who are diagnosed early compared to those who found their cancer later are convincing reasons to follow the basic guidelines for colon cancer screening. The National Cancer Institute recommends that all people over 40 years old should have annual digital rectal exams and fecal occult blood tests. People over 50 years old should have a sigmoidoscopy every 3 to 5 years. Regular colonoscopies are not recommended unless there is reason to suspect the growth of abnormal tissues higher in the colon.[1]

If a polyp is found to be cancerous, the next step is to determine how far the cancer has progressed. Although most cancers are rated from Stage 0 to Stage IV, colon cancer has a slightly different tradition in its staging sequence, called Duke's Classification. This method refers to the cancer in Stages A through D.

---

[1] Colon cancer. National Cancer Institute/PDQ: Patient Statement. Last modified September 1997. URL: http://rex.nci.nih.gov/INTRFCE_GIFS/INFO_PATS_INTR_DOC.htm. Accessed fall 1997.

- *Stage A* colon cancer means that the tumor hasn't penetrated any deeper than the mucosa of the colon.
- *Stage B* colon cancer means that the growth has affected the muscular layer of the bowel wall.
- *Stage C* colon cancer means that the cancer has metastasized to nearby lymph nodes.
- *Stage D* colon cancer means that tumors have invaded distant organs.

TREATMENT

Treatment for colon cancer depends on the stage at which it is identified. Stage A or B cancer is generally treated with surgery to remove the affected section of bowel. The remaining bowel may be reconnected, if possible, or the healthy section may be connected to a colostomy bag for exterior storage and disposal of wastes. Colon cancers treated in Stage A or B show a 90% survival rate.

Stage C colon cancer will require surgery to remove the affected length of bowel, as well as chemotherapy to reduce the chance of metastasis through the lymph system.

Stage D colon cancer is treated in much the same way as Stage C, but with more aggressive chemotherapy, and perhaps radiation to limit growths at distant sites. Stage D colon cancer is generally considered to be practically incurable, and has a 5-year survival rate of less than 10%.

MASSAGE?

Circulatory massage is contraindicated for clients who are fighting active cancer, although other bodywork techniques can offer many of the benefits of massage without the potential hazards. Decisions must be made on a case-by-case basis, with as much information as possible, so that clients, therapists, and doctors can work together to make an informed and compassionate decision.

Colon cancer survivors are good candidates for massage. If a colostomy bag is present, massage therapists should be aware that oil may dissolve the adhesive that holds the bag to the skin.

Diverticulosis/Diverticulitis

DEFINITION: WHAT IS IT?

Diverticular disease is a condition of the colon in which the inner, or mucosal, layer of the colon bulges through the outer muscular layer to form a small sac or diverticulum. It happens most often in the descending section or sigmoid bend of the colon.

DEMOGRAPHICS: WHO GETS IT?

Diverticular disease is very common in the United States. About 300,000 cases are diagnosed every year, but the actual incidence is probably quite a bit higher since most cases of diverticulosis are identified when a patient is undergoing diagnosis for some other problem. It is estimated that although this condition is rare in people under 40 years old, 50% or more of all people over 60 have one or more diverticular pouch.

Diverticulosis is related to a diet high in animal fats and low in fiber and bulk. It is common in Western

DIVERTICULUM
This is a Latin word from *deverto,* meaning "to turn aside." Diverticula are byroads or detours in the large intestine.

DIVERTICULOSIS/DIVERTICULITIS IN BRIEF

What is it?
Diverticulosis is the development of small pouches that protrude from the colon. Diverticulitis is the inflammation of these pouches when they become infected.

How is it recognized?
Diverticulosis is usually symptomless. When inflammation is present, lower left-side abdominal pain, cramping, bloating, constipation, or diarrhea will occur.

Is massage indicated or contraindicated?
Deep abdominal massage is locally cautioned if the client knows diverticula are present. Massage is systemically contraindicated in the presence of active infection.

countries, but is significantly rarer in Asia and Africa, where diets are differently balanced.

ETIOLOGY: WHAT HAPPENS?

Diverticula form during segmentation, a special type of smooth muscle contraction in the large intestine. These contractions are very strong, and if enough bulk isn't present to press against, the pressure will cause colon walls to bulge. The mucosal, or inner, layer will protrude right through the outer muscular layer. These sacs may be filled with fecal matter and bacteria, and the potential for infection is high. (See Figure 7.4.) About 20% of

DIVERTICULOSIS: CASE HISTORY

Cathy S., 50 years old

"Try warm prune juice."

Cathy is a 50-year-old speech and language pathologist with a number of problems involving a hyperreactive immune system. She suspects she may have rheumatoid arthritis and/or lupus. Although she has never been formally diagnosed for either condition, her blood tests indicate that she is prone to autoimmune dysfunction. In addition to systemic arthritis, Cathy has spondylosis: a degeneration of the articular facets between L5 and S1 resulting in hypermobility of the low back, chronic pain, and a fragile state of balance that is easily disrupted by a minor force such as a cough or sneeze.

My husband's mother had colon cancer. We knew what it was like to have to deal with this disease, so last August we all got checked. I had a Colo-Rectal scope that revealed a very large diverticulum; the doctor said it was big enough that he could double up the scope hose into it. I had no pain, and there was no infection. I didn't think much more about it.

For the last 10 years, I've had problems with bowel movements, just being regular. I didn't think much of it. I had a hysterectomy 5 years ago, and at that time, I asked what would be the best way to become regular. I was told to take warm prune juice. I did it, and that took care of the problem for quite a while.

I didn't really know there was anything wrong until last April, on Good Friday, as a matter of fact. It was a day worse than most days at work. I didn't have time to eat properly, so I snacked on graham crackers all day. By 2:00, I was just about bent over double—still charting patients, mind you, but bent over double. I just couldn't get any relief.

I continued to work until 6:00, at which point I was just about screaming. (But, of course, not telling anybody.) I went to the after-hours clinic, and they gave me prescription-strength Zantac and an antibiotic. Within half an hour the pain went away—or at least resolved to the point where I could stand myself.

Having had that experience, I decided I better see a gastroenterologist. I had the upper and lower scope, a colonoscopy and endoscopy, and that's when they found the diverticulum again, although there was no longer any infection.

I was diagnosed with diverticulosis along with "chronic inflammatory disease," which may go along with my generally hyperactive immune system.

These days I stick with a low fat diet, and I drink *lots* of water—64 ounces a day, minimum. I eat small meals. I take Zantac every night, along with Relafen for arthritis pain, and I've never had another episode. I receive massage regularly. Deep psoas work can often help to relieve my lower back pain, but I can't do it every time because some days I'm just too tender.

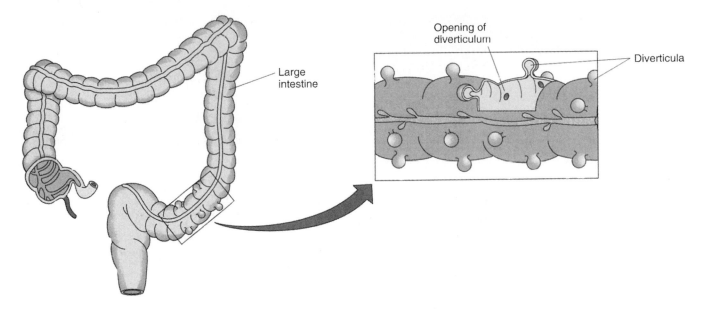

Figure 7.4. Diverticulitis, diverticulosis

people diagnosed with diverticulosis will go on to develop diverticulitis, or inflammation of the diverticula.

SIGNS AND SYMPTOMS

Symptoms of diverticulosis may be nonexistent. When infection is present, however, symptoms include nausea, fever, cramping, and severe pain on the lower left side of the abdomen. The severity and length of time symptoms are present vary greatly from one person to another.

COMPLICATIONS

In very extreme cases of diverticulitis, inflammation may create an obstruction in the colon. Occasionally the pouches can erode the wall of the nearby bladder, causing chronic severe bladder infections (see *urinary tract infection*, chapter 8, page 318). When the inner layer of the colon is damaged, passing stools may scrape and erode blood vessels, causing bleeding with bowel movements. Abscesses may form in the diverticula, with the danger of rupture, which would release bacteria into the peritoneal space (see *peritonitis*, this chapter, page 301).

TREATMENT

Treatment for diverticulosis isn't usually necessary because the symptoms are so mild or don't exist at all. Although the diverticula are not reversible, further growths can be prevented with changes toward a higher fiber diet and exercise.

Acute diverticulitis sometimes mimics symptoms of colon cancer, so it is often diagnosed very thoroughly with barium enemas, sigmoidoscopes or colonoscopes, CT scans, and ultrasounds. Treatment for active infection starts with antibiotics and a strictly controlled diet. If substantial tissue damage, a bowel obstruction, or uncontrolled bleeding has occurred, surgery may be performed to resolve the situation.

MASSAGE?

A client probably won't know if he or she has diverticulosis or not. If the condition has been diagnosed, conduct deep abdominal work with caution; the muscular wall

IRRITABLE BOWEL SYNDROME IN BRIEF

What is it?
Irritable bowel syndrome (IBS) is a collection of signs and symptoms related to a functional problem of the digestive system. It is aggravated by stress and diet.

How is it recognized?
The symptoms of IBS include alternating bouts of constipation and diarrhea, bloating or abdominal distension, and moderate to severe abdominal cramps that are relieved with defecation.

Is massage indicated or contraindicated?
Massage is indicated for IBS with caution against aggravating an already hypersensitive GI tract.

of the colon is already structurally impaired. Swedish massage is systemically contraindicated for acute diverticulitis.

Irritable Bowel Syndrome

DEFINITION: WHAT IS IT?

Irritable bowel syndrome (IBS) is a recently acknowledged and little understood condition. It has also been known as spastic colon, irritable colon, mucus colitis, and functional bowel syndrome. Up to an estimated 15 million Americans have this condition, although only about 20% of them have sought medical help.

ETIOLOGY: WHAT HAPPENS?

Exactly how IBS problems start is probably different for each individual, but some general observations include that the digestive tract as a whole, and the colon in particular, are hyperreactive in IBS patients. That is, small stimuli can create major contractions for no discernible reason. In IBS, peristalsis, which should be smooth and rhythmic, becomes uncoordinated and irregular.

IBS very often occurs hand in hand with anxiety and stress. Most people with this condition report flare-ups in conjunction with threatening situations: job interviews, exams, major life changes, and so on. The development of IBS probably has little to do with the presence of stress per se, and more to do with how the individual handles it. Learning new coping strategies for how to deal with stress through psychotherapy is a frequent treatment recommendation. This becomes especially important as depression, a complication of many long-term disorders, can exacerbate symptoms.

SIGNS AND SYMPTOMS

IBS can manifest in a variety of ways: cramps, abdominal pain, gas, bloating, constipation and diarrhea (usually in cycles), and a frequent need to defecate, although often with a feeling of incomplete evacuation. Abdominal pain is usually relieved after bowel movements.

IRRITABLE BOWEL SYNDROME: CASE HISTORY

Debbie T., 29 years old

"It's just something you ate."

I had my first attack of IBS in January 1991. I woke up out of a dead sleep. I thought I had appendicitis or something. I had diarrhea, I was throwing up, I had never hurt that bad. There was no warning, no buildup, it was just there. I hurt so bad I passed out. My husband called the ambulance and I went to the hospital. In the ambulance, they asked about my sunburn—I was completely covered with a red rash. The rash only happened the first time.   *(continued)*

IRRITABLE BOWEL SYNDROME: CASE HISTORY, cont.

At the hospital they gave me something through an IV that was supposed to coat my stomach. They said I probably had food poisoning.

Four months later, it happened again. I woke up out of a dead sleep and ended up in the hospital. Four months later, there I was again. It was so painful, I was really noisy, but I didn't care. They took a bunch of blood samples, but they didn't show anything. "It's just something you ate," they kept saying. It got to where they would recognize me coming in, and know exactly what to do.

When the attacks started happening more and more frequently, I finally went to see a gastroenterologist. He said, "Write down everything you eat, and call me from the hospital the next time it happens." I knew it wasn't anything I was eating—I'd get attacks after a bowl of cereal! And I didn't want another attack to happen. People said it was lactose intolerance, but I have milk all the time, and my attacks didn't happen all the time.

The next time was 2 months later. I was in the hospital, and they decided to do a blood gas test; they have to stick the needle into an artery to do that. It is no fun. I couldn't have any medication, and I was supposed to lie completely still. Well, they couldn't get the needle in. My gastroenterologist said, "If you can't get the blood gas, I won't see you again." That's when I switched to a different doctor.

I told my new doctor what was happening, and he scheduled me for a colonoscopy right away. He looked at that for ulcers or tumors or something, but there was nothing, and he diagnosed me with irritable bowel syndrome. He put me on 25 milligrams of amitriptyline, a mild antidepressant, and it cleared right up.

The only problem with the medicine was that I wanted to get pregnant again. I tried to go off it, but found I couldn't go more than one day without another attack.

It was only after all this that I was finally told that IBS is a stress-related disease. I had sort of noticed a pattern; for instance, every time I had company, I would have an attack. Whenever my sister came to visit, she would stay with my son while my husband would take me to the hospital. Every time I went on vacation, I'd get so stressed because I didn't know where the hospital was, and sure enough, I'd need to go to one. My doctor said, "Get biofeedback." Well, I'd never even heard of biofeedback, and my insurance company wouldn't cover it. I didn't know what to do.

When I went through a divorce, I stopped taking the amitriptyline, and I didn't have any more major attacks. I went to counseling for a long time to help with other things, and now I'm taking a different antidepressant. I haven't seen my gastroenterologist in over a year.

These days I will occasionally have a mild episode. Very greasy food tends to aggravate my stomach. I have found that if I can wake up before my stomachaches get too bad, and if I can make myself breathe slow and deep, I can make them go away—it takes about 20 minutes. But if I get all worked up and I lose control, they just get worse and worse, and I have to go to the hospital. I haven't had to do that for a long time.

DIAGNOSIS

Several serious digestive system conditions can produce similar symptoms to IBS. In particular, *colon cancer* (this chapter, page 282) and inflammatory conditions such as *ulcerative colitis* (this chapter, page 290), and Crohns disease must be eliminated as possibilities. Other GI tract problems that can look like IBS include parasitical infestations (i.e., Giardia), food allergies, inflammatory bowel disease, and chronic infections.

No definitive test exists for IBS; it is diagnosed in the absence of other conditions that may cause similar symptoms. Fortunately, with the advent of colonoscopes, this isn't a difficult process. A colonoscope can confirm the absence of structural change or damage to the colon, and it can also show the characteristic uncoordinated contraction of the colon to aid in diagnosis.

TREATMENT

Treatment for IBS depends on the individual. The first recourse is to consider dietary and stress factors. Caffeine and alcohol have been found to be particularly irritating, but no particular food or drink is a definitive trigger for IBS attacks for all patients. Fiber supplementation is recommended by some doctors; the addition of bulk to the diet can fill the colon more completely and help to limit spasm.

Drug intervention usually involves anti-spasmodics, anti-diarrheals, antacids, and antidepressants. Although these medicines may offer some relief, IBS is generally considered a life-long condition, and so patients are encouraged to find their own best ways to cope through therapy, relaxation techniques, and even hypnotism.

MASSAGE?

Massage may be appropriate, depending on how each individual takes in this stimulus. It is important to work on these clients very conservatively, especially with any mechanical work around the abdomen, but many of them will respond well to the autonomic balancing massage provides.

Ulcerative Colitis

ULCERATIVE COLITIS IN BRIEF

What is it?
Ulcerative colitis is a condition in which the inner layer of the colon becomes inflamed and develops ulcers.

How is it recognized?
Symptoms of acute ulcerative colitis include abdominal cramping, pain, chronic diarrhea, blood and pus in stools, weight loss, and mild fever.

Is massage indicated or contraindicated?
Massage is locally contraindicated for acute ulcerative colitis, and systemically contraindicated in the presence of fever. In subacute situations, gentle (not deep) abdominal massage may be helpful, but only within the tolerance of the client.

DEFINITION: WHAT IS IT?

Ulcerative colitis is a disease of the colon involving progressive inflammation and ulceration. It begins in the rectum and may travel up the length of the bowel. The inflammation is limited to the large intestine, however, which distinguishes it from Crohns disease, a closely related inflammatory disease.

ETIOLOGY: WHAT HAPPENS?

The actual cause of ulcerative colitis is a subject of some debate. Although no definitive trigger has been identified, most people now agree that it is an autoimmune condition. It occurs in unpredictable flares followed by periods of remission: a pattern similar to other autoimmune conditions such as multiple sclerosis or rheumatoid arthritis.

SIGNS AND SYMPTOMS

Symptoms of ulcerative colitis depend largely on how much of the bowel is affected: the greater the extent of inflammation, the worse the symptoms will be. During flare-ups, the primary symptom will be painful, chronic diarrhea, with blood and pus in the stools. Abdominal cramping, loss of appetite, and mild fever may also occur during acute episodes. During remission, however, all symptoms will disappear.

COMPLICATIONS

One of the most dependable complications of long-term ulcerative colitis is *anemia* (chapter 4, page 178), from the slow, constant blood loss. For reasons not well understood but probably related to the autoimmune nature of the condition, ulcerative colitis is associated with other inflammations, notably in the liver, where it can cause *cirrhosis* (this chapter, page 291), and in the joints, where it can cause arthritis. These secondary inflammations generally subside during remission or when the colitis is treated. Probably because of the prolonged cellular irritation and cellular replacement, patients with ulcerative colitis involving the whole colon are significantly more at risk of developing *colon cancer* (this chapter, page 282) than the general population. In very rare situations, the colon may swell to the point that it is in danger of rupture. This is called *toxic megacolon*, and it is a medical emergency.

TREATMENT

Treatment options for ulcerative colitis begin with a class of medications that lessen the severity of flare-ups and prolong periods of remission. If these don't control the inflammation satisfactorily, corticosteroids may be prescribed for short periods. Immune suppressive drugs and, surprisingly, nicotine patches have also been found to improve symptoms.

If a patient is still not relieved with these options, or if inflammation of the colon has progressed to a dangerous degree, surgery is the only permanent solution for ulcerative colitis. Several surgical options have been developed, but all of them involve the removal of the entire bowel. External colostomy bags, internal colostomy bags, or the joining of the small intestine to the muscles of the rectum are options for ways to replace the main functions of the colon.

MASSAGE?

Deep abdominal work is definitely contraindicated for a client with ulcerative colitis in any stage; so is any kind of work that would reflexively increase blood flow to the pelvic cavity. Massage is systemically contraindicated if a fever is present. In periods of remission, gentle massage to the abdomen may be useful, within the client's tolerance, and any other work to balance the autonomic nervous system is highly called for.

Disorders of the Accessory Organs

Cirrhosis

DEFINITION: WHAT IS IT?

Cirrhosis is a symptom, rather than a disease itself; it involves the replacement of healthy liver cells with nonfunctioning scar tissue. Remember all those absolutely vital and important things the liver does? Cirrhosis can interfere with virtually every function of the liver, with potentially fatal repercussions.

DEMOGRAPHICS: WHO GETS IT?

Cirrhosis and other liver diseases affect some 25 million Americans per year, and it kills about 25,000 of them. It is the eighth leading cause of death in the United States.

CIRRHOSIS

This is a Greek word from the roots *kirrhos* (yellow) and *osis* (condition). Thus it is easy to see the association between cirrhosis and a related condition, jaundice, which comes from the French word for yellow.

CIRRHOSIS IN BRIEF

What is it?

With cirrhosis normal liver cells are replaced with scar tissue.

How is it recognized?

The symptoms of cirrhosis can be subtle until the disease is very far advanced. Early symptoms include loss of appetite, nausea, vomiting, and weight loss. Later symptoms include jaundice, ascites, and vomiting blood.

Is massage indicated or contraindicated?

Massage is contraindicated for people with advanced cirrhosis.

ETIOLOGY: WHAT HAPPENS?

The liver is peculiar in its blood supply: it has the portal vein and the hepatic artery going in, but only the hepatic vein going out. Consequently, it must be able to process huge amounts of blood. In cirrhosis, this ability is greatly impaired by an accumulation of scar tissue where functioning cells should be. The scar tissue will permanently scramble what should be highly organized cells, blood vessels, and tiny bile ducts. The cirrhotic deposits of fat and scar tissue have a characteristically knobby, bumpy appearance, hence the nickname "hobnailed liver." In the early stages, cirrhosis causes a liver to enlarge. But as the connective tissue contracts, the liver sometimes returns to a normal size, though not to normal function.

CAUSES

In the United States *alcoholism* (chapter 10, page 356) is the leading cause of cirrhosis. It can also arise from types B, C, D, drug-related, and autoimmune *hepatitis* (this chapter, page 296). Any obstruction of the bile duct, some inherited liver diseases, long-term exposure to environmental toxins, and *congestive heart failure* (chapter 4, page 206) are all causes of cirrhosis. In Africa, cirrhosis is usually caused not by alcoholism, but by exposure to a specific parasite called *schistosoma*, or blood fluke.

SIGNS AND SYMPTOMS

Cirrhosis is often a silent disease until it is quite advanced. Early symptoms are vague and can be attributed to any number of other common disorders. They include nausea, vomiting, weight loss, and the development of red patches on the skin of the upper body. At this point, blood tests may still be normal; no clear signs may point to cirrhosis. Later symptoms are usually identified by the complications discussed below.

COMPLICATIONS

As blood in the portal system backs up from the congested liver, the repercussions will be felt throughout the body.

- Splenomegaly. The spleen enlarges in a condition called *splenomegaly*, because it can't get rid of its by-products from red blood cell breakdown. Furthermore, impairment of spleen function will reduce blood clotting action: easy bruising and bleeding are common complications of cirrhosis.
- Jaundice. Bilirubin (a by-product of the recycling of dead red blood cells) is produced in the spleen, and it is supposed to be broken down in the liver. When this is impossible because of cirrhosis, water-soluble components of bilirubin will accumulate in the bloodstream. It is strongly pigmented and turns the sclera of the eyes and the skin a yellowish color (see *jaundice*, this chapter, page 299).
- Ascites. When blood pressure in the portal system increases, plasma filtrates out of the venous capillaries into the peritoneal space, causing the abdominal distension known as *ascites*. (See Figure 7.5.) Sometimes the bacteria that normally inhabit the abdomen will set up an infection in this fluid, causing spontaneous bacterial peritonitis, a life-threatening infection.
- Systemic edema. Cirrhosis can limit blood flow leaving the liver as well as blood flow going in. One of the critical proteins for maintaining fluid balance in the body, albumin, is significantly lowered in advanced cirrhosis. Without albumin, the body can-

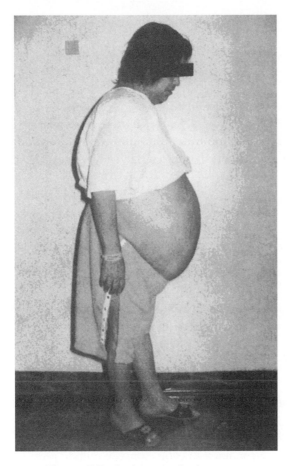

Figure 7.5. Cirrhosis can lead to ascites

not maintain proper fluid levels. Edema will accumulate, not only in the abdomen (ascites), but systemically in all interstitial spaces. (See *edema*, chapter 5, page 224.)

- Internal varices. Pressure in abdominal veins grows as fluid backs up through the system. This can lead to internal venous distensions and varicosities. Pressure in the esophageal veins also accumulates; sometimes they will bulge into esophageal varices, or varicose veins of the esophagus. These can hemorrhage during vomiting, leading to bloody vomit, shock, and even death.

- Hormone disruption. Men with cirrhosis have livers that will no longer inactivate their normal low levels of estrogen; feminizing characteristics such as breast development, loss of chest hair, impotence, and atrophy of the testicles soon follow. For women, hormonal changes will include the cessation of menstrual periods. Both men and women can expect decreased sex drives.

- Encephalopathy. When cirrhosis is very advanced, the detoxifying agents in the liver are out of commission. Protection no longer exists from the chemicals—ammonia, for instance—produced whenever protein is metabolized. These toxins accumulate in the blood and eventually cause brain damage. Symptoms here include somnolence, confusion, tremors, hallucinations, and coma.

- Kidney failure. Advanced cirrhosis can affect blood flow to the kidneys, resulting in kidney failure. *Hepatorenal syndrome* is an emergency situation that requires a liver transplant in order for a person to survive.

TREATMENT

The prognosis for someone in the early stages of cirrhosis caused by alcoholism is excellent, *if* the damage can be stopped. That is the main treatment objective: *stop the damage*.

Medication is sometimes administered to counteract the complications of the disease: diuretics for edema; antacids for intestinal discomfort; levulose, an undigestible sugar, to bind with ammonia so that it can be excreted. Vitamins are recommended to guard against malnutrition.

Cirrhosis due to hepatitis is treated with interferon as an antiviral measure. Steroids for inflammation due to autoimmune hepatitis are occasionally prescribed.

New advances with transplant surgery are making it possible to restore normal health to people in end-stage cirrhosis. Transplants are recommended for alcoholic patients only when they have not suffered extensive damage to other organs, and when they are in long-term recovery (6 months or more).

MASSAGE?

Massage is contraindicated for advanced cirrhosis because the circulatory system is simply not equipped to handle the changes this work brings about. If a client has had cirrhosis in the past, and if he or she has medical clearance, massage may be appropriate, although care must be taken not to overchallenge the circulatory system's adaptability.

Gallstones

DEFINITION: WHAT ARE THEY?

The technical term for gallstones is cholecyst. The formation of tiny crystals or stones in the gall bladder is also called cholelithiasis.

DEMOGRAPHICS: WHO GETS THEM?

This is a fairly common condition, affecting some 20 million people in the United States, with about 1 million new cases reported each year. Obesity and pregnancy are both predisposing factors, but it seems that just being a woman creates the biggest risk of developing gallstones. Twenty percent of all women autopsied have gallstones when they die. The same statistic is nearer 5% for men.

Specific risk factors for developing gallstones have been identified: being overweight or having recently lost a lot of weight; hormonal disruptions such as being pregnant, taking birth control pills, or being on estrogen replacement therapy; being elderly; having a family history of gallstones; or being Native American are all situations that show statistically higher rates of gallstone development.

ETIOLOGY: WHAT HAPPENS?

Bile is primarily made up of water, bile salts (which help in fat digestion), bilirubin from recycled red blood cells, and cholesterol filtered out of the bloodstream by the liver. Gallstones themselves are composed either of cholesterol (80% of all gallstones) or bilirubin (20% of all gallstones). For reasons that are not yet clear, these substances become highly concentrated in the gall bladder, and either become large deposits or remain in hundreds of discreet little pieces that surgeons refer to as "gravel" or "bile sludge."

SIGNS AND SYMPTOMS

It is estimated that up to 80% of all people who have gallstones experience no symptoms. The only reason a person

---

GALLSTONES IN BRIEF

What are they?
Gallstones are crystallized formations of cholesterol or bile pigments in the gall bladder. They can be as small as grains of sand or as large as a golf ball.

How are they recognized?
Most gallstones do not cause symptoms. When they do, long-term or short-term pain occurs in the upper right side of the abdomen, which may refer to the back and right scapula. Gallstones stuck in ducts may cause jaundice or pancreatitis.

Is massage indicated or contraindicated?
Massage is appropriate for symptom-free gallstones although draining strokes over the liver are contraindicated.

would have symptoms would be if a stone got lodged, either in the cystic duct or lower down in the common bile duct. (See Figure 7.6.) In this situation the pain, referred to as *biliary colic*, is excruciating. (*Colic* is the spasmatic contraction of involuntary muscle, in this case in the common bile duct.) This extreme local pain will often last for hours, building to a peak and then gradually subsiding when the stone moves either back into the gall bladder sack or into the duodenum. The pain may be intense enough to induce nausea and vomiting. If the stone gets immovably stuck, the patient may require hospitalization to have it surgically removed.

COMPLICATIONS

Gallstones in themselves are not a serious threat, but they can create some unpleasant complications. The most obvious is an obstruction of the cystic or common bile duct, which can lead to *jaundice* (this chapter, page 299). If the clog is distal to where the pancreas adds its secretions to the common bile duct, the pancreas can also sustain damage from a backup of its highly corrosive digestive juices; this is acute pancreatitis, and gallstones are the leading cause of this disorder. The pooling of stagnant bile can also lead to infection of the gallbladder, or cholecystitis.

TREATMENT

Some drugs will soften gallstones, but these can take months or years to break down large deposits. Surgery is a more common intervention to remove the gall bladder, thereby preventing the formation of future gallstones. Traditionally, open surgery has been used for this purpose, but recent advances in laparoscopic surgery have made it possible to remove the gallbladder through a very small incision. This reduces general trauma to the body, and radically reduces recovery time. About half a million gall bladder surgeries are performed every year; 80% are by laparoscopy.

    If a person should lose her gallbladder, she will still produce bile, but it will be dripped into the duodenum in a steady stream, rather than being saved up for high-fat meals. The only real concern is that she may lose some access to important fat-soluble vitamins. Fortunately, some digestive supplements are available that can aid in the digestion of fats.

MASSAGE?

Massage is contraindicated for someone who is experiencing acute biliary colic; that is, a gallbladder attack. If a client knows she has gallstones, consider the costal angle on the

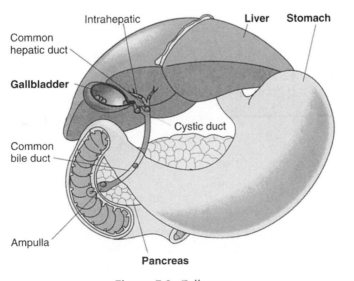

Figure 7.6. Gallstones

right side a local contraindication. Otherwise, massage is appropriate. It is also important to remember the referred pain patterns for the gallbladder (right shoulder and between scapulae) because less acute attacks will sometimes create pain here rather than at the site of injury, and, mysteriously, all the massage in the world won't make the pain go away.

Hepatitis

DEFINITION: WHAT IS IT?

Hepat-itis means liver inflammation. It can be caused by drug reactions and exposure to certain toxins, but it is most often one of a variety of viral infections that can mildly or severely impair liver function. Seven types of viral hepatitis have been identified so far: hepatitis A through hepatitis G. Hepatitis A, B, and C will be discussed here because they are by far the most common, and the other types are just being identified and explored.

Hepatitis A

DEFINITION: WHAT IS HEPATITIS A?

This used to be called infectious hepatitis. It is a short, acute infection, which usually causes no lasting damage and creates life-long immunity. This virus is transmitted through food or water contaminated with fecal matter. Shellfish grown in contaminated water can spread the disease to humans. Hepatitis A is also the reason for those huge signs about hand washing in restaurant bathrooms.

DEMOGRAPHICS: WHO GETS HEPATITIS A?

Anyone can get this disease, although it is most common in children. It occurs between 125,000 and 200,000 times in the United States every year, and is responsible for about 100 deaths. Every ten years or so, a nationwide outbreak of hepatitis A occurs; the last one was in 1989. Up to 30% of Americans have antibodies to hepatitis A, showing that they've been exposed to this infection.

HEPATITIS IN BRIEF

What is it?
Hepatitis is inflammation of the liver, usually due to viral infection.

How is it recognized?
All types of hepatitis produce the same symptoms, with variable severity. Symptoms, when any exist, include fatigue, jaundice, abdominal pain, nausea, and diarrhea. Sometimes no symptoms are present.

Is massage indicated or contraindicated?
Massage is systemically contraindicated for acute hepatitis. For clients with chronic hepatitis, the appropriateness of massage will depend on their general health.

SIGNS AND SYMPTOMS OF HEPATITIS A

Symptoms of hepatitis A are similar to those of the rest of the hepatitis family, but they tend to be more acute and have a shorter life span. They include weakness, nausea, fever, anorexia, and possible *jaundice* (this chapter, page 299), that will be accompanied by dark urine and pale stools. This virus incubates for 2 to 6 weeks before symptoms appear, but it is contagious during the incubation period. Then the virus is present in the system for another 2 to 3 weeks, although a person may not feel fully restored to health for up to 6 months.

TREATMENT FOR HEPATITIS A?

Treatment for hepatitis A is a combination of rest, fluids, good sense, and in some cases, gamma globulin shots. These injections can provide short-term protection when a specific source of infection has been identified, such as a contaminated restaurant. A life-long vaccine exists against this infection for people traveling, working, or living in places where the virus is prevalent.

MASSAGE FOR HEPATITIS A?

Massage is contraindicated for any kind of acute hepatitis. Not only is the therapist at risk of catching the disease, but he or she could put a client at risk for more serious complications, such as permanent liver damage or enlarged spleen from blood backing up into the portal system.

Hepatitis B

DEFINITION: WHAT IS HEPATITIS B?

This is a different virus entirely, and the risks and possible complications of this disease are much more serious than those associated with hepatitis A.

DEMOGRAPHICS: WHO GETS HEPATITIS B?

About 200,000 new infections of the hepatitis B virus (HBV) occur every year. Most of them (90%) will resolve within 6 months, and the virus will be completely eradicated from the body. But about 10% of the people who get hepatitis B never successfully shed the virus. These people will be life-long carriers of the disease, and they can spread it to other people. About one million people carry HBV in the United States.

Specific populations are especially at risk for contracting hepatitis B: any person who comes in contact with someone else's body fluids—not just blood—runs the risk of exposure to this virus. High-risk groups include healthcare workers, intravenous drug users, anyone who is sexually active with more than one partner, newborn babies of infected mothers, adoptive families of children from parts of the world where the disease is endemic, and travelers to those same parts of the world.

COMMUNICABILITY OF HEPATITIS B

HBV is transmitted through body fluids: blood, semen, even saliva and tears. The virus is quite sturdy and remains viable for many hours outside of a human body. It also requires very little exposure to spread the infection. A teaspoon of blood from a person with an active HBV infection will contain 500 million viral particles. In comparison, the same amount of blood from a person with an active AIDS infection will contain only 5 to 10 viral particles.

SIGNS AND SYMPTOMS OF HEPATITIS B

Symptoms of hepatitis B are basically the same as those of hepatitis A, but the onset is slower, and they last for a much longer time. The incubation period is 2 to 6 months in this case (it is contagious during that time), and it can stay in the system for months or years. The severity and duration of the viral attack is largely determined by the general health of the infected person. Long-term carriers of HBV have no symptoms at all.

COMPLICATIONS OF HEPATITIS B

About 10% of the people who get hepatitis B will go on to have some kind of chronic liver disease. Chronic hepatitis is one possibility, along with *cirrhosis* (this chapter, page 291) and liver cancer. The high incidence of hepatitis B in the tropics is thought to be at least partly related to the high rate of liver cancer in those areas.

TREATMENT FOR HEPATITIS B

Hepatitis B is sometimes treated with interferon, but it is successful for only a small percentage of patients, and they often experience relapses after treatment is ended.

PREVENTION OF HEPATITIS B

An effective vaccine series exists against HBV. Massage therapists are not required to be vaccinated against this disease, although many may choose to be vaccinated just in case.

MASSAGE FOR HEPATITIS B?

Massage is out of the question for a client who is currently ill with hepatitis of any sort. Furthermore, a hepatitis B patient is contagious for months or years at a time. But if someone has a history of HBV and he's in good health and has clearance from his doctor, massage could be appropriate, administered conservatively.

Hepatitis C

DEFINITION: WHAT IS HEPATITIS C?

Before the viruses D, E, F, and G were discovered, this disorder was called hepatitis non-A non-B. Although it's been investigated since the late 1970s, the causative virus was just identified in 1989.

DEMOGRAPHICS: WHO GETS HEPATITIS C?

For being such a new disease, hepatitis C is relatively common. About 150,000 new infections occur each year in this country. Hepatitis C becomes a chronic disease up to 85% of the time; about 3.5 million Americans have chronic hepatitis C infections. This number is falling, however, thanks to better screening mechanisms for blood and organ donors.

COMMUNICABILITY OF HEPATITIS C

This type of hepatitis has spread most easily through transfusions; no effective screening mechanism existed until very recently. Blood-to-blood contact is the most reliable way to transmit the disease, though in some cases the mode of transmission is unclear.

SIGNS AND SYMPTOMS OF HEPATITIS C

Symptoms of hepatitis C are weakness, fever, nausea, and possible jaundice, but they are generally milder than those seen with hepatitis A or B. However, hepatitis C has a much greater chance of complicating into chronic hepatitis or cirrhosis.

TREATMENT FOR HEPATITIS C

Treatment of hepatitis C is good sense (rest, fluids, and good nutrition), and close monitoring to watch for signs of complications. No vaccine exists for this virus. Hepatitis C responds slightly better to interferon than HVB; however, most patients still experience a relapse when treatment is withdrawn.

MASSAGE FOR HEPATITIS C?

As with other hepatitis infections, massage is contraindicated in the presence of acute disease.

Chronic Hepatitis

DEFINITION: WHAT IS CHRONIC HEPATITIS?

Chronic hepatitis is usually a complication of hepatitis B or C, characterized by liver inflammation that persists for 6 months or longer. Sometimes chronic hepatitis can develop without any episode of acute hepatitis, for instance, as a consequence of a drug reaction.

The two classes of chronic hepatitis are *chronic persistent hepatitis* and *chronic active hepatitis*. In chronic persistent hepatitis, progress is very slow and the patient usually remains in good health. Chronic active hepatitis is much less predictable, varying greatly from person to person. It leads to cirrhosis in some, and mild, symptomless liver inflammation in others.

Chronic hepatitis of either sort can cause permanent damage to liver cells. The risk of developing cirrhosis (which in itself can be life-threatening) or liver cancer is much higher than for the general population.

MASSAGE FOR CHRONIC HEPATITIS?

The appropriateness of massage for chronic hepatitis depends on the situation. If the client is in good health and symptom-free, conservative massage with medical clearance may be appropriate, always remembering that the liver has a big job and isn't functioning at its peak capacity.

Jaundice

DEFINITION: WHAT IS IT?

Jaundice, from the French *jaune* (yellow), is not a disease in itself, but a symptom of some underlying pathology.

ETIOLOGY: WHAT HAPPENS?

One of the functions of the liver is to accept the by-products of dead red blood cells delivered from the spleen. It recycles the hemoglobin and synthesizes the bilirubin into bile. Bile then drips from the liver into a storage tank: the gall bladder. Bile is used for the digestion and absorption of fats and fat-soluble vitamins. Leftover bilirubin gets into the digestive tract and is a coloring agent for feces, which makes it a useful diagnostic tool.

If the liver or the gall bladder malfunctions, bilirubin accumulates in the bloodstream, leading to the yellowish tinge it gives to skin, mucous membranes, and the sclera of the eyes.

Several types of jaundice are possible, each one categorized by the pathology that created the problem. Jaundice is treated according to the underlying causes.

- Neonatal jaundice. This is a fairly common condition for newborns. Their livers are not yet mature and cannot handle the release of fetal red blood cells. It takes a few days to process this extra load. Treatment is usually exposure to "bili-lights."
- Hemolytic jaundice. This rare condition is specifically related to hemolytic anemia. In this situation, red blood cells are dying off at a tremendous rate, and though the liver may be functioning at normal levels, it can't keep up with the volume, so bilirubin backs up into the system. (See *anemia*, chapter 4, page 178.) Hemolytic jaundice may be caused by infection or incompatible blood transfusions.
- Hepatic jaundice. This covers any jaundice caused by other liver dysfunction: *cirrhosis* (this chapter, page 291), *hepatitis* (this chapter, page 296), malaria, or

---

JAUNDICE IN BRIEF

What is it?
Jaundice is a symptom of liver dysfunction, involving the presence of excess bilirubin in the blood, which is then dissolved in subcutaneous fat, mucous membranes, and the sclera of the eyes.

How is it recognized?
Jaundice gives the skin, eyes, and mucous membranes a yellowish cast.

Is massage indicated or contraindicated?
Massage is contraindicated for jaundice, which is usually a sign of significant congestion and dysfunction in the liver or gall bladder.

more rarely, a congenital malfunctioning of liver enzyme systems. In any case, the liver is compromised by scar tissue or inflammation and is incapable of processing the bilirubin delivered from the portal system.

- Extrahepatic jaundice. This is jaundice caused by a mechanical obstruction somewhere outside the liver: gallstones, or pancreatic or colon tumors. Advanced pregnancy can also constrict the gall bladder in a way that may prevent the drainage of bile. The pooling of fluid because of blockage can lead to infection and permanent liver damage. Extrahepatic jaundice not caused by pregnancy may require surgery to excise the obstruction.

SIGNS AND SYMPTOMS

Jaundice indicates that for some reason, the liver cannot complete its many tasks. The bilirubin, instead of passing from the liver into the duodenum, backs up into the blood stream. It dissolves in subcutaneous fat. Skin, mucous membranes, and sclera take on a characteristic yellow color, and urine gets unusually dark as more bilirubin is excreted by the kidneys. But fecal matter gets lighter instead of darker. One of the symptoms of jaundice is light, or "clay colored" stools, because the bilirubin isn't reaching the digestive tract.

COMPLICATIONS

Although jaundice is simply a signal of some other problem, it can itself create some difficulties. If the body is absorbing little or no fat, important fat-soluble vitamins have no access to enter the body. One of the worst short-term consequences of this problem is bleeding disorders caused by a shortage of Vitamin K.

MASSAGE?

Jaundice indicates that the liver is not functioning under a normal circulatory flow. To increase that flow, even indirectly by massage, would only make the situation worse. Circulatory massage is systemically contraindicated for jaundice until liver function is fully restored.

Liver, Enlarged

DEFINITION: WHAT IS IT?

Just as it sounds, enlarged liver is a condition in which the liver grows to large proportions, although it does not increase in functioning capacity.

ETIOLOGY: WHAT HAPPENS?

Hepatomegaly, or enlarged liver, could be caused by any number of things including *alcoholism* (chapter 10, page 356), *gallstones* (this chapter, page 294), *hepatitis* (this chapter, page 296) or *cirrhosis* (this chapter, page 291). The liver is an enormous filter with huge amounts of blood pouring into it every minute of the day. If that filter is clogged or somehow obstructed with fat or scar tissue, it will not function as well as necessary. Enlarged livers may also be connected with leukemia or advanced general circulatory problems, such as *congestive heart failure* (chapter 4, page 206) or congenital heart defects.

SIGNS AND SYMPTOMS

In a mild situation, no symptoms of hepatomegaly may appear. But in more advanced cases, the person often experiences some abdominal discomfort, especially on palpation, and possibly some distension of the abdomen from ascites (the seepage of plasma into the peritoneal space when blood flow into the liver is backed up). X-rays of people with enlarged livers often show the shadow of the colon out of place, since it has been displaced by the liver.

TREATMENT

Treatment for hepatomegaly depends entirely on the underlying causes.

MASSAGE?

As with other conditions related to liver dysfunction, circulatory massage is contraindicated when the liver is enlarged because of underlying disease.

Other Digestive System Conditions

Peritonitis

DEFINITION: WHAT IS IT?

This is an infection that has found its way into the peritoneal space, where it is dark, moist, and just about 100 degrees: a perfect growth medium. Bacteria may also thrive in the peritoneal space because some key immune devices are absent: there is no direct contact with white blood cells, nor are there any corrosive fluids such as digestive juices to impede bacterial expansion. (See Figure 7.7.)

ETIOLOGY: WHAT HAPPENS?

The bacteria that cause peritonitis can gain access to the peritoneal space through a variety of sources:

- *Rupture or perforation of an organ* is one possibility. This is a complication of *appendicitis* (this chapter, page 280), perforated *ulcers* (this chapter, page 278), and *diverticulitis* (this chapter, page 285).
- *Abdominal abscesses*, such as those seen with *pelvic inflammatory disease* (chapter 9, page 346), can release bacteria into the bigger space for systemic infection.
- *Mechanical perforation of the abdomen* can introduce bacteria from the outside, with a knife wound, for instance. This is an occasional complication of intestinal or colon surgery, and the possibility of peritonitis is the reason behind the heavy doses of antibiotics prescribed before such surgeries take place.
- *Cirrhosis* (this chapter, page 291) in an advanced stage can sometimes cause spontaneous peritonitis because ascites, the seepage of plasma into the abdomen, may carry bacteria along.
- *Peritoneal dialysis* is a particular method of kidney dialysis for people with advanced kidney failure. It uses the peritoneal membrane as a filter to clean the blood. One of the risks of peritoneal dialysis is the contamination of the tubing that connects to the peritoneum; this can cause peritonitis.

SIGNS AND SYMPTOMS

The symptoms of peritonitis vary, depending on the original cause. Abdominal pain is always part of the picture.

ENLARGED LIVER IN BRIEF

What is it?
Enlarged liver, or hepatomegaly, is a condition in which the liver becomes distended and may displace other internal organs.

How is it recognized?
Hepatomegaly may have no symptoms, but it can sometimes cause abdominal discomfort or ascites: fluid accumulation in the abdomen.

Is massage indicated or contraindicated?
Massage is contraindicated for persons whose livers are distended because of internal dysfunction.

PERITONEUM
This is a Latin word derived from a Greek root. *Periteino* means "to stretch over," an apt description of the peritoneum, which stretches over all the abdominal contents.

PERITONITIS IN BRIEF

What is it?
Peritonitis is inflammation, usually due to bacterial infection, of the peritoneal lining of the abdomen.

How is it recognized?
Acute peritonitis shows the signs of systemic infection: fever and chills, along with abdominal pain, distension, nausea, and vomiting.

Is massage indicated or contraindicated?
Massage is contraindicated for acute peritonitis, which is a medical emergency.

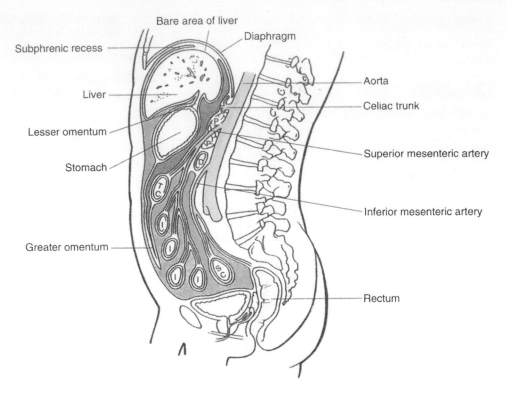

Figure 7.7. Peritonitis is an infection in the peritoneal space.

It usually begins as diffuse pain, but it will localize at the original site of infection. Usually nausea and vomiting are present, and if the infection is untreated, severe dehydration may result. Many patients experience reduced urine output and difficulty passing gas or bowel movements. After 2 or 3 hours, the abdomen will swell and pain may subside, but this is not a sign of improvement; rather, it is an indication that the intestines have gone into paralysis. At this point, death is not far away, unless the patient receives immediate hospital care.

TREATMENT

Treatment for peritonitis varies according to cause and severity. At the very least, antibiotics are called for. Emergency situations will require abdominal surgery to remove or repair the ruptured organ and to wash out the peritoneal cavity as fully as possible. When peritonitis is caught early, it usually responds well to treatment, but if it is left too long, it can be deadly.

MASSAGE?

Massage is systemically contraindicated for any form of acute peritonitis until all signs of infection have passed.

CHAPTER REVIEW QUESTIONS: DIGESTIVE SYSTEM CONDITIONS

1. Describe how ongoing stress can result in digestive system problems.

2. Why is the appendix no longer routinely removed in the course of other abdominal surgery?

3. What is ascites? How can liver dysfunction cause it?

4. Why might someone with ulcerative colitis be at a higher risk of developing colon cancer than the general population?

5. Describe the leading theory behind the development of colon cancer.

6. What is the difference between diverticula and colon polyps?

7. Most people with gallstones never have symptoms. What finally causes symptoms to occur?

8. Why are antibiotics ineffective for dealing with a bacterial infection of the gastrointestinal tract?

9. What is a possible cause of ulcers that does not involve the Helicobacter pylori bacterium?

10. A client is recovering from a bout with hepatitis A. His skin has a yellowish tone and the sclera of his eyes is yellow, too. What condition is probably present? Is this client a good candidate for massage? Why or why not?

BIBLIOGRAPHY, DIGESTIVE SYSTEM CONDITIONS

General References, Digestive System

1. Carmine D. Clemente. Anatomy: A regional atlas of the human body. 3rd ed. Baltimore: Urban & Schwarzenburg, 1987.

2. I. Damjanou. Pathology for the health-related professions. Philadelphia: Saunders, 1996.

3. Giovanni de Dominico, Elizabeth Wood. Beard's massage. Saunders: Philadelphia, 1997.

4. Jeffrey R. M. Kunz, Asher J. Finkel, eds. The American Medical Association family medical guide. New York: Random House, Inc., 1987.

5. Elaine M. Marieb. Human anatomy and physiology. Redwood City, CA: Benjamin/Cummings Publishing Co., Inc., 1989.

6. Ruth Lundeen Memmler, Dina Lin Wood. The human body in health and disease. 5th ed. Philadelphia: JB Lippincott Co., 1983.

7. Mary Lou Mulvihill. Human diseases: A systemic approach. 2nd ed. East Norwalk, CT: Appleton &Lange, A publishing division of Prentice-Hall, 1987.

8. Stedman's medical dictionary. 26th ed. Baltimore: Williams & Wilkins, 1995.

9. Taber's cyclopedic dictionary. 14th ed. Philadelphia: F.A. Davis Company, 1981.

10. Gerard J. Tortora, Nicholas P. Anagnostakos. Principles of anatomy and physiology. 6th ed. New York: Biological Sciences Textbook, Inc., A&P Textbooks, Inc. and Elia-Sparta, Inc.; Harper & Row Publishers, Inc., 1990.

11. Janet Travell, David G. Simons. Myofascial pain and dysfunction: The trigger point manual. Baltimore: Williams & Wilkins, 1983.

Gastroenteritis

1. Bacterial gastroenteritis. Copyright 1998 ADAM Software, Inc., all rights reserved. Copyright 1998 CommuniHealth. URL: www.healthanswers.com. Accessed winter 1998.

2. E. coli enteritis. Copyright 1998 ADAM Software, Inc., all rights reserved. Copyright 1998 CommuniHealth. URL: www.healthanswers.com. Accessed winter 1998.

3. Mark A. Graber, Rhea J. Allen. Acute diarrhea. In University of Iowa Family Practice Handbook: Chapter 4: Gastroenterology. University of Iowa, 1992–1997. URL: http://www.vh.org/Providers/ClinRef/FPHandbook/Chapter04/01-4.html. Accessed fall 1997.

4. Mark A. Graber, Rhea J. Allen. Chronic diarrhea. In University of Iowa Family

Practice Handbook: Chapter 4: Gastroenterology. University of Iowa, 1992–1997. URL: http://www.vh.org/Providers/ClinRef/FPHandbook/Chapter04/02-4.html. Accessed fall 1997.

5. Mark A. Graber, Rhea J. Allen. Dyspepsia/peptic ulcer disease. In University of Iowa Family Practice Handbook: Chapter 4: Gastroenterology. University of Iowa, 1992–1997. URL: http://www.vh.org/Providers/ClinRef/FPHandbook/Chapter04/09-4.html. Accessed fall 1997.

6. Viral gastroenteritis. Copyright 1998 ADAM Software, Inc., all rights reserved. Copyright 1998 CommuniHealth. URL: www.healthanswers.com. Accessed winter 1998.

Ulcers

1. Digestive diseases statistics. National Institute of Diabetes and Digestive and Kidney Diseases. NIH Publication No. 95-3873. February 1995. URL: http://www.niddk.nih.gov/DD_Statistics/DD_Statistics.html. Accessed fall 1997.

2. B.J. Marshall. Diseases related to helicobacter pylori. December 10, 1995. URL: http://www.helico.com/web/infoweb.html. Accessed fall 1997.

3. Sally Squires. A saliva test for H. Pylori? Washington Post Health, January 31, 1995.

4. Stomach and duodenal ulcers. National Institute of Diabetes Digestive and Kidney Diseases. NIH Publication No. 95-38. January 1995. URL: http://www.niddk.nih.gov/StomachUlcers/Ulcers.html. Accessed fall 1997.

Appendicitis

1. K Handal. Acute appendicitis. URL: http://www.parentzone.com/health/apped.htm. Accessed fall 1997.

2. MedicineNet: Power points about appendicitis. Information Network, Inc., 1995–1997. URL: http://www.medicinenet.com. Accessed fall 1997.

Colon Cancer

1. Caresheet™ of the month: Colon cancer. Palo Alto Medical Publishing, Inc., 1995, 1996. URL: http://www.infolane.com/pamp/coloncancer/coloncancer.html. Accessed fall 1997.

2. Colon cancer. Copyright 1998 ADAM Software, Inc., all rights reserved. Copyright 1998 CommuniHealth. URL: www.healthanswers.com. Accessed winter 1998.

3. Colon cancer. National Cancer Institute/PDQ: Patient Statement. Last modified September 1997. URL: http://rex.nci.nih.gov/INTRFCE_GIFS/INFO_PATS_INTR_DOC.htm. Accessed fall 1997.

4. J. Randolph Hecht. Colon cancer and polyps: Frequently asked questions. Version 1.0, Modified March 31, 1996. URL: http://www.ddc.org/pat/faqs/cancer_faq.html. Accessed fall 1997.

5. MedicineNet: Colon cancer: Screening and surveillance. Information Network, Inc., 1995–1997. URL: http://www.medicinenet.com. Accessed fall 1997.

6. MedicineNet: Power points about colorectal cancer. Information Network, Inc., 1995–1997. URL: http://www.medicinenet.com. Accessed fall 1997.

Diverticulosis/Diverticulitis

1. Diverticulosis and diverticulitis. National Digestive Diseases Clearinghouse, Healthtouch. NIH Publication No. 92-1163, October 1991. URL: http://www.mediconsult.com/frames/stoma/shareware/divertic/ Accessed fall 1997.

Irritable Bowel Syndrome

1. Karl Hempel. Irritable Bowel Syndrome. The Health Gazette. URL: http://www.freenet.scri.fsu.edu/HealthGazette/ibs.html. Accessed fall 1997.

2. Irritable bowel syndrome (functional bowel). Copyright 1998 ADAM Software, Inc., all rights reserved. Copyright 1998 CommuniHealth. URL: www.healthanswers.com. Accessed winter 1998.

3. Irritable Bowel Syndrome. National Institute of Diabetes Digestive and Kidney Dieases. NIH Publication No. 95-693, October 1992. URL: http://www.niddk.nih.gov/IBS/IBS.html. Accessed fall 1997.

4. Laura Zurawski, Anthony Lembo. Irritable bowel syndrome. Version 3.1.1, October 30, 1996. URL: http://qurlyjoe.bu.edu/cducibs/ibsfaq.html. Accessed fall 1997.

Ulcerative Colitis

1. MedicineNet: Power points about ulcerative colitis. Information Network, Inc., 1995–1997. URL: http://www.medicinenet.com. Accessed fall 1997.

2. Sally Squires. Deft exploration of the colon. Washington Post Health, November 1, 1994; p. 9.

3. Ulcerative colitis. National Institute of Diabetes and Digestive and Kidney Diseases. NIH Publication No. 95-1597, April 1992. URL: http://www.niddk.nih.gov/UlcerativeColitis/UlcerativeColitis.html. Accessed fall 1997.

4. Ulcerative colitis: Manageable, with a brighter outlook. Originally published in Mayo Clinic Health Letter, December 1995. Mayo Foundation for Medical Education and Research, 1996. URL: http://www.mayo.ivi.com/mayo/9512/htm/ulcercl.htm. Accessed fall 1997.

Cirrhosis

1. Cirrhosis: Many causes. The American Liver Foundation, 1997. URL: http://sadieo.ucsf.edu/alf/alffinal/infocirrh.html. Accessed fall 1997

2. Howard J. Worman. What is cirrhosis? Columbia University Department of Gastroenterology, 1995. URL: http://cpmcnet.columbia.edu/dept/gi/cirrhosis.html. Accessed fall 1997.

Gallstones

1. Cholelithiasis. Copyright 1998 ADAM Software, Inc., all rights reserved. Copyright 1998 CommuniHealth. URL: www.healthanswers.com. Accessed winter 1998.

2. Gallstones. National Institute of Diabetes and Digestive and Kidney Diseases. NIH Publication No. 95-2897, March 1993. URL: http://www.niddk.nih.gov/Gallstones/Gallstones.html. Accessed fall 1997.

3. Gallstones: A national health problem. The American Liver Foundation, 1997. URL: http://gi.ucsf.edu/alf/info/infogallstones.html. Accessed fall 1997.

Hepatitis

1. Chronic hepatitis. The American Liver Foundation, 1997. URL: http://gi.ucsf.edu/alf/info/infochronhep.html. Accessed fall 1997.

2. Hepatitis A. The American Liver Foundation, 1997. URL: http://gi.ucsf.edu/alf/info/hepa.html. Accessed fall 1997.

3. Hepatitis B. The American Liver Foundation, 1997. URL: http://gi.ucsf.edu/alf/info/infohepb.html. Accessed fall 1997.

4. Hepatitis C. The American Liver Foundation, 1997. URL: http://gi.ucsf.edu/ALF/hcv_fact.html. Accessed fall 1997.

5. Hepatitis A. New York State Department of Health Communicable Disease Fact Sheet, March 1996. URL: http://www.health.state.ny.us/nysdoh/consumer/hepat.htm. Accessed fall 1997.

Jaundice

1. Jaundice—Associated conditions. Copyright 1998 ADAM Software, Inc., all rights reserved. Copyright 1998 CommuniHealth. URL: www.healthanswers.com. Accessed winter 1998.

Peritonitis

1. Peritonitis. Copyright 1998 ADAM Software, Inc., all rights reserved. Copyright 1998 CommuniHealth. URL: www.healthanswers.com. Accessed winter 1998.

2. Peritoneal dialysis: Is it the best choice for me? Baxter International, Inc., 1995–1998. URL: http://www.baxter.com/www/remal/resource/thereduc/Periton1.htm. URL: http://www.baxter.com/www/remal/resource/thereduc/Periton2.htm. URL: http://www.baxter.com/www/remal/resource/thereduc/Periton3.htm. Accessed fall 1997.

Urinary System Conditions

OBJECTIVES

After reading this chapter, you should be able to tell . . .

- What the disorder is.
- How to recognize it.
- Whether massage is indicated or contraindicated for that condition.
- Whether a contraindication is local or systemic, or refers to a specific stage of development or healing.
- Why those choices for massage are correct.

In addition to this basic information, you should be able to . . .

- Name four structures that comprise the urinary system.
- Name three problems that could be present if red blood cells are found in the urine.
- Name the difference between interstitial cystitis and urinary tract infection.
- Name four possible causes for kidney stones.
- Name the organism most often responsible for the development of pyelonephritis.
- Name one common cause for acute renal failure, and one common cause for chronic renal failure.

INTRODUCTION

FUNCTION AND STRUCTURE OF THE URINARY SYSTEM

The urinary system is a relatively small system in the body, comprised of the kidneys, the ureters, the bladder, and the urethra. The huge renal artery comes directly off the aorta to enter the kidneys. It rapidly decreases in diameter to form thousands of capillaries. Each of these is entangled with another type of epithelial tube: the nephron, which starts as the knot-like glomerulus, and winds a torturous route all around the blood capillary. (See Figure 8.1.) The constant force of blood pressure from the renal artery causes movement of fluids between circulatory capillaries and the nephrons.

Chemical exchanges are made back and forth at this point. Waste products and water are squeezed out of the capillaries and into the nephrons, and then later in the loop, the capillaries reabsorb whatever water and salts are needed to keep the blood properly diluted. The nephron then takes its load of wastes and excess water to the renal pelvis, where it delivers everything from the blood that the body needs to expel. The renal pelvis

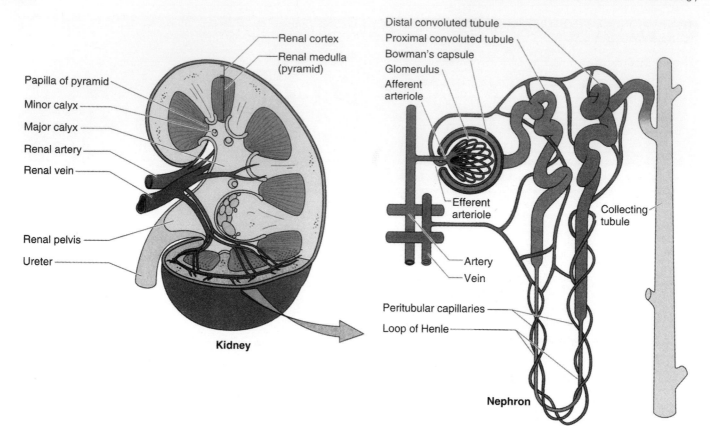

Figure 8.1. Overview of kidney function

empties into the ureters. They lead to the bladder, which acts as a holding tank. When enough urine has accumulated, it is expelled through the urethra. The cleansed blood, now relieved of excess water, nitrogenous wastes, uric acid, and other debris, exits the kidney through the renal vein.

The kidneys have another function that is not directly involved in the filtering of waste products from the blood. *Erythropoietin*, a hormone that is important in red blood cell production, is produced in the kidneys. Damage to these delicate organs can therefore sometimes be identified by changes in red blood cell production.

Kidneys are constructed primarily of epithelial tissue, which makes them very vulnerable to injury. This is why tapotement along the inferior edge of the rib cage is contraindicated: it is unlikely, but possible to injure the kidneys here. When the tissues in the kidneys have been damaged, red blood cells will leak from capillaries into the nephrons. This will show as blood in the urine, and is evidence of a potentially dangerous situation in the kidneys.

Filtration, the movement of substances through a membrane by external mechanical pressure—in this case the blood pressure—is the mechanism by which most substances are exchanged between the circulatory system and the urinary system. It is clear how carefully intertwined blood pressure and kidney health must be. If blood pressure is consistently high (see *hypertension*, chapter 4, page 199), then the delicate tissues of the kidneys will be damaged and become less efficient. Conversely, if the kidneys are not functioning adequately, the body will accumulate excess fluid, which forces blood pressure up. Some of the conditions discussed in this chapter have to do with the complicated relationship that exists between the urinary system and circulatory health. Other conditions considered here are related to the vulnerability of the urinary system organs to infection.

URINARY SYSTEM CONDITIONS

Kidney Disorders

Glomerulonephritis

Kidney Stones

Pyelonephritis

Renal Failure

Bladder and Urinary Tract Disorders

Interstitial Cystitis

Urinary Tract Infection

Kidney Disorders

Glomerulonephritis

DEFINITION: WHAT IS IT?

Glomerulonephritis is a relatively rare but serious situation, involving the inflammation and deterioration of the glomeruli: microscopic capsules of epithelial tissue that surround tiny knots of blood capillaries and help to absorb blood plasma for cleansing. Several types of glomerulonephritis exist. Many of them have no known cause, some are related to other specific diseases, and some are complications of or autoimmune reactions to other infections in the body.

DEMOGRAPHICS: WHO GETS IT?

Different age groups are at risk for different types of glomerulonephritis. Children may experience this disease as a complication of some other infection, but most cases of glomerulonephritis are experienced by adults.

ETIOLOGY: WHAT HAPPENS?

This disease causes the glomeruli to be badly inflamed, increasing permeability to the extent that red blood cells, and even vital blood proteins, can leave the circulatory system and be excreted with the urine. Depending on what type of glomerulonephritis is present, fibrosis may develop within the nephron, which further limits the ability of the kidneys to process fluids and filter wastes.

CAUSES

Glomerulonephritis can take many forms. Many cases of it are idiopathic: they have no known origin, and they may occur in people with no personal or familial history of kidney problems. Some cases are linked to other diseases, specifically *lupus* (chapter 5, page 241) and *diabetes* (chapter 4, page 210). Sometimes infections elsewhere in the body can lead to an autoimmune reaction in the kidneys, and other infections can simply complicate into kidney involvement.

PROGNOSIS

Depending on the cause, glomerulonephritis can be a short-term acute infection with complete recovery, or a

GLOMERULUS

This is the diminutive form of the Latin word *glomus*, for "ball of yarn," which is an excellent description of the tufts of capillary loops that allow for diffusion and filtration in the kidneys.

GLOMERULONEPHRITIS IN BRIEF

What is it?

Glomerulonephritis is a condition in which the glomeruli (small structures that are part of nephrons) become inflamed and cease to function efficiently.

How is it recognized?

Early symptoms of glomerulonephritis include dark or rust-colored urine, foamy urine, or blood in the urine. Later symptoms indicate chronic renal failure: systemic edema, fatigue, headaches, decreased urine output, discoloration of the skin, and general malaise.

Is massage indicated or contraindicated?

Massage is systemically contraindicated for glomerulonephritis. This inflammatory condition impairs the body's ability to manage fluid exchanges.

long-term progressive condition in which the kidneys are slowly destroyed, leading to end-stage renal failure and dependence on dialysis. At this time, no preventive or curative measures are known. Some varieties of this disease have been known to recur, even after the kidneys have been replaced.

SIGNS AND SYMPTOMS

When the kidneys function inefficiently, the repercussions are felt throughout the rest of the body, but it may take a long time to see the results. Early symptoms of glomerulonephritis are abnormalities in the urine: high protein levels or the presence of red blood cells. Hematuria, or blood in the urine, can be observed as dark or rust-colored urine, or as urine that looks pink or foamy; the location of the bleeding determines the color. Occasionally, no observable signs show up at all. Glomerulonephritis is sometimes suspected only when a routine analysis reveals higher than normal levels of protein or blood in the urine.

Another indicator of glomerulonephritis is *hypertension* (chapter 4, page 199). This is both a symptom and a complication of most chronic kidney disorders, since a disruption in urine output will cause fluid retention and external pressure on all blood vessels. Hypertension that does not respond to normal interventions can sometimes lead to a diagnosis of glomerulonephritis.

Later symptoms of glomerulonephritis are indicators of *renal failure* (this chapter, page 314), including general malaise, skin discoloration, itching, fatigue, low urine output, systemic edema, and in very severe cases, lethargy, confusion, and coma.

COMPLICATIONS

Permanent damage to the glomeruli opens the door to chronic renal failure. Disruption in the processing of blood in the kidneys can also lead to clot formation: glomerulonephritis is associated with the formation of renal vein thrombi, which can then cause disturbances elsewhere in the circulatory system.

TREATMENT

The treatment for this disease depends entirely on the cause and is generally geared toward symptom abatement. Controlling high blood pressure associated with this condition is the first priority. If the glomerulonephritis is a complication of a general infection, antibiotics may lead to a complete recovery. If it is an autoimmune or other inflammatory problem, corticosteroids may be employed to limit damage to the nephrons. Cytotoxic drugs are also used to inhibit the damaging effects of an immune system attack against the kidneys.

MASSAGE?

With this condition, the kidneys are inflamed from a pathogen, an autoimmune reaction, or some unknown cause. The affected person may have an infection, probably has high blood pressure, and is incapable of processing fluids under normal conditions, much less under the increased volume that massage can produce. Circulatory massage is systemically contraindicated for glomerulonephritis, although many techniques can yield important benefits without increasing fluid return.

Kidney Stones

DEFINITION: WHAT ARE THEY?

Also called renal calculi, or nephrolithiases, kidney stones are crystals that sometimes develop in the renal pelvis. Big ones can completely obstruct the kidney, preventing the movement of urine into the bladder. Some stones even grow into the cortex of the kidney, forming what's called a staghorn calculus. (See Figure 8.2.)

Most large kidney stones become lodged in the body of the kidney itself, but others may progress as far as the ureters before they get stuck. The technical name for them in this location is ureterolithiases.

> **KIDNEY STONES IN BRIEF**
>
> **What are they?**
>
> A kidney stone is a deposit of crystalline substances inside the kidney or the ureters.
>
> **How are they recognized?**
>
> Small stones may show no symptoms at all, but larger stones can cause extreme pain that may be accompanied by nausea and vomiting. Pain may refer from the back into the groin and hips.
>
> **Is massage indicated or contraindicated?**
>
> Massage is contraindicated for someone experiencing renal colic (a kidney stone attack) although it is appropriate for people with a history of stones, but no current symptoms.

DEMOGRAPHICS: WHO GETS THEM?

Kidney stones usually form in the absence of adequate fluids. Thus, they are very common in tropical environments where people tend to lose more liquid through sweat than they replace. Peak months for the diagnosis of kidney stones in this country are June through August, for the same reason.

Four out of five people diagnosed with kidney stones are men. The incidence in this country ranges from between 7 to 21 out of every 10,000 people; every year about one million people pass a stone. Most people experience their first kidney stone between 20 and 30 years of age, and 75% of them will experience at least one repeat stone sometime in their life.

Calcium
Magnesium
uric acid

ETIOLOGY: WHAT HAPPENS?

Kidney stones can be composed of many different substances, but the vast majority (up to 80%) are made of calcium oxalate. The rest are composed of struvite (magnesium, ammonium, and phosphate), uric acid (by-products of kidney infections), or other substances. The composition of a person's kidney stones is an important piece of information, because it indicates what the metabolic disruption was that caused the stone in the first place.

Parathyroid disorder
regulates C in bl.

CAUSES

In the case of calcium oxalate stones, the cause is almost always super-saturation of the urine. Most people have the potential to form these stones, and anything that increases urine concentration may lead to their development. Another factor is the environment inside the patient's kidney; a normal environment inhibits the growth of stones, but if this environment is somehow disrupted, the chance of developing kidney stones is much higher.

Because calcium is a common element in most kidney stones, it is a common misconception that taking in too much calcium increases the chance of forming the stones. In fact, kidney stones usually have much more to do with how calcium is processed in the body than with how much is actually consumed. A disorder of the parathyroid glands can cause a particular class of kidney stones; these glands regulate how much calcium needs to be available in the bloodstream for chemical reactions throughout the body. Another version of this problem is an excess of Vitamin D, which helps to determine how much calcium is absorbed in the digestive tract.

Some statistical evidence suggests that kidney stones may run in families. This is most likely related to inherited metabolic problems with how calcium is used, the pH balance of the blood, and other factors that may increase the chance of developing renal calculi.

Other causes of kidney stones include certain foods that can change the internal environment (these foods will be different for different patients); the presence of *gout* (see chapter 2, page 74), which indicates difficulty with the processing of uric acid; a mechanical blockage of the urinary tract; chronic *pyelonephritis* (this chapter, page 313); and the use of some diuretics, which serve to concentrate the urine.

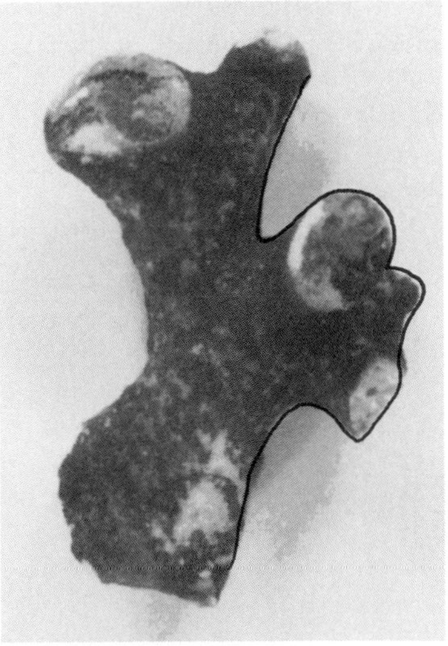

Figure 8.2. Staghorn calculus

KIDNEY STONES: CASE HISTORY

Walter B., age 77

"Once you've had a kidney stone, you never forget what it feels like."

I've had kidney stone attacks in 1939, then in 1944, and so on and so forth. The first time, I was 19 years old. I'd been horseback riding the day before, so when the pain started, we figured I had just thrown my back out somehow. The director of the hospital finally detected what it really was.

In 1944, I had an attack at night, in bed. I was in the army, stationed in Europe. Once you've had a kidney stone attack, you never forget what it feels like. I knew immediately what was happening, and they rushed me via command car to the military hospital, 20 miles away from the Battle of the Bulge. The renal surgeon authorized an attempt to remove the stone with a uteroscopic tube. Back in those days, the tube was metal, not flexible—hence the discomfort, which I've never forgotten. The procedure was unsuccessful because somehow I had already passed the stone. The doctor said I had "anomalous kidneys." "What the hell does that mean?" I asked. "It just means they're unlike any kidneys I've ever seen," he said.

After these two incidents, I wasn't given any further treatment or medication. I was just told to drink plenty of liquids.

I had another attack in the 1960s. I was visiting a friend in Swampscott and had to drive into Boston without killing myself or anyone else, which was quite an ordeal. But I never passed a whole stone; they all turned to gravel.

Then during the Blizzard of 1978, I had my last attack. Boston was digging out from a huge snow storm. No one was allowed to drive; the streets had to be clear for ambulances and fire trucks. The pain was God-awful, just unbearable. They always say it's like having a baby—you just wouldn't believe it. I couldn't get to the hospital right away, so the doctor told me to drink some whiskey to dull the pain. Finally, I was given special dispensation to take a taxicab to the hospital.

In the hospital, they put a tube up the urethra to try to "basket" the stone. That was the only one they ever got. I remember, I was laying on my side with the sheet like a big tent draped over me. I just had a local anesthetic, and when the doctor finally got the stone, he dropped it on my sheet. It sounded just like a pebble dropping.

When the stone was basketed at the hospital, it was sent to the kidney stone lab where it was identified as a calcium stone. The medication consisted of Allopurinol tablets and Hydrochlorothiazide pills taken daily. There's been no sign of an attack since then.

About 4 years ago, I had another uteroscopic procedure, as part of a regular examination. The urologist used a new flexible tube (not like the metal one from 1944!). The whole thing took about 4 minutes, and involved a minimum of discomfort. Several of my friends, though, have had attacks within the past year or two, and their treatment and recovery seemed to be much more painful and prolonged than mine, in spite of all the new techniques available.

SIGNS AND SYMPTOMS

Kidney stones typically cause an extreme "grabbing pain" when they become stuck in the ureters. The ureters contract in irritation, causing renal colic. The pain has a sudden onset, and can be so severe that it causes nausea and vomiting as a sympathetic reaction. The pain often refers into the groin area. Occasionally, the stone may be caused by, or may lead to, an infection in the kidneys; in these instances, a fever and chills will accompany severe pain.

COMPLICATIONS

Most kidney stones big enough to cause problems are excruciatingly painful, but they do eventually pass into the bladder and out in the urine, without causing long-lasting damage to the urinary system. Occasionally, however, a stone can grow to be of a size to seriously disrupt kidney function. This leads to chronic or acute *renal failure* (this chapter, page 314).

DIAGNOSIS

The large majority of all kidney stones are "silent"; that is, they are too small to cause any pain or symptoms, although they may be discovered during routine x-rays for other problems. When they are big enough to get lodged in some spot in the urinary tract, the typical flank pain occurs, often accompanied by signs of blood in the urine. The precise size and location of the stones can be determined by x-ray or sonogram.

TREATMENT

The pain of kidney stones is so intense that long ago people operated on them without anesthesia; "cutting for stone" was considered worth living through, just to get rid of them. Nowadays, kidney stone patients have several other options, and only a small percentage have to go through major surgery. Three main interventions are used for kidney stones, depending on their size, location, and the general health of the patient:

- Percutaneous nephrolithotomy. This surgery is conducted through a tiny tunnel in the back leading to the offending stone. When the stone is reached, it is either extracted or subjected to sonic waves that reduce it in size.
- Uteroscopic stone removal. This technique uses a flexible tube that is inserted into the urethra, and snakes up to where the stone is lodged to remove it from the ureters.
- Extracorporeal shock-wave lithotripsy. This is the use of sound waves to break up stones into a size that can be passed through the ureters without pain. This has been a highly successful procedure, although it can leave the patient feeling bruised and battered, from the extremity of the shock waves that are required to break up stones.

Other treatments for kidney stones depend on what the stones are made of, which is why it is necessary for patients to catch their stones as they pass with the urine. The stones are then analyzed, and a treatment program will be developed based on those findings.

Some interventions include surgery to remove the parathyroid glands, medication to regulate metabolism, dietary adjustments, and most importantly, adequate hydration. Kidney stone patients need to drink up to a gallon of water everyday, in order to keep stones moving through the system, *before* they become big enough to cause problems.

MASSAGE?

Massage for people with a history of kidney stones, but no present symptoms, is perfectly appropriate. However, a person with or without a history of kidney stones who is experiencing any symptoms of renal colic should not receive massage. Because circulatory massage has a profound influence on how fluids flow through the body, a client who is under medication for recurrent stones needs medical clearance before receiving this work.

Pyelonephritis

DEFINITION: WHAT IS IT?

As the name implies, pyelonephritis is an infection of the nephrons in the kidney, although the renal pelvis may also be involved.

Yes indicated [handwritten margin note]

PYELONEPHRITIS IN BRIEF

What is it?

Pyelonephritis is an <u>infection of the kidney and/or renal pelvis</u>.

How is it recognized?

Symptoms of pyelonephritis include <u>cystitis</u>, <u>back pain</u>, <u>fever</u>, <u>chills</u>, <u>nausea</u>, and <u>vomiting</u>.

Is massage indicated or contraindicated?

Massage is <u>systemically contraindicated for</u> a person with a <u>kidney infection</u>, until the infection has been eradicated.

ETIOLOGY: WHAT HAPPENS?

Most kidney infections are a complication of an E. coli infection in the urinary tract that travels up the ureters to set up an infection in the kidneys themselves. Other kidney infections can be caused by more obscure pathogens; they can be pregnancy-related; they can arise from a neurogenic bladder (a bladder that has no motor control and so empties passively into a bag); or they can come from surgical or medical instrumentation such as catheters or cystoscopes. Some kidney infections can be related to the development of *kidney stones* (this chapter, page 310).

SIGNS AND SYMPTOMS

Pyelonephritis can be a chronic situation with few or no symptoms, or it can be acute with high fever, nausea, vomiting, painful urination, and cloudy urine from the pus being released into the ureters.

COMPLICATIONS

Regardless of whether it's an acute or chronic situation, if pyelonephritis is recurrent, it can cause scarring and long-lasting kidney damage. Insufficient kidney activity will lead to *hypertension* (see chapter 4, page 199) and *renal failure* (this chapter, page 314). Another possible complication of a very acute infection is sepsis: blood poisoning from the infection leaking into capillaries. This life-threatening situation can lead rapidly to dangerously low blood pressure and death.

DIAGNOSIS

A urinalysis to look for signs of infection, combined with symptoms that describe pain higher and more extreme than found with a typical urinary tract infection, is usually enough information for a diagnosis of kidney infection. If the infectious agent is something unusual, more tests may be needed. CT scans are sometimes used to look for kidney stones that might be causing problems or abscesses on the kidneys that can create similar symptoms.

TREATMENT

Most kidney infections clear up satisfactorily with antibiotic therapy. If the infection is very extreme, the patient may need to be hospitalized in order to monitor how the kidneys are processing fluids.

PREVENTION

Acute pyelonephritis is almost always related to bacteria that enter the body at the urethral opening. Let this be a lesson, ladies: always wipe front to back.

MASSAGE?

Massage is systemically contraindicated for acute pyelonephritis, until the infection has been completely eradicated from the body. For clients with chronic kidney infections that flare and recede, noncirculatory massage between episodes of the problem may be appropriate, but only with a doctor's approval.

Renal Failure

DEFINITION: WHAT IS IT?

Renal failure means that, for whatever reasons, the kidneys are not functioning adequately to do their jobs of concentrating urine, excreting wastes, conserving electrolytes,

[handwritten notes at top of page:] Pre real - heart failure / Hemorage / damage kidney tissue LEADS TO - Renal failure

and producing erythropoietin. If the kidneys shut down suddenly, in response to shock or systemic infection, for instance, this is referred to as acute renal failure. If they sustain gradual damage over the course of many years, this is called chronic renal failure. In either case, although the name implies that they have ceased functioning altogether, the truth is that they are still working but they are simply unable to keep up with the body's demands.

ETIOLOGY: WHAT HAPPENS?

Although the kidneys are able to heal from most short-term abuse, any chronic or severe recurrent problems will eventually cause permanent damage to the delicate tissues, thereby interfering with kidney function. Fortunately, the human body is equipped with about twice as much kidney as is really needed, so people can tolerate a lot of damage before they run into problems.

Acute renal failure is generally a short-term problem, and unless the patient also suffers from heart disease, lung problems, or stroke, it generally has a good prognosis. It may last days or weeks, but if the contributing factors are controllable, kidney function may be restored.

Chronic renal failure is an impairment in kidney function that may last for years before it becomes serious or causes any symptoms. It occurs in three stages.

- *Diminished renal reserve* is the first stage of chronic renal failure. During this stage, scar tissue gradually replaces nephrons injured in recurrent infections, from recurring stones, or from chronic high blood pressure, often related to *diabetes* (chapter 4, page 210). Up to 75% of the nephrons will be lost before any symptoms of this stage show.
- *Renal insufficiency* is the second stage of chronic renal failure. At this point the kidneys are functioning at about 25% of normal levels. Blood levels of nitrogenous wastes, uric acid, and creatinine increase. Tests for protein in the urine will be positive at this time, although no other specific symptoms may present.
- *End stage kidney failure* is the last stage of the disease. In this situation, up to 90% of the nephrons have been lost. Patients must rely on hemodialysis to process wastes out of the blood. They are candidates for a kidney transplant, if the rest of their body is in strong enough health to withstand the surgery.

CAUSES

Both types of renal failure are brought about by other diseases that happen to affect how fluid is processed in the body. Thus, both acute and chronic renal failure are not diseases in and of themselves, but complications of other disorders that can have life-threatening repercussions.

- Acute renal failure. This is a short-term problem that is usually associated with severe ischemia from a lack of blood flow (which could happen for any number of reasons); a reaction to toxic levels of metabolic waste products; a tube blocked by a *kidney stone* (this chapter, page 310) or a tumor; direct damage to the kidney; or severe hemorrhaging. When blood pressure drops dangerously low (hypotension), an insufficient amount of blood will enter the kidneys through the renal artery. The body goes into "kidney shock" and starts retaining water. Urine output dries to a trickle within a matter of hours. High levels of waste products may accumulate in the blood, leading to vomiting, confusion, even convulsions or coma. Acute kidney failure is treated

[sidebar, right column:]

RENAL FAILURE IN BRIEF

What is it?
Renal failure is a situation in which the kidneys are incapable of functioning at normal levels. It may be an acute or a chronic problem, but it can be life-threatening.

How is it recognized?
Symptoms of acute and chronic renal failure differ in severity and type of onset, but they have in common reduced urine output, systemic edema, and changes in mental state brought about by the accumulation of toxins in the blood.

Is massage indicated or contraindicated?
Massage is systemically contraindicated for both acute and chronic renal failure.

[handwritten notes, right margin:] may produce Arrhythmias erythropoitan

according to the underlying cause. This is an emergency situation, and requires immediate medical attention.

Other causes of acute renal failure include acute tubular necrosis, in which a part of the kidney dies from oxygen deprivation. This is similar to a stroke or heart attack in the kidney tissue. Hemolytic uremic syndrome will also cause kidney failure; it is an infection of E. coli bacteria from undercooked meats, which will produce enough toxins to interfere with kidney function.

- Chronic renal failure. This condition affects about 200,000 people in the United States every year, and it is increasing by about 8% per year. It is directly linked to chronic *hypertension* (see chapter 4, page 199). African Americans are about twice as likely as Caucasians to progress from hypertension to chronic renal failure. The reason is unclear, but it may have something to do with the fact that while a Caucasian's blood pressure significantly drops during sleep, an African American's blood pressure does not.[1]

Other causes for chronic renal failure include *glomerulonephritis* (this chapter, page 309), polycystic kidney disease, *diabetes* (chapter 4, page 210), and physical obstruction of the kidneys by a stone or tumor.

SIGNS AND SYMPTOMS

Symptoms of renal failure, chronic or acute, will appear in the form of decreased urine output, systemic *edema* from salt and water retention (chapter 5, page 224), arrhythmia from potassium retention, anemia (chapter 4, page 178) from the lack of erythropoietin (the kidney hormone that stimulates red blood cell production), and osteomalacia (bone thinning), from the lack of Vitamin D which is necessary for calcium metabolism.

Renal failure through uremia (an excess of urea and other nitrogenous wastes in the blood) can also cause lethargy, fatigue, headaches, itchiness, loss of sensation in the hands and feet, discolored (yellowish or brownish) skin, tremors, seizures, easy bruising and bleeding, muscle cramps, and changes in mental and emotional states, as the accumulation of wastes in the blood affects the brain.

COMPLICATIONS

Both acute and chronic renal failure are potentially life-threatening complications of other disorders or trauma. But they in turn can cause further problems in the body. These have already been addressed under "Signs and Symptoms" and include anemia, osteomalacia, edema, and dementia from the toxic levels of metabolic wastes affecting the brain.

TREATMENT

Treatment for acute and chronic renal failure is determined by whatever underlying pathologies caused the damage. Treatment goals are to control the symptoms, prevent further complications, and slow the progress of the disease. Often this means getting blood pressure and blood sugar levels (if diabetes is part of the picture) under control. Medication to control potassium levels in the blood is important to avoid heart problems. Fluid and salt intake may be restricted until kidney function can keep up with the body's demands. Diuretics are sometimes prescribed to help the kidneys process fluids.

If a patient's kidneys are simply incapable of handling his or her needs regardless of these interventions, dialysis may become necessary. This routes the blood through a machine that does essentially the same job as the kidneys. Approximately 200,000 people in the United States currently use kidney dialysis machines today.

---

[1]Sandy Rovner. High blood pressure and kidney disease: How two medical problems can make each other worse. Washington Post Health News, April 5, 1994:7.

Kidney transplants will replace a damaged organ with a healthy kidney from an appropriate donor. They can be successful surgeries, if the new tissue isn't rejected. Unfortunately, the shortage of suitable donated organs means that among the 27,000 people waiting for kidney transplants today, only 11,000 operations will be performed.

MASSAGE?

Circulatory massage is systemically contraindicated during any stage of renal failure. If a client has a history of acute renal failure, he must receive medical clearance before receiving massage.

[handwritten: Receive Medical clearance. Light effleurage]

Bladder and Urinary Tract Disorders

Interstitial Cystitis

DEFINITION: WHAT IS IT?

Interstitial cystitis is a condition in which the walls of the bladder become permeated with scar tissue, and the bladder can become smaller and less elastic. It is not to be confused with ordinary cystitis, which is a complication of a *urinary tract infection* (this chapter, page 318).

DEMOGRAPHICS: WHO GETS IT?

Statistics on interstitial cystitis have been difficult to gather, but it is estimated that up to 500,000 people suffer from it each year. Of those, 90% are women, 10% are men; interstitial cystitis is rare in children. The population group most at risk are women between 20 and 50 years old.

ETIOLOGY: WHAT HAPPENS?

The bladder, a hollow organ, is designed to shrink when it's empty and expand when it's full. A healthy bladder holds about 1½ cups of urine when it's full. The average adult passes about 1½ quarts of urine every day, depending on how much liquid has been consumed, and a number of other factors.

[handwritten: Sun Shiny Day]

[handwritten: Prolonge months to years]

Normal urine is composed of water, excess salts extracted from the blood, nitrogenous wastes such as urea and uric acid, and other debris. It should not contain any living microorganisms; fragments of white blood cells or pathogens indicate an infection somewhere in the urinary system (see *urinary tract infection*, this chapter, page 318). The bladder itself is shielded from the highly acidic urine by a lining of protective material.

The leading theory behind interstitial cystitis is that an autoimmune response results in inflammation. This shield then becomes "leaky," allowing irritating chemicals from urine to infiltrate and irritate the walls of the bladder.

Prolonged irritation of this sort will substantially change the bladder. It becomes stiff, thickened, and fibrotic; scar tissue permeates layers of epithelium and smooth muscle, making the organ inflexible and inelastic. Unable to contract or expand, the bladder loses capacity. Irritated capillaries may bleed into the cavity. In some cases, characteristic star-shaped ulcers may appear on the walls.

INTERSTITIAL CYSTITIS IN BRIEF

What is it?
Interstitial cystitis is a chronic inflammation of the bladder, involving scar tissue, stiffening, decreased capacity, bleeding, and sometimes ulcers in the bladder walls.

How is it recognized?
Symptoms of interstitial cystitis are similar to those of urinary tract infections: burning, frequency, urgency of urination; decreased capacity of the bladder may become a problem, along with pain, pressure, and tenderness.

[handwritten: Painful intercourse]

Is massage indicated or contraindicated?
Massage is only locally contraindicated for interstitial cystitis, as long as no signs of generalized infection (i.e., fever, chills, malaise) are present.

CAUSES

The causes of interstitial cystitis are unknown. The fact that people have widely different combinations and severities of symptoms, as well as the fact that this condition will respond to very different treatment options in different people, indicates that it may actually be several distinct diseases that happen to have similar symptoms.

It is not uncommon for interstitial cystitis to follow antibiotic treatment for a basic urinary tract infection (UTI). This leads to a theory that prolonged antibiotic therapy may somehow damage the lining of the bladder. This theory has not held up under laboratory testing, however. Another theory is that interstitial cystitis is an autoimmune complication of a UTI: once the original infection has been conquered, the body continues to fight, in this case against the bladder itself. At this point, no general consensus exists on the specific causes for this disease.

SIGNS AND SYMPTOMS

Symptoms of interstitial cystitis are much the same as those for urinary tract infections: pain and burning on urination, frequency, urgency, painful intercourse. The difference is that symptoms can persist much longer than for UTIs, sometimes for months or years. Also, UTIs seldom result in serious long-term effects, while interstitial cystitis can cause permanent damage to the bladder. Interstitial cystitis may even eventually require surgery to remove the organ.

DIAGNOSIS

No definitive diagnostic test for interstitial cystitis has been developed; it is diagnosed in the absence of other conditions that cause similar symptoms. Conditions that must be ruled out for a positive diagnosis include urinary tract infections (with interstitial cystitis, symptoms will persist while the urine is no longer infected with bacteria, fungus, or parasites), vaginitis, bladder cancer, *kidney stones* (this chapter, page 310), *endometriosis* (chapter 9, page 328) for women, and prostatitis for men. Once these have been ruled out, a cystoscopic examination may be conducted to look for ulcers or bleeding spots.

TREATMENT

Because this disease has no known cause, it also has no known cure. Treatment for interstitial cystitis is generally aimed at symptomatic relief. Often the diagnostic tool of bladder distension can give relief, as can a "distillation," or bladder wash, done with dimethyl sulfoxide (DMSO), which can pass into the bladder wall to act as an anti-inflammatory and block pain sensation. This is done weekly, for up to 12 weeks. Aspirin and other painkillers may be recommended, as are exercise, stopping smoking, and dietary changes. No single intervention has permanent success, however. Interstitial cystitis may recur after months or even years of remission.

MASSAGE?

Massage is only locally contraindicated for interstitial cystitis, as long as no other signs of systemic infection are present. Because so little is known about the causative factors of this disease, massage should be conducted under a doctor's supervision.

Urinary Tract Infection

DEFINITION: WHAT IS IT?

This infection attacks the urethra, and sometimes the bladder, which results in inflammation.

DEMOGRAPHICS: WHO GETS IT?

UTIs are the cause of about eight million visits to the doctor every year; one woman in five will have an episode at least once in her life. It is almost always a women's disorder, because the female urethra is short, and located close to the anus, where bacteria that are harmless in the digestive tract can cause havoc if they gain access to the urinary tract. Urinary tract infections are not unheard of in men, however, and are sometimes the warning sign of something quite serious, like prostate problems. (See *prostate cancer*, chapter 9, page 344.)

ETIOLOGY: WHAT HAPPENS?

Under normal circumstances, the environment in the bladder is sterile. The urine contains waste products to be expelled from the body, but should contain no living microorganisms. Furthermore, the bladder is lined with a protective layer that works to prevent infectious agents from infiltrating the bladder walls.

Sometimes, however, foreign microorganisms are introduced into the urethra. If the circumstances are right, they can set up an infection. This infection may remain localized, or it may travel further into the urinary system.

Another type of inflammation of the urinary tract is not an infectious condition, but rather one of chronic irritation: this is also known as "honeymoon cystitis."

CAUSES

Most UTIs are caused by E. Coli and are not sexually transmitted. But in some cases, infection by chlamydia or mycoplasma organisms can cause infections in the urinary tract. These need to be diagnosed carefully; they don't respond to the same treatments as more typical bacterial infections do.

A sympathetic nervous system component probably plays a part in the development of UTIs; much anecdotal evidence exists concerning stress and bladder infections. Living in a sympathetic state may cause reduced blood flow to this internal organ, which, in turn, may make it more susceptible to infection. However, clinical evidence to date shows that, while stress may aggravate symptoms of UTIs, it has not been proven to cause them.

RISK FACTORS

Some women are found to be more susceptible to UTIs than others, although the reasons for this are not completely clear. Some factors, however, can reliably predict the chance of contracting a UTI:

- Blood types. Some blood types are more prone to this disorder than others; slight differences in internal chemistry seem to make it easier for invading bacteria to cling to the bladder walls.
- Spermicides. Spermicide foams have been shown to raise the risk of UTIs in some women.
- Diaphragm use. Women who use diaphragms show statistically higher rates of UTIs than women who don't.
- Pregnancy. Pregnant women have reduced immune activity (to prevent a reaction against the new tissue they're growing), and this, along with changes in the architecture of the pelvic cavity, make them prone to UTIs.

URINARY TRACT INFECTION IN BRIEF

What is it?

A urinary tract infection (UTI) is an infection of the urinary tract, usually by bacteria that live normally and harmlessly in the digestive tract.

How is it recognized?

Symptoms of UTIs include pain and burning sensations during urination, frequency, urgency, and cloudy or blood-tinged urine. In the acute stage, fever and general malaise may also present.

Is massage indicated or contraindicated?

Circulatory massage is systemically contraindicated during acute UTIs, as it is for all acute infections. Massage may be appropriate in the subacute stage, although deep work on the abdomen is still locally contraindicated until all signs of infection are gone.

June 19, 2002
Bonnaroo

- Diabetes. Elevated sugar levels in the urine make a hospitable environment for bacteria to grow in the bladder.
- Neurogenic bladder. If a bladder has lost motor function, it may not empty as completely as normal. This raises the potential for infection, as does the presence of catheter tubes, which are often used for people with limited bladder function.
- Menopause. Lower levels of estrogen will also decrease lactobacillus, which increases susceptibility to UTIs.
- Antibiotics. Being on long courses of antibiotics can raise the risk of contracting this disease. Long-term antibiotic use kills off protective bacteria and can lead to the birth of new, more resistant strains of bacteria.

SIGNS AND SYMPTOMS

The symptoms of UTIs are painful, burning urination; a feeling of frequency; reduced bladder capacity; urgency; blood-tinged or cloudy urine; back pain; fever; and achiness. Men suffering from UTIs may also experience pain in the penis or scrotum.

COMPLICATIONS

Almost all cases of urinary tract infections are caused by microorganisms that live in the digestive tract and have easy access into the short female urethra, where the infection usually begins as urethritis. If the bacteria travel up the system, they may set up an infection in the bladder. This is cystitis, which is not to be confused with *interstitial cystitis* (this chapter, page 317). If the infection remains unchecked, it may move all the way up the ureters into the kidneys, causing *pyelonephritis* (this chapter, page 313).

TREATMENT

The first step in self-treatment of a UTI is to drown it: radically increasing fluid intake gives the body a much needed opportunity to fully and frequently empty the bladder—not only of urine, but of bacteria as well. Drinking highly acidic liquids such as orange or cranberry juice is helpful for many women, as an acidic environment inhibits bacterial growth. For subacute situations, hydrotherapy in the form of hot and cold sitz baths may be recommended.

A short course of antibiotics is frequently prescribed for UTIs. In this case, 3 to 5 days' worth of medication is more appropriate than 2 weeks' worth, because the body concentrates antibiotics in the urine, and the risks of long-term antibiotic use have already been discussed.

The exceptions to this rule are women who experience low-grade chronic UTIs that don't clear up with normal treatments; they are sometimes successfully treated with long-term low doses of antibiotics.

PREVENTION

Some basic precautions can help prevent UTIs, especially for women who are especially vulnerable to them. These include drinking lots of water and acidic juices; urinating whenever necessary rather than holding it for a more convenient time; wiping from front to back after a bowel movement to prevent the introduction of digestive bacteria into the urethra; taking showers rather than baths; emptying the bladder after sex; and avoiding feminine hygiene sprays and douches, which can aggravate the urethra.

MASSAGE?

Acute cystitis will sometimes be accompanied by *fever* (see chapter 5, page 232), a systemic contraindication. Also, a small but significant risk of spreading the infection to the kidneys exists. Even in the postacute stage (after signs of acute infection have subsided), the lower abdomen is a local contraindication until all signs of infection have been eradicated.

CHAPTER REVIEW QUESTIONS: URINARY SYSTEM CONDITIONS

1. Describe how high blood pressure can lead to kidney dysfunction.

2. Describe how kidney dysfunction can lead to high blood pressure.

3. Why do people get kidney stones more often in hot environments than in other places?

4. Why are women more likely to suffer from urinary tract infections than men?

5. How can renal failure lead to disconnected symptoms such as itching or mental incapacitation?

6. Describe the relationship between long-term stress and urinary tract infections.

7. A client describes an accident in which she was sliding into home base and collided with the catcher. She complains of extreme pain on one side of her midback. Her muscles are not particularly tender, and she shows no signs of infection. What condition is likely to be present?

BIBLIOGRAPHY, URINARY SYSTEM CONDITIONS

General References, Urinary System

1. Carmine D. Clemente. Anatomy: A regional atlas of the human body. 3rd ed. Baltimore: Urban & Schwarzenburg, 1987.
2. I. Damjanou. Pathology for the health-related professions. Philadelphia: Saunders, 1996.
3. Giovanni de Dominico, Elizabeth Wood. Beard's massage. Saunders: Philadelphia, 1997.
4. Jeffrey R. M. Kunz, Asher J. Finkel, eds. The American Medical Association family medical guide. New York: Random House, Inc., 1987.
5. Elaine M. Marieb. Human anatomy and physiology. Redwood City, CA: Benjamin/ Cummings Publishing Co., Inc., 1989.
6. Ruth Lundeen Memmler, Dina Lin Wood. The human body in health and disease. 5th ed. Philadelphia: JB Lippincott Co., 1983.
7. Mary Lou Mulvihill. Human diseases: A systemic approach. 2nd ed. East Norwalk, CT: Appleton &Lange, A publishing division of Prentice-Hall, 1987.
8. Stedman's medical dictionary. 26th ed. Baltimore: Williams & Wilkins, 1995.
9. Taber's cyclopedic dictionary. 14th ed. Philadelphia: F.A. Davis Company, 1981.
10. Gerard J. Tortora, Nicholas P. Anagnostakos. Principles of anatomy and physiology. 6th ed. New York: Biological Sciences Textbook, Inc., A&P Textbooks, Inc. and Elia-Sparta, Inc.; Harper & Row Publishers, Inc., 1990.

Glomerulonephritis

1. Glomerulonephritis. Copyright 1998 ADAM Software, Inc., all rights reserved. Copyright 1998 CommuniHealth. URL: www.healthanswers.com. Accessed winter 1998.

Kidney Stones

1. Kidney stones in adults. National Institute of Diabetes Digestive and Kidney Disorders. URL: http://www.niddk.nih.gov/ KidneyStones/kidney.html. Accessed fall 1997.
2. The kidney stones network newsletter. Intelligent Information Resource, Inc., 1995–1997. URL: http://www.readersndex. com/fourgeez/news/. Accessed fall 1997.
3. Prevention and treatment of kidney stones. NIH Consesus statement online. March 28–30, 1988; 7(1):1–23. URL: http://text.nlm.nih.gov/nih/cdc/www/ 67txt.html. Accessed winter 1998.

Pyelonephritis

1. Cornell Peters. Pyelonephritis. In University of Iowa Family Practice Handbook: Chapter 11: Genitourinary. University of Iowa, 1992–1997. URL: http://www.vh. org/Providers/ClinRef/FPHandbook/ Chapter11/03-11.html. Accessed fall 1997.

Love has been Lost!

Renal Failure

1. Acute renal failure. Copyright 1998 ADAM Software, Inc., all rights reserved. Copyright 1998 CommuniHealth. URL: www.healthanswers.com. Accessed winter 1998.
2. Chronic renal failure. Copyright 1998 ADAM Software, Inc., all rights reserved. Copyright 1998 CommuniHealth. URL: www.healthanswers.com. Accessed winter 1998.

Interstitial Cystitis

1. Interstitial cystitis. National Institute of Diabetes, Digestive and Kidney Diseases. NIH Publication No. 94-3220, August 1994. Last updated June 3, 1997. URL: http://www.niddk.nih.gov/InterstitialCystitis/InterstitialCystitis.html. Accessed fall 1997.

Urinary Tract Infection

1. MedicineNet: Power points about urinary tract infections. Information Network, Inc., 1995–1997. URL: http://www.medicinenet.com. Accessed fall 1997.
2. Sally Squires. Insights on bladder infections. The Washington Post Health, March 15, 1994:9.
3. When your diagnosis is cystitis. MedHelp International, 1995–1997. URL: http://www.medhelp.org/. Accessed fall 1997.

Reproductive System Conditions

O B J E C T I V E S

After reading this chapter, you should be able to tell . . .

- What the disorder is.
- How to recognize it.
- Whether massage is indicated or contraindicated for that condition.
- Whether a contraindication is local or systemic, or refers to a specific stage of development or healing.
- Why those choices for massage are correct.

In addition to this basic information, you should be able to . . .

- Know where in the reproductive system fertilization usually occurs.
- Name the two most common types of breast cancer.
- List four treatment options for breast cancer.
- Know the connection between endometriosis and anemia.
- Name four risk factors for the development of ovarian cancer.
- Know why ovarian cancer is so dangerous.
- Name two types of ovarian cysts.
- Know the most dangerous complication of pelvic inflammatory disease.
- Name three serious conditions associated with pregnancy.
- Know why one of the major signs for prostate cancer is difficulty with urination.

INTRODUCTION

This chapter is mostly devoted to women's health problems, except for prostate cancer. Therefore, the only anatomical review will be of the female reproductive system, with an eye on where these conditions fit in. (See Figure 9.1.)

Terminology for structures in the reproductive system can sometimes be confusing. Recently, a movement toward calling items by their location or function has become common, rather than by their traditional names, which often refer to the physicians or anatomists who first recorded them. Thus, fallopian tubes, named for sixteenth century anatomist Gabriele Fallopio, may now be called uterine tubes, which is more descriptive. Traditional names are still in common use, however. In this chapter, structures will be referred to by both traditional and functional/locational names, so that practitioners trained in either terminology will feel comfortable.

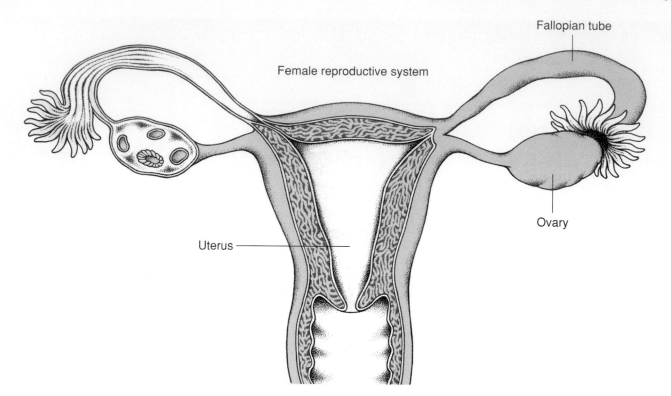

Figure 9.1. Overview of the female reproductive system

FUNCTION AND STRUCTURE

Low in the female pelvis, two small structures called the *ovaries* are located. They are attached via the ovarian ligament to the uterus. The ovaries produce hormones, which are released into the bloodstream, and they produce eggs, usually one each month during ovulation, which are released into the peritoneal space. The fimbriae of the fallopian (uterine) tubes gently caress the ovaries, coaxing the egg toward them. Once inside the tubes, the eggs make the 5-day journey to the uterus itself. If an egg is going to be fertilized, it will usually happen inside the uterine tube.

When the egg reaches the uterus, it finds itself inside a hollow organ built of crisscrossed layers of muscle. The inside surface of the uterus, the *endometrium*, is made of delicate epithelial tissue that holds vast, billowy supplies of blood to provide a nest for that fertilized egg. If the released egg is not fertilized, the uterus will shed the blood and the egg with it in the menses. Then it will begin the process of building a new nest for next month's candidate.

The timing of the ripening and release of eggs from the ovaries, and the building and shedding of the endometrial nest, is under the control of the endocrine system. Hormones secreted from the ovaries themselves, as well as the pituitary gland, determine when and how these various events will happen. Birth control pills work because they introduce artificial hormones into the blood. These trick the pituitary into believing that the woman is always pregnant, so she never ovulates.

Reproductive conditions of significance for massage therapists generally have to do with growths or local tenderness deep in the abdomen. Although working deeply in the vicinity of the uterus or ovaries is not generally practiced, sometimes these conditions can displace internal organs, making them vulnerable in places they wouldn't ordinarily be found.

REPRODUCTIVE SYSTEM CONDITIONS

Disorders of the Uterus

Abortion, Spontaneous and Elective

Dysmenorrhea

Endometriosis

Fibroid Tumors

Disorders of Other Reproductive Structures

Breast Cancer

Ovarian Cancer

Ovarian Cysts

Disorders of the Male Reproductive System

Prostate Cancer

Other Reproductive System Conditions

Pelvic Inflammatory Disease

Pregnancy

Disorders of the Uterus

Abortion, Spontaneous and Elective

DEFINITION: WHAT ARE THEY?

An elective abortion is the intentional termination of a pregnancy; a spontaneous abortion is an unintentional termination.

ETIOLOGY OF ELECTIVE ABORTION: WHAT HAPPENS?

A pregnancy can be terminated in different ways, depending on the stage. Within the first 12 weeks, an elective abortion will probably be accomplished by a vacuum suction. The walls of the cervix are dilated to allow a flexible tube into the uterus, which removes the fetal tissue. Between weeks 13 and 15, a D&C, or *dilatation* and *curettage*, may be performed; this more complicated procedure requires more anesthetic and sometimes a hospital stay. Later terminations involve inducing premature labor. They can be very difficult and always require hospitalization.

ETIOLOGY OF SPONTANEOUS ABORTION: WHAT HAPPENS?

Sometimes a fertilized egg never firmly establishes itself in the uterine lining. Structural problems in the uterus, such as *fibroid tumors* (this chapter, page 330), or a band of tissue called a *uterine septum*, may prevent a fertilized egg from implanting. Sometimes an anomaly occurs in the development of the fetus, making it nonviable. Up to 61% of fetuses spontaneously aborted in the first trimester have genetic chromosomal abnormalities. If the mother has a hormonal condition such as *diabetes* (see chapter 4, page 210) or thyroid problems, it may interfere with the chemical changes pregnancy demands. In other cases, inappropriate immune responses to the growing tissue will cause it to detach and die. All these events are called spontaneous abortions, or *miscarriages*, and

---

ABORTION, SPONTANEOUS AND ELECTIVE IN BRIEF

What are they?

Spontaneous and elective abortions are pregnancies that are ended, unintentionally or intentionally, before the fetus is born naturally.

How are they recognized?

Generalized or pelvic pain and bleeding may be present, but often no outward signals indicate a woman is recovering from a spontaneous or elective abortion.

Is massage indicated or contraindicated?

Massage is locally contraindicated (no deep abdominal work) for women recovering from a recent spontaneous or elective abortion, until her bleeding has stopped, and she is free of any signs of infection.

they usually happen within the first 14 weeks of pregnancy. If the fetus dies after week 20, it is no longer called a spontaneous abortion; it is a *stillbirth*, but the principles are the same.

The frequency of spontaneous abortions is a subject of debate. It is estimated that up to 50% of all fertilized eggs are expelled, for one reason or another, before women even know that they are pregnant at all. Of recognized pregnancies, anywhere from 10 to 20% of all fetuses are spontaneously aborted.

The causes of the majority of spontaneous abortions are never fully determined. It is known, however, that the risk of miscarrying a fetus is significantly higher for women who are over 35, who have systemic diseases such as diabetes or thyroid problems, and who have experienced three or more spontaneous abortions in the past.

SIGNS AND SYMPTOMS

When the endometrial lining of the uterus is disrupted in any way besides a normal menses, left behind is a large surface area of raw, bleeding epithelium. This is true for elective and spontaneous abortions as well as childbirth. Symptoms of this trauma can include pain (local and referred), bleeding, and cramping. These are generally self-limiting; that is, the symptoms resolve themselves with time, unless complications occur.

COMPLICATIONS

Complications of abortions or miscarriages include infection from incomplete shedding of the uterine lining and possible hemorrhaging. Depression is also a frequent complication of these events.

TREATMENT

The best treatment for a woman recovering from an abortion, a miscarriage, or successful childbirth is tender, loving care. If any infection is present, or if an incomplete shedding of the uterine lining occurs, a D&C and antibiotics may be necessary.

MASSAGE?

Deep abdominal massage is locally contraindicated for women recovering from spontaneous and elective abortions, and postpartum situations, at least until any bleeding has stopped. Massage elsewhere is very much indicated, although the risk of blood clotting for postpartum women is quite high, so it is wisest to stick with noncirculatory modalities until she receives medical clearance.

Dysmenorrhea

DEFINITION: WHAT IS IT?

Dysmenorrhea is a technical term for painful menstrual periods. Generally, a woman is said to have dysmenorrhea if she has to limit her regular activities or requires medication in order to function for 1 day or more every month.

DEMOGRAPHICS: WHO GETS IT?

Most women will have severe menstrual pain at least once in their lives. It is estimated that 42 million women suffer from repeated painful periods in the United States, and dysmenorrhea is the leading cause of lost time from school or work for women of childbearing age. It usually affects women in their late teens or early twenties, and subsides as a woman grows older. It is generally not changed by childbearing.

ETIOLOGY: WHAT HAPPENS?

Dysmenorrhea can be primary (i.e., it starts within the first 3 years of menstruation in an otherwise healthy woman) or secondary to some underlying pathology.

Several different factors can contribute to primary dysmenorrhea. At the top of the list are *prostaglandins*: chemicals produced throughout the body, especially in the uterus. They cause smooth muscle contractions, but they also sensitize the body to pain. Prostaglandins are found in higher concentrations in women who have menstrual pain than in women who do not. Progesterone, a hormone involved in the menstrual cycle, inhibits the action of prostaglandins, but just before menstruation begins, progesterone levels plummet, leaving the prostaglandins to do their work unchecked. Also, when the uterus is in sustained contraction, oxygen cannot easily supply the muscle, so ischemia will contribute to the pain-spasm-pain cycle. And finally, the uterine ligament, which anchors the uterus to the pelvic wall, can be pulled and irritated when the uterus is in spasm.

It is easy to see how physical or emotional stress fits into the picture of menstrual pain. Sympathetic reactions in the body will exacerbate uterine ischemia, leading to pain, which reinforces spasm. The emotional state of dreading the pain and discomfort of menstrual periods can then become a self-fulfilling prophecy: the stress of anticipating an unpleasant event works to make that event even more unpleasant.

Secondary dysmenorrhea is a complication of some other reproductive disorder such as *endometriosis* (this chapter, page 328), *pelvic inflammatory disease* (this chapter, page 346), *fibroid tumors* (this chapter, page 330), *ovarian cysts* (this chapter, page 341), or irritation from an IUD.

SIGNS AND SYMPTOMS

Symptoms of dysmenorrhea vary. They can include dull aches in the abdomen and low back, or sharp pains and cramping in the pelvis and abdomen. Headaches, nausea, vomiting, diarrhea, and constipation are all possibilities, along with a frequent need to urinate.

DIAGNOSIS

Ongoing, severe menstrual pain is important to investigate, because it could be indicative of serious underlying problems. Diagnosis will often involve a laparoscopy to check for endometriosis, which is the leading cause of secondary dysmenorrhea. Ultrasounds may be performed to look for fibroid tumors. Cultures of vaginal secretions may also be examined, to look for signs of PID, chlamydia, syphilis, or gonorrhea. In the absence of these conditions, painful periods can be treated without fear of ignoring some important underlying causes.

TREATMENT

For most cases of dysmenorrhea, painkillers such as ibuprofen and naproxen work by inhibiting the secretion of prostaglandins. A thorough nutritional analysis often also reveals strategies for dealing with menstrual pain; this is a useful course for many women, but no specific nutritional adjustments have been found to alleviate all cases of dysmenorrhea. Certain exercises and stretches can also relieve the pain caused by the irritated uterine ligament being tugged on by a uterus in spasm.

DYSMENORRHEA IN BRIEF

What is it?
Dysmenorrhea is the technical term for menstrual pain that is severe enough to interfere with and limit the activities of women of childbearing age.

How is it recognized?
The symptoms of dysmenorrhea are dull aching or sharp severe lower abdominal pain, preceding and/or during the early stages of menstruation. Nausea and vomiting may accompany very severe cases.

Is massage indicated or contraindicated?
Massage is appropriate for dysmenorrhea that is not linked to underlying pathology, although the abdomen is locally contraindicated for deep work during days of heavy menstrual flow.

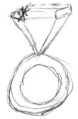

For more serious situations where painkillers, heat, and stretching don't help the pain, more aggressive interventions may be considered. Taking low-dose birth control pills will prohibit ovulation, which in turn prohibits the secretion of prostaglandins in the uterus. If a mechanical problem, such as a fibroid tumor, is found, surgery may be an option. Also, medications or laparoscopic surgery for endometriosis may alleviate symptoms.

MASSAGE?

Deep abdominal massage is a local contraindication for the first 2 days of a painful period, but reflexive work to relax the uterus is perfectly appropriate, as is work anywhere else on the body.

Endometriosis

DEFINITION: WHAT IS IT?

Endometriosis is a condition in which cells from the endometrium, the inner lining of the uterus, become established elsewhere in the body. They usually begin in the pelvic cavity, but may spread further into the abdomen and even above the diaphragm.

DEMOGRAPHICS: WHO GETS IT?

Endometriosis is probably fairly common. It is estimated that up to five million American women deal with this problem, but statistics are difficult to gather, since it cannot be diagnosed without surgery. It affects women as young as 11 years old, but is most common in women between the ages of 20 and 40, most of whom have not had children. Women of Asian descent and Caucasians are the most vulnerable to endometriosis; African-American women and Hispanics are less likely to be affected.

ETIOLOGY: WHAT HAPPENS?

The endometrium is the innermost lining of the uterus. The part that holds the soft cushion of blood for a fertilized egg is shed each month in the menstrual period. It should all exit the body through the uterine cervix into the vagina, but sometimes it does not.

During normal menstruation, the entire endometrial lining may *not* completely exit the uterus through the cervix. Bits of endometrium can implant wherever they land: on the outside of the ovaries, the uterine tubes, the bladder, the colon, nearby lymph nodes, or elsewhere. (See Figure 9.2.) Endometrial growths have been found as far away from the uterus as the lungs and even the brain. Wherever they land, they will continue to grow in accordance with the hormonal commands in the body. Because these growths cannot be shed, the body attempts to isolate them by surrounding the deposits with fibrous connective tissue. Eventually, multitudes of fibrous "blood blisters" will form on whatever surfaces the endometrium can find.

Endometrial growths found early resemble clear vesicles on whatever structures they have colonized. Later, these vesicles become bright red. Over a course of 10 or more years they will appear thick, black, and scarred.

This is one theory behind the development of endometriosis, though the true etiology has not been confirmed.

ENDOMETRIOSIS IN BRIEF

What is it?
Endometriosis is the growth of endometrial cells in the peritoneal cavity (and possibly elsewhere). The cells swell and subside with the menstrual cycle.

How is it recognized?
Endometriosis often has no symptoms. When it does, they are generally infertility and abdominal pain during menstruation.

Is massage indicated or contraindicated?
Massage is a local contraindication for diagnosed cases of endometriosis.

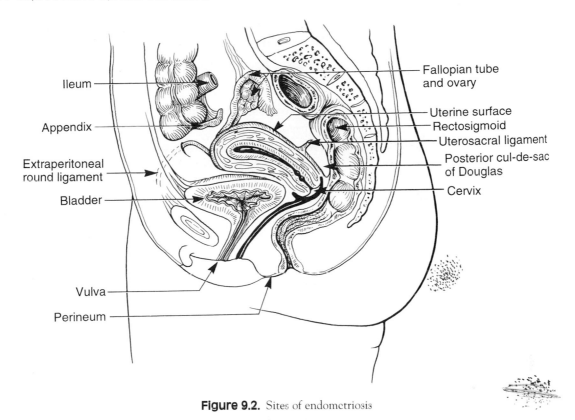

Figure 9.2. Sites of endometriosis

CAUSES

Studies of peritoneal fluid reveal that all women have endometrial cells outside of the uterus during menstruation. Several theories have been developed about *why* these cells sometimes implant outside of the uterus; none of them fully explain this phenomenon for all women. As more about this disorder is discovered, it will probably be found that it is actually several different kinds of closely related problems.

The main theory for the development of endometriosis is that the endometrial cells back up from the uterus through the uterine tubes. From there, they leak onto the surface of the ovaries, the uterus, or other structures in the pelvis. Other theories involve specific changes in the peritoneal lining that will support endometrial cells, and the exudation of cells through the uterine veins or the lymphatic vessels.

SIGNS AND SYMPTOMS

Very often, infertility will be the symptom that brings a woman with endometriosis to a doctor for an initial diagnosis. Other symptoms of endometriosis are often nonexistent, at least in the early stages, but some women may experience premenstrual spotting, a sensation of urinary urgency and painful urination, diarrhea, and rectal bleeding during menstruation. Advanced cases may show severe *dysmenorrhea* (this chapter, page 326) before, during, and *after* periods. Sometimes, but not always, menstrual bleeding will be very heavy for a woman with endometriosis.

COMPLICATIONS

Accumulations of bloody deposits and fibrous connective tissue can cause a lot of damage in the pelvic cavity. The process of building the fibrous coverings for the deposits can cause scarring and adhesions in or on the fallopian (uterine) tubes and ovaries, which will cause infertility. The stagnant pools of endometrium are also a good growth medium for bacteria, raising the possibility of *pelvic inflammatory disease* (this chapter, page 346).

Finally, the collecting of blood in these extra, unintentional deposits routes blood away from where it can be useful, resulting in *anemia* (see chapter 4, page 178).

DIAGNOSIS

At present, only one dependable diagnostic technique exists for endometriosis: laparoscopic surgery. Research to confirm a diagnosis through blood tests is underway, but nothing definitive has yet been found.

Endometriosis is often left undiagnosed, or misdiagnosed as another problem. Conditions that are sometimes diagnosed instead of endometriosis are *irritable bowel syndrome* (chapter 7, page 288), *ulcerative colitis* (chapter 7, page 290), or primary dysmenorrhea.

TREATMENT

Treatment for endometriosis depends on what outcome the woman desires. At present, the only permanent solution to the problem is the removal of the ovaries and uterus, so if a woman wants to treat her endometriosis in order to become pregnant, that is obviously not an option.

Three main avenues exist for treating this condition without a full hysterectomy:

- Pain relief. Analgesics for pain relief are all the treatment some women will pursue. These may be NSAIDs or, for more severe pain, narcotic painkillers.
- Hormone therapy. This is sometimes employed as a treatment in itself, and sometimes in order to shrink the growths in preparation for removal. This can backfire, though, when growths shrink so thoroughly that they are invisible during surgery, but grow again later. Hormone therapy options include birth control pills that minimize the amount of menstrual buildup that occurs, progesterone or testosterone-like compounds, and a drug that inhibits the release of gonadotropic hormone, thus inducing an artificial menopause. The complications of this therapy include loss of bone density and other menopause-related problems. None of the hormonal therapies are permanent solutions to the problem of endometriosis; the growths will recur when medication is stopped.
- Surgery. Several surgical techniques have been developed to remove endometrial growths, including cauterization, vaporization, employing lasers or electrosurgery, and excising the growths from the organs they're attached to. None of these are permanently successful if any part of the growths are missed.

Removing the ovaries and the uterus is the only permanent solution for endometriosis to date. This condition is responsible for the majority of hysterectomies (uterectomies) performed on women younger than 56 years of age.

MASSAGE?

Endometriosis locally contraindicates massage. Deep abdominal work is not appropriate for someone who may have blood blisters in her pelvic cavity, *especially* when she is menstruating. Be aware also that endometriosis can sometimes displace the pelvic contents. In other words, the ovaries of a woman with endometriosis may not be in exactly the same place as they are for other women. But outside of this area, massage is appropriate.

Fibroid Tumors

DEFINTION: WHAT ARE THEY?

Fibroid tumors, or *leiomyomas*, are benign tumors that grow in or around the uterus. They can grow within the smooth muscle walls or, more rarely, they can be suspended from a stalk into the cavity of the uterus. Some even hang down into the vagina. (See Figure 9.3.) They

HYSTERECTOMY
This comes from the Greek root *hystera*, which means womb or uterus. The word hysteria comes from the same root. In the early days of medicine, hysteria was assumed to be a woman's complaint, associated with womb-related disturbances.

vary in size from being microscopic to weighing several pounds and completely filling the uterus.

DEMOGRAPHICS: WHO GETS THEM?

Approximately 20 to 30% of women between 30 and 50 years old have fibroids, but this number is largely postulation because they are mostly symptomless, and therefore, go unreported. Fibroid growth seems to be stimulated by estrogen; after menopause they tend to shrink and ultimately disappear. Fibroids are far more common in African-American women than they are in Caucasians.

SIGNS AND SYMPTOMS

Usually fibroids create no symptoms at all. In very extreme cases, the fibroid may grow large enough to put pressure on the sensory nerves inside the uterus, or press on nearby structures such as the bladder, which can cause urinary frequency. If they press on the fallopian (uterine) tubes, they may interfere with pregnancies. They can also cause particularly heavy menstrual bleeding, and occasionally bleeding between menstrual periods.

FIBROID TUMORS IN BRIEF

What are they?
Fibroid tumors are benign growths in the muscle or connective tissue of the uterus.

How are they recognized?
Most fibroid tumors are asymptomatic. Some, however, cause increased menstrual bleeding or may put mechanical pressure on other structures in the pelvis.

Is massage indicated or contraindicated?
Deep abdominal massage is locally contraindicated for large, diagnosed fibroid tumors. However, most fibroids are quite small and virtually symptomless. In these cases, massage is appropriate.

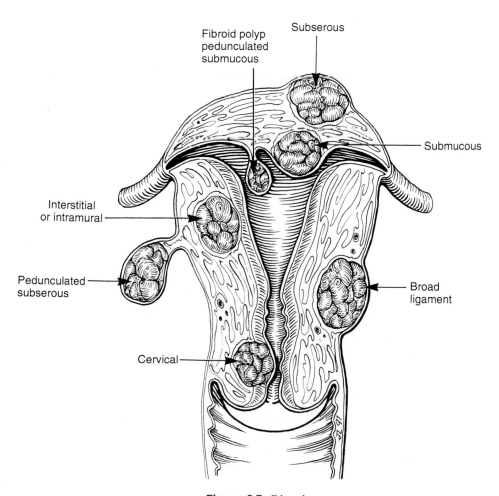

Figure 9.3. Fibroid tumors

COMPLICATIONS

Fibroids are very seldom a serious condition, but they can lead to some troubling consequences. The heavy menstruation they cause sometimes leads to *anemia* (see chapter 4, page 178) from excessive blood loss. They occasionally cause infertility by obstructing fallopian tubes or interfering with the implantation of a fertilized ovum. They may also interfere in pregnancies brought to term: if a fibroid is large, it may crowd the growing fetus or block the exit through the cervix. These problems can lead to premature births and cesarean sections.

Pedunculate fibroids, the type that dangle into the uterus or vagina, are known to become twisted, which causes extreme pain and requires removal by surgery. It is also possible for very large fibroids to outgrow their blood supply. This leads to a process called *degeneration*, in which tissue, deprived of oxygen, dies. The necrotic mass usually is slowly reabsorbed by the body, but can be painful in the process; more often, surgery is required to remove the fibroid.

DIAGNOSIS

Fibroids are generally found during pelvic exams, when it is noted that the uterus is enlarged or irregularly shaped. The diagnosis can usually be confirmed by ultrasound, but occasionally it is difficult to tell whether it is the uterus that is distended, or if a cyst or tumor has grown on the ovaries—a much more dangerous situation. If it is not clear what kind of growth is present, a CT scan or laparoscopy may be recommended to rule out *ovarian cancer* (this chapter, page 338).

TREATMENT

Fibroids seldom require treatment, unless they are causing pain and bleeding. Hormone therapy can shrink them, but they will grow back when medication is stopped. Surgery generally isn't recommended unless the fibroid is larger than a grapefruit, or is otherwise endangering the woman by placing pressure on other structures. In those cases, they can be surgically excised or, if the whole uterus is infiltrated with them, a hysterectomy (uterectomy) may be recommended.

MASSAGE?

Diagnosed fibroids locally contraindicate deep abdominal work. Undiagnosed fibroids (which are probably present in about 30% of all women anyway) indicate massage, although deep abdominal work shouldn't be done in the vicinity of the uterus, regardless. Anywhere else on the body, massage of any kind is perfectly appropriate.

Disorders of Other Reproductive Structures

Breast Cancer

DEFINITION: WHAT IS IT?

Breast cancer is the development of malignant tumors in the epithelial tissue of the breast.

DEMOGRAPHICS: WHO GETS IT?

Over 180,000 new cases of breast cancer are diagnosed in women, and about 1,000 cases in men, every year in this country. Most women with breast cancer are mature; 77% of them are over 50 years old when diagnosed. Before 1980, the lifetime risk of contracting breast cancer was 1 in 11. Now it is 1 in 8, but some significant factors may be influencing the higher number, including women's increasing longevity (the chance of getting breast cancer increases significantly with age alone), and the fact that breast cancer is being found and diagnosed earlier than ever before.

Breast cancer is the second most common cause of death by cancer for women in this country (lung cancer is the first). It is responsible for the deaths of some 44,000 women each year, as well as over 200 men.

ETIOLOGY: WHAT HAPPENS?

With breast cancer, as with all other cancers, cellular replication grows out of control. Malignant cancer growths, unlike the fluid-filled cysts that are fairly common in breast tissue, are not self-limiting; they will continue to grow and invade neighboring tissues. Some cells may move into the lymph system in the chest or axillary area. They can grow in the lymph nodes themselves, or travel through the system to invade distant organs; the liver, bones, and lungs are the most common sites of secondary tumors.

Although several different types of breast cancer have been identified, two types are by far the most common: *lobular* and *ductal carcinoma*. Lobular carcinoma begins in the lobules: small structures clustered around breast ducts

---

BREAST CANCER IN BRIEF

What is it?
Breast cancer is the growth of malignant tumor cells in breast tissue; these cells can invade skin and nearby muscles. If they invade lymph nodes, they can metastasize to the rest of the body.

How is it recognized?
The first sign of breast cancer is a small painless lump or thickening in the breast tissue or near the axilla. The lump may be too small to palpate, but may show on a mammogram. Later, the skin may change texture, the nipple may change shape, and the nipple may release discharge.

Is massage indicated or contraindicated?
This is a topic of some controversy. It is impossible to make a blanket statement; advantages and disadvantages of massage for the breast cancer patient must be weighed on a case-by-case basis.

BREAST CANCER: CASE HISTORY

Carol E., 60 years old

"When you have had breast cancer, the thought of possible recurrence is always with you. It makes you look at what is really important in life."

It was in July, right before my 57th birthday, when I found a lump in my left breast while doing a breast exam in the shower. We were just getting ready to leave on a vacation with friends, so I did not say anything. My annual mammogram was already scheduled in about 3 weeks.

When I went in for my mammogram, I told the doctor about the lump. He said he couldn't feel a lump. The mammogram was normal. A subsequent ultrasound did not reveal anything, and the technician also could not feel what I felt. So, even though I knew better, because of a medical background, this gave me a sense of security that all was well.

Until January. I could still feel the lump and by now my husband could also— so I was not imagining it. I talked with our daughter, an RN involved in risk management. She said, "You could have a normal mammogram and ultrasound and still have breast cancer. You have to go by what you know is normal for you." So, I made an appointment with a surgeon for the week I returned from a previously planned trip to Florida.

I returned on Valentine's Day, and my appointment was on February 16th. The surgeon not only felt what I had felt (which was a thickening, more than a lump), but in checking my previous mammogram, he found pinpoints of calcium in the right breast, which are sometimes indicators of cancer. Three days later I had bilateral biopsies.

(continued)

BREAST CANCER: CASE HISTORY, cont.

During the biopsies, a frozen section was done on the thickening on the left side, which meant the pathologist could tell right away whether the tissue was malignant. (The tissue from the right breast biopsy went through routine pathology, and I had to wait several days for those results). So there I was, in the recovery room, when the doctor came in and told me that the left breast biopsy was malignant. Then he left to talk to my husband and I was by myself. The most noticeable feeling I had was just incredible sadness. I don't know why I wasn't angry or anything else; I was just so sad. After a few minutes, I was able to join my husband and we both cried.

When something like this happens to you, you begin by wondering, how bad is it? Are you going to die soon? Then you go home and do the waiting game again, for the results of the other biopsy, and this was absolutely, incredibly stressful. You are already facing surgery on one breast, and now you are wondering if you will lose both breasts. After 3 days, the call came saying the second biopsy was not malignant. By that time I was thankful that only one breast had a malignancy. Strange thing for which to be thankful.

My diagnosis was a Stage 1 infiltrated ductal carcinoma, upper medial quadrant, left breast. After getting a second opinion, surgery was scheduled for the following Monday. Before that, I had to have chest x-rays, bone scan, and a radiation oncology consult, as I had opted to have conservative surgery (a lumpectomy followed by 6 weeks of radiation).

The surgeon performed a lumpectomy and also did an axillary dissection—removal of some lymph nodes in the armpit. During this surgery, a nerve in the armpit may be either severed or damaged. This produces numbness in the underarm and inner upper arm that can be permanent. The lymph nodes removed (16 in my case) were tested for malignancy, and later I learned that they showed no cancer. Chances were that the cancer had been confined to the breast tissue. Good news indeed!

However, the next Thursday, the surgeon called and said that the margins of the tissue removed were not clean—meaning that there were still some cancer cells in the breast. So, back to surgery the next Monday for a re-resection of the breast. My surgeon did not usually do this, but he felt that there was very little cancer left, and a mastectomy could still be avoided.

After a few days of recuperation, I returned home from being out to find my husband in bed with a bad headache. This was very rare, so I didn't bother him. The telephone rang and it was my surgeon again, saying (in a very upset and sad tone) that the margins on the last tissue sample still were not clean. He had spoken with the radiation oncologist, and she felt she could kill the remaining cancer cells with radiation. However, the surgeon felt he could give me even better odds by performing a total mastectomy. Of course, I opted for the better odds against recurrence, and the following Monday again found me in surgery having a total mastectomy. Three major surgeries in three weeks with general anesthetic each time is a lot to cope with, but you do what you have to do.

Because I had a mastectomy, I did not have to have any radiation, and because my lymph nodes were negative for cancer cells, I also did not have to have chemotherapy. A big relief!

I do take Tamoxifen, an anti–breast cancer drug used in certain circumstances to guard against recurrence. The standard commitment to this is 5 years. I also

(continued)

BREAST CANCER: CASE HISTORY, cont.

take amitriptyline, a mild antidepressant, to help break the cycle of chronic nerve pain that I have had in my left arm—an unusual and difficult complication. About 8 months ago, I also started on Neurontin, an anti-seizure drug that can also work on nerve pain, and in my case it has really helped. So, after almost 2 years, the pain in my arm is under control. I have no lymphedema (swelling of the arm due to a compromised lymph system). However, this could happen at any time.

I feel that the doctors do not emphasize enough how vulnerable the affected arm is. Infections can develop very easily and I have to be very careful, especially working in the garden. It seems that little burns and scratches take forever to heal. I should not lift more than 10 pounds with the affected arm and should not have any needle sticks or have blood pressure taken on that arm. Once I awoke after minor surgery to find a blood pressure cuff on my left arm, and was I upset! I thought that I had taken enough precautions that this should not have happened. The prescription for post-surgery medication had been clipped over the warning note! The next time I had an anesthetic, I wrote on my left arm with a surgical pen, and that did not come off!

When you have had breast cancer, the thought of possible recurrence is always with you. Breast cancer does not follow the 5-year rule; it can come back at any time. It is a lifelong commitment to always be on the watch and take really good care of yourself. This makes you look at what is really important in life. You try not to put off things that you want to say or do. Life is precious and I am glad to still have it!

*As a part of her recovery process, Carol became active in several breast cancer support groups. One of the groups of **Bosom Buddies**, which she helped to co-facilitate, still meets every month to have fun and encourage support for each other. Through **Reach to Recovery**, Carol does hospital and home visits to new breast cancer patients, teaching them about their options, telling them what they might expect, and giving them guidance to get more information. She would like to see women become their own advocates as they deal with the complexities of this disease.*

for the secretion of milk. Ductal carcinoma begins in the duct linings. Both lobules and ducts are surrounded by loose arrangements of connective tissue and fat; there is plenty of room for a tumor to develop before it causes noticeable symptoms.

The progression of breast cancer, like other types of cancer, is categorized by stages.

- Stage 0 breast cancer describes in situ tumors, which are small growths detected before they are large enough to displace tissue or travel to other parts of the body.
- Stage I involves discrete tumors under 2 centimeters in diameter, with no indication of spreading to nearby lymph nodes.
- Stage II involves tumors that are still under 2 centimeters in diameter, but with axillary node involvement, or larger tumors (up to 5 centimeters) with no lymph node involvement.
- Stage III describes tumors larger than 5 centimeters that may have invaded nearby tissue—the chest wall, musculature, skin, and local lymph nodes—but without signs of distant metastasis.
- Stage IV involves large tumors, axillary nodes, and distant metastasis.

Although the progression of cancer from stage to stage has been categorized for the sake of convenience, it is impossible to predict accurately exactly how this disease progresses in each person. Every person who develops breast cancer undergoes a unique disease process, unlike anybody else's.

RISK FACTORS

Breast cancer is not strongly linked to diet or environmental factors as are lung, colon, and skin cancer. One of the most frustrating things about this disease is the lack of a dependable profile of a woman who is likely to develop it. Statistically, women who began menstrual periods early in life, who had children later in life or not at all, and who are obese are at a somewhat greater risk; however, the majority of women with some or all of these features may never develop breast cancer, and 25% of all women who develop breast cancer show none of these tendencies.

Considerable interest has been raised over the recent isolation of two breast cancer genes. The presence of these genes can identify some women with particularly high risk of developing breast cancer. These women may then be more alert to identify their disease early in the process, which yields a better chance of survival. Unfortunately, women with these genes comprise only about 10% of all the women who are diagnosed with breast cancer every year. For the other 90%, no dependable risk profile exists, other than age.

SIGNS AND SYMPTOMS

Early symptoms of breast cancer are subtle. Breast tissue is soft, so tumors have ample room to grow without causing pain. Sometimes self examination will detect hard spots or lumps before a mammogram shows them, and sometimes a mammogram will reveal thickenings too subtle to feel. As with all cancers, the sooner breast cancer is treated, the better chance the patient has for survival. Advanced cases of breast cancer show asymmetrical breast growth, inverted nipples that may have discharge, and sometimes a characteristic "orange peel" texture of the skin on the breast. Advanced cases may also create symptoms in other parts of the body that are under attack: bone pain, weight loss, and swelling in the arms may be the result of tumors far from the site of the original cancer.

DIAGNOSIS

Breast cancer is usually detected first by self exam, and then confirmed by mammogram (see Figure 9.4), ultrasound, and tissue biopsy. These procedures will rule out the small

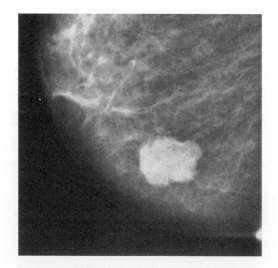

Figure 9.4. Mammogram of breast cancer

fluid-filled cysts that occasionally appear in breast tissue without posing a serious threat.

PREVENTION

At this point in time, breast cancer is not a preventable disease. The two most dependable risk factors, age and familial history, are not controllable. Therefore, efforts toward prevention are targeted at early detection, which significantly increases the life expectancy of the breast cancer patient. Three main courses exist for early detection: self exam, breast exam by a professional, and mammograms, which use radiation to look for unusually dense masses in the breast tissue.

Considerable controversy exists over how frequently mammograms should be performed. This stems from the fact that the breast tissue of many women is too dense to yield dependable results before the age of 40, or even older. Therefore, as yet, no specific time of life is ideal for every woman to include regular mammograms as a part of her healthcare; the age differs according to each woman's particular tissue. This is not to say that mammograms are unnecessary, however. They are responsible for identifying up to 85% of all breast cancers and also for finding atypically soft growths that self exams may miss. Monthly self exams, however, carry no risks, no expense, and may find typical tumors long before a mammogram.

TREATMENT

Treatment for breast cancer depends entirely on what stage the disease is in when it is diagnosed. Whatever treatment strategy is followed, every cancer patient should have access to support groups to benefit her healing process.

Four main options for treatment have been developed. These are often used in various combinations for best results.

- Surgery. Lumpectomies, partial mastectomies, total mastectomies, and modified mastectomies are surgical options for removing tumors and nearby lymph nodes. Lymph nodes are then examined for signs of further metastasis.
- Radiation. Radiation is aimed at tumors to slow or stop growth, or to shrink tumors in order to make them easier to remove surgically. Radiation may be applied externally or internally, with radioactive pellets that are surgically placed around the tumors and then removed later.
- Chemotherapy. Chemotherapy is the treatment of cancer with highly toxic drugs to slow or stop the growth of tumors.
- Hormone therapy. Some breast cancer tumors are sensitive to estrogen; they need access to this hormone in order to grow. A medication called *tamoxifen* binds up the estrogen receptors on tumors, which then prevents them from growing.

COMPLICATIONS OF TREATMENT

Cancer is a life-threatening disease that aggressively invades the body. Options to deal with cancer are similarly aggressive and often create serious side effects, which, though not as deadly as the disease itself, can be debilitating.

Surgery to remove part of the breast tissue and lymph nodes can also injure brachial plexus nerves, resulting in chronic pain in the shoulder and arm. If enough lymph nodes are removed, lymphedema, the accumulation of interstitial fluid in the arm, can be a serious problem. A variety of pumps and drainage devices have been developed, but all have limited success. Manual Lymph Drainage techniques can deal with this problem, but this is a very different approach than Swedish massage, and is not appropriate to practice without rigorous training.

Radiation therapy, if conducted over a long period of time, can cause skin problems from drying and itchiness to burns and even localized ulcerations.

Chemotherapy introduces highly toxic drugs into the body. These drugs can kill cancer cells, but they also cause hair loss, nausea, mouth sores, and immune suppression. Extremely high doses of chemotherapy can be successful to treat advanced cases of cancer, but must be followed by bone marrow transplants to replace damaged tissue there as well.

Tamoxifen can be effective at keeping hormone-sensitive tumors under control, but it is associated with several side effects, including menopause-like symptoms, an increased chance of uterine cancer, and for some women, a tendency to form blood clots.

PROGNOSIS

If breast cancer is caught and removed before it spreads into the axillary lymph nodes, a patient has a 96% chance to live 5 years or more. Overall, the 5-year survival rate is 83%, the 10-year survival rate is 65%, and the 15-year survival rate is 56%. Not surprisingly, women in whom cancer cells have been found in the lymph nodes have a much higher recurrence rate.

MASSAGE?

This is an issue of heated debate. Some people say the circulatory effects of massage make it systemically contraindicated for anyone with a condition that can be spread through the bloodstream or lymphatic flow; breast cancer certainly fits this description. Others suggest that the stress-balancing effects and immune system support offered by massage make it a valuable adjunct to traditional cancer therapies, as long as the tumors themselves are locally avoided. Massage is shown to ameliorate some of the worst side effects of cancer treatments by reducing pain and perceived stress and by inducing a general parasympathetic state.

The safest and most responsible thing a massage therapist can do is to consult with the client and the client's doctors, thoroughly explaining both the benefits and possible risks that massage may offer, and allowing the people involved to make the choice that is best for them. Ultimately, however, the responsibility rests on the shoulders of the massage therapist, and the decision to work with a client who has cancer must be a personal one.

If a decision is made to include massage as part of a treatment program for a cancer patient, certain cautions must be observed: radiation and tumor sites are local contraindications; chemotherapy will compromise immune system reactions, making the client vulnerable to a variety of infections that may contraindicate massage; changes in the health of the tissues may make clients susceptible to bruising or other damage that healthy people would not sustain.

Regardless of whether massage therapists choose to work with women who have breast cancer, one thing they *can* do is encourage their women clients to perform monthly self exams. It is not within the scope of practice to do this for clients, or even to teach them how, but stressing the importance of self exams is a meaningful way for all massage therapists to support their clients.

Ovarian Cancer

DEFINITION: WHAT IS IT?

Ovarian cancer is the growth of malignant tumors on the ovaries. Several varieties of ovarian cancer have been found, but most of them begin in the epithelial lining of these organs. The tumors may take a long time to become established, but once they do, they can grow quickly and metastasize readily to other organs in the abdomen.

DEMOGRAPHICS: WHO GETS IT?

Ovarian cancer usually strikes women who live in industrialized areas. Caucasians are the highest risk group for this disease. It can occur at any age, but is most common in women who are 60 years old or older. It affects 20,000 women in the United States every year (1 in every 70), and is responsible for about 14,000 deaths every year.

CAUSES

The precise causes of ovarian cancer are unknown. A close look at high-risk populations indicates that at least one predisposing factor is no history of childbirth or other interruption in menstruation, such as that provided by birth control pills. Since cancer often affects tissues subject to a lot of wear and tear (for example, lung cancer in smokers, or skin cancer in people who get a lot of sun exposure), it is postulated that the ovaries of women who never experience an interruption in their ovulatory cycle are "overstressed" and consequently vulnerable to the formation of tumors.

OVARIAN CANCER IN BRIEF

What is it?
Ovarian cancer is the development of malignant tumors on the ovaries; they rapidly metastasize to other structures in the abdominal cavity.

How is it recognized?
Symptoms of ovarian cancer are generally extremely subtle until the disease has progressed to life-threatening levels. Early symptoms include a feeling of heaviness in the pelvis, vague abdominal discomfort, occasional vaginal bleeding, and weight gain or loss.

Is massage indicated or contraindicated?
As with all cancers, the appropriateness of massage depends on whether a client wishes to include it in a treatment program. Massage for ovarian cancer patients must be done under medical supervision.

PROGRESSION

Once the tumors have formed on the ovaries, they can grow very quickly. Cancerous cells may be shed into the peritoneal space, where they then will land on and colonize other organs. Common sites of metastasis of ovarian cancer are the uterus, colon, diaphragm, stomach, and lymphatic system. The biggest danger with ovarian cancer is that metastasis often happens before anyone suspects an original tumor.

RISK FACTORS

Although it's not known what triggers the formation of tumors on the ovaries, some of the most important risk factors for developing the disease have been identified.

- Familial history. Perhaps the greatest risk factor for ovarian cancer is having it in the family. Women who have a first-degree relative (mother, sister, daughter) with ovarian cancer could have up to a 50% chance of developing the cancer themselves. Having a second-degree relative (grandmother, aunt, half-sister) with ovarian cancer also increases the chance of developing the disease. Families with a history of *breast cancer* (see this chapter, page 332) also have statistically higher rates of ovarian cancer than the general population.
- Reproductive history. Any woman who has never had a child or taken birth control pills, or who has experienced multiple miscarriages, is at increased risk for developing ovarian cancer. In addition, women who have taken fertility drugs without conceiving and bearing a child may also be at increased risk, although the statistics for these women have been a bit inconsistent.
- Health history. Women who have a history of breast cancer themselves have approximately twice the chance of developing ovarian cancer as the rest of the population.
- Estrogen replacement therapy. Women who have employed ERT against *osteoporosis* (chapter 2, page 62) have a higher chance of developing ovarian cancer than others.
- Other. Other risks involve exposure to radiation or asbestos, the use of talcum powder on the genitals, a high fat diet, and age; the chance of developing ovarian cancer increases considerably between ages 40 and 60.

SIGNS AND SYMPTOMS

Ovarian cancer is such a dangerous disease because early symptoms are practically nonexistent, or they are so subtle, they are easily passed over. When the cancer is finally identified, it has often metastasized beyond the point of control.

Early symptoms of ovarian cancer include a feeling of heaviness in the pelvis, vague abdominal discomfort, vaginal bleeding, a change in menstrual cycles, and weight gain or loss. Later symptoms can include a palpable abdominal mass, increased girth around the abdomen, ascites, and gastrointestinal signs such as gas, bloating, loss of appetite, nausea, and vomiting.

DIAGNOSIS

Ovarian cancer is difficult to diagnose early. A pelvic exam may reveal unusual abdominal masses, but only a fourth of these turn out to be cancerous. Other tests that may be conducted include special ultrasound tests, CT scans, and MRIs. Barium enemas and pyelograms (a process that stains urine in the kidneys to see how it moves down the ureters into the bladder) may be conducted to look for structures pressing on other abdominal organs. A test called CA-125 looks for a particular tumor marker in the bloodstream. This has been useful in confirming a diagnosis, but it occasionally yields both false positive and false negative results, so it is not a definitive test. Ultimately, a laparotomy must be conducted to take a tissue sample from the ovaries for analysis.

TREATMENT

If the test results from a laparotomy are positive, further abdominal exploration is conducted to see how far (if at all) the cancer has progressed. Samples from nearby lymph nodes, the diaphragm, and peritoneal fluid will be examined for signs of metastasis.

Ovarian cancer is generally treated with surgery and chemotherapy. Surgery removes the ovaries (oophorectomy) and sometimes the uterine tubes and uterus as well. If a woman has a malignant tumor on one side and still wants to have children, only one ovary may be taken, but the chances that she will develop cancer later in life are fairly high.

Chemotherapy can be conducted orally at home or intravenously in a hospital. A new method is being developed to deliver the cytotoxic drugs directly into the peritoneum, where it can immediately access malignant tumors.

Radiation therapy is not usually used for ovarian cancer.

PROGNOSIS

Ovarian cancer is a relatively rare disease, but it is the fifth highest cause of death from cancer for all women. It is the number one cause of death from gynecologic diseases. Because it is so hard to diagnose early, the prognosis is generally poor. More than 50% of women diagnosed have already experienced some metastasis. The 5-year survival rate overall is 35 to 38%, but if the disease is identified early, that statistic rises to 85%.

PREVENTION

Many women who get ovarian cancer don't fit the profile outlined in the known risk factors. But women who *do* fit that profile (i.e., women with a familial history of ovarian cancer, a familial or personal history of breast cancer, and especially women who are 40 to 60 years old), need to be especially vigilant to take note of the subtle symptoms that early ovarian cancer can cause. Prophylactic oopheorectomy (surgical removal of the ovaries) is sometimes recommended for women who have ovarian cancer in their immediate family and who have completed their childbearing.

MASSAGE?

As with breast cancer, the appropriateness of massage for ovarian cancer is a matter of personal choice. A client who is recovering from ovarian cancer may find massage to ameliorate the unpleasant side effects of chemotherapy, but deep abdominal massage is contraindicated. If a client wishes to include massage in her treatment program, she and her massage therapist should consult with her oncologist for the best and safest results.

Ovarian Cysts

DEFINITION: WHAT ARE THEY?

Ovarian cysts are fluid-filled sacs that develop on the ovaries, usually at the site of egg release.

ETIOLOGY: WHAT HAPPENS?

A *follicle* is a small sac or cavity that produces a secretion. Usually follicles are discussed in the context of the skin, where they produce lubrication for hairs, but ovaries have follicles, too, from which the ova emerge. Every time an egg is released from the ovary, it leaves a tiny pock mark at the follicle. By the time a woman reaches menopause, her ovaries are completely covered with these little pock marks. The follicles, or the pock marks left after ovulation, are the sites for the development of most ovarian cysts.

TYPES OF CYSTS

Several types of cysts can form on the ovaries. Three of the most common kinds will be discussed here.

- Follicular cysts. Occasionally, the follicle holding an egg never ruptures to release it. In this case, a blister forms and the fluid isn't immediately reabsorbed into the body. Follicular cysts rarely become bigger than 2 to 3 inches across, and they are generally resolved within a few months. (See Figure 9.5.)

OVARIAN CYSTS IN BRIEF

What are they?
Ovarian cysts are benign, fluid-filled growths on the ovaries.

How are they recognized?
Ovarian cysts may exhibit no symptoms, or they may cause a change in the menstrual cycle. Also possible are constant pain in the pelvis, pain with intercourse, or symptoms similar to early pregnancy: nausea, vomiting, and breast tenderness.

Is massage indicated or contraindicated?
Massage is locally contraindicated for diagnosed ovarian cysts.

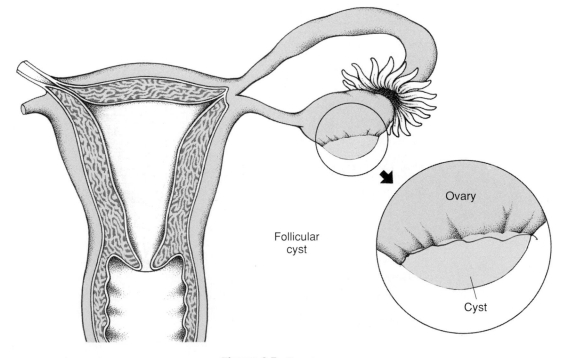

Follicular cyst

Ovary

Cyst

Figure 9.5. Ovarian cyst

OVARIAN CYSTS: CASE HISTORY

Sarah R., age 11

"Just knock me out with a chair!"

Sarah: I had some pains when I was 6. It kind of felt like someone was twisting something inside me. It hurt a lot. These pains happened at night. My mom took me to the hospital, but they thought I just had a cramped bowel.

I didn't have any pains again, until one day when I was 10. I told my mom that I was having some pains in my stomach, but she didn't believe me because I wasn't doing well in school, and I would do anything to get out of going. So I went to school, and I had them until about 9:00 or so. Then I told my teacher, and she said I could call my mom.

My mom was a little hesitant to take me home, because she still didn't believe me. She had a neighbor come pick me up. My mom took me to the doctor. They thought it was my appendix, but they said they couldn't do anything until there were more symptoms. They gave me muscle relaxants, and told me only to eat liquids. That frustrated me a lot.

The next day I had the pains again really bad, so my mom took me to urgent care. They took some blood tests, but they didn't find anything. All the tests were clear.

The next day, I was writhing in pain. I begged my mom to knock me out with a chair—that's when she really believed me. We went to the hospital. On the way there, I twisted myself upside down in the seat, the pain was so bad.

When we got to the hospital, the nurse gave us a room. We were there for 8 hours all together, before we got any help. First they came in and gave me 3 blood tests. I hate needles really bad, but I didn't even care.

Sarah's mother: The head surgeon came in and checked her. He wasn't sure what was wrong and he said to go home and watch her overnight, because he suspected appendicitis. I wasn't about to take her home again. I said, "Would you consider doing an ultrasound just to check, since you'll probably do one tomorrow anyway?"

Sarah: I got to ride on this cool table with wheels, all the way to the ultrasound place. They put this weird cold stuff all over my skin over my ovaries. It hurt when they were pressing down really hard. They got some other people to come in and look at it.

I was feeling really drowsy but I remember hearing the words: "She almost definitely will immediately need surgery." I got to ride the bed back to the emergency room.

Sarah's mother: An Ob-GYN said, "There's a large mass on the ovary. We don't know what it is yet. We anticipate at least a two-hour surgery."

Sarah: They gave me a mask to breathe into. Everything went black. Then a minute later I was awake, and my mom and Grandma were holding my hand and crying.

Sarah's mother: An hour and a half into the surgery, the doctor came out and said, "It's not a tumor, it's not cancer. It's the kind of cyst where a cell begins to grow teeth and hair and so on." The cyst was turned twice around the ovary, which is what caused so much pain.

They gave her a full bikini cut; she was too small for a laparoscopy. They removed two-thirds of the ovary, but said it shouldn't affect her puberty or ability to have children at all.

- Corpus luteum cysts. After a follicle releases an egg, it is then referred to as the *corpus luteum*. Blisters can form over these structures, which will change the balance of hormones being secreted from the ovaries. Corpus luteum cysts delay subsequent ovulations and produce pregnancy-like symptoms (nausea, vomiting, breast tenderness), until they spontaneously resolve, usually within a month or two.
- Polycystic Ovaries. Also called *Stein-Leventhal Syndrome*, this condition involves enlarged ovaries, with multiple small cysts. This condition creates an interference in hormone secretion, which causes obesity, loss of menstrual cycle, and increased body hair.

Other cysts appearing on the ovaries may be a part of *endometriosis* (this chapter, page 328); cystadenomas, which are usually benign tumors but can occasionally become cancerous; and dermoid cysts or *teratomas*. In these cysts, some primitive cells have been isolated from the rest of the body and have developed into different types of tissues. Dermoid cysts have been found to contain teeth, hairs, bone fragments, and other types of tissue. They are harmless in women. Men can develop them, too, but for males, teratomas are a much more serious condition that can involve testicular cancer.

SIGNS AND SYMPTOMS

Usually, no symptoms of ovarian cysts appear until the cyst is injured in some way. Some women, however, will experience a constant dull ache in the lower abdomen on the affected side. A firm, painless swelling in the pelvis may occur, and occasionally an ovarian cyst will cause pain with intercourse. Large cysts may create low back pain or, through pressure on the lumbar plexus, pain into the legs. Corpus luteum cysts and polycystic ovaries have special symptoms of their own, which are described above. In the absence of these signs, a person might never know a cyst is present, unless it grew big enough to interfere with other functions or if it ruptured.

COMPLICATIONS

Size is the major factor that determines whether or not ovarian cysts are going to cause any trouble. They can become big enough to interfere with blood flow; they may also rest on the bladder. In rare cases, they grow to incredible dimensions. An ovarian cyst that hangs from a stalk may sometimes become twisted. If that happens, a woman will have acute abdominal pain, nausea, and fever, necessitating medical intervention. The same symptoms will present themselves if the cyst ruptures; in this situation, the woman is at risk for *peritonitis* (see chapter 7, page 301).

Perhaps the most serious complicating factor of ovarian cysts is that their early symptoms, subtle as they may be, mimic an *advanced* case of *ovarian cancer* (this chapter, page 338). This is a highly dangerous cancer that has few early symptoms. By the time a person feels a firm, painless swelling in her pelvis, the disease will be quite far along. Therefore, if a client displays any of these symptoms, but has not been examined, urge her to see a doctor as soon as possible.

DIAGNOSIS

Ovarian cysts are frequently found as a swelling or mass during a routine pelvic exam. Ultrasound pictures generally confirm the diagnosis. If, for any reason, it is suspected that the cyst may be cancerous, a laparoscopy may be performed to take a tissue sample for analysis. It is important to follow up on cyst-like symptoms that last for more than 60 days, since follicular and corpus luteum cysts, the two most common and benign varieties, usually resolve within this period.

TREATMENT

Ovarian cysts that don't spontaneously resolve may be treated by draining the fluid out, but more often surgery is performed to remove them. The affected ovary is usually taken as well. In some cases, a complete removal of the ovaries and uterus will be recommended, because some types of cysts tend to recur, and can develop into cancer.

MASSAGE?

Ovarian cysts are a local contraindication for massage. Ovarian cysts can also displace the pelvic contents. Because of this, deep abdominal work, done in an area that is safe for women without cysts, may lead to bruising of the ovaries or even rupturing of the cyst for someone who has this condition. Massage elsewhere on the body is appropriate.

Disorders of the Male Reproductive System

Prostate Cancer

DEFINITION: WHAT IS IT?

Prostate cancer is the growth of malignant tumor cells in the prostate gland. This cancer is usually slow-growing, but can metastasize to other parts of the body, most often the bladder, rectum, and bones of the pelvis.

DEMOGRAPHICS: WHO GETS IT?

Over 300,000 cases of prostate cancer are diagnosed in this country every year. This rate is up 65% from 1980, mainly because early detection of this cancer is easier than ever before. Prostate cancer is rarely found in men under 40, but microscopic tumors are found in about 30% of men over 50. By the age of 90 years, 90% of men have this disease.

Prostate cancer is directly responsible for over 40,000 deaths every year. African Americans are affected more than any other population group, with a 37% higher incidence rate than Caucasians.

ETIOLOGY: WHAT HAPPENS?

The prostate is a donut-shaped gland that lies inferior to the bladder and encircles the male urethra. (See Figure 9.6.) It produces the fluid that makes up the bulk of semen and allows for the motility and viability of sperm. The prostate also controls release of the urine from the bladder. Some enlargement of the prostate in later years is almost a guarantee for men. Simple enlargement with no malignant cells is called BPH, or *benign prostatic hyperplasia*, and to some degree, it affects 80% of men over 40 and 95% of men over 80. But sometimes the growth and thickening of the prostate gland is not benign; it indicates prostate cancer.

CAUSES

The precise causes of prostate cancer are unknown. It has been observed, however, that in order for tumors to grow, they must have access to testosterone from fully functional testes. This disease is unknown in men who have been castrated, and castration has also been shown to shrink cancerous tumors.

A specific gene for prostate cancer has not been identified, but it does show statistically higher rates in fami-

PROSTATE CANCER IN BRIEF

What is it?
Prostate cancer is the growth of malignant cells in the prostate gland. The tumors may then metastasize, usually to nearby bones.

How is it recognized?
Symptoms of prostate cancer include problems with urination: weak stream, frequency, urgency, nocturia, and other problems arising from constriction of the urethra.

Is massage indicated or contraindicated?
Massage may be appropriate in the presence of slow-growing prostate cancer, when medical clearance has been obtained.

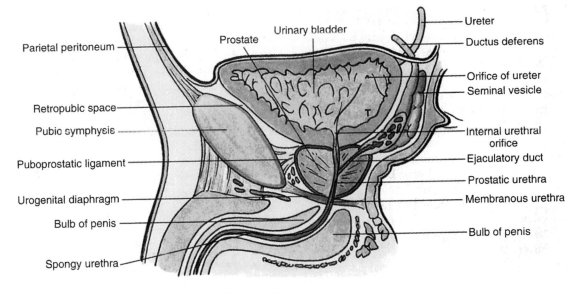

Figure 9.6. Prostate cancer

lies with a history of the disease, so heredity is probably one factor involved in its development.

PROGRESSION

When cancerous cells begin to form a tumor in the prostate, direct pressure is exerted on the urethra. This can lead to a number of different problems, from difficulty urinating to urgency, frequency, nocturia (the need to urinate frequently during the night), and bladder infections. Because the symptoms of prostate cancer are so similar to those of BPH, these signs may be ignored until the urethra is seriously restricted. Prostate cancer grows slowly, but it can stay silent long enough for cells to metastasize before it is detected. This feature of the disease makes it potentially lethal; it is the second leading cause of death by cancer for all men.

RISK FACTORS

Possible risk factors, besides having functional testes and a family history of prostate cancer, are still under investigation. Some possibilities include a diet high in fats, having had a vasectomy, and exposure to some environmental chemicals.

SIGNS AND SYMPTOMS

Symptoms of prostate cancer are exactly the same as those for BPH: an enlarged, hard prostate; obstruction of the urethra with resulting difficulty in urination; and susceptibility to *urinary tract* and *kidney infections* (see chapter 8, pages 318 and 313).

DIAGNOSIS

Prostate cancer is not usually an aggressive disease until quite late in life. Consequently, until recently, it has not been easily diagnosable until it had metastasized into the rectum, bladder, or bones, where it is no longer operable. It is also difficult to distinguish prostate cancer from BPH in the earliest stages, so it is very important to monitor it carefully. Fortunately, some very accurate methods have been developed to watch the growth of tumors in the prostate. Palpation through the wall of the rectum is the first step. Blood tests to look for elevated levels of certain prostate secretions are another tool. And ultrasonic pictures of the prostate can actually reveal tumors as small as a grain of rice. These tumors are then biopsied to look for malignant cells.

TREATMENT

If the disease is found before it has metastasized, it is usually manageable. The 5-year survival rate for prostate cancer is 98%. Treatment options include radiation from internal or external sources, surgery to remove the prostate or the testes, and hormone therapy: estrogen counteracts elevated levels of testosterone. Chemotherapy is not generally successful with prostate cancer.

Choosing the best treatment options for prostate cancer can be somewhat controversial. Because it tends to grow so slowly, and doesn't interfere with prostate or urinary tract function in early stages, sometimes a patient and doctor opt to simply keep small tumors under observation until they become more threatening.

MASSAGE?

Massage therapists who have elderly men among their clientele probably have some clients who live with the threat of prostate cancer. It is important to know if the disease is under observation, and if any danger of metastasis exists. The best way to do this is to consult with the client's doctor. As long as the growth is slow and the client's healthcare team is informed, massage may be appropriate for these clients.

For more information on massage and *cancer* in general, see chapter 10, page 358.

Other Reproductive System Conditions

Pelvic Inflammatory Disease

DEFINITION: WHAT IS IT?

The arrangement of female reproductive organs unfortunately makes women prone to a variety of infections with which men don't have to be concerned. Inflammation of the uterus, the fallopian tubes, or the ovaries can lead to serious long-term consequences. Although the term *salpingitis* (inflammation of the fallopian tubes) is sometimes used to refer to pelvic inflammatory disease (PID), infection of any of the reproductive structures is included under this umbrella.

DEMOGRAPHICS: WHO GETS IT?

PID is usually a disorder of young women. It is most common among women between 16 and 25 years old who have had multiple sexual partners; it is rare in women over 35. Over 1 million cases of PID are reported in the United States every year; 20,000 of them are among teenagers. It's impossible to estimate how many cases of PID remain unreported and untreated every year.

ETIOLOGY: WHAT HAPPENS?

Pelvic inflammatory disease is usually the result of a bacterial or fungal infection that begins in the uterus. The infectious agents are almost always chlamydia or gonorrhea, but irritation from an IUD, or incomplete elective or spontaneous abortions can also be precipitators for PID.

PELVIC INFLAMMATORY DISEASE IN BRIEF

What is it?
Pelvic inflammatory disease, or PID, is a bacterial infection of female reproductive organs. It starts at the cervix and can move up to infect the uterus, fallopian (uterine) tubes, ovaries, and entire pelvic cavity.

How is it recognized?
Symptoms of acute PID include abdominal pain, fever, chills, headache, lassitude, nausea, and vomiting. Chronic PID may produce no symptoms, or may involve chronic pain, pain on urination, and pain with intercourse.

Is massage indicated or contraindicated?
Massage is systemically contraindicated for any active pelvic infection.

Although it begins in the uterus, the infection may spread up the fallopian tubes and into the pelvic cavity.

SIGNS AND SYMPTOMS

Two types of PID have been identified. *Chronic PID* has low-grade, long-term symptoms that seldom flare up into an acute situation, but which can ultimately cause the same kind of internal damage as acute PID. Its symptoms include mild abdominal pain, backache, heavy menstrual periods, painful intercourse, and general lethargy. *Acute PID* is, as its name implies, more serious and more severe. Its symptoms include abdominal pain, low back pain, fever, chills, nausea, vomiting, painful intercourse, heavy periods, and heavy, pus-laden vaginal discharge.

COMPLICATIONS

If an infection infiltrates from the vagina to the uterus to the fallopian tubes, it *can* spread across to the ovaries, but it can just as easily start growing in the open pelvic cavity; this is *peritonitis* (see chapter 7, page 301), a potentially life-threatening situation. Another complication of PID is the abscesses that sometimes grow on the ovaries or fallopian tubes. The body isolates these infections with fibrous connective tissue, but the growth of that scar often leads to a blockage of the tubes and sterility. Up to one-half of all women who get PID become infertile; the more often a woman gets an infection, the higher her chances of permanent sterility. Even if the tubes remain partly functional, a history of PID raises the chances of an ectopic pregnancy: implantation of a fertilized egg in the uterine tubes instead of in the uterus itself. Ectopic pregnancies can lead to rupture of the fallopian tubes, killing the fetus, and endangering the life of the mother.

DIAGNOSIS

Diagnosis of this disorder is based on several different signs: abdominal tenderness, pain at the uterine cervix, ovaries, and fallopian tubes. These are palpated during a standard pelvic exam. In addition to these symptoms, a high white blood cell count, possible pelvic abscesses, and analysis of vaginal or cervical secretions may indicate an infection. A laparoscopy may be performed to look for abscesses and internal adhesions that may interfere with reproductive function.

TREATMENT

Most of the time, PID is a fairly simple bacterial infection. If it's caught early, it responds well to antibiotics and bedrest, although 20 to 40% of women require hospitalization and IV antibiotics. Sexual activity needs to be curtailed for several weeks. If internal abscesses are found, they may need to be surgically removed.

MASSAGE?

PID is a potentially life-threatening infection that can complicate into peritonitis. Massage is systemically contraindicated in the presence of generalized infections, until the client has completed a course of antibiotics and has been cleared by her doctor.

Pregnancy

DEFINITION: WHAT IS IT?

Obviously, pregnancy is the condition a woman is in when she is carrying a fetus. Most of the general information about pregnancy (etiology, etc.) will be skipped in this discussion, but it's worthwhile to look at some of the aspects of this condition in the context of massage.

PREGNANCY IN BRIEF

What is it?
Pregnancy is the state of carrying a fetus.

How is it recognized?
The symptoms of advanced pregnancy are obvious, but symptoms that specifically pertain to massage include swelling, loose ligaments, muscle spasms, clumsiness, and fatigue.

Is massage indicated or contraindicated?
Massage is indicated for all stages of uncomplicated pregnancy, with specific cautions relating to each trimester.

SIGNS AND SYMPTOMS

Some of the symptomatic complaints of pregnant women that massage therapists can help with include:

- Loose ligaments. One of the hormones secreted during pregnancy is *relaxin*. Its job is to loosen the ligaments so that the pelvis is elastic enough to allow the baby to emerge. But relaxin starts working practically from day one, making all the ligaments in the body looser and more mobile. This can cause all kinds of problems, from unstable vertebrae to asymmetrical sacroiliac joints. Muscles then tighten up to stabilize the joints, causing *spasms* (chapter 2, page 57) and pain.
- Fatigue. Pregnant women carry around a lot of extra weight. The baby itself is only a tiny part of the whole load, which includes the placenta, amniotic fluid, 40% more blood, and any extra body fat cells accumulated during her pregnancy.
- Shifting proprioception. Pregnant women change in size every day. This is especially true in the last trimester, when the baby grows at an astounding rate. The result is that the pregnant woman never knows exactly how much room she takes up. Her sense of where in space her body ends, and the rest of the world begins, becomes very shaky. This tends to make a pregnant woman clumsy and somewhat prone to injury. Massage provides an extraordinary sense of where bodies are in space. It can improve proprioceptive senses by giving continuous and positive feedback about boundaries.

COMPLICATIONS

In the vast range of things that could possibly go wrong in a pregnancy, massage therapists especially need to watch out for three specific conditions:

- Gestational diabetes. Pregnancy-related diabetes develops in about 2% of all pregnancies. It is diagnosed through a glucose tolerance test, in which the woman drinks a sweet beverage, and then her urine is examined for elevated levels of glucose.

  If diabetes develops because of pregnancy, risks to the baby and mother increase. The incidence of birth defects and stillbirths with diabetic mothers is three times greater than with non-diabetic mothers, and the rerouting of nutrients in the blood makes for abnormally large babies. A woman who develops prenatal diabetes *must* be under a doctor's care, and she should receive clearance before receiving massage; her blood pressure may be higher than is otherwise healthy.
- Pregnancy-induced hypertension. This condition generally starts mildly but can quickly become life-threatening both for the baby and the mother. It occurs in three categories: hypertension alone; *preeclampsia*, which is hypertension along with elevated proteins in the urine and possible systemic edema; and *eclampsia*, which is the same situation in addition to convulsions.

  The exact causes of pregnancy-induced hypertension are unknown. Some postulate that it may be an autoimmune problem, or even an allergic reaction to the baby; others suggest that in processing waste products for two people, the mother's system is simply overloaded. In any case, increased blood pressure drastically reduces the efficiency of the placenta for delivering nutrients to the baby. Pregnancy-induced hypertension tends to affect women in their first pregnancy, especially those with a personal or family history of hypertension. Treatment includes medication to bring down the blood pressure, strict bedrest, and where appropriate, cesarean section.

- Ectopic pregnancy. An ectopic pregnancy is any pregnancy that develops outside of the uterus. Most ectopic pregnancies develop in the fallopian tubes. Some estimates indicate that 1 to 5% of all pregnancies in the United States are ectopic. Risk factors include intrauterine device (IUD) use, a history of *pelvic inflammatory disease* (this chapter, page 346), *endometriosis* (this chapter, page 328), and adhesions from previous abdominal surgeries. Ectopic pregnancies cannot come to term; the fallopian tube will eventually rupture, killing the fetus and endangering the life of the mother. The only treatment is surgery to remove the fetus, placenta, and any damaged tissue, including the affected fallopian tube.

MASSAGE?

For pregnancies that are *not* complicated, massage is a wonderful gift for someone whose body doesn't quite belong to herself anymore. Special training is available to learn pregnancy and prenatal massage, but for more general purposes, here are some guidelines and cautions to preserve the pregnant woman's comfort and safety:

- First trimester. From the moment a woman knows she's pregnant, to several days after she's delivered, deep abdominal work is contraindicated. The first and last trimesters are the times when the fetal attachment is most fragile, and massage therapists must respect that fragility. Practitioners of Eastern techniques add that other cautions for massage in the first trimester include deep specific point work on the heels and Achilles tendons (reflexology abortion points) and on the *hoku* point in the web of the thumb.
- Second trimester. This is the safest, easiest part of the pregnancy. Very often a woman's energy levels will be up, while her nausea levels will be down. She probably has not yet gained enough weight to be very uncomfortable. *But* the connective tissue changes begin to show up during this time. Massage at this stage centers upon making sure she is comfortable. Bolsters and other physical support tools are very useful. Somewhere in this trimester, often around week 22, she will no longer want to be face down; then the therapist is limited to doing work from the side or supine.
- Third trimester. A midwife once said, "God invented the third trimester of pregnancy to make labor look like a pretty good deal." Massage therapists are more limited in what they do in this trimester than any other, but their work is more important than ever. Prone work is out of the question at this point, and supine work probably needs to be limited or modified, according to the mother's comfort. Being fully reclined allows the fetus to rest directly on the big abdominal blood vessels, which may either limit blood flow to the legs, leading to cramping in the gastrocnemius, or limit blood flow up the vena cava, leading to dizziness and possible unconsciousness. (See Figure 9.7.) It may be best to do a lot of side work, unless the client can be in a semi-reclined position.

Another caution for this stage is limited blood return from the legs, leading to edema. Watch for varicose veins as well. These, in combination with long-standing edema and the increased number of red blood cells that play a normal part in pregnancy, are ideal environments for clot formation. Some people suggest that to be completely safe, the medial calf and thigh (in other words, the

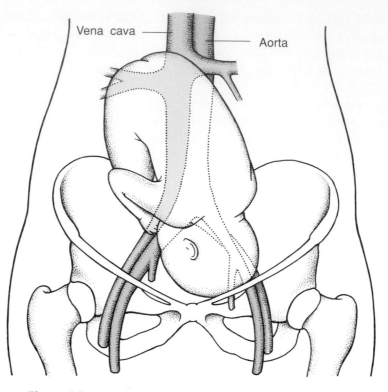

Figure 9.7. Pregnancy: A late-term fetus can obstruct blood flow.

area around the great saphenous vein) should be a local contraindication for massage during the third trimester, regardless of whether edema or varices are present.

- If *pitting* edema, coupled with fever, dizziness, headache, and nausea are present, the client may be in preeclampsia and may need immediate medical referral. Massage is contraindicated until she has medical clearance.

CHAPTER REVIEW QUESTIONS: REPRODUCTIVE SYSTEM CONDITIONS

1. Describe how birth control pills work.

2. Is the risk factor profile a very useful guideline for breast cancer? Why or why not?

3. What are prostaglandins, and how are they involved in dysmenorrhea?

4. Describe how stress can exacerbate menstrual pain.

5. Under what circumstances may fibroid tumors cause symptoms?

6. How can endometriosis or pelvic inflammatory disease lead to sterility?

7. Ovarian cancer is the leading cause of death from gynecological diseases, yet it is a relatively rare condition. How can this be true?

8. Discuss the relationship between certain hormonal changes that occur in pregnancy and muscle spasm.

9. Why may it be uncomfortable for a late-term pregnant woman to receive massage in a fully supine position?   *(continued)*

CHAPTER REVIEW QUESTIONS:
REPRODUCTIVE SYSTEM CONDITIONS, cont.

10. A client has been diagnosed with endometriosis, but has no particular symptoms at the time of her appointment. In order to help with her low back pain, her massage therapist works deeply on the psoas. Within a few hours the client has sharp shooting pains low in her abdomen and can't stand up straight. What may have happened?

BIBLIOGRAPHY, REPRODUCTIVE SYSTEM CONDITIONS

General References, Reproductive System

1. Carmine D. Clemente. Anatomy: A regional atlas of the human body. 3rd ed. Baltimore: Urban & Schwarzenburg, 1987.
2. I. Damjanou. Pathology for the health-related professions. Philadelphia: Saunders, 1996.
3. Giovanni de Dominico, Elizabeth Wood. Beard's massage. Saunders: Philadelphia, 1997.
4. Jeffrey R. M. Kunz, Asher J. Finkel, eds. The American Medical Association family medical guide. New York: Random House, Inc., 1987.
5. Elaine M. Marieb. Human anatomy and physiology. Redwood City, CA: Benjamin/Cummings Publishing Co., Inc., 1989.
6. Ruth Lundeen Memmler, Dina Lin Wood. The human body in health and disease. 5th ed. Philadelphia: JB Lippincott Co., 1983.
7. Mary Lou Mulvihill. Human diseases: A systemic approach. 2nd ed. East Norwalk, CT: Appleton &Lange, A publishing division of Prentice-Hall, 1987.
8. Stedman's medical dictionary. 26th ed. Baltimore: Williams & Wilkins, 1995.
9. Taber's cyclopedic dictionary. 14th ed. Philadelphia: F.A. Davis Company, 1981.
10. Gerard J. Tortora, Nicholas P. Anagnostakos. Principles of anatomy and physiology. 6th ed. New York: Biological Sciences Textbook, Inc., A&P Textbooks, Inc. and Elia-Sparta, Inc.; Harper & Row Publishers, Inc., 1990.

Abortion, Spontaneous and Elective

1. Abortion—elective or therapeutic. Copyright 1998 ADAM Software, Inc., all rights reserved. Copyright 1998 CommuniHealth. URL: www.healthanswers.com. Accessed winter 1998.
2. Abortion, spontaneous. Copyright 1998 ADAM Software, Inc., all rights reserved. Copyright 1998 CommuniHealth. URL: www.healthanswers.com. Accessed winter 1998.
3. Miscarriage. Information Network, Inc., 1995–1997. URL: http://www.medicinenet.com. Accessed fall 1997.

Dysmenorrhea

1. Menstrual Cramps. McKinley Health Center, The Board of Trustees of the University of Illinois, 1995. Modified May 26, 1996. URL: http://www.uiuc.edu/departments/mckinley.health-info/womenhlt/mencramp.html. Accessed fall 1997.
2. Menstruation, painful. Copyright 1998 ADAM Software, Inc., all rights reserved. Copyright 1998 CommuniHealth. URL: www.healthanswers.com. Accessed winter 1998.

Endometriosis

1. Endometriosis update. Mark Perloe, 1995. URL: http://www.ivf.com/endomp.html. Accessed fall 1997.
2. Endometriosis 2000 meeting focuses on research agenda. National Institute of Child Health and Human Development, July 1995. URL: http://www.ivf.com/endo2000.html. Accessed fall 1997.
3. MedicineNet: Power points about endometriosis. Information Network, Inc., 1995–1997. URL: http://www.medicinenet.com. Accessed fall 1997.

Fibroid Tumors

1. J. Glenn Bradley. Uterine fibroids—what every woman should know. Copyright 1997 www.obgyn.net. URL: http://www.obgyn.net/english/pubs/features/fibroids.htm. Accessed fall 1997.
2. Uterine fibroids. Copyright 1998 ADAM Software, Inc., all rights reserved. Copyright 1998 CommuniHealth. URL: www.healthanswers.com. Accessed winter 1998.

Breast Cancer

1. Breast cancer. National Cancer Institute/PDQ: Patient Statement. Last modified May 1997. URL: http://cancernet.nci.nih.gov/clinpdq/pif/Breast_cancer_Patient.html. Accessed fall 1997.
2. Breast cancer. Copyright 1998 ADAM Software, Inc., all rights reserved. Copyright 1998 CommuniHealth. URL: www.healthanswers.com. Accessed winter 1998.
3. Can breast cancer be prevented? American Cancer Society, Breast Cancer Network. URL: http://www.cancer.org/bcn/brmenu.html. Accessed winter 1998.
4. Can breast cancer be found early? American Cancer Society, Breast Cancer Network. URL: http://www.cancer.org/bcn/brmenu.html. Accessed winter 1998.
5. How is breast cancer diagnosed? American Cancer Society, Breast Cancer Network. URL: http://www.cancer.org/bcn/brmenu.html. Accessed winter 1998.
6. How is breast cancer staged? American Cancer Society, Breast Cancer Network. URL: http://www.cancer.org/bcn/brmenu.html. Accessed winter 1998.
7. How is breast cancer treated? American Cancer Society, Breast Cancer Network. URL: http://www.cancer.org/bcn/brmenu.html. Accessed winter 1998.
8. What are the key statistics about breast cancer? American Cancer Society, Breast Cancer Network. URL: http://www.cancer.org/bcn/brmenu.html. Accessed winter 1998.
9. What are the risk factors for breast cancer? American Cancer Society, Breast Cancer Network. URL: http://www.cancer.org/bcn/brmenu.html. Accessed winter 1998.
10. What is cancer? American Cancer Society, Breast Cancer Network. URL: http://www.cancer.org/bcn/brmenu.html. Accessed winter 1998.
11. What will happen after treatment for breast cancer? American Cancer Society, Breast Cancer Network. URL: http://www.cancer.org/bcn/brmenu.html. Accessed winter 1998.
12. Annette Chamness. Massage therapy and persons living with cancer. Massage Therapy Journal; 32(3): pp. 53–64.
13. Annette Chamness. Massage and breast cancer. Massage Therapy Journal; 35(1): pp. 44–46.
14. Rick Weiss. Breast cancer gene's impact limited. Washington Post, September 20, 1994; p. 7.

Ovarian Cancer

1. Gilda Radner familial ovarian cancer registry. Newsletter 1996–97. URL:http://rpci.med.buffalo.edu/clinic/gynonc/grnl.html. Accessed fall 1997.
2. MedicineNet: Power points about ovarian cancer. Information Network, Inc., 1995–1997. URL: http://www.medicinenet.com. Accessed fall 1997.
3. Ovarian cancer. Copyright 1998 ADAM Software, Inc., all rights reserved. Copyright 1998 CommuniHealth. URL: www.healthanswers.com. Accessed winter 1998.
4. Ovarian Cancer. US Healthcare, 1995. Last updated January 1995. URL: http://noah.cuny.edu/illness/cancer/ushc/ovariancan.html. Accessed fall 1997.
5. Health Magazine. Washington Post, April 19, 1994; pp. 3–23.

Ovarian Cysts

1. Ovarian Cysts. National Women's Health Resource Center, The Bod Squad. Wire Networks, Inc., 1995–1997. Last updated December 13, 1995. URL: http://more.women.com/wwire/archives/html/qabod/951213.qa.bat.html. Accessed fall 1997.
2. Ovarian cysts. Med Help International, 1995–1997. URL: http://www.medhelp.org/. Accessed fall 1997.
3. Ovarian cyst. Copyright 1998 ADAM Software, Inc., all rights reserved. Copyright 1998 CommuniHealth. URL: www.healthanswers.com. Accessed winter 1998.

Prostate Cancer

1. Benign prostatic hyperplasia. Copyright 1998 ADAM Software, Inc., all rights reserved. Copyright 1998 CommuniHealth. URL: www.healthanswers.com. Accessed winter 1998.
2. MedicineNet: Power points about prostate cancer. Information Network, Inc., 1995–1997. URL: http://www.medicinenet.com. Accessed fall 1997.
3. Prostate cancer. American Cancer Society. URL: http://www.cancer.org/cidSpecificCancers/prostate/index.html. Accessed winter 1998.

Pelvic Inflammatory Disease

1. Pelvic inflammatory disease. McKinley Health Center, The Board of Trustees of the University of Illinois, 1995. Modified April 7, 1996. URL: http://www.uiuc.

edu/departments/mckinley.health-info/
womenhlt/pid.html. Accessed fall
1997.

2. Pelvic inflammatory disease and vaginitis. Peer Health, Williams College,
Williamstown, MA. URL: http://wso.
williams.edu/peerh/sex/std/pid.html.
Accessed fall 1997.

3. Watch out for PID (pelvic inflammatory
disease). Joel R. Cooper, 1995. The Medical Reporter, June 1995, 1(3). URL:
http://medicalreporter.health.org/tmr0695/
pid0695.html. Accessed fall 1997.

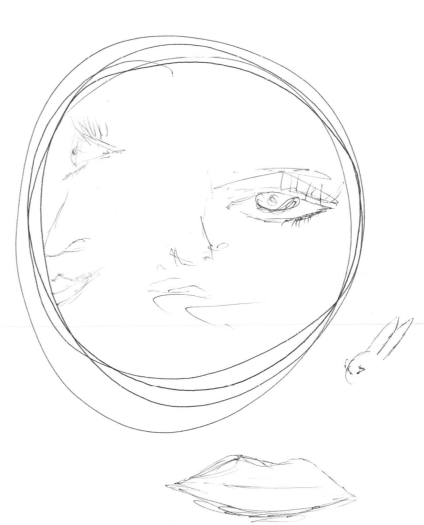

Miscellaneous Conditions

10

OBJECTIVES

After reading this chapter, you should be able to tell . . .

- What the disorder is.
- How to recognize it.
- Whether massage is indicated or contraindicated for that condition.
- Whether a contraindication is local or systemic, or refers to a specific stage of development or healing.
- Why those choices for massage are correct.

In addition to this basic information, you should be able to . . .

- Name three criteria for a diagnosis of alcoholism.
- Name two external factors and two internal factors in the development of cancer.
- Name five common signs that indicate the possibility of cancer, as presented by the American Cancer Society.
- Name four suggestions for helping to prevent cancer, as presented by the National Research Council.
- Name three types of cysts.
- Know what conditions may be suspected if ongoing fatigue is not relieved by normal amounts of rest.
- Name three contributing factors to insomnia.
- Name three consequences of sleep deprivation.
- Name two major cautions for working with clients who are recovering from major surgery.
- Define "abuse" as in "substance abuse."

MISCELLANEOUS CONDITIONS

Alcoholism

Cancer, General

Cysts

Edema Due to Inactivity

Fatigue

Insomnia

Postoperative Situations

Substance Abuse

Miscellaneous Conditions

Alcoholism

DEFINITION: WHAT IS IT?

Most people have a general idea of what alcoholism is, but the line between having a problem and not having one is different for every person. One generally accepted definition for when alcohol *use* becomes *abuse* is when the patient must drink in order to feel "normal." This may mean different quantities, and different frequencies, for each person.

Other criteria to determine the presence of alcoholism include:

- an increasing tolerance to the effects of alcohol;
- the cessation of alcohol use creates withdrawal symptoms, including tremors, increased heart rate and sweating, insomnia, nausea and vomiting, anxiety, hallucinations, and seizures;
- self-imposed efforts to limit or stop alcohol use are repeatedly unsuccessful;
- significant amounts of time are spent in alcohol use and recovery from hangovers;
- responsibilities to family members, jobs, and personal health are neglected because of alcohol use;
- denial that alcohol is seriously impeding in or damaging the user's life.

DEMOGRAPHICS: WHO GETS IT?

Alcohol addiction research indicates that a genetic factor may exist in alcoholism, but environmental influences are impossible to ignore. Statistics vary, but estimates in the United States suggest that slightly more than 7% of adults are alcoholics. Although two-thirds of all American adults report using alcohol, only 10% of them drink one-half of all the alcohol consumed in this country. Up to 43% of adults have been exposed to alcoholism in the family.

ETIOLOGY: WHAT HAPPENS?

Alcohol use affects virtually every system of the body. Here is a brief synopsis.

The Digestive System

Alcohol is highly irritating to the stomach lining, and high levels of consumption are responsible for a specific type of *gastroenteritis* (see chapter 7, page 276). It is also very rapidly absorbed through the gastric mucosa, into the portal system. The portal vein dumps the alcohol directly into the liver, from whence it enters the rest of the bloodstream. The effects of alcohol are felt until the liver has finished neutralizing the poison.

People who have preexisting gastrointestinal problems are especially vulnerable to the worst effects of alcohol. It is implicated in the development of *cancer* (see this chapter, page 358) in the upper gastrointestinal tract, especially in the esophagus, pharynx, larynx, and mouth. Alcoholism can cause *ulcers* (see chapter 7, page 278), internal hemorrhaging, and pancreatitis. About 20% of long-term drinkers will go on to develop *cirrhosis* (see chapter 7, page 291).

ALCOHOLISM IN BRIEF

What is it?
Alcoholism is the dependence on alcohol use to feel "normal" and the lack of ability to limit or stop consumption.

How is it recognized?
Symptoms of alcoholism include increased tolerance to the effects of alcohol, solitary drinking, memory loss (blackouts), and the neglect of responsibilities and personal health.

Is massage indicated or contraindicated?
Massage can be appropriate for persons recovering from alcohol use in rehabilitative settings, under medical supervision. Massage is always appropriate for alcoholics who no longer consume alcohol, providing they have no other contraindicating conditions. Massage is contraindicated for persons under the influence of alcohol at the time of their appointment.

The Cardiovascular System

Alcohol use decreases the force of cardiac contractions, and can lead to irregular heart-beats, or arrhythmia. Alcohol is also toxic to myocardial tissue, and can lead to *alcoholic cardiomyopathy*. Alcohol tends to agglutinate red blood cells, making them stick together. This leads to the possibility of *thrombi*, (see chapter 4, page 182) not only in the brain (see *stroke*, chapter 3, page 161), but in the coronary arteries as well (see *atherosclerosis*, chapter 4, page 193). Alcohol use can also have the opposite effect: liver damage can lead to poor vitamin K synthesis, which may result in uncontrollable bleeding.

Moderate alcohol consumption may actually help prevent cardiovascular disease by increasing HDL levels (the "good" cholesterol) in the blood.

The Nervous System

Memory loss frequently occurs for biochemical reasons, as well as from agglutinated red blood cells becoming stuck in the cerebral capillaries, causing brain cells to starve to death. Even some "social drinkers" will sustain measurable brain damage from repeated agglutination. In the short term, alcohol slows reflexes, slurs speech, impairs judgment, and compromises motor control. In the long term, the same effects can happen on a permanent basis, in a condition known as *organic brain syndrome*. In advanced stages of cirrhosis, the blood has toxic levels of metabolic wastes that can cause brain damage, and several other brain disorders associated with alcohol use are possible, although they won't be discussed here.

The Immune System

Prolonged alcohol use severely impedes resistance, especially to respiratory infections. Alcoholics are especially vulnerable to *pneumonia* (see chapter 6, page 252).

The Reproductive System

Alcoholism can cause reduced sex drive, erectile dysfunction, menstrual irregularities, and infertility. Babies of alcoholic women are susceptible to fetal alcohol syndrome (FAS): the most common type of environmentally caused mental retardation in the United States. FAS affects 4,000 to 12,000 newborns every year.

Other Complications

Alcohol is a factor in almost half of all automobile fatalities. It is involved in 40% of all industrial accidents and up to 65% of adult drownings. It costs about $96.4 billion a year in lost productivity, health care, and death costs. It contributes to about 100,000 deaths every year.

TREATMENT

The good news is that not all alcoholics experience irreversible damage; the liver has great powers of regeneration. Much of the cellular damage from alcoholism can be undone or compensated for, *if* the behavior stops. Treatment success rates for alcoholism vary greatly. The one common denominator is that an alcoholic person must be convinced that he or she really has a problem. Without that step, most treatment interventions are unsuccessful.

A variety of treatment styles are available, but all have to do with taking personal initiative to stop the use of alcohol. Nothing but total abstinence limits the damage alcohol use inflicts on the body.

MASSAGE?

Massage is being used successfully in some rehabilitation clinics as a substitute or a complement to tranquilizers or sedatives that are prescribed to ameliorate the effects of withdrawal. It is especially important to be working under a physician's direction, because the complications of alcoholism and liver damage can have important influence on general circulation, the tendency to form clots or spontaneously bleed, and immune function, all of which will determine the appropriateness of massage therapy.

Massage for successfully recovering alcoholics who have no long-lasting health problems is very much indicated. Massage is contraindicated if a client is intoxicated at the time of his or her appointment.

Cancer, General

Cancer is a big topic, and it would be impossible to cover it all here. Some basic information about the process of the disease will be discussed, along with the most commonly chosen treatment options. This will allow therapists to "talk shop" with their clients who are cancer patients or survivors and any doctors that might be consulted about the appropriateness of massage.

DEFINITION: WHAT IS IT?

Cancer is a variety of over one hundred different diseases that have one thing in common: for some reason, body cells mutate slightly and begin to replicate uncontrollably. Most cancers involve tumors: localized growths of new cells that infiltrate and damage nearby tissues.

DEMOGRAPHICS: WHO GETS IT?

Over the course of a lifetime, one in every three people will develop cancer or a precancerous condition. The overall rate is slightly higher for men than for women. Cancer can strike anyone at any age, but people over 65 years old account for half of all cancers in this country. About 1.5 million new cases are diagnosed, and more than half a million deaths occur from cancer every year. Cancer survivors living in the United States number about eight million today.

Skin cancer is the most common variety of cancer reported (and these statistics don't even reflect the countless moles removed as a safeguard against developing melanoma), but lung cancer is the leading cause of death by cancer for both men and women. Other leading causes of death include breast and ovarian cancer for women, prostate cancer for men, and cancer of the pancreas, colon, and rectum for both genders.

ETIOLOGY: WHAT HAPPENS?

No one is positive about how a healthy cell first begins to change into a cancer cell. One thing all cancers have in common is that the DNA of a cell mutates in a way that the cell acquires certain growth properties. This first step is called *initiation*. The second step occurs when the mutated cell begins to proliferate, which is called *promotion*. And the third step in the development of cancer is *progression*, in which the new cells develop malignant characteristics. Progression is the dividing line between cancerous and noncancerous growths.

When cancer begins, the mutated cell starts to behave differently. The cell replicates mutated versions of itself. As replication continues, the cancer cells resemble the parent cells less and less; they become less specialized and more generic in appearance. At first, these new cells remain localized, piling up on each other until they are a

CANCER IN BRIEF

What is it?
Cancer is the growth of malignant cells into tumors that invade tissues and spread throughout the body.

How is it recognized?
Cancer in early stages is often difficult to detect. Early signs depend on what part of the body is affected.

Is massage indicated or contraindicated?
The decision of whether to include massage as part of a treatment plan with cancer is a complicated one. Many benefits are possible, along with some risks. Circulatory massage that is not vigorous may be appropriate for persons dealing with cancer, but it should be performed with medical approval.

distinguishable neoplasm. At some point they start to vary from each other slightly, but enough to make treatment difficult, because within a well-developed tumor, *some* cells will respond to *some* kinds of treatment, but others won't. The only kind of treatment that *all* the cells will respond to is excision, which is not always possible or practical.

At some point, the cells in the neoplasm travel to other places in the body. They may simply flake off and float to another site, as ovarian tumors do to the bladder or rectum, or they may travel through the lymph or blood vessels to become established in distant sites. This process is called *metastasis*. "Meta" means "beyond" (e.g., the metacarpals are *beyond* the carpals). "Stasis" means "staying the same." Meta-stasis means "beyond staying the same"; in other words, *changing what shouldn't be changed.*

Some of the cells in a malignant tumor will act to metastasize the cancer. Called *metastasizers*, they break away and establish in some other location in the body. There they begin replicating into more new tumors. Or, they could simply spread into another part of the organ in which they start. Through some mysterious chemical conversations between cells, metastasizers seem to be able to convince healthy cells to make room for them. When enough of them have grown together, they release another chemical, which triggers the growth of new blood vessels to feed the tumor.

The first tumor that grows in the disease process is called the *primary tumor*; tumors that grow from metastasis of the primary tumor are called *secondary tumors*. In other words, a tumor in the bladder that metastasized from the ovary is not bladder cancer; it's secondary ovarian cancer in the bladder.

In the difficult field of diagnosis and survival-predicting for cancer patients, the tendency for some types of tumors to grow blood vessels before others is attracting attention. Counting the number of blood vessels in excised tumors is proving to be a dependable way to predict whether the tumors are likely to reappear elsewhere. Obviously, the more blood vessels that have grown, the more access mutated cells have to the rest of the body. Thus, if a tumor is removed that is heavily invested with blood vessels, that is a sign that the cancer should be attacked very aggressively.

No one knows for sure how often various kinds of cancers get started in a body. Mutated cells are different enough from healthy ones that the immune system, usually through natural killer cells, often tags and destroys them before they become established. This raises some interesting questions about the connections between cancer, stress, and immune system efficiency.

One of the most dangerous things about cancer is that it is practically painless until the tumors have grown and healthy tissue has been destroyed; therefore, it's often too late to fight back. Even so, the cancer itself often doesn't kill the patient. Opportunistic infections such as *pneumonia* (chapter 6, page 252) are responsible for a large percentage of cancer deaths.

CAUSES

Causes of cancer are slowly being narrowed down to some identifiable factors. Generally these are discussed as internal or external factors.

INTERNAL FACTORS

Every cell in the body has a built-in capacity for self destruction. This is a natural and healthy process called *apoptosis*, or *programmed cell death*. Cancer researchers are now investigating this phenomenon because a specific gene has been found to inhibit it. Therefore, cancer may be as much caused by cells that *refuse to die*, as it is by new cells coming to life. The opposite end of the spectrum would be diseases in which cells die off too soon: Alzheimer's and Parkinson's are two examples of what may be apoptosis taken too far.

Some cancers are brought about by or connected to genetic features. This may mean that a specific gene is likely to cause cellular mutations sometime in the future (such genes have been identified for a small percentage of breast cancers), or genetic susceptibility to factors may be present in one person that wouldn't be a threat to other people. Sometimes hormonal problems or immune system dysfunctions also increase the risk for developing cancer.

EXTERNAL FACTORS

Carcinogens are chemical or environmental agents identified as cancer-causers. The hydrocarbons in cigarette smoke are carcinogens, as is UV radiation from the sun, especially for fair-skinned people. Viruses have long been known to cause cancer in some animals, but only recently has HIV been shown to actually *cause*, not just open the door for, Kaposi's sarcoma. Other viruses have statistical connections to cancers but have not yet been proven to *cause* them:

- *HTLV-1*, a virus in the same family as HIV, has been linked to leukemia and lymphoma.
- *Hepatitis B* (HBV) has been linked to liver cancer.
- *Epstein Barr Virus* (EBV) has been linked to Burkitt's lymphoma and Hodgkin's disease. Recently, it was observed that EBV will actually switch off its host cell's "suicide apparatus," rendering it immune to natural killer and other immune system cells.
- *Human papilloma virus* is implicated in nearly all cases of cervical cancer.
- *Herpes Simplex Type II* (genital herpes) has been linked to cervical and uterine cancer.

Other external factors that contribute to cancer are radiation from excessive x-rays and exposure to certain substances, such as asbestos, benzene, nickel, cadmium, uranium, and vinyl chloride.

Often a combination of external and internal factors tips the scales in favor of developing cancer. Exposure to carcinogens in certain combinations can also be dangerous: heavy smoking combined with excessive alcohol consumption is an especially potent combination for developing cancers of the mouth or upper gastrointestinal tract, for instance. Very often many years, even decades, elapse between the initial exposure to a carcinogen and the development of distinguishable tumors. This makes it very difficult to pin down precise causes of cancer that will be consistent from person to person.

SIGNS AND SYMPTOMS

Symptoms of cancer vary widely, depending on the site. Cancer is often painless until it's too late to do anything about it—one of the most insidious features of this disease. Tumors will begin to cause pain when they place pressure on nerve endings, or when they cause a blockage in a tube or duct, which will in turn put pressure on nerve endings. The American Cancer Society has compiled a list of common signs that are red flags for the possibility of cancer.[1] They include:

- a change in bowel or bladder habits;
- a sore that does not heal;
- unusual bleeding or drainage;
- thickening or lump in the breast or elsewhere;
- indigestion or swallowing difficulty;
- a change in a wart or mole;
- persistent cough or hoarseness.

---

[1]Medicine Net: Cancer, detection, and treatment. Information Network, Inc., 1995–1997. URL:http://www.medicinenet.com. Accessed fall, 1997.

DIAGNOSIS

Cancers are found by a variety of methods, depending on the affected part of the body. Many cancers are found by either self or clinical exams: this is true for breast, cervical, rectal, and prostate cancers. Other tumors are found by imaging techniques such as x-rays, CT scans, MRIs, endoscopies, and ultrasound. Barium swallows and enemas can reveal tumors in the gastrointestinal tract.

If suspicious changes are noted, tissue samples are taken and analyzed for the presence of malignant cells. If these tests are positive, further exams of the patient follow to determine the stage of the cancer's progression.

Because most types of cancer develop in predictable patterns, they can be "staged," or given a label to indicate how advanced the cancer is. Different systems for staging cancer have been developed; it depends somewhat on what types of tissues are being affected. Breast cancer, for instance, tends to progress very differently than colon cancer. Two widely recognized systems for staging cancer are used. They can be used independently or together to rate the degree of progression of the disease.

The TNM classification system rates tumors by:

- Tumor size (*T*);
- Nodal involvement (*N*);
- Extent of metastasis (*M*).

The numerical staging system gives a number to indicate the degree of progression.

- *Stage* 0 means some malignant cells are present, but they are isolated and show no signs of spreading. Stage 0 cancer is sometimes called cancer *in situ*.
- *Stage* I cancer involves a small tumor.
- *Stage* II means the tumor may be larger, or signs indicate metastasis to nearby lymph nodes.
- *Stage* III indicates larger tumors and further signs of metastasis.
- *Stage* IV generally means that the cancer has metastasized to distant parts of the body.

TREATMENT

Decisions for how to treat cancer depend on what kind of cancer is present, the stage it's in, and the age and general health of the patient. Within each tumor, different kinds of cells may require different modes of attack. This makes the successful treatment of cancer a matter of finding the correct combination of chemotherapy drugs, hypothermia, radiation, hormones, and surgery.

- Chemotherapy. A variety of cytotoxic drugs have been developed for use in cancer treatment. These drugs specifically target any fast-growing cells in the body, so in addition to killing cancer cells, they may also attack the skin (resulting in hair loss), the gastrointestinal tract (leading to chronic nausea and mouth sores), and the blood cells (causing easy bruising and bleeding disorders as well as white blood cell suppression).
- Radiation. With this type of therapy, high-energy rays are focused on tumors to kill them or at least slow their growth. The radiation may be applied from an external machine, which requires daily outpatient visits for several weeks, or it may come from small radioactive pellets implanted close to the tumor; this method is performed in a hospital setting.
- Surgery. Cancer surgeries are performed to remove malignant tumors when possible. A sample of nearby lymph nodes is often taken as well, to examine for signs of metastasis.
- Hormones. Breast cancer and prostate cancer tumors both depend on the presence of certain hormones to grow. Therapies to limit the secretion of these hormones, or to change the way they affect the body, are used in the treatment of these cancers.
- Hypothermia. In some cases, specifically with cervical cancer, malignant cells may be killed by being frozen off the affected structure.

- Other treatments. Recent research on tumors and blood vessel growth has revealed promising new prospects for simply starving the tumors to death. This would be accomplished by limiting new blood vessel growth with *anti-angiogenic* ("anti–blood vessel growing") drugs.

Another treatment being tried with cancers that don't respond to traditional interventions is *autologous bone marrow transplant*. In this procedure, some bone marrow from the patient is harvested and stored. Then a very extreme course of cytotoxic drugs is administered, which kills the cancer cells, but kills white blood cells as well. After the chemotherapy, the stored bone marrow is replanted in the patient, where it will replace the immune system cells killed off by the chemotherapy. This procedure is for use only in very extreme cases; it has a number of dangerous side effects and serious complications, but it can be a lifesaver if nothing else works.

PREVENTION

By looking at who gets cancer and some of the causes involved, the National Research Council published a list with suggestions for how to stay cancer-free.[2] Not surprisingly, this list could be applied to any number of disorders.

- Eat more fruit, vegetables, and whole grain breads and cereals.
- Reduce dietary fat.
- Control weight.
- Exercise regularly.
- Use sunscreen.
- Stop smoking and other tobacco use.
- Limit alcohol consumption.

MASSAGE?

This is a controversial topic. Massage that directly affects blood and lymph flow carries the risk of aiding the process of metastasis. However, research conducted on cancer patients who received massage from nurses confirms that massage assists in pain control, decreases perceived stress levels, and creates a general parasympathetic state through reduced blood pressure and decreased muscle tension. In addition, massage has been seen to boost natural killer cell activity, which can be part of the body's own defense against cancer cells.

If a cancer patient wishes to include massage as part of a cancer treatment program, that person and his or her doctors need to be well informed of the possible risks and benefits that massage can offer. Massage should be administered to cancer patients under medical supervision.

For more information about cancer, see *breast cancer* (chapter 9, page 332), *lung cancer* (chapter 6, page 266), *colon cancer* (chapter 7, page 282), *ovarian cancer* (chapter 9, page 338), and *prostate cancer* (chapter 9, page 344).

Cysts

DEFINITION: WHAT ARE THEY?

When something gets inside or grows inside the body that doesn't really belong, a remarkable reaction occurs. Like an oyster covering a grain of sand with layers of pearl, humans cover their "grains of sand" with layers of connective tissue, making an easily discernible and isolated *cyst*. The notable exception to this habit is *cancer* (this chapter, page 358).

---

[2]Cancer prevention: tips to lead a healthy life. Cancer Research Foundation of America. URL:http://www. preventcancer.org/tipps.html. Accessed winter, 1998.

A variety of types of cysts can develop in the body. *Baker's cysts* (chapter 2, page 92) are outpouchings of the synovial joint in the popliteal fossa. *Ganglion cysts* (chapter 2, page 98) are pouches formed by tendonous sheaths. *Ovarian cysts* (chapter 9, page 341) are usually harmless, self-limiting growths on the ovaries at the site of egg release. Layers of connective tissue will also form around any foreign material that gets into the body. Unremoved shrapnel will be encysted, for example, and so will localized infections of *tuberculosis* (chapter 6, page 259).

The most common kinds of cysts that massage therapists encounter are *sebaceous cysts*, which will be the focus of the rest of this discussion. Sebaceous cysts are a bit like a pimple gone bad. (See *acne*, chapter 1, page 19.) A sebaceous gland has filled with pus and waste, but instead of draining or being consumed by macrophages, the debris from this localized infection is walled off and "removed" from the body by a tough layer of dense connective tissue. It generally stays there until it is surgically removed or the body eventually (and this can take months or years) gets around to reabsorbing it.

> ### CYSTS IN BRIEF
>
> **What are they?**
> Cysts are layers of connective tissue surrounding and isolating something that shouldn't be in the body, e.g., a piece of shrapnel or a localized infection.
>
> **How are they recognized?**
> Palpable cysts are generally small, painless, distinct masses that move slightly under the skin.
>
> **Is massage indicated or contraindicated?**
> Massage is locally contraindicated for cysts.

SIGNS AND SYMPTOMS

Sebaceous cysts are small, usually painless bumps under the skin that may move slightly, depending on the mobility of the fascia. They are most common on the scalp, neck, or shoulders: sites of acne infections.

COMPLICATIONS

Sebaceous cysts sometimes are attacked by staphylococcus bacteria, resulting in an acute infection. Other cysts are generally not vulnerable to infection, but may be situated in a place to become snagged or irritated by normal day-to-day activities.

TREATMENT

Most cysts require no treatment, unless they are in a place that causes pain, or they're removed for cosmetic reasons. If the wrapping of connective tissue has isolated the cyst adequately, it can generally be removed with a simple surgery. Infected sebaceous cysts are treated with systemic antibiotics.

MASSAGE?

Cysts locally contraindicate massage. In the extremely unlikely event that a massage therapist pops one, its contents would empty into the body and cause a dangerous immune reaction. It is more likely, though, that massage would simply irritate the surrounding tissues and causes soreness. If a client has a questionable or new cyst that hasn't been diagnosed, recommend that she get it diagnosed before the next appointment. Most painless bumps under the skin are not dangerous, but diagnosis is not within the scope of practice of massage therapy.

Edema Due to Inactivity

The most important question a massage therapist can ask a person in a bedridden state is, "Why are you here?" If the answer is, "I'm pregnant and I have high blood pressure," the decision about whether massage is appropriate will obviously be different than if the answer is, "I am recovering from bunion surgery."

EDEMA DUE TO INACTIVITY IN BRIEF

What is it?
Edema is the accumulation of excess interstitial fluid. It can be highly localized, as with a sprained ankle, or systemic, as with renal failure.

How is it recognized?
Fluid levels need to be 30% higher than normal for signs of edema to show. Tissue may be puffy or boggy; it can also be hot, cold, or clammy. Discoloration may or may not be present.

Is massage indicated or contraindicated?
It entirely depends on what condition led to inactivity. Some situations require bedrest or immobility for reasons that contraindicate massage; others will not be negatively impacted by massage at all.

ETIOLOGY: WHAT HAPPENS?

Imagine what is happening to the tissues of an immobilized person at a cellular level. Tissue cells—muscles, for instance—are bathed in muddy, waste-laden interstitial fluid that is utterly stagnant in the absence of muscular contraction. Those muscle cells are starving for oxygen and glucose, but the supplying capillaries are far away, and moving further away with the accumulation of more interstitial fluid. The amount of time it takes for nutrients to diffuse from capillaries to tissue cells increases exponentially with every micron of distance. To complicate things even further, muscle cells are surrounded by sheaths of connective tissue which, in response to the buildup of fluid, are themselves becoming thicker and harder for nutrients to penetrate.

COMPLICATIONS

Long-term immobility can have long-lasting repercussions. Muscles deprived of exercise develop fibrosis and atrophy; skin similarly cut off from blood supply starves to death and ulcerates. (See *decubitus ulcers*, chapter 1, page 36.) Circulation may become sluggish, and eventually clotting factors may accumulate enough to create the danger of *thrombi* (see chapter 4, page 182).

MASSAGE?

Exercise is the best proven method of moving lymph fluid through most tissues, but when exercise isn't an option, massage is a strong second-best. Passive and active range-of-motion exercises and other Swedish gymnastics are recognized for their positive impact on immobilized people. Bodies are use-it-or-lose-it propositions; without movement for any length of time, the strength of muscles, the elasticity of connective tissues, and the mobility of joints are all compromised. The damage doesn't have to be permanent, but it can be very difficult to reverse. In circumstances where massage is indicated, the worst effects of long-term edema can be avoided. It's important, however, to receive medical clearance from a physician who understands the circulatory impact of massage, in order to prevent the risk of dislodging clots.

Fatigue

FATIGUE IN BRIEF

What is it?
Fatigue is a state of less than optimal performance because the body has had inadequate rest and recovery time.

How is it recognized?
A person suffering from mental or physical fatigue feels tired, moves inefficiently, and may be more prone to injury.

Is massage indicated or contraindicated?
In the absence of other contraindicated conditions, massage is systemically indicated for fatigue.

DEFINITION: WHAT IS IT?

Most people are familiar with this condition. Fatigue is a state in which the body doesn't function at its best level because of lack of recovery time. For the purposes of simplicity, the world of fatigue is divided here into two types: *mental/emotional* fatigue and *physical* fatigue brought about by overexertion.

ETIOLOGY: WHAT HAPPENS?

The two varieties of fatigue are usually inextricably blended together. For example, living in chronic stress (mental/emotional fatigue) can throw the neck muscles into an ongoing contraction (physical fatigue). This person always feels more tired than if those muscles were able to release their unnecessary tension. The feeling of always being tired is a self-fulfilling prophecy; the perception that a person is tired causes him to move less efficiently, which exacerbates that loss of energy.

COMPLICATIONS

Fatigue is often related to *insomnia* (this chapter, page 365), which can create long-lasting problems in the body. Fatigue can cause a person to move inefficiently or clumsily, thus increasing the chance of accident or injury. If fatigue is not relieved with a reasonable amount of rest and recovery time, it may be a warning sign of some other conditions. *Chronic fatigue syndrome* (see chapter 5, page 229) is a possibility, as is *anemia* (see chapter 4, page 178).

MASSAGE?

Fatigue, be it mental or physical, is very much indicated for massage. After a good session, a client can get off the table and feel like he'd just been infused with several hours' worth of sleep. That's the extra measure of energy available when it's not being wasted on counterproductive muscular contractions. Massage also provides an hour-long vacation from the stress that was stimulating the contractions to begin with.

For fatigue brought on by mental or emotional stress, massage can reestablish the lost balance between sympathetic and parasympathetic reactions. Massage sessions provide a rare opportunity for clients to listen and pay attention to what's happening in their body, which provides tools for avoiding similar problems in the future.

For physical fatigue from exhaustion or overexertion, massage works on a mechanical level by reducing hypertonicity, flushing out waste products, improving local circulation, and speeding recovery time.

Ultimately, ongoing fatigue is a continuous circle between emotions reflected in bodies through muscular tension, and muscular tension that interferes with rest and recovery and causes emotional upset. For massage therapists, it's a chicken and egg proposition: frankly, it doesn't matter which one came first. The massage therapist's job is to address whatever symptoms are present, and to be sensitive to the more subtle signals about underlying tensions that may exacerbate those symptoms.

Insomnia

DEFINITION: WHAT IS IT?

Insomnia is a condition in which, for a variety of reasons, a person is unable to get sufficient restorative sleep. It may be difficult for someone to fall asleep, or sleep may be interrupted by bouts of wakefulness in the night. Whatever the pattern, insomnia can become a debilitating condition that leaves a person vulnerable to accidents, injuries, poor healing, and a number of serious secondary problems.

Insomnia is only 1 of over 100 different sleep disorders that range from trouble falling or staying asleep, to trouble staying awake (narcolepsy), to trouble keeping with a consistent sleeping schedule, to any number of physical prob-

---

INSOMNIA IN BRIEF

What is it?
Insomnia is the inability to attain adequate amounts of sleep.

How is it recognized?
Signs of insomnia include general fatigue, reduced mental capacity, and slow healing processes.

Is massage indicated or contraindicated?
Massage is systemically indicated for insomnia.

lems that cause sleep disruptions. Insomnia may be a transient problem that lasts for a week or less, or a chronic situation that goes on for months or even years.

DEMOGRAPHICS: WHO GETS IT?

Insomnia can affect anyone, including children, but most sleep studies have been conducted among adults. A survey of 1000 adults showed that up to one-half of them report having difficulties with sleep. Men generally have insomnia more often than women, and people over 65 years old are especially prone to this problem.

ETIOLOGY: WHAT HAPPENS?

The potential to lead long lives in healthy bodies depends on the ability to recover from the shocks and insults the human body tolerates every day. That ability is provided in part by good nutrition and in part by adequate high-quality sleep.

A healthy sleep cycle shows a consistent blend of REM (rapid eye movement) and non-REM sleep. REM sleep is a surprisingly active sleep phase; blood pressure, heart rates, and respiratory rates during REM sleep are quite close to those during wakefulness. During non-REM sleep, activity is much lower, although in this phase, the hormones that stimulate healing from injury or infection are released and circulated. If a person is deprived of either type of sleep, she will soon show signs of fatigue and distress.

Every day the human body suffers innumerable subtle and severe insults. A person twists an ankle getting out of the car, or scrapes a knuckle on the cheese grater, or introduces new viruses into the body. Under normal circumstances, these little incidents are hardly even noticed: the ankle feels better in a day or two; the skin grows back over the knuckle overnight; people conquer and expel many viruses without even knowing they've been exposed.

None of this can happen without high-quality sleep. It is during the deepest cycles of sleep that the immune system is refreshed and rejuvenated. *Somatotrophin*, the hormone that stimulates the action of fibroblasts for wound healing, is secreted primarily during deep sleep. In the absence of somatotrophin, people have very limited ability to heal from any kind of injury. Furthermore, lack of sleep depletes immune system activity. If the immune system isn't functioning well, the pathogens that live on the skin could turn into a life-threatening infection through any tiny hangnail or scrape.

CAUSES

Causes of sleeplessness are fairly easy to predict; the triggers for individual people show wide variations. The causes for insomnia include:

- Stress and anxiety. A precipitating event may begin the cycle of insomnia, but a pattern of sleeplessness can outlive the stress of the initial event. Eventually it can explode into a vicious circle, in which a person lays awake, stressed about not being asleep, which increases stress, which decreases the ability to sleep, ad infinitum.
- Depression. Clinical depression is both a cause and a symptom of chronic insomnia.
- Counterproductive habits. These can include changing time zones or sleep cycles frequently, napping, consuming caffeine close to bedtime, heavy smoking, or excessive alcohol consumption.
- A poor sleeping environment. This includes a room that is too cold or hot, too much noise, too much light, or being forced to get adequate sleep during daylight hours.
- Physical pain. If a person experiences pain when lying down, this can interfere with adequate sleep. This becomes a vicious circle, as not getting adequate sleep can hinder the injury-repair process, thus prolonging the pain.
- Mechanical pressure on the sympathetic trunk. If any cervical vertebrae are even slightly subluxated anteriorly, they can put pressure on the sympathetic trunk, the

chain of ganglia that connect sympathetic neurons. This constant stimulus can literally lock someone into a fight-or-flight state that will not be relieved until the mechanical pressure on the trunk is removed.

- Other problems. Other factors that can interfere with sleep include *sleep apnea*, a breathing disorder; *nocturia*, the need to urinate frequently at night; and *nocturnal myoclonus*, a condition in which the legs involuntarily twitch during sleep, repeatedly waking the person.

SIGNS AND SYMPTOMS

Symptoms of insomnia include general *fatigue* (see this chapter, page 364), reduced ability to focus on mental tasks, slowed reflexes, memory loss, and impaired healing. Prolonged deprivation of REM sleep (the dreaming stage) can even lead to varieties of psychosis.

COMPLICATIONS

Sleep deprivation is a situation that seems harmless enough, but if it is prolonged, it can cause a number of serious consequences. In the short term, lack of sleep creates measurable changes in reflexes, memory capacity, reasoning skills, and the ability to do simple math problems. Lack of sleep is implicated in 200,000 automobile accidents every year, and costs the United States approximately $150 billion every year in costs from absenteeism.

In the long run, insomnia and other sleeping problems are part of the syndromes accompanying clinical depression, *fibromyalgia* (chapter 2, page 50), *chronic fatigue syndrome* (chapter 5, page 229), and chronic pain and injury patterns.

TREATMENT

Treatment for insomnia emphasizes the need for self-help measures: creating a dependable bedtime routine; creating an environment that is conducive to high-quality sleep; and reducing counterproductive activities such as taking caffeine in the afternoon or evening, drinking, or smoking heavily. Sleep-aid medications are considered a last option, because they can be habit forming (see *substance abuse*, this chapter, page 368), and they don't always provide the proper blend of REM and non-REM sleep.

MASSAGE?

Massage is very much indicated for a person experiencing insomnia. One of the finest gifts massage can offer is a good night's sleep, brought about by the restoration of balance between the sympathetic and parasympathetic nervous systems. For insomniac conditions brought about by pain, massage can serve the dual purpose of soothing the sympathetic reaction, while helping to set the stage for optimum healing of the injury, as long as the pain-causing problem does not contraindicate massage.

Postoperative Situations

DEFINITION: WHAT IS IT?

Not so very long ago, most surgeries involved systemic anesthesia, large incisions, and major trauma to the body. These were followed by prolonged hospital stays, and a wide variety of possible complications ranging from infection, to blood clots, to the discovery that a sponge or clamp had been left inside the body.

Today the whole world of surgery has changed with lasers, balloons, and procedures that are conducted with miniature tools through tiny incisions in the skin. Many surgeries that used to involve general anesthesia and hospital stays are now being performed on an outpatient basis, with patients leaving for home on the same day.

POSTOPERATIVE SITUATIONS IN BRIEF

What are they?
Postoperative situations are conditions in which a client is recovering from any kind of surgery.

How are they recognized?
Surgeries may be major and invasive, or they may be conducted through tiny holes in the abdomen or through long tubes inserted into blood vessels to get to a destination far away.

Is massage indicated or contraindicated?
Massage can be appropriate for persons recovering from surgery, depending on the reason for the surgery, and the danger of possible complications.

MASSAGE?

The rapid development of new, less invasive surgical techniques is good news for massage therapists, because the risks involved with open surgery are very serious, and frequently they make doing massage impractical. Obviously, the appropriateness of massage for someone recovering from any kind of surgery depends on the scope and predisposing cause of the surgery, and how much of the body has been affected.

Two major cautions for massage exist with major surgery: immunosuppressant drugs and blood clots (see *thrombi*, chapter 4, page 182). Immunosuppressant drugs are usually used with patients recovering from organ transplants or cancer surgery. Persons taking these drugs are at risk for infection from anyone else's pathogens. It is best to wait until the course of medication is completed before preforming massage.

Blood clots are a lurking threat for anyone who has just been through major surgery. A safe plan is to wait for 6 weeks after the procedure, and to receive clearance from a physician who is familiar with the circulatory impact of massage, before doing any circulatory-based bodywork. Reflexive and energetic work up until then is not only safe and appropriate, but is very welcomed as well.

In the absence of contraindications, carefully applied frictions around the edges of a new scar can have tremendous impact on the localized healing process. It's important not to stretch the skin beyond tolerance, or to work near an open wound. Therapists can also teach their clients how to mobilize their own scar tissue, to minimize hypertrophy and adhesions.

Substance Abuse

DEFINITION: WHAT IS IT?

SUBSTANCE ABUSE IN BRIEF

What is it?
Substance abuse is the use of a material (not necessarily a drug) in methods or dosages for which it was never intended; this use results in damage to the user and other people whom the user contacts.

How is it recognized?
Symptoms of substance abuse depend entirely on what substances are being consumed.

Is massage indicated or contraindicated?
Massage is indicated, with medical supervision, for people who are recovering from substance abuse, under medical supervision. Massage for people with a history of substance abuse but no lasting health problems is also indicated. Massage is contraindicated for people who are intoxicated at the time of their appointment.

Here is a controversial topic: Just what *is* abuse? Are caffeine or sugar inherently less damaging than an illegal substance like cannabis? What's more "abusive," smoking a cigarette or eating a cheese danish? And if a person can get addicted to nasal decongestants (which is very possible), can that be called drug abuse?

The official definition of substance abuse makes no particular distinction between legal and illegal substances. Abuse is simply the use of a substance in ways or dosages that were never intended for that product. The substance is used to modify or control mood or state of mind in a way that is potentially harmful to the user or to other people.

ETIOLOGY: WHAT HAPPENS?

The process of becoming addicted to a particular substance is different for everyone, and is dependent on a long list of risk factors, including genetic predisposition, availability of the substance, peer pressure, coping mechanisms for stress, depression, environmental factors, and the chemical makeup of the substance in question. Typically it begins as experimentation that leads to increasing tolerance, requiring more and more of a particular substance to achieve the same results.

Drug dependence can also arise from the use of substances for medical reasons. The patient's need for the medication sometimes outlives the injury or problem that required the initial prescription. Addiction to painkillers or sleeping pills are examples of this phenomenon.

Substance use becomes dependence when the user continues to take the drug in order to seek out the pleasurable sensations it offers, or to avoid the negative effects of withdrawal, or both. *Psychological* addiction is a dependency on some pleasurable or satisfying sensations that some substance provides. *Physical* addiction is a dependency arising from the need to avoid withdrawal symptoms. Substance abuse is usually a combination of these two factors.

A couple of issues are important to bear in mind in any discussion of substance abuse. One is that even easy-to-get, over-the-counter drugs can change body chemistry, which makes it very hard to cope without them. Nasal decongestants are an excellent example: why should a body's antihistamines do any work if some externally supplied nasal decongestant will do it for them? The difficulty lies in how long it takes to convince the body that no more decongestants will be consumed. The same kinds of dependency can develop with the use of sleeping pills, muscle relaxants, and even some kinds of painkillers.

The other thing to remember is that the body builds up chemical tolerances to most kinds of drugs. That is, it will take more and more decongestant to clear up that stuffy nose, more sleeping pills, more painkillers, more caffeine, and so on. The higher the doses a person needs to feel satisfied, the harder it will be to shake off the dependency.

COMPLICATIONS

Complications of substance abuse depend on the substance in question. They can range from paranoid delusions, to coma, or even to death. Some of the worst effects of drug use are not limited to the users, however. People close to substance abusers also suffer tremendously. Car accidents, industrial accidents, and impaired judgment leading to the spread of AIDS are other complications of substance abuse that affect many people beyond the user.

TREATMENT

As with *alcoholism* (this chapter, page 356), the first and most important step in treating any kind of substance abuse is recognizing that a problem exists. Once a person has reached that point, a number of treatment programs have various rates of success. It often seems to be a matter of finding which program best fits the personality of the patient. Most programs begin with a detoxification process, during which the drugs are expelled from the body. This may be ameliorated with sedatives, tranquilizers, or even less potent versions of the drug in question, until all chemical remnants have been processed out of the body. The length of time this requires varies according to the substance in question.

Detoxification is then followed by a process of rehabilitation, during which the patient is educated about the effects of drug use, and often trained in avoidance behaviors to provide some ammunition against the temptation to return to old habits.

Aftercare may be the most important part of treatment for substance abuse: this gives the patient a support system that will carry him or her throughout a lifetime choice of total drug abstinence. This is the only successful conclusion to drug abuse treatment.

MASSAGE?

In the context of drug abuse, massage has the same rules as it does for alcoholism. Always work under a supervising physician and beware of complications associated with "hard" drug use: staph or strep infections, hepatitis B, AIDS, and heart problems.

Clients who are in long-term recovery and have had no lasting contraindications are good candidates for massage therapy.

Clients who are under the influence at the time of their appointment are contraindicated for massage.

CHAPTER REVIEW QUESTIONS: MISCELLANEOUS CONDITIONS

1. Pick two body systems and describe the effects of alcohol on organs of those systems.

2. Briefly describe the staging process for cancer: what are the stages, and what do they mean?

3. What are the possible risks of massaging a client who is living with cancer?

4. What are the possible benefits of massaging a client who is living with cancer?

5. Describe the circular relationship between mental/emotional fatigue and physical fatigue.

6. Describe the relationship between inadequate sleep and limited capacity to heal from injury.

7. What makes the difference between substance use and substance abuse?

8. Describe the difference between physical addiction and psychological addiction.

9. How have recent innovations in surgical techniques changed the way massage applies to postoperative patients?

10. A client has a small (5 cm) undiagnosed lump on her upper back. It is dense but not painful, and it moves slightly on palpation. What is it most likely to be, and what should a responsible massage therapist do about it?

BIBLIOGRAPHY, MISCELLANEOUS CONDITIONS

General References, Miscellaneous Conditions

1. Carmine D. Clemente. Anatomy: a regional atlas of the human body. 3rd ed. Baltimore: Urban & Schwarzenburg, 1987.

2. I Damjanov. Pathology for the health-related professions. Philadelphia: Saunders, 1996.

3. Giovanni de Dominico, Elizabeth Wood. Beard's massage. Saunders: Philadelphia, 1997.

4. Jeffrey R. M. Kunz, Asher J. Finkel, MD, eds. The American Medical Association family medical guide. New York: Random House, Inc., 1987.

5. Elaine M. Marieb. Human anatomy and physiology. Redwood City, CA: Benjamin/Cummings Publishing Co., Inc., 1989.

6. Ruth Lundeen Memmler, Dina Lin Wood. The human body in health and disease. 5th ed. Philadelphia: JB Lippincott Co., 1983.

7. Mary Lou Mulvihill. Human diseases: a systemic approach. 2nd ed. East Norwalk, CT: Appleton & Lange, 1987.

8. Stedman's medical dictionary. 26th ed. Baltimore: Williams & Wilkins, 1995.

9. Taber's cyclopedic dictionary. 14th ed. Philadelphia: F.A. Davis Company, 1981.

10. Gerard J. Tortora, Nicholas P. Anagnostakos. Principles of anatomy and physiology. 6th ed. New York: Biological Sciences Textbook, Inc., A&P Textbooks, Inc. and Elia-Sparta, Inc., Harper & Row Publishers, Inc., 1990.

Alcoholism

1. Alcoholism. Applied Medical Infomatics Inc., Orbis-AHCN, L.L.C., 1997. URL: http://www.healthanswers.com/health_answers/search_get_answer/scroll_frame. html. Accessed winter 1998.

2. Alcohol dependence, American description. Phillip Long, MD, 1995-1997. URL: http://www.mentalhealth.com/fr04.html. Accessed fall 1997.

3. Alcohol and other drugs in the workplace. National Council on Alcoholism and Drug Dependence, 1996/97/98. Updated March 3, 1998. URL: http://www.ncadd. org/workplac.html. Accessed winter 1998.

4. Alcoholism and alcohol-related problems: A sobering look. National Council on Alcoholism and Drug Dependence, 1996/97/98. Updated March 3, 1998.

URL: http://www.ncadd.org/problems.html. Accessed winter 1998.

Cancer

1. Annette Chamness. Massage therapy and persons living with cancer. Massage Therapy Journal 32(3):53–65.
2. Cancer. Applied Medical Infomatics Inc., Orbis-AHCN, L.L.C., 1997. URL: http://www.healthanswers.com/health_answers/search_get_answer/scroll_frame.html. Accessed winter 1998.
3. MedicineNet: Power points about cancer, causes. Information Network, Inc., 1995-1997. URL: http://www.medicinenet.com. Accessed fall, 1997.
4. MedicineNet: Cancer, detection and treatment. Information Network, Inc., 1995-1997. URL: http://www.medicinenet.com. Accessed fall, 1997.
5. Cancer prevention: Tips to lead a healthy life. Cancer Research Foundation of America. URL: http://www.preventcancer.org/tipps.html. Accessed winter 1998.
6. Rick Weiss. Cancer's vulnerable support system. Washington Post Health Magazine, March 29, 1994, p. 8.
7. Boyce Rensberger. A healthy strain of cannibalism runs through every body. Washington Post, January 1, 1995, p. A3.
8. Gayle MacDonald. Massage for cancer patients: a review of nursing research. Massage Therapy Journal 34(3):53–56.

Insomnia

1. Sleep Disorders. Applied Medical Infomatics Inc., Orbis-AHCN, L.L.C., 1997. URL: http://www.healthanswers.com/health_answers/search_get_answer/scroll_frame.html. Accessed winter 1998.

Substance Abuse

1. Drug abuse and dependence. Applied Medical Infomatics Inc., Orbis-AHCN, L.L.C., 1997. URL: http://www.healthanswers.com/health_answers/search_get_answer/scroll_frame.html. Accessed winter 1998.
2. Diagnosis and treatment of drug abuse in family practice. National Institute on Drug Abuse. Updated January 13, 1998. URL: http://www.nida.nih.gov/Diagnosis_Treatment/Diagnosis1.html. Accessed winter 1998.

Taking a Client History

Appendix 1

Taking a thorough client health history is a delicate art, especially if it's to be done in something under an hour. Many people have uncomplicated backgrounds and simple complaints and disorders, but as massage moves into the medical mainstream, therapists need to be prepared to deal responsibly and professionally with people whose lists of diseases, conditions, accidents, surgeries, and medications can make a person's head swim.

Massage therapists go to school to learn how to touch people in ways that are beneficial to their health. But they also go to massage school to learn whom *not* to touch, or at least not to touch in certain ways. The health history is the first conversation a therapist has with a potential client about his or her body. This is the time to make that all-important judgment about the appropriateness of massage. At some point, most therapists will have to turn someone away, at least temporarily. It's not easy to do, but knowing that, above all, it is for the client's safety and benefit makes it an easier task.

A successful client-therapist relationship is a partnership in which both parties work together toward specific goals. The most important quality for massage therapists to cultivate as they learn how to establish this relationship is careful, patient listening. This skill is a rare one, but it is critical for a successful practice. A massage therapy client puts herself in a very vulnerable, intimate relationship with a virtual stranger. If the therapist is a good listener, who takes in and shows he understands her experiences, that relationship can be one of warmth, safety, and productivity rather than disconnection or even anxiety.

What follows is a sample client history form that might be used in a massage clinic specializing in circulatory-based bodywork. Relevant questions are discussed to see how some answers might influence the decision-making process. Finally, some ideas for creating possible treatment plans are offered.

This is a longer, more detailed intake form than many therapists use, but it can provide a lot of valuable information not only about a client's present status, but about her past and her attitudes about her own health. It is often a good idea to schedule an extra-long appointment for a therapist and client to go through this form together.

It is utterly impossible to create comprehensive guidelines for taking client histories; there are simply too many variables. The way some conditions connect to or hint at others; whether a client is taking various kind of medications; a client's occupation, working conditions, and living conditions; the way sleep, diet, and exercise habits influence overall health; these things may influence the decision about whether certain types of massage may be appropriate, or if, perhaps, the client should seek help elsewhere.

Sample Client History Form

Name
Address
Billing Information

General Information
Age
Occupation
Describe your exercise habits:
Describe your general diet:
Describe how well you sleep:
Describe your general health:

Health History
Describe any surgery or hospitalization:
   More than 10 years ago:
   5 to 10 years ago:
   Less than 5 years ago:
Describe any injuries or accidents:
   More than 10 years ago:
   5 to 10 years ago:
   Less than 5 years ago:
What kind of care did you receive?
Do you consider that you have recovered from these events? Please explain:
Do you have any chronic, ongoing conditions that you deal with on a regular basis?
   Please explain:
Are you taking any medication? Please explain:
Are you currently seeing a doctor for any reason? Please explain:
Do you have any skin rashes or other skin problems right now?
Check off any of the following conditions that you have experienced:

Integumentary	*Musculoskeletal*	*Nervous*
Boils	Fibromyalgia	Multiple sclerosis
Fungal infections	Rheumatoid arthritis	Peripheral neuropathy
Herpes simplex	Osteoarthritis	Post polio syndrome
Warts	TMJ dysfunction	Headaches
Eczema	Strains, sprains or tendinitis	Stroke
Psoriasis	Carpal tunnel syndrome	Seizure disorders
Skin cancer	Thoracic outlet syndrome	Reduced sensation
	Cramping, spasms, soreness	

Circulatory	*Lymph and Immune*	*Digestive*
Anemia	Edema	Cirrhosis
Thrombophlebitis	Hodgkin's disease	Ulcerative colitis
Heart disease	AIDS, HIV	Diverticulosis
High blood pressure	Chronic fatigue syndrome	Gallstones
Varicose veins	Lupus	Hepatitis
Diabetes		Irritable bowel syndrome
Clotting disorders		Ulcers

Respiratory
Asthma
Emphysema
Sinusitis
Tuberculosis

Urinary
Kidney stones

Reproductive
Breast cancer
Endometriosis
Ovarian cysts
Prostate cancer
Painful menstruation
Are you pregnant?

Miscellaneous
Insomnia
Cancer, other than specified above
Alcoholism/substance abuse

Other

Explanation

Treatment plan
Why are you here? What do you hope to accomplish?
Please indicate where you have pain:
(line drawing of human body, front and back)
Describe what you do that causes pain, and what activities tend to make it worse.
What questions do you have about massage or this massage session?
(Disclaimer)
Subjective findings:
Objective findings:
Assessment:
Plan:

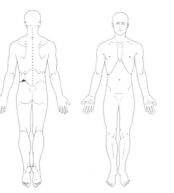

General Questions

Age

Age is a pertinent question because some conditions are particularly prevalent in certain age groups. Of course, it's fairly easy to tell if a client is within a reasonable age expectation for these conditions just by sight, but it's a good idea to get it in writing anyway.

Occupation

This is a key piece of information, particularly for clients who come in with specific pain patterns or injuries they want addressed. This question can lead to a brief discussion of the physical demands that a job may place on a person. The massage therapist should not hesitate to try to "act out" any repetitive or stressful motions a client describes, in an attempt to understand how these activities might contribute to pain and dysfunction.

Exercise, Sleeping, Eating Habits

These descriptions reveal how clients sees their health efforts. This is not the time to pass judgment or make recommendations; it's just a chance to add information to the whole picture.

General Health Description

Many people describe themselves as basically healthy, but seek massage to help them cope with ongoing difficult physical situations. How clients perceive their own health is a useful piece of information.

Health History

Surgeries and Hospitalizations

For convenience, these are broken into three time periods. It's useful to know about past events, because they may influence what's currently happening. However, it's usually more crucial to know what has been going on in more recent history.

Injuries and Accidents

As with surgeries and hospitalizations, recent events are usually more pertinent than ancient history, but the complete picture can reveal important patterns. This question should elicit information about on-the-job injuries, sports injuries, car accidents, and any other kinds of trauma that caused significant pain or loss of function.

Care and Recovery

Follow-up questions about accidents and injuries provide information about clients' perspectives of their healing processes.

Ongoing, Chronic Conditions

This question is asked again in a different way under the check-off list of diseases, but it's always desirable to give clients an extra chance to reveal important information.

Taking Medication

If the answer to this question is yes, it is vitally important to know *why*. If a client is unsure why, then the therapist should arrange a consultation with the primary care physician.

Medications for cardiovascular problems, high blood pressure, and kidney dysfunction, as well as antibiotics, painkillers, muscle relaxants, and antidepressants all have implications for massage. A discussion of why a client may need them, and how to fit massage into the picture, keeps both client and therapist on safe ground.

Seeing a Doctor

If a client is under a doctor's care, she probably has at least a moderately serious condition that massage may influence for better or worse. It is never a bad idea to inform a primary care physician that a particular patient wishes to include massage as part of her healthcare.

Skin Rashes

This self-defensive question for massage therapists is an important part of the health picture. If the answer is yes, again, it's important to know *why*. A skin rash may be just a local caution, or it may suggest that a client needs to reschedule.

Check-Off List

If everything has gone well, nothing will appear on this list that hasn't already been discussed. This is by no means a complete list of every condition a person may contract; the conditions included are chronic, ongoing, or repetitive situations, or they have special significance to massage therapists. This list is simply a model. A therapist's own client history form may include other conditions and may leave out some listed here.

Disclaimer

Many people recommend including a disclaimer explaining that a massage therapist does not diagnose conditions or treat them medically. They may also state that it is the client's responsibility to seek medical care appropriately and to keep the therapist updated on his or her health status.

Treatment Plan

The difference between an outstanding massage therapist and a mediocre one is intention. Good massage therapists always know why they're doing what they're doing, and though those goals and methods may change from moment to moment, the consciousness of working with purpose should always be present. Treatment plans are important tools for therapists and clients. They provide a basis for "before and after" comparisons and reminders of intentions for future work. Even clients who seek massage as a once-in-a-while treat can benefit from the clarification of goals offered by a treatment plan.

A drawing of a human figure that a client can mark with painful spots is a useful visual guide to accompany a therapist's own sensitivities. Some people recommend that a client mark this figure with numbers from 1 to 10, indicating the amount of pain found in certain areas.

Problem areas can change, move, and even disappear. Treatment goals may also change as a person's health status evolves. Having clients redo this portion of the history form every few appointments provides useful progress reports for the client-therapist team.

Some massage therapists use a standard "SOAP" format, outlined below, in addition to the general health information included on a client history. This form can be updated with each appointment or as needed. The format follows:

Subjective Findings

What does the client report: what hurts, where, when, and under what circumstances?

Objective Findings

What does the therapist find compared to the client's descriptions? Does the tissue have varying qualities of elasticity and resilience in different areas? Are hot spots present? Cold areas? Limited range of motion?

Assessment

This is the therapist's interpretation of findings. It is *not* a diagnosis, but rather a pulling together of information to create an understanding of why a client is experiencing particular symptoms.

Plan

This strategy is what the client and therapist will use together to achieve their goals. It might be as simple as, "Swedish massage for relaxation of muscles, improved circulation, and pain relief in upper back," or as complex as, "Cross fiber friction to specific tendon insertions with range of motion gymnastics, followed by ice and a referral to a physical therapist for strengthening exercises in order to overcome chronic tendinitis."

Plans should be updated frequently as the client's needs change.

An Example of a Completed Client History Form

An example of a client intake form follows. This client is a real person, whose past problems recurrently influence her everyday living.

Sample Client History Form

Name *Janet M.*

General Information
Age *34*

Occupation *Accounting. I sit at the computer and am on the phone for 8 hours a day. I have a cordless headset.*

Describe your exercise habits: *I walk 2 times a day, for 15 minutes. Some days are more vigorous than others. From July to October, I coach cheerleading, and I never ask the girls to do something I'm not willing to do.*

Describe your general diet: *I have a quick breakfast: a bagel or something like that. Lunch depends on how busy I am. It could be some yogurt or a microwave meal. Sometimes I have leftovers from last night's supper. Dinner is always a sit-down meal. We eat lots of fruit and veggies.*

Describe how well you sleep: *I usually sleep for 6 hours, but I never feel rested. I can always remember my dreams. I never seem to get past the dream stage.*

Describe your general health: *It's pretty good. I seldom get sick, although it's happened more this year than ever before. I have to make myself do a lot of things; I have very low energy. And depression is a factor in all of this too.*

Health History
Describe any surgery or hospitalization:

   More than 10 years ago: *1988: childbirth, followed by cryosurgery for dysplasia.*

   5 to 10 years ago: *1990: I had a kidney stone while I was pregnant. I finally passed it, soon before my daughter was born. If I hadn't, they would have taken it out right after labor.*

   Less than 5 years ago: *Four years ago I had two surgeries for thoracic outlet syndrome. In the first one they went in through the axilla on the left side. They took out the cervical rib and the first rib. A month later, they did the same thing on the right side, but they only took the first rib. The cervical rib was too small to worry about.*

Describe any injuries or accidents:

   More than 10 years ago: *I was in a VW bug in the middle of a five-car pile up. My little car ended up looking like an accordion.*

   5 to 10 years ago:

   Less than 5 years ago:

What kind of care did you receive?
No care for the whiplash following the car wreck. Lots of physical therapy following my surgeries.
Do you consider that you have recovered from these events? Please explain:
Oh, yes. Before I had surgery, I couldn't even hold my hands above my shoulders.
Do you have any chronic, ongoing conditions that you deal with on a regular basis?
Please explain:
Sure. I have pain, fatigue, stress, depression. Several months ago I was diagnosed with fibromyalgia.
Are you taking any medication? Please explain:
I take Zoloft, an antidepressant.
Are you currently seeing a doctor for any reason? Please explain:
Yes, I see an MD for fibromyalgia and a chiropractor as needed.
Do you have any skin rashes or other skin problems right now?
No.
Check off any of the following conditions that you have experienced:

Integumentary
Boils
Fungal infections
Herpes simplex
Warts
Eczema
Psoriasis
Skin cancer

Musculoskeletal
✓ Fibromyalgia
Rheumatoid arthritis
Osteoarthritis
TMJ dysfunction
Strains, sprains or tendinitis
Carpal tunnel syndrome
✓ Thoracic outlet syndrome
✓ Cramping, spasms, soreness

Nervous
Multiple sclerosis
Peripheral neuropathy
Post polio syndrome
✓ Headaches
Stroke
Seizure disorders
Reduced sensation

Circulatory
Anemia
Thrombophlebitis
Heart disease
High blood pressure
Varicose veins
Diabetes
Clotting disorders

Lymph and Immune
Edema
Hodgkin's disease
AIDS, HIV
✓ Chronic fatigue syndrome
Lupus

Digestive
Cirrhosis
Ulcerative colitis
Diverticulosis
Gallstones
Hepatitis
✓ Irritable bowel syndrome
Ulcers

Respiratory
Asthma
Emphysema
Sinusitis
Tuberculosis

Urinary
✓ Kidney stones

Reproductive
Breast cancer
Endometriosis
Ovarian cysts
Prostate cancer
Painful menstruation
Are you pregnant?

Miscellaneous
Insomnia
Cancer, other than specified above
Alcoholism/substance abuse

Other: *My hands swell up at night. I had severe dizziness and headaches for several months at the onset of the fibromyalgia.*

Explanation: *Chronic fatigue and irritable bowel syndrome are part of the fibromyalgia.*

Treatment plan:
Why are you here? What do you hope to accomplish?
I was told this would help with stress and muscle pain.

Please indicate where you have pain:
(See attached figure.)

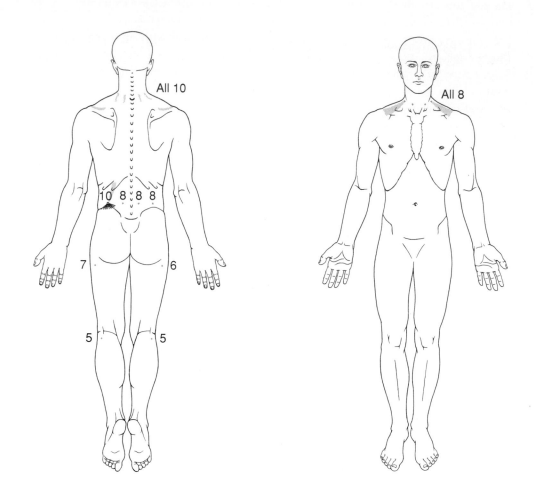

Describe what you do that causes pain, and what activities tend to make it worse:
At the onset of my fibromyalgia, I was working full time, I went to school two nights a week, I was on the PTA and helped to run Brownies. I've found that overdoing in general makes everything much worse, but so does doing nothing. I also have to be careful about over-exercising.
What questions do you have about massage or this massage session?
How bad is it going to hurt, and how often should I do it?

Subjective Findings

These are recorded on the image of the human body, above.

Objective Findings

Janet's tissues are generally mobile and elastic superficially, although there is a sense of brittleness or fragility when the deeper layers are palpated. Circulation is good. The area over and above the scapula on the right side is particularly unyielding; it feels like a piece of cardboard under skin. By the end of our time together, it had begun to give, but just a little.

When she lies supine, Janet's shoulders rise up off the table by several inches. The tissue on the anterior aspect of the shoulder girdle is tender and not clearly definable through touch.

Assessment

I suspect that as a result of Janet's thoracic outlet surgery, her pectoralis minor and major are bound up with significant scar tissue. This accounts for the rolling of the shoulders anteriorly, and the chronic pain she feels in her upper back—she marked these areas with "10"s on her chart. I wouldn't be at all surprised if her diagnosis of fibromyalgia is related to the muscular imbalances caused by her surgeries, although the headaches and dizziness she experienced may be connected to a different aspect of that disease.

Plan

I recommend regular sessions (every week or every other week, depending on time constraints) of gentle Swedish massage, focusing on the muscular relationships surrounding the shoulder girdle: pec minor and major, the deltoid, trapezius, rhomboids, levator scapulae, etc.

I encourage Janet to do the exercises taught by her physical therapist to stretch the anterior shoulder girdle muscles.

I plan to focus on the paraspinals and quadratus lumborum, perhaps in relationship to the iliopsoas, in future appointments.

I plan to work slowly and conservatively, and to encourage Janet to drink a lot of water following each appointment to minimize any soreness that may follow.

Massage therapists work with a physical intimacy unmatched by practically any other healthcare professional. How many health professionals, outside of surgeons, spend an hour or more devoting the sum total of their concentration and focus, as well as their touch, to the well-being of their clients?

Working in physically intimate circumstances carries the risk of spreading infection. Infection can move from the therapist to the client, but also from the client to the therapist (who can transfer it to the next client and so on). For this reason, massage therapists should be familiar with the most common types of infectious agents, in order to recognize them when possible, and to guard against always.

The Centers for Disease Control (CDC) developed a series of criteria to prevent the spread of AIDS and other communicable diseases for people working in close contact with others. These guidelines, called Universal or Standard Precautions, provide instructions regarding the use of disposable gloves, gowns, and masks, as well as protocols for dealing with needles and the disposal of blood-contaminated items.

Most massage therapists are not working with bleeding wounds, hypodermic needles, or mouth-to-mouth resuscitation. It's not practical to use gloves every time we work with a client, nor is it desirable. But, in order to be prepared for every eventuality, massage therapists should be well-conversant with the principles of Universal Precautions. Because these protocols are subject to frequent change, the best place to get up-to-date information is from a local Health Department or Board of Health.

The guidelines given in this section may be more conservative than most practicing therapists currently observe. Massage is a quickly growing profession, however, and massage therapists will be increasingly at risk for professional liability if stringent standards for cleanliness and professionalism are not followed.

This discussion focuses on three aspects of keeping therapists and clients healthy: the infectious agents to guard against, methods by which to keep free of infection, and practical applications for massage therapists.

Infectious Agents

Millions of pathogens exist to make people sick. The groups discussed here are not comprehensive, but this section covers the most common agents in industrialized countries. They include bacteria, viruses, fungi, and animal parasites.

Bacteria

Colonies of bacteria grow on everyone's skin. Hosts don't usually become sick, because their immune system develops resistance to resident pathogens, and intact skin is a powerful barrier. But clients, especially clients who are in any way immune-suppressed, won't be so resistant to a therapist's personal colonies of bacteria. Therefore, it is important to avoid touching areas where the skin is not intact: these lesions are an infection waiting to happen.

Bacteria are divided into *saprophytes* (the "good guys" that live off of dead material) and *parasites* (the "bad guys" that live off of living material, such as human bodies). Parasitical bacteria include the following groups:

Cocci

Cocci, round-shaped bacteria, appear in these configurations:

* *Staphylococcus* bacteria are shaped like bunches of grapes. They are responsible for most local skin infections, boils, and acne.
* *Streptococcus* bacteria occur in chains. They cause many systemic infections such as strep throat and blood poisoning.
* *Gonococcus* bacteria cause gonorrhea.
* *Diplococcus* bacteria cause bacterial pneumonia.

Staphylococcus and streptococcus are the two most important cocci-type bacteria to know about. These have mutated into thousands of tough varieties that can be difficult to treat.

Other Bacteria

Other types of bacteria are less common, but it's a good idea to be familiar with them. They include:

* Bacilli. These rod-shaped bacteria are spore-makers. They have a tough outer shell to protect them from the environment and many chemicals that would kill other bacteria. Bacilli bacteria are responsible for tuberculosis, typhoid, tetanus, and diptheria.
* Spirochetes. This group of spiral-shaped bacteria includes the agent that causes syphilis.

Viruses

Viruses are not, technically speaking, alive. They are tiny (much smaller than bacteria) collections of proteins with genetic coding. Once inside a host cell, the virus changes the cell to function as a virus factory. When that factory becomes full of inventory, it ruptures, releasing the new viruses to search for new host cells.

Viruses outside of bodies usually disintegrate fairly quickly. Some of them, however, are tougher to get rid of than others. The two main adversaries of massage therapists are herpes simplex and hepatitis B.

* *Herpes simplex* causes oral and genital herpes. A sturdy virus, it can linger on tables, doorknobs, and other surfaces for several hours. It is highly contagious in the acute (blistering) stage. If a client has fever blisters or suspicious sores around the thighs and buttocks, consider them at least a local contraindication, and isolate sheets, face pads, or other equipment in a special laundry container for bleaching.
* *Hepatitis B* is not easy to catch (it requires some sort of intimate contact or fluid exchange), but it has a serious impact on the body and is strongly associated with liver cancer. Hepatitis B is transmissible through shared fluid, including saliva, lymph, and blood. The virus is extremely sturdy and very virulent. It is the leading killer of nurses in this country. In some places, it's considered to be an epidemic.

A vaccine for hepatitis B is available. People in blood-exposure professions are required to get it, and massage therapists can, too.

Fungi

Chief fungal enemies are dermatophytes, specifically the fungi that cause tinea corporis (body ringworm), tinea capitis (head ringworm), or tinea cruris (jock itch). Tinea lesions appear as red, slightly raised rings on the skin. They are very common, and very contagious, especially for people with weak immune systems.

Fungal infections can have a gestation period of 2 to 3 weeks, during which time the infected person can transmit the fungus to others. This means if a massage therapist is exposed to ringworm, he or she may have to take a 3-week vacation, to prevent the possibility of spreading the infection to other clients.

Athlete's foot is a different type of fungal infection and is also at least a local contraindication for massage.

Animal Parasites

Three main species of animal parasites are important to consider:

- Head lice. These arthropods live on the scalp. They spread from one person to another very easily, either by jumping from one head to the next, or by lurking on coat hooks, chair backs, or in shared hats. Lice are often identified by the presence of nits, the white lice eggs, which cling to hair shafts.
- Crab lice. These are close relatives of head lice. They usually live in pubic hair, but can also be found in body hair, eyebrows, and lashes. They drink blood and cause a lot of itching. Crab lice usually spread through intimate contact, as in sharing a bed or massage sheets.
- Scabies. These lesions are caused by microscopic mites that burrow under the skin, drinking blood, laying eggs, and leaving behind irritating wastes. They can be hard to diagnose because the actual parasites are not always picked up in skin samples. Scabies lesions are itchy, especially at night, and they often appear in warm, sweaty places such as the groin, armpits, crooks of elbows and knees, and between fingers and toes.

Consider the sheets and other linens of any client who shows signs of parasitical infestation as "hot." Separate them from other sheets, wash them in hot water with extra bleach (1 cup per wash), and dry them in a hot dryer, rather than hanging them on a line.

Aseptic Methods: Keeping Free from Infection

Asepsis means absence of infection. Aseptic methods are techniques to keep massage therapists and their clients as safe as possible from infectious agents.

Antiseptics

Antiseptic substances are the weakest of the aseptic methods. They create a hostile environment for many bacteria, but they may not actually kill them. Antiseptics are ineffective against bacteria encased in spores as well as many viruses. Antiseptics are safe to use on skin. Some antiseptics (rubbing alcohol, iodine, hydrogen peroxide) used to be considered disinfectants (a stronger class of germ-killer), but now, because germs have become so much tougher, they no longer dependably kill what they used to.

Antiseptics include:

- Hand soap. Some hand soaps include special germ-killers in their formulae. These may increase the soap's effectiveness at killing easily accessible pathogens, but this doesn't mean hands washed with special "antiseptic soap" are completely germ-free.
- Rubbing alcohol. Rubbing alcohol works best in a 70% solution (as it is packaged) because a 100% solution makes the germs' membranes thicker and less permeable. Rubbing alcohol is effective against bacteria, but not viruses or spores.
- Hydrogen peroxide. This mild antiseptic is used in 3% solution for skin and mucus membranes.

Disinfectants

These agents should be effective against all viruses and bacteria except those with spores, e.g., tuberculosis. Many disinfectants are marketed with target pathogens. They can also be called *germicides* or *bactericides*.

Disinfectants and disinfecting methods are too strong to use on skin, but as a rule, they *don't* kill spores. Examples include:

- Bleach. A 10% solution for surfaces, 1 cup per wash for laundry. Bleach is effective against staph, strep, fungus, hepatitis, HIV, and herpes. It is still the industry standard for disinfecting most surfaces.
- Phenol. A 10% solution of phenol can be used for surfaces. It is caustic to skin and lungs. Phenol is effective against bacteria, fungus, herpes, and flu virus.
- Quats, or Quaternary Ammonium Compounds. These substances are available through medical or janitorial supply outlets. Although they are useful for killing pathogens, they don't necessarily remove dirt or other debris. Quats are used for "cold sterilization" of items that can't be subjected to an autoclave.
- Boiling. When boiling, an item should be completely immersed in water at 212°F for 20 minutes. Even this may not kill all spores and heat-resistant microbes, which is why it's considered a disinfectant measure rather than a sterilizer.

Sterilization

These methods kill every living thing within a field. Massage therapists cannot sterilize themselves or their clients, but they can sterilize some of their tools and work surfaces, if absolutely necessary. Sterilization methods include:

- Baking. 350°F, one hour.
- Autoclave (steam cabinet). Items should be under 15 p.s.i., at 250°F for 30 minutes.

Note: Microwave ovens don't sterilize items because the heat is unevenly distributed.

Practical Applications for Massage Therapists

Massage therapists should be especially aware of the dangers of pathogens and parasites. They carry the risk of contracting disease themselves, and of spreading disease from client to client. It is important for massage therapists to use aseptic methods wisely and regularly.

Personal Cleanliness

- Washing hands. It's impossible to say this too often. Hands should be washed between clients and after handling tissues or other bodily fluid–bearing items. Remember, cold and flu viruses are transmitted by hands far more efficiently than by floating randomly in the air.
- Liquid soap is easier to dispense hygienically than bar soap, which can harbor pathogens. The *friction* of hands rubbing together is the most important part of handwashing; this should occur for 15 seconds or more (some people recommend singing a chorus of "Yankee Doodle" to be sure that adequate time is spent). The faucet should then be turned off with a clean paper towel.
- Keep fingernails short and clean. Imagine receiving a massage from someone with longish or slightly dirty nails. How relaxed could a person be, imagining all those cooties crawling around on his skin?
- Attend to clothing. Uniforms, jackets, or aprons should be scrupulously clean. If during a massage, the client's skin comes in contact with the therapist's clothing (for instance, when arms are being treated), then that clothing should be treated in the same way as sheets. Care should be taken so that one client doesn't come in contact with cloth or materials that may have been contaminated by a previous client.
- Broken skin. Broken skin is an open invitation to infection. Massage therapists should avoid it on their clients and keep it covered on themselves. Rubber "finger cots" are extremely useful items when a therapist has a scraped knuckle or a hangnail. Of course, these coverings should be changed with each client.

Linen

Laws regarding linen storage for healthcare professionals vary from state to state. Some states require professionals to store their dirty linen in closed containers, and clean linen in closed cabinets. It's a good idea to have a second container available for "hot" sheets that need to be treated with special care. In addition to sheets, a massage therapist's laundry may include uniforms or aprons, pillowcases, face hole covers, heating pad covers, towels, bolster covers, and anything else that touches a client's skin.

Beware of stuffing oily sheets into baskets or boxes and letting them sit; oil will go rancid and smell, and it has been known to spontaneously combust. The moral: wash sheets promptly!

Some massage therapists or clinics hire a laundry service to take care of their linens. In this case, sheets will probably be rented from the service. These sheets are typically washed and rinsed repeatedly at 180°F. They are bleached and then subjected to antibleachers to reduce the chemical aftermath. Even so, some people may have a reaction to the chemicals left in the fabric.

Extra blankets, mattress pads, sheepskins, and so forth, don't need to be washed every time *unless* they come in direct contact with clients. It's a good idea to wash them once a month or so anyway, just for freshness.

Storage and Dispensation of Oil, Lotion, Creams, and Other Lubricants

All lubricants need to be kept in clean containers, and dispensed in a way that prevents contamination. For instance, if a therapist has a tub of coconut oil, she must dip out what she's going to use into a paper cup (using a spatula, not her fingers). Then she must *not* put the leftovers back into the tub—they are contaminated and must be thrown away.

Remember, if a client has a contagious condition (herpes, for example), the therapist may transmit the virus to the outside of her oil bottle. That same oil bottle may be used for the next client, and the virus is lurking on the surface just waiting for a chance to get back on another potential host's skin. In other words, it's a good idea to wash oil bottles while washing hands.

Care of Massage Tables and Other Equipment

If a client who shows signs of a communicable disease has been on a table, it's time to swab. Some states and municipalities mandate swabbing a table after every client anyway; check with the local Board of Health. Rubbing alcohol or a 10% bleach solution are the standards, though they can be drying to vinyl and of questionable impact against sturdy viruses such as herpes and hepatitis B. (They will remove those annoying oily handprints, though.) Regardless, it's a good habit to swab the table once a week, especially the face cradle. Rinsing the table with water afterwards may save the vinyl from the worst effects of the chemical wash.

Any other surfaces that clients contact should be regularly cleaned. Most things, for example, heat or cold packs, are probably covered by cloth that can be laundered, but therapists must be ever-vigilant against possible contaminated surfaces.

Endangerments

Endangerment sites are locations where massage therapists can cause damage to some of the body's most delicate tissues. Structures particularly at risk are nerves, blood vessels, organs, and lymph nodes. This list covers the most basic endangerment sites, although if a massage therapist is not careful, he or she could cause injury to almost any part of the body.

The easiest way practitioners can damage delicate tissues is to pin or pinch them against some hard surface, usually a bone. Called "entrapment," this can result in bruising, irritating, or otherwise damaging a vulnerable structure.

Nerves

Pinning or compressing nerves will cause sharp shooting, tingling, electric, or hot sensations. It's important to know the pathways of the most vulnerable nerves because, unfortunately, massage therapists can't always count on clients, some of whom *expect* massage to hurt, to give accurate feedback about whether the pain they're feeling is good pain or bad pain.

Blood Vessels

The general risk of arterial entrapment is the blocking of circulation, causing numbness, discomfort, and even blackouts. Entrapment of veins, since they are weaker, can injure them, creating varicosities, hemorrhages, or clots.

Organs

A few organs can be trapped and impaired by massage therapy. They are generally at risk because they are close to the surface, or they are anchored in a way that makes them vulnerable to being pinned or compressed.

Lymph Nodes

Lymph nodes are constructed of epithelial cells within a connective tissue framework. They are especially palpable when they are inflamed. The ability to feel lymph nodes, especially around the neck or the back of the head, often indicates that they are working overtime, and the client may be fighting off an infection.

Head and Face Endangerments

Eyes

Obviously, eyes are a local caution for massage. Special care must also be taken with clients who wear contact lenses. If a client wears hard lenses, the therapist should suggest that they be removed during a treatment (potential problems include drying out and lacerations to the sclera). If a client wears soft or extended wear contacts, removing them usually isn't necessary.

Some therapists keep a bottle of distilled water and a lens case in their office, just in case a client decides to remove his or her contact lenses while there.

Nerve Foramina

The skull has three pairs of foramina where the *mental*, the *infraorbital*, and the *supraorbital* nerves exit to supply the face with sensation and motor control. Heavy pressure on these spots can be extremely painful, and may even damage the nerves as they emerge. See Figure End-1.

Temporomandibular Joint (TMJ)

Branches of both the trigeminal and the facial nerves are accessible near the TMJ. Whether or not massage therapy could actually *cause* an attack of Bell's palsy or trigemi-

Figure End-1. Head profile

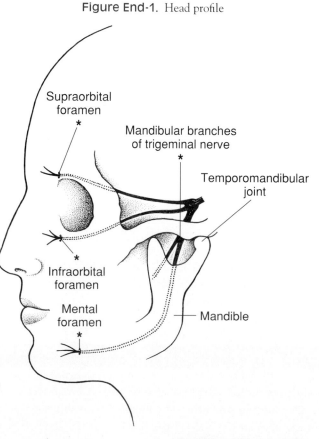

*Possible endangerment

nal neuralgia is not clear, but every therapist is responsible to know how to avoid even the possibility of putting a client at risk for these problems.

This is not to imply that the whole TMJ area and jaw muscles are off limits to massage. On the contrary, massage can be important to reduce habitual muscle tone in persons prone to jaw-clenching. But massage practitioners who work in this area must know where the nerves are vulnerable, and how to avoid putting them at risk. See Figure End-1.

Anterior Trunk and Neck Endangerments

For all structures in the anterior triangle of the neck and the anterior trunk, see Figure End-2.

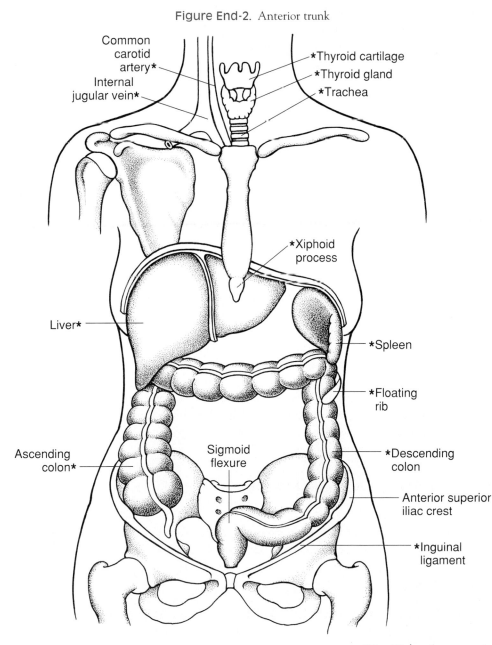

Figure End-2. Anterior trunk

Common carotid artery*

Internal jugular vein*

*Thyroid cartilage
*Thyroid gland
*Trachea

*Xiphoid process

Liver*

*Spleen

*Floating rib

Ascending colon*

Sigmoid flexure

*Descending colon

Anterior superior iliac crest

*Inguinal ligament

*Possible endangerments

Anterior Triangle of the Neck

The anterior triangle of the neck is defined by the sternal fibers of the left and right sternocleidomastoid muscles, and the mandible. Many structures contained in this area are vulnerable to damage, and most musculature is not easily accessible for massage. Some therapists make a specialty of working on the muscles of the anterior neck with good results, but they, along with all other massage practitioners, must be very familiar with the complicated anatomy of this area in order to stay out of harm's way. Structures in the anterior triangle of the neck that must be respected include:

Common Carotid Artery

This huge artery runs deep to the sternocleidomastoid muscles and carries most of the blood supply to the head. About level with the thyroid cartilage, the common carotid artery splits into the internal and external carotid artery. The point of division, the *carotid sinus*, is equipped with special sensory nerves that measure blood pressure in order to maintain appropriate blood flow to the head. External pressure applied here can alter that blood flow, leading to dizziness and faintness.

Jugular Vein

The jugular vein lies superficial to the common carotid. It is less vulnerable to damage, but still should not be stretched or compressed in any way.

Trachea

This cartilaginous tube is part of the respiratory system, and leads to the lungs. It is quite strong and resilient, but pressure directly on the tube will cause a choking sensation for the client.

Thyroid Cartilage

The thyroid cartilage is a moveable piece of material that bobs up and down with swallowing. The most prominent part of the thyroid cartilage is the laryngeal prominence, or "Adam's apple."

Thyroid Gland

The thyroid gland is a butterfly-shaped organ that wraps around the trachea. It is an endocrine gland, secreting hormones that control metabolism. Embedded within the thyroid gland are much smaller parathyroid glands. This whole structure is primarily epithelial, with little connective tissue protection.

Brachial Plexus: Neck and Shoulder

The brachial plexus is made up of spinal nerves C_5 to T_1. They crisscross and interweave with each other before separating into the different nerves that supply the arm. Specific pathways of the brachial plexus are discussed in the "Arm Endangerments" section of this appendix.

Xiphoid Process

The inferior edge of the sternum has a small piece of bone that protrudes out over the liver. This prominence, the xiphoid process, can be broken off if sharp, downward pressure is exerted on it.

Floating Ribs

Massage is unlikely to actually damage floating ribs. Tracing or outlining the ribcage can cause ticklishness or even pain if a therapist doesn't know exactly where the floating ribs are, and how to avoid pinning soft tissue against them.

Liver

A massage therapist would have to be working much too deep and much harder than is usually called for in order to bruise a healthy liver. However, it's good to know both where it's located and its size.

Spleen

The spleen is tucked up way under the left ribs. For most people, the spleen isn't a significant endangerment, but if it is enlarged for any reason, the whole area may be uncomfortable.

Colon

The colon is at special risk for entrapment and bruising, because it is anchored at the flexures, and cannot simply move out of the way like the small intestine can. Care must be taken, when doing deep abdominal work, to respect both that the colon can be pinned, and that material should move through it in a clockwise direction. Pressure should not be exerted contrary to this direction of flow.

Ovaries

Normally, the ovaries are located low and central in the pelvis and are inaccessible to massage therapists. Sometimes, though, endometriosis, an ovarian cyst, or other anomaly causes the ovaries to move into areas where they may be pinned and bruised.

Posterior Trunk and Neck Endangerments

See Figure End-3.

Kidneys

The kidneys are vulnerable to damage because they are only partially protected by the rib cage. The right kidney sits a bit lower than the left; an easy way to remember this is that it looks like the right kidney is pushed downward by the liver. Both can be bruised if vigorous tapotement is performed over the midback area.

Spinous Processes

These are listed as endangerments because massage therapists can cause pain by pressing on or causing friction to paraspinal muscles in *toward* the spinous processes, rather than out and away from them. Pressure toward the spine can be appropriate, as long as soft tissues aren't being impaled or ground into hard ones.

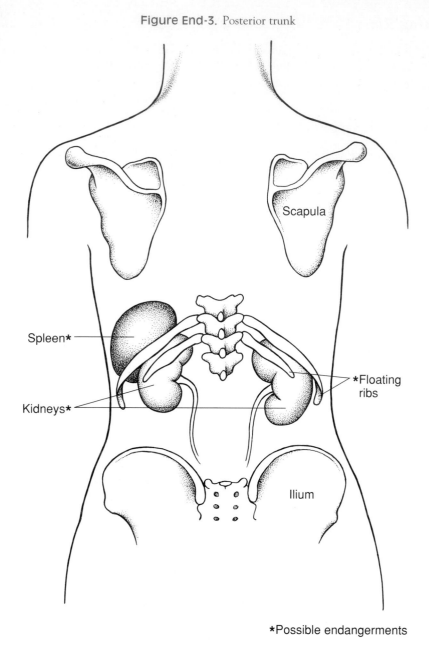

Figure End-3. Posterior trunk

Spleen*

*Floating ribs

Kidneys*

Scapula

Ilium

*Possible endangerments

Arm Endangerments

See Figure End-4

Brachial Plexus: Neck

The brachial plexus nerves emerge from C₅ to T₁ and intercommunicate with each other before separating into the five different nerves. Most of this interweaving happens between the neck and the shoulder. The nerves run between the medial and posterior scalene muscles, under the clavicle and coracoid process, and then wrap around the humerus. They are larger than they seem; coming out of the neck, they are actually about as thick as shoelaces. They can be pinned against several different bones or other tissues on their way to the arm, so massage therapists should be familiar with the pathways of the brachial plexus nerves.

Figure End-4. Anterior arm/shoulder

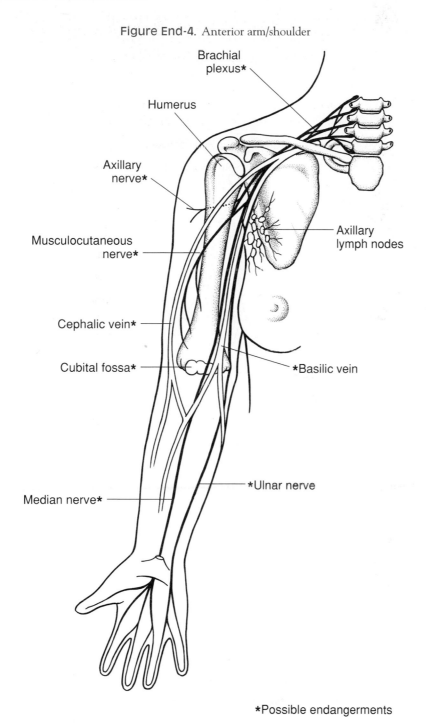

Brachial
plexus*

Humerus

Axillary
nerve*

Musculocutaneous
nerve*

Cephalic vein*

Cubital fossa*

Median nerve*

Axillary
lymph nodes

*Basilic vein

*Ulnar nerve

*Possible endangerments

Brachial Plexus: Arm

By the time the brachial plexus has reached the arm, it has separated into its five different components: the *axillary, musculocutaneous, radial, median,* and *ulnar* nerves. It is useful to know the basic pathways of all these structures, although they may vary slightly
from one person to another. Specific endangerment spots include the axilla, the medial
aspect of the upper arm, and the cubital fossa. The ulnar nerve is vulnerable around the
olecranon: it causes the "funny bone" sensation when it's knocked or irritated. See Figure End-5.

Figure End-5. Posterior arm/shoulder

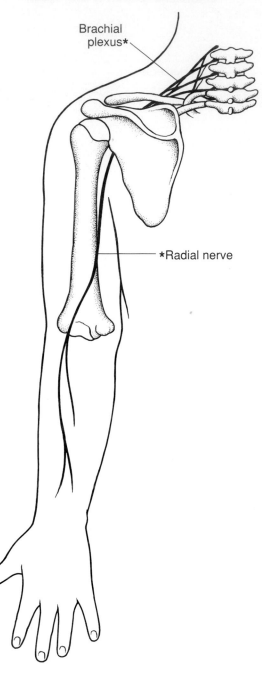

Brachial plexus*

*Radial nerve

Axillary Lymph Nodes

Lymph nodes should not be specifically isolated or massaged. They have the important job of filtering pathogens from the tissues, and should be left alone.

Cephalic and Basilic Veins

Veins, perhaps more than any other structure discussed, run in unique pathways from one person to the next, so it is impossible to state categorically where they might be vulnerable. One thing is consistent, however: they run at least partway up the medial side of the upper arm. Conveniently, this is an area inappropriate for deep, specific massage because some of the brachial plexus nerves are also vulnerable here. The cephalic vein can also be trapped with specific pressure where it runs along the edges of the anterior deltoid and pectoralis major.

Leg Endangerments

Femoral Triangle

The femoral triangle, defined by the inguinal ligament, the sartorius muscle, and the medial aspect of the leg, is a particularly rich area for vulnerable structures. The femoral artery and vein are both accessible here, as are the inguinal lymph nodes and the femoral nerve. Deep, specific work on the adductors must be conducted with special care in order to avoid damaging these structures. See Figure End-6.

Sciatic Nerve

The sciatic nerve, the thickest nerve in the body, runs through the deep lateral rotators and down the back of the leg where it splits into the common peroneal nerve and the tibial nerve. The sciatic nerve is difficult to pin or damage because the musculature sur-

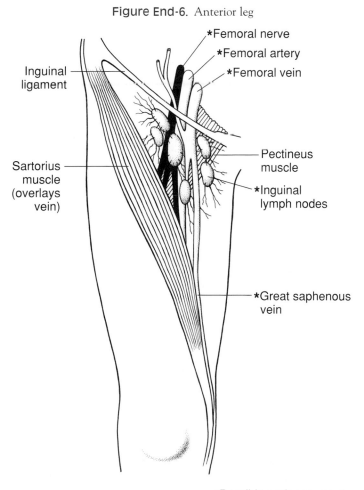

Figure End-6. Anterior leg

Inguinal ligament

*Femoral nerve
*Femoral artery
*Femoral vein

Sartorius muscle (overlays vein)

Pectineus muscle

*Inguinal lymph nodes

*Great saphenous vein

*Possible endangerments

rounding it is so thick, but if the nerve is irritated for any reason, massage may exacerbate the situation. See Figure End-7.

Popliteal Fossa

The popliteal fossa is the area on the posterior aspect of the knee that is defined by the heads of the gastrocnemius below, and the edges of the biceps femoris and the semitendinosus above. Several vulnerable structures exist in this hollow, including the small saphenous vein, the popliteal vein, the popliteal artery, and the lower branches of the sciatic nerve: the tibial and common peroneal nerves. See Figure End-7.

Figure End-7. Posterior leg

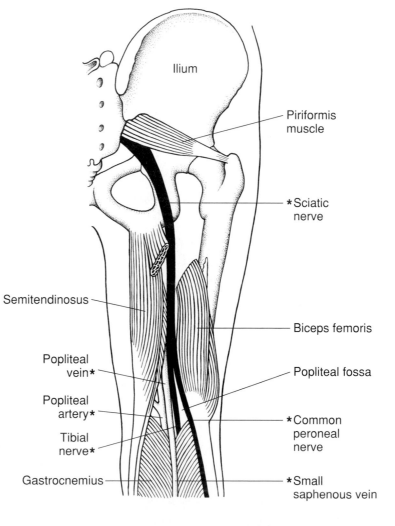

Ilium

Piriformis muscle

*Sciatic nerve

Semitendinosus

Biceps femoris

Popliteal vein*

Popliteal fossa

Popliteal artery*

*Common peroneal nerve

Tibial nerve*

Gastrocnemius

*Small saphenous vein

*Possible endangerments

Great Saphenous Vein

The great saphenous vein runs up the medial side of the calf where nothing protects it from being pinned to the tibia. On the upper leg, the vein runs along the edge of the sartorius, but the quadriceps are bulky enough that pinning the great saphenous to the femur is not generally possible. See Figure End-6 and Figure End-8.

Figure End-8. Medial leg

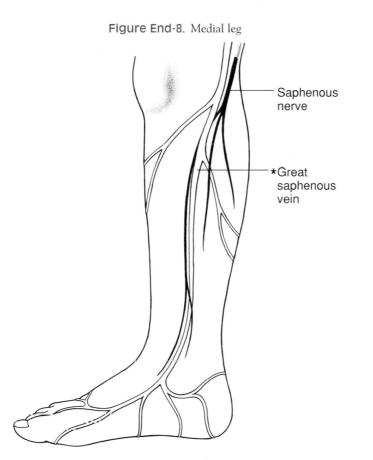

Saphenous nerve

*Great saphenous vein

*Possible endangerments

Common Peroneal Nerve

The common peroneal nerve is vulnerable for a short distance, just inferior to the head of the fibula. Specific pressure or friction on the peroneus longus can sometimes irritate this nerve, which will send shocky, electrical sensations down into the foot. See Figure End-9.

Figure End-9. Lateral leg

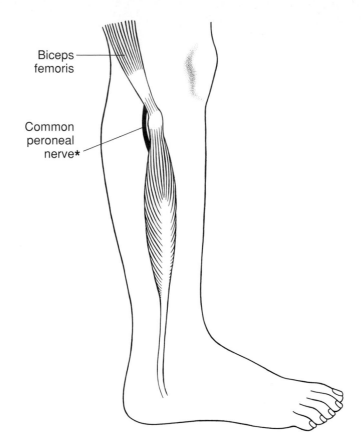

Biceps femoris

Common peroneal nerve*

*Possible endangerments

Chapter Objectives and Chapter Review Answers

Appendix 4

Introduction

Taking tests and answering questions can be a stressful business. Although it may be hard to remember sometimes, the chapter objectives and review questions have been included in this text to make your lives easier, not more difficult. They do not require comprehensive knowledge of every conceivable fact. Instead, they are a means to determine if you have achieved a basic level of mastery of this material.

The answers provided in this appendix are drawn directly from the text and include all of the applicable information found there. For example, if a question reads, "List four causes of kidney stones," many more than four possibilities are discussed in the text, and the answer provided here has more than four variations.

Please be aware, however, that the text itself is not a comprehensive discussion of every possible variation of every conceivable disease or condition. Perfectly correct answers may exist for some of these questions even though they are not specifically addressed in the text. They may not be listed here, but that doesn't make them less accurate.

Chapter Objectives: Integumentary System Conditions

Tell why massage is contraindicated in the presence of broken skin.

Broken skin indicates a compromise in the immune "shield." Even lesions covered by scabs are vulnerable to infection.

Name three differences between a boil and acne.

Like acne, boils are staphylococcus infections of sebaceous glands clogged by dirt, dead skin cells, and/or other debris. But in this case, the staph is not simply taking advantage of a stagnant pool of oil, but actively attacking living tissue. Boils tend to occur one at a time instead of being spread over large areas. And finally, boils are much more contagious than acne.

Name three variations on fungal infections of the skin.

Tinea corporis (body ringworm); tinea capitis (head ringworm); tinea cruris (jock itch); and tinea pedis (athlete's foot) are all fungal infections.

Name what kind of bacteria are usually associated with boils and acne.

The staphylococcus family bacteria are primarily responsible for boils and acne.

Name what kind of bacteria are usually associated with erysipelas.

The streptococcus family of bacteria are primarily responsible for erysipelas.

Name two dangers associated with widespread burns.

If a significant amount of skin is damaged by burns, it will be unable to accomplish its protective tasks: it *won't* provide a shield from microbial invasion; it *won't* help to maintain a stable temperature; and perhaps most importantly, it *won't* provide protection from fluid loss. This opens the door to a number of complications, including loss of water, plasma, and plasma proteins, which will lead to shock.

Name three dangers associated with long-term use of corticosteroid creams.

Steroid creams can cause their own "steroid rash," or they can quell macrophage action, which makes users prone to boils.

Also, a "backlash" effect may occur: after the use of steroidal creams is stopped, the original complaint can come back in a more extreme version.

If steroid creams are used over a long period of time (several months), permanent changes will be brought about by exposure to a substance that melts connective tissue: the skin can become thin, delicate, and easily damaged.

Finally, in a worst case scenario, the adrenal glands can suffer damage, which can be life-threatening.

Name the ABCDEs of melanoma.

A: Asymmetrical: Most benign moles are circular or oval. A melanoma has an indeterminate shape.

B: Border: The borders of melanomas are irregular and may be indistinct as it goes into the skin.

C: Color: The colors of most moles are consistent: they are brown or black, but not both. Melanomas are typically multicolored, with brown, black, and even purple all mixed together.

D: Diameter: Melanomas are large. Any mole that is bigger than 5 mm across should be examined by a dermatologist.

E: Elevated: Melanomas are usually at least partly elevated from the skin. They may even be big enough to snag on things and bleed.

Name the cardinal sign of non-melanoma skin cancer.

The most important sign of non-melanoma skin cancer is a sore or lesion on the skin that never completely heals. A scab may form and fall off to reform again, but the wound never closes.

Name a feature that distinguishes plantar warts from calluses.

Plantar warts are distinguishable from corns and calluses because they tend *not* to be bilateral, and they tend to have a speckled appearance from blood in their dilated capillaries. Corns and calluses have no blood source, so they are just white.

Chapter Review Questions:
Integumentary System Conditions

1. Describe the relationship between cortisol depletion and allergies.

   When people undergo long-term stress, their cortisol supplies can become depleted. When cortisol is depleted, limited resources within the body are available to quell the inflammatory reaction. For the person subject to allergies, this means that they have a difficult time de-inflaming from immune system attacks against non-threatening stimuli, such as wheat, pollen, cat dander, or anything else.

2. A client has eczema on her hands that is extremely dry and flaky. Does this condition indicate or contraindicate massage? Why?

   Dry, flaky eczema indicates massage locally as long as the skin is intact: that is, no cracking or oozing is present. It's a good idea, with clients like this, to use a hypoallergenic type of oil.

3. A client has severe ichthyosis that is cracked and oozing. Does this condition indicate or contraindicate massage? Why?

   Any kind of skin condition that results in cracking or oozing at least locally contraindicates massage.

4. What does psoriasis have in common with cancer?

   Psoriasis and cancer both involve cells replicating for no useful reason.

5. When working with a client who is prone to acne, is it a good idea to follow massage with an alcohol rinse to remove the oil? Why?

   Wiping down a client who is prone to acne with alcohol after an oily treatment makes sense because the alcohol cuts right through and removes *all* the oil from the skin. But the human body has a habit of lashing back from such extreme changes in environment: it will work overtime to replace all the natural oils the alcohol just removed and more.

6. A client has white flakes that cling to hair shafts and don't brush out. What condition is probably present?

   This client probably has head lice. Separate these sheets from others, and bleach them.

7. A client has a circle-shaped, reddish-pink mark on the back of his upper thigh. What condition may be present?

   This client may have tinea cruris, or jock itch.

8. What should be done with this client's massage sheets?

   These sheets need to be isolated from all others and bleached or otherwise disinfected.

9. In what stage of the development of a decubitus ulcer is massage appropriate?

   If a client is at risk for developing bedsores (and is not otherwise contraindicated for massage), the improved skin nutrition provided by massage could be an excellent preventative measure. Massage is only appropriate *before* decubitus ulcers begin to form.

10. In what situation would an open sore be a systemic rather than simply a local contraindication?

    If an open sore indicates a systemic dysfunction, such as diabetes mellitus, it systemically contraindicates massage.

Chapter Objectives: Musculoskeletal System Conditions

List three differences between osteoarthritis and rheumatoid arthritis.

Rheumatoid arthritis (RA) is not a result of age and joint wear and tear; osteoarthritis is. RA does not target the weight-bearing joints; osteoarthritis does. RA tends to act symmetrically on the body, rather than simply where the most use has worn down a joint. Osteoarthritis may be asymmetrical; it simply depends on which joints have suffered the most cartilage and bone damage.

Name what Paget's disease and osteoporosis have in common.

Paget's disease and osteoporosis are both diseases of calcium metabolism. They both cause bones to be thin, brittle, and prone to breakage.

Name the leg muscles most involved with pes planus and pes cavus.

The "stirrup muscles" of the lower leg are most involved with the arch of the foot: the tibialis anterior and the peroneus longus.

Name four types of fractures.

Fractures can be simple, incomplete, or compound. In addition to these classifications, other fractures include greenstick, march, stress, comminuted, and impacted.

Name the medical emergency situation associated with shin splints.

It is possible for shin splints to complicate into anterior compartment syndrome, in which the fascial sheaths of the anterior leg muscles become so packed and inflamed that the enclosed tissue can starve and die.

Name two causes for patellofemoral syndrome.

Patellofemoral syndrome can be caused by the presence of thin cartilage on the patella, which eventually erodes and leads to joint damage, or by a patella that doesn't track correctly, leading to uneven wear and tear on the cartilage.

Describe the difference between structural and functional problems in postural deviations.

In the early stages of these conditions, the soft tissues pull the spine out of alignment: this is a *functional* problem. If the soft tissues are left untreated and the bones are constantly pulled in one direction or another, they will actually change shape to adapt to those stressors. At this point, the condition becomes a *structural* dysfunction.

Name three possible causes of thoracic outlet syndrome.

Cervical misalignment, cervical ribs, spondylosis, rib misalignment, tight muscles, and atrophied muscles around the shoulder girdle can all contribute to thoracic outlet syndrome.

Name two diseases associated with advanced gout.

The complications of gout are actually complications of having too much uric acid in the bloodstream, which indicates kidneys that are not functioning at adequate levels. Uric acid crystals can also cause kidney stones. If the kidneys become sufficiently clogged by kidney stones, renal failure will result. Impaired kidneys can't process adequate fluid. This stresses the rest of the circulatory system, causing high blood pressure, which can result in coronary artery disease or stroke. All of these problems—hyperuricemia, kidney insufficiency, gout, high blood pressure, and cardiovascular disease—are closely related.

Name three structures the brachial plexus passes through, around, or under on the way to the arm.

The brachial plexus nerves travel from intervertebral foramina through the anterior and medial scalenes, between the clavicle and the first rib, under the pectoralis minor and around the humerus.

Chapter Review Questions: Musculoskeletal System Conditions

1. What is the relationship between fibromyalgia and sleep disorders?

   One theory states that fibromyalgia begins as a sleep disorder. Persons with fibromyalgia may get adequate hours of sleep, but they don't reach Stage IV sleep, wherein the body's tissues are healed and rejuvenated. This leads to chemical imbalances in the central nervous system, the muscles, and the blood. These imbalances slow healing and decrease pain tolerance. In essence, poor sleep makes a person vulnerable to the syndrome of fibromyalgia.

2. What does "hernia" mean? Name three kinds of abdominal hernias.

   "Hernia" means hole. In this case, it means specifically, "hole through which contents that are supposed to be contained are protruding." Abdominal hernias include epigastric (above the navel), paraumbilical (at or below the navel), inguinal (through the inguinal ring for men), and femoral (through the femoral ring for women).

3. Why are herniated discs in the thoracic spine rare?

   Intervertebral discs seldom herniate in the thoracic spine because the thoracic vertebrae connect to the ribs. This makes them much more stable and resistant to the kinds of injury that cause a disc to herniate.

4. Where do massage therapists often suffer from osteoarthritis?

   Massage therapists are particularly prone to arthritis at the saddle joint of the thumb where the first metacarpal articulates with the trapezium. This joint experiences the bulk of the stress exerted when the thumb is pressed into a client's tissues.

5. Why are women more prone than men to osteoporosis?

   Both women and men can suffer from osteoporosis. Women are more prone to it for two reasons: the process of childbearing takes enormous reserves of calcium off the bones, and women generally have less dense bones to begin with.

6. Describe how pes planus can lead to headaches.

   Pes planus can contribute to headaches in many ways. Here is just one example: Fallen arches on one side cause the knee of the affected side to track off center. The pelvis slightly twists to accommodate the knee. The paraspinals are chronically tight because the pelvis isn't centered. The tightness of the postural muscles continues up into the neck, leading to tension headaches.

7. What kind of muscle spasm is actually an important part of the healing process?

   Muscles that are protecting an injured joint from potentially dangerous movement are *splinting* the joint. Although their tightness may outlive the injury, in the acute phases, this type of muscle spasm is an important protective device.

8. What is more serious: sciatica from a problem inside the spinal cord or from a problem outside the spinal cord? Why?

   If sciatica is being caused inside the spinal cord, it is due to spondylosis, bone spurs, a herniated disc, or something even more serious such as a tumor or bone chip. Irritation to the sciatic nerve outside the spinal cord is more likely to be caused by a soft tissue injury, like a ligament sprain or muscle spasm: conditions that are often easily resolved by massage.

9. In which stage of healing do soft tissue injuries generally contraindicate massage? Why?

   Soft tissue injuries generally contraindicate in the acute stage because at this point the tissues are just beginning to marshal their resources for healing. Capillaries and blood vessels need time to seal off and limit bleeding. Connective tissues and muscle fibers may be vulnerable to further tearing. It is inappropriate to disrupt the tissues during this time.

10. What does ICE stand for?

   Ice, compression, and elevation. This also appears as RICE: rest, ice, compression, and elevation.

11. Define "specific weakness."

   "Specific weakness" refers to a pattern of muscular degeneration that follows the path of motor nerve supply.

12. Describe the pain-spasm-ischemia cycle.

   This is a circular situation in which muscles experience pain and tighten in response, limiting blood flow (ischemia), which causes pain, which reinforces the spasm, further limiting blood flow, and so on.

13. Describe the differences between strains, sprains, and tendinitis.

   Strains are injuries to muscles. Sprains are injuries to ligaments. Tendinitis is inflammation from injury to tendons. These injuries are all similar in that they involve the fraying of longitudinal fibers and the development of scar tissue in the form of randomly laid down collagen fibers.

   These injuries differ because of the structures they affect and the time it takes to recover from them. Of the three, ligament sprains are often the slowest to heal because of low blood supply. Sprains also tend to swell much more than tendon or muscular injuries.

14. Describe the relationship between stress and chronic injury.

   The hormone most closely linked to long-term stress is cortisol. Although cortisol can be a beneficial substance in many circumstances, chronically high levels of it systemically weaken all types of connective tissue, raising the chances for injury and ongoing pain.

Chapter Objectives: Nervous System Conditions

Know which nerve is involved in Bell's palsy.

Bell's palsy is a result of damage to the facial nerve.

Name three classes of headaches.

Vascular headaches. These include classic and common migraines, cluster headaches, and possibly sinus headaches. They account for a total of about 6 to 8% of all headaches.

Muscular contraction headaches. By far the most common type of headache people experience (90 to 92%), these are brought about by muscular tension, bony misalignment, TMJ disorders, fibromyalgia, or other muscular problems.

Traction-inflammatory headaches. These account for 2% of the headaches people experience, and they are indicative of severe underlying pathology such as tumors, aneurysm, or infection in the central nervous system.

Name two signs that a headache could be indicative of a life-threatening situation.

The time to become concerned is when headaches are accompanied by extreme fever; when they are severe, repeating, and have a sudden onset; or when they have a gradual onset but no remission.

Name two types of seizures.

Over 30 classes of seizures are listed now, including absence seizures, tonic-clonic seizures, partial, general, and static seizures.

Know the causative agent for shingles.

The causative agent for shingles is the chicken pox virus: varicella zoster.

Know the difference between myelin and neurilemma.

Most neurons in the peripheral and central nervous system have a waxy, insulating coating called myelin. This layer of material speeds nerve conduction along the fiber and prevents the jumping of electrical impulses from one fiber to another. In the peripheral nervous system, neurons have another protective feature in *neurilemma*: an outside covering of special cells that can help to regenerate damaged tissue.

Name three diseases that may be confused with multiple sclerosis.

Several conditions may produce MS-like symptoms. Part of a thorough diagnosis is ruling these out:

- Lyme disease
- AIDS
- Scleroderma
- Vascular problems in the brain
- Herniated or ruptured disc
- Lupus
- CNS tumors
- Fibromyalgia

Know the target tissue of the polio virus.

The polio virus targets intestinal mucosa first, and anterior horn nerve cells later.

Name six symptoms of stroke.

Unilateral weakness, numbness, or paralysis on the face, arm, or leg, or any combination of the three.

Suddenly blurred or decreased vision in one or both eyes; asymmetrical dilation of pupils.

Difficulty in speaking or understanding simple sentences.

Dizziness, clumsiness, vertigo.

Sudden, extreme headache.

Possible loss of consciousness.

Know the difference between transient ischemic attack and stroke.

In a transient ischemic attack (TIA), a tiny blood clot creates a temporary blockage in the brain, but it quickly breaks apart and disperses before causing any lasting damage. Symptoms of TIA are similar to those of stroke, except that they last only a few minutes or hours. They are, however, like the muffled rumblings of an incipient eruption; about one-half of all people who experience a TIA will have a major stroke within 5 years.

Chapter Review Questions: Nervous System Conditions

1. What's the difference between spastic and flaccid paralysis? Where in the nervous system does each indicate damage?

   Spastic paralysis indicates *central nervous system* damage. Spastic paralysis combines aspects of hypertonia, hypokinesia, and hyperreflexia.

   Flaccid paralysis is typically a sign of *peripheral nerve* damage. Flaccid paralysis involves muscles in a state of *hypo*tonicity.

2. How can a person who has experienced spinal cord damage at C_6 still have control of his head and neck?

   The arrangement of the cranial nerves, which are not vulnerable to spinal cord injury, allows a person with severe neck injuries to maintain motor function in the neck, head, and internal organs.

3. Why is massage indicated for Bell's palsy, when it is contraindicated for most other types of paralysis?

   Bell's Palsy is a flaccid paralysis with sensation left intact. Massage is appropriate for flaccid paralysis because flaccid muscle fibers are less vulnerable to damage than spastic ones, and because the client has sensation and can give feedback about his or her comfort. Massage keeps the facial muscles elastic and the local circulation strong. This sets the stage for a more complete recovery when nerve supply is eventually restored

4. Is post polio syndrome contagious? Why or why not?

   Post polio syndrome is *not* a resurgence of the original polio infection. Instead, it seems to be the result of normal aging combined with the loss of some percentage of anterior horn cells from the initial polio attack.

5. Describe the safest course of action for a client who experiences an epileptic seizure during a massage.

   It is inappropriate to try to massage someone who is in the midst of a seizure of any kind. In this situation, the practitioner's job is to make sure the client is safe, call 911 or the local emergency number, and then wait until the seizure has subsided.

6. A client who has multiple sclerosis comes for massage. The therapist performs a rigorous sports-massage type treatment and then recommends a soak in a hot tub. Is this a good idea? Why or why not?

   This is probably not a good idea. Most MS patients are hypersensitive to extreme types of sensation. They may have a spasmodic reaction to both the vigorous, fast-paced massage, and the hot bath. A more appropriate course with most (although perhaps not all) MS patients is a gentler, less stimulating type of massage that may or may not be followed by hydrotherapy depending on that person's tastes and tolerance.

7. Can a person who has had chicken pox catch herpes zoster from another person? Why or why not?

   Although the fluid in zoster blisters is filled with virus, shingles isn't particularly contagious to a person who has had chicken pox, unless he comes in contact with it while his own immune system is depressed.

8. Name three conditions that can result in hyperesthesia.

   Hyperesthesia can accompany any nervous system disorder that involves irritated nerve endings; herpes simplex and zoster are perfect examples. Other possibilities include herniated discs, carpal tunnel syndrome, and any kind of neuritis. Hyperesthesia can also be the by-product of stress or an emotional reaction to touch.

9. What is neuritis? Name two conditions that can cause it.

   Neuritis means any inflammation of a peripheral nerve.

   Nerve inflammation is often caused by some mechanical injury to the nerve. With a herniated disc or sciatica, a hard object presses against the nerve root, irritating and inflaming it. Neuritis is also common with major body trauma such as bone fractures because the nerves in the periosteum are inflamed, suffer bruises, or penetrating injuries.

A host of other conditions include neuritis among their symptoms or complications: herpes simplex and zoster, systemic lupus erythematosus, and peripheral neuropathy all involve neuritis.

Exposure to some chemicals can also cause neuritis: carbon monoxide and carbon tetrachloride can cause this disorder, as can exposure to heavy metals, and some kinds of drugs and alcohol. A deficiency in thiamin can also result in nerve inflammation.

10. A client is recovering from a major stroke. What are some of the key criteria on which to base a judgment about the appropriateness of Swedish massage?

    The vast majority of stroke patients also have other circulatory problems. Therefore, it's *very important* to receive medical clearance before proceeding with massage. Also, if the client has experienced hemiplegia, it's important to remember that spastic paralysis carries specific cautions for Swedish massage.

Chapter Objectives: Circulatory System Conditions

Describe the three tissue layers of most blood vessels.

Arteries and veins share the same basic properties of most of the tubes in the body. They have an internal layer of epithelium (called *endo*thelium here, because it's on the inside); a middle layer of smooth muscle; and an external layer of tough, protective connective tissue. This combination of tissues makes these tubes strong, pliable, and stretchy.

Describe the structural differences between veins and arteries.

Arteries have to deal with much higher blood pressure than veins do, and they have a thicker layer of smooth muscle tissue to help them do it. Veins help blood to return, usually against gravity, to the heart. They have flaps or valves to ensure that blood flows through them in only one direction.

Name four ways in which the circulatory system works to maintain homeostasis.

Delivery of nutrients and oxygen. The blood carries nutrients and oxygen to every cell in the body. If for some reason the blood can't reach a specific area, cells in that area will starve and die. This is the situation with many disorders, including stroke, myocardial infarction, and decubitus ulcers.

Removal of waste products. While dropping off nutrients, the blood, along with lymph, picks up the waste products generated by metabolism. These include carbon dioxide and other more noxious compounds that, left to stew in the tissues, can cause problems. Again, if blood and lymph supply to an area is limited, the affected cells can "drown" in their own waste products and become damaged or even die.

Temperature. Superficial blood vessels dilate when it's hot, and they constrict when it's cold. Furthermore, blood prevents the hot places (the heart, the liver, working muscles) from getting too hot by flushing through and distributing the heated blood throughout the rest of the body. By keeping a steady temperature, the circulatory system maintains a stable internal environment .

Clotting. This is an often overlooked but truly miraculous function of the circulatory system, without which people would quickly die. Every time a rough place occurs in the endothelium of a blood vessel, a whole chain of chemical reactions happen that cause the spinning of tiny fibers to catch cells to plug any possible gaps. Unfortunately, under certain circumstances, this reaction is sometimes more of a curse than a blessing.

Protection from pathogens. Without white blood cells, the body would have no defense against the hordes of microorganisms that are longing to gain access to the body's precious (and precarious) internal environment.

Chemical balance. A narrow margin of tolerance exists for variances in internal chemistry. A person can actually die if his or her blood becomes even fifteen one-hundredths too alkaline or too acidic. Happily, blood components, including red blood cells, are supplied with enzymes and other mechanisms specifically designed to keep pH balance within the safety zone.

Name three varieties of anemia.

Varieties of anemia include: idiopathic anemias, nutritional anemias, iron deficiency anemia, folic acid deficiency anemia, B_{12} deficiency anemia, pernicious anemia, hemorrhagic anemias, hemolytic anemias, sickle cell anemia, and aplastic anemia.

Name two types of aortic aneurysm.

Aneurysms come in a variety of shapes and sizes, some of which are particular to where the lesion occurs.

Saccular. These are usually thoracic or abdominal aortic aneurysms. The aortal wall bulges like a small (or large) rounded sack that throbs and pushes against neighboring organs and other structures.

Fusiform. This is also common for aortic aneurysms; in this case, the bulge is less round and more tubular, as if the aorta were widened like a sausage for a few inches.

Berry. This is a term for several small aneurysms clustered together in the brain.

Dissecting. This is the least common and most painful type of aneurysm. It happens again with the aorta, and in this situation, the blood pressure actually *splits* the layers of the aorta. It can happen between the tunica intima (innermost layer) and the tunica media (muscular layer), or between the tunica media and the adventitia (outer layer). In some cases, this type of aneurysm seals itself off when the blood trapped inside the split coagulates and solidifies.

Name four risk factors for developing atherosclerosis.

Modifiable risk factors for atherosclerosis include smoking, high cholesterol levels, high blood pressure, and a sedentary lifestyle. Unmodifiable risk factors include a family history of cardiovascular disease, kidney disorders, and diabetes.

Name three common symptoms of diabetes.

Three defining "polys" are common for all types of diabetes. *Polyuria,* or frequent urination, results from elevated blood sugar, which acts as a diuretic; it pulls water from the cells in the body, then pulls excess water into the kidneys and urine. *Polydipsia* means excessive thirst, which accompanies the loss of water with polyuria. *Polyphagia* refers to increased appetite, since diabetics must get all their energy from fats and proteins instead of carbohydrates, which are the most efficient kind of fuel.

Other symptoms of diabetes include fatigue, weight loss, nausea, and vomiting.

Describe the difference between primary and secondary Raynaud's syndrome.

Raynaud's syndrome can be a primary problem or a secondary one, when it appears as a symptom of another disease. As a primary problem, that is, unconnected to underlying pathology, it is called *Raynaud's disease.*

Occasionally extreme vasoconstriction is a complication of some other disorder such as diabetes, lupus, or cardiovascular disease. In this case, the condition is called *Raynaud's phenomenon.* It will generally have a much faster onset than Raynaud's disease, and can become quite a lot worse before it responds to treatment.

Name the primary danger for complications of deep vein thrombosis.

Fragments that detach from blood clots in leg veins will land in the lungs, causing pulmonary embolism. The seriousness of this condition depends on the size of the clot and where in the lung it lands.

Name three causative factors for varicose veins.

Many things can damage the valves in the veins. It could be simple wear and tear: being on one's feet for many hours a day, especially if the legs' muscles are not allowed to fully contract and relax during that time, will weaken the veins. It could also be a mechanical obstruction to returning blood: knee socks that are too tight, for instance, or a fetus which presses on the femoral vein. Systemic congestion from kidney problems or liver backups has caused problems, too. Finally, it could be simply congenitally weak veins.

Chapter Review Questions: Circulatory System Conditions

1. Describe the process of the development of atherosclerosis.

   Different theories exist about the development of atherosclerosis. One of them goes like this:

   1. *Endothelial damage*. The inside layer of arteries is subject to a lot of abuse. Regardless of the source, endothelial damage may begin the process of developing atherosclerosis.
   2. *Monocytes arrive*. These small white blood cells are attracted to any site of damage in the body. The monocytes infiltrate the epithelial layer, and turn into *macrophages*—big eaters.
   3. *Macrophages take up LDL (low density lipoproteins)*. Now they are called foam cells. This is the beginning of the development of fatty streaks that characterize atherosclerosis.
   4. *Foam cells infiltrate the next layer*. Foam cells secrete growth factors; this causes the smooth muscle cells in the arterial wall to proliferate all around them. Furthermore, these foam cells can release enzymes that damage arterial walls and cause bleeding and clot formation.
   5. *Platelets arrive*. Attracted by the changing texture of the arterial wall, platelets come and release their chemicals, which secrete growth factors, form clots, and cause vascular spasm.

2. What indication of diabetes might a massage therapist be the first person to notice?

   Diabetic clients, particularly those who have not been diagnosed, may have reduced sensation in the extremities along with severely impaired circulation. The tissue on their feet may die from starvation or become infected with pathogens that are impossible to fight off, forming characteristic diabetic ulcers.

3. Where will all venous emboli go? Why?

   All venous emboli go to the lungs because the venous system is routed through the right side of the heart to the pulmonary circuit.

4. Name three places arterial emboli can go to cause significant damage.

   The arteries of the brain, the heart, the kidneys, and the legs are statistically the most common sites for arterial emboli to lodge.

5. Heart attacks involve blockages where: in the heart itself or in the coronary arteries?

   Heart attacks involve blockages in the coronary arteries, which supply the cardiac muscle with oxygen. In the absence of oxygen, portions of the cardiac muscle will die; this is a myocardial infarction.

6. Which chamber of the heart is the worst place to experience a myocardial infarct? Why?

   The left ventricle is a particularly dangerous place to experience the loss of cardiac function, because the contractions of the left ventricle push blood all the way through the systemic circuit. Other chambers of the heart do not have to work as hard, so a loss is not so dangerous.

7. Why is hypertension called the "Silent Killer"?

   Hypertension is an almost symptomless problem, yet it can cause major damage to the circulatory system. A person with uncontrolled hypertension is at risk for a variety of life-threatening cardiovascular problems.

8. Describe the relationship between high blood pressure and kidney dysfunction.

   Hypertension can cause atherosclerotic plaques to form in the renal arteries, which are subject to *tremendous* blood pressure. This causes reduced blood flow into the kidney, which will impair kidney function, leading to kidney damage and systemic edema, which will exert even more pressure on the outsides of blood vessel walls.

   Hypertension can also cause kidney dysfunction through direct pressure on the delicate kidney tissues. Injury to the nephrons decreases kidney function. This results in systemic fluid retention, which increases blood pressure and puts even more stress on the kidneys.

9. Describe how a person may experience any three of the following conditions at the same time: high blood pressure, chronic renal failure, edema, atherosclerosis, diabetes, aortic aneurysm, stroke.

   These conditions can all be closely interrelated. Following are a few of the many ways in which a person may experience some combination of these disorders.

   1. A person has high blood pressure. The constant pressure in his vessels has damaged them to the point that he has developed atherosclerotic plaques in his coronary arteries and in other major arteries as well, including the common carotid. A plaque fragment from the carotid breaks loose and goes to the brain, causing a stroke.
   2. A person has diabetes. The disturbances in metabolism have put a particular stress on the kidneys, and she has developed chronic renal failure as a result. The systemic edema she experiences because her kidneys are not functioning well, along with the atherosclerotic plaques that accumulate because of the diabetes, have raised her blood pressure to dangerous levels.
   3. A person has high blood pressure, which gradually complicates into atherosclerosis. The combination of blood pressure and narrow, brittle arteries has resulted in a bulge in the abdominal aorta: an aneurysm.

10. A client has ropey, distended varicose veins on the medial aspect of the right knee. Distal to the knee, the tissue is clammy and slightly edematous. Pressing at the ankle leaves a dimple that takes several minutes to disappear. What cautions must be exercised with this client? Why?

    This client is at very high risk for thrombophlebitis or deep vein thrombosis. He or she should not receive circulatory massage at all until the edema has been resolved and he or she has been cleared of all danger of blood clots by a physician.

Chapter Objectives: Lymph and Immune System Conditions

Name five ways that lymph can be moved through the body.

Gravity. Gravity will help move lymph if the limb is elevated.

Muscle contraction. When muscle fibers squeeze down around lymphatic vessels, they push fluid through as though a hand is squeezing around a tube of toothpaste.

Alternating hot and cold. Hydrotherapy applications can create contractions in the smooth muscle tissue of lymphatic vessels, which then moves fluid along.

Breathing. Deep breathing draws lymph up the thoracic duct (like an expanding bellows) during inhalation, and squeezes it muscularly during exhalation.

Massage. Big, mechanical, manipulative strokes, such as petrissage and deep effleurage, can increase lymph flow, but even small, extremely superficial reflexive strokes can cause stagnant fluid to be drawn into lymphatic capillaries.

Name the type of immunity supplied by T cells and by B cells.

T cells and B cells supply "specific immunity." They are designed to fight specifically identified pathogens, rather than offering the same protective devices against any possible invader, as agents of nonspecific immunity do.

Name three places in the body where macrophages are concentrated for immune system defenses.

Macrophages are distributed generously all through the blood and interstitial fluid, but they are concentrated in the superficial fascia, lymph nodes, lungs, and liver, where the chances of meeting pathogens are especially high.

Name two "indicator diseases" for AIDS.

Pneumocystis carinii pneumonia (PCP) is a protozoal infection of the lungs.

Cytomegalovirus (CMV) can cause retinitis and blindness, colitis, pneumonia, and infection of the adrenal glands.

Kaposi's sarcoma (KS) is a type of skin cancer.

B-cell lymphomas: HIV has recently been found to specifically initiate the cancer cell replication with a variety of lymphomas, as well as KS.

Name three criteria, besides fatigue, necessary for a positive diagnosis of chronic fatigue syndrome.

At least four of the following symptoms must be present. They must *not* predate the onset of fatigue, and they must be a consistent problem for 6 months or more:

- short term memory loss;
- tender lymph nodes;
- pain that exceeds 24 hours after mild exercise;
- confusion;
- muscle pain;
- nonrestorative sleep;
- sore throat;
- joint pain without signs of inflammation;
- headaches of a new type or pattern since the onset of symptoms.

Name two examples of edema that contraindicate circulatory massage, and one example of edema that indicates massage.

Edemas that contraindicate massage: If the heart is overtaxed and is not pumping the volumes it should be, fluid will accumulate in the tissues. Vigorous massage will not improve this situation, and could quite possibly make it worse by putting an even greater load on the system.

If the kidneys are not filtering blood fast enough or completely enough because of chemical imbalance or mechanical obstruction, edema will develop and massage could make the situation much worse.

If the liver is congested, the puffiness and bogginess of typical edema may be less visibly apparent, but the same rules apply: pushing blood through a system that is chemically or mechanically impaired will do only damage.

If edema is due to local infection, massage is contraindicated because of the risk of pushing bacteria into the lymphatic and circulatory systems before the body has had a chance to tag it and marshal appropriate defenses.

If a chance of mechanical blockage exists anywhere in the circulatory system, massage is contraindicated, because it can damage delicate structures in the circulatory system; or worse, it could break loose an embolism or thrombus. Some examples of mechanical blockages include edema associated with pregnancy, blood clots or emboli, and elephantiasis.

Edemas that indicate massage: If a client has fluid retention related to a subacute musculoskeletal injury, skilled massage is *very* indicated, and in fact, could be vital to the healing process. Likewise, if a client is temporarily confined to bed or is even partially immobilized for some condition that does *not* otherwise contraindicate massage, massage can be valuable to the health of the injured tissues, as long as the risk of blood clotting has been ruled out.

Name three good reasons to let a mild fever run its course without interference.

The presence of interleukin-1 and other cytokines not only help to reset the body's thermostat, but also stimulate T-cell production. Increased T-cell production then stimulates B cells and antibodies.

In the presence of fever, a powerful antiviral agent called *interferon* is much more active.

Increased temperature limits iron secretion from the liver and spleen, starving off and slowing bacterial and viral activity.

Increased temperature will raise the heart rate (10 beats per minute per degree), which in turn increases the distribution of white blood cells throughout the body.

Increased temperature increases cell wall permeability and speeds chemical reactions. This promotes faster recovery for damaged tissues.

Name the four cardinal signs of inflammation. What is a fifth possible sign?

The four cardinal signs of inflammation are heat, pain, redness, and swelling. A fifth sign, loss of function, may sometimes be present, especially if the inflammation is in a joint.

Name what lupus can do to the musculoskeletal system organs.

Of people with lupus, 80 to 90% eventually develop arthritis. Some even experience necrosis (tissue death) of bone and joint tissue, especially in the hips and shoulders.

Nonspecific muscle pain is another common symptom, and some overlap often occurs between lupus and fibromyalgia.

Name the most dangerous complication of lymphangitis.

Lymphangitis is an infection of the *lymph* system, not the circulatory system. However, if even a few bacteria get past the filtering action of the lymph nodes, the infection *will* enter the bloodstream at the right or left subclavian veins. The situation then changes to a more serious one: septicemia, or blood poisoning, which is life threatening.

Chapter Review Questions: Lymph and Immune System Conditions

1. What is an allergy?

   An allergy is an immune-system attack against a stimulus that is not necessarily dangerous, such as pollen, cat dander, or mildew.

2. What is an autoimmune disease? Give two examples.

   An autoimmune disease is a situation in which the immune system attacks parts of the patient's own body. Several autoimmune diseases are well documented, and other conditions exist for which an autoimmune dysfunction is one possibility for their etiology.

   Examples of autoimmune diseases include rheumatoid arthritis, chronic fatigue syndrome, allergies, lupus erythematosus, rheumatic heart disease, and Sjögren's syndrome. Other conditions that have shown evidence of an autoimmune component include type I diabetes, ulcerative colitis, and multiple sclerosis.

3. What are lymphokines, and what do they do?

   Lymphokines are chemicals secreted by cells, and they carry specific messages and instructions. These chemical messages are beginning to be deciphered, and some of them say things like, "act like me," "come over here," and "eat this."

4. What type of cell is the primary target for HIV?

   The primary target of HIV is the helper T cell (also called CD4 cells) and some other nonspecific white blood cells.

5. Who is most at risk for getting sick when a massage therapist works with an AIDS patient? Why?

   The person most at risk for getting sick when an AIDS patient receives massage is the patient. Therefore, the practitioner must take care not to carry active pathogens that may put the AIDS client at risk.

6. What is the link between chronic fatigue syndrome and the immune system?

   The CFS patient was probably infected at one time with some pathogen that initiated a normal immune response. Long after that infectious agent was cast out of the body, the immune system still tries to fight it. This condition is very similar to an ongoing allergic reaction: the body is trying desperately to fight something, *even though no danger is present*. The symptoms of CFS are *not* caused by the original infectious agent, but by immune system hyperactivity.

7. Describe how the inflammatory process causes pain, heat, redness, and swelling.

   Vasodilation brings about the redness, heat, and swelling by drawing extra blood to a small area. Pain and itching are the result of several factors: edemic pressure, damaged nerve endings, irritating pathogenic toxins, even irritating chemicals released by other cells. If the inflammation limits joint movement, the patient experiences loss of function.

8. What are the dangers of working with a client who is taking anti-inflammatories?

   Anti-inflammatories may hide the results of overtreatment, thus raising the risk of massage causing an injury.

9. How is lupus generally treated medically? Why?

   Lupus is a disease with no known cause and no known cure. It is treated palliatively; medications are prescribed to control symptoms as much as possible. It starts with nonsteroidal and then steroidal anti-inflammatories. Immunosuppressive drugs are sometimes used to quell the needless attacks on the connective tissues.

10. Why are massage therapists particularly at risk for lymphangitis?

    This condition is an occupational hazard for bodywork professionals because repeated immersions of the hands in soapy water may lead to hangnail formation and drying and cracking of nail beds.

Chapter Objectives:
Respiratory System Conditions

Describe the basic mechanics of breathing, listing the main muscles involved.

The lungs are two sacs that inflate or deflate according to the air pressure inside and outside of them. Changes in air pressure result from the changing shape of the thoracic cavity. If the cavity is made larger, the air pressure inside is low until air rushes in to equalize it. In other words, the act of inhaling is simply filling a vacuum. When the pressure inside and outside the lungs has been equalized, air eases out again: exhalation.

Ideally, about 75% of the change in internal air pressure is caused by the contraction and flattening of the diaphragm muscle. The intercostals do most of the rest of the work, with a bit of help from the scalenes and serratus posterior muscles in a type of breathing called *paradoxical inspiration*.

Describe where in the lungs gaseous exchange occurs and what structures are involved.

The air passages in the lungs subdivide into smaller and smaller tubes until they terminate in microscopic alveoli. These little grape-shaped clusters of epithelium, like tiny balloons, are surrounded by blood capillaries. Gaseous exchange occurs through the alveoli.

Name two possible factors behind the recent rise in asthma statistics.

Asthma is on a distinct rise in the United States. Theories to explain this increase include higher levels of air pollution and more airtight houses and office buildings where dust, dander, and other allergens concentrate in the air.

Name two differences between influenza and the common cold.

Influenza is worse than a cold. It involves a fever up to 104°F. Also, instead of being segregated to the upper respiratory tract like a cold, flu can cause swollen lymph nodes and joint and muscle pain. Cold viruses, although contagious, are not as virulent as flu viruses.

Know how Type A flu viruses can reinfect the same person.

Type A flu viruses mutate quickly, therefore causing repeated infections in the same person.

Name three risk factors for the development of emphysema.

More than 80% of emphysema cases are traced to cigarette smoking. Others may be due to occupational hazards: working with grain dust, in coal mines, or quarries increases risk. A small percentage of emphysema patients have a genetic lack of the alpha-1 anti-trypsin (AAT) protein that protects alveolar walls.

Briefly describe stages 0 through IV of lung cancer.

Staging for small cell and non–small cell carcinomas follow the same basic pattern: from Stage 0 to Stage I the cancer is localized. In Stage II, it has invaded nearby lymph nodes in the mediastinum. In Stage III, the tumors may have invaded the chest wall, the diaphragm, and lymph nodes in the neck. Stage IV lung cancer is systemic throughout the body; it can affect the brain and spinal cord, the bones, and abdominal organs, particularly the liver and pancreas.

Tell which is more common, primary or secondary pneumonia, and why.

Primary pneumonia is relatively rare. In this case, no predisposing factor exists; it is simply a bacterial attack directly on the lungs.

Secondary pneumonia is by the far the most common situation. In this case, a virus or bacterium assaults the lung tissue because the body's immune system is weakened by another disease.

Name three possible causes for sinusitis.

Viruses. The most serious types of sinusitis begin as a viral infection. Then, when defenses are low, the bacteria that normally colonize the skin and mucous membranes take advantage of the situation and begin to multiply.

Allergic rhinitis. Hay fever also causes inflammation of the sinus membranes, but since no underlying infection is present, neither is danger of infectious complications.

Structural problems. A deviated septum or the growth of nasal polyps can obstruct the flow of mucous out of the sinuses. This is not an infectious situation in the beginning. But because mucous held back from normal flow is a perfect growth medium for bacteria, what begins as a structural anomaly can become a true infection.

Fungal infections. These are particular dangers for persons who are immune-suppressed. Fungi such as Aspergillus or Curvularia are not threats to most people, but can cause sinus infection in AIDS patients or others whose immune systems are compromised.

Medicine intolerance. Occasionally, a reaction to aspirin or ibuprofen can produce inflammation in the mucous membranes of the sinuses.

Know the prevalence of tuberculosis worldwide.

The World Health Organization reports that tuberculosis affects one-third of the world's population. Eight million people become sick with it every year, and three million people die.

Chapter Review Questions: Respiratory System Conditions

1. What is the purpose of mucous membranes? Where are they found?

   Mucous membranes line any cavity in the body that communicates with the outside world: the respiratory, digestive, reproductive, and urinary systems.

   In the respiratory system, the mucous membranes start inside the nose and mouth, continue down the sinuses and throat, all the way into the smaller tubes in the lungs. The wet, sticky mucous membranes in the respiratory system are re-sponsible for warming, moistening, and filtering the air that passes by. Mucous membrane secretions also trap pathogens and other particles. Then the "mucous blanket" slowly creeps toward the mouth and nose for expulsion.

2. How does the structure of the lungs work to limit the spread of infection?

Each lung has two or three lobes, and within each of those lobes are smaller seg-ments. This isolation of different areas makes it difficult for pathogens to infect the whole structure.

3. Explain the sympathetic/parasympathetic swing that occurs with asthma.

When the appropriate stimulus occurs, the bronchioles first dilate (a sympa-thetic reaction), and then the body overcompensates by sending them into spasm. The irritated membranes lining these tubes then swell up and secrete extra mucous.

4. What is the best defense against catching or spreading the cold virus?

The best way to prevent the spread of colds and other infectious diseases is by frequently washing the hands, focusing on the cuticles and nails, using soap or detergent, and scrubbing for 15 seconds or more before rinsing.

5. What is the danger associated with taking broad spectrum antibiotics for a cold, "just in case"?

Only about 20% of colds will develop into bacterial infections. The frequent ad-ministration of needless antibiotics doesn't improve recovery time, but can con-tribute to the creation of new and more drug-resistant strains of bacteria.

6. What are the repercussions of having alveoli fuse together, as happens with em-physema?

With emphysema, the alveolar walls eventually break down and the alveoli merge together, forming larger sacs, called bullae. These sacs have less volume and less surface area for gaseous exchange than the uninjured alveoli did.

7. Why is the prognosis for lung cancer generally so poor?

The difficulty with lung cancer is identifying the early symptoms in time to catch the tumors while they're still isolated. Only 15% of all lung cancers are found this early. Once they spread, the disease becomes difficult to treat successfully.

8. What feature of the tuberculosis bacterium distinguishes it from most other pathogens?

The mycobacterium tuberculosis is a microorganism with a peculiar waxy coat that gives it many advantages over regular bacteria. This pathogen exists quite happily outside of the body. The saliva or mucous that might initially surround it eventually dries up, but the bacteria wait on, often suspended in the air, until a rich growth medium comes its way again. Ordinary antiseptics and disinfectants don't kill it. Even boiling isn't dependable. The only thing that always kills my-cobacterium tuberculosis is direct sunlight.

9. What happens when prescriptions of antibiotics for tuberculosis (or other bacterial infections) are not completed as directed? Why is this a particular danger for TB?

If antibiotics are not used exactly as prescribed, the tuberculosis bacterium quickly mutates into a form drugs can't affect. Whoever is infected with this new strain will be resistant to treatment.

10. A client has sinusitis. Her mucous is thick, opaque, and sticky. She has had a headache and a mild fever for several days. Is she a good candidate for massage? Why or why not?

This client needs to reschedule her appointment. Her symptoms indicate a possible sinus infection. Thick, opaque mucus is usually indicative of pus, and fever, however mild, always contraindicates circulatory massage.

Chapter Review Questions: Digestive System Conditions

1. Describe how ongoing stress can result in digestive system problems.

   When a person is under stress, digestion becomes a low priority. Circulation is routed elsewhere, and the digestive organs have to function with insufficient blood flow. If this state of affairs continues for a long time, problems will develop.

2. Why is the appendix no longer routinely removed in the course of other abdominal surgery?

   These days it is recognized that the lymphatic follicles lining the appendix may help to produce some types of immunoglobulins, so the appendix is only taken out when leaving it in poses significant danger.

3. What is ascites? How can liver dysfunction cause it?

   When liver dysfunction causes blood pressure in the portal system to increase, plasma filtrates out of the veins into the peritoneal space, causing the abdominal distension known as ascites.

4. Why might someone with ulcerative colitis be at a higher risk of developing colon cancer than the general population?

   Because of prolonged cellular irritation followed by cellular replacement, patients with ulcerative colitis are at significantly more risk of developing colon cancer than the general population.

5. Describe the leading theory behind the development of colon cancer.

   One theory about the development of colon cancer is that high-fat foods linger in the colon longer than others, and some of their by-products are carcinogenic, or cancer-causing. The presence of these chemicals may contribute to chromosome damage in the polyps, causing them to reproduce at even more abnormal rates. This theory also suggests that diets high in fiber cause matter to move through the colon faster and more completely, "scrubbing" the bowel walls of damaging or irritating materials.

6. What is the difference between diverticula and colon polyps?

   Diverticula are small sacs, possibly filled with fecal matter, that protrude out from the colon. Colon polyps are masses of epithelial cells that protrude into the colon; they may be precursors of colon cancer.

7. Most people with gallstones never have symptoms. What finally causes symptoms to occur?

   Estimates suggest that up to 80% of all people who have gallstones experience no symptoms. A person will have symptoms if a stone becomes lodged in either the cystic duct or lower down in the common bile duct.

8. Why are antibiotics ineffective for dealing with a bacterial infection of the gastrointestinal tract?

   Antibiotics for bacterial infections tend to make intestinal inflammation worse. Gastroenteritis generally is not treated with anything more sophisticated than rest and fluid replacement.

9. What is a possible cause of ulcers that does not involve the Helicobacter pylori bacterium?

Helicobacter pylori is found in much, but not all, ulcer tissue. About 20 to 30% of ulcers have nothing to do with bacteria; they result from the use of aspirin and other nonsteroidal anti-inflammatory drugs (NSAIDs) for aches and pains, or to avoid the risks of heart attack or stroke.

10. A client is recovering from a bout with hepatitis A. His skin has a yellowish tone and the sclera of his eyes is yellow, too. What condition is probably present? Is this client a good candidate for massage? Why or why not?

This client probably has jaundice. He is not a good candidate for circulatory massage, as his condition indicates that his liver is not functioning at full capacity. His appointment should be rescheduled for a time when his liver has recovered full function, and he has been cleared for massage by a physician.

Chapter Objectives: Digestion System Conditions

Name three functions of the liver.

The liver receives all the vitamins, amino acids, and glucose not immediately needed in the body. By storing glucose as glycogen until it is called for, the liver also acts as a sugar buffer, preventing some of the radical swings in blood glucose levels that would occur if no intermediate stop existed for sugar. The liver is also the site for much of the most vital protein synthesis in the body. Many of the enzymes that sponsor cellular activity are born here; this is also the origin of blood proteins that regulate intracellular fluid and blood clotting.

Name three conditions that mimic symptoms of appendicitis.

Appendicitis is extremely difficult to diagnose. It resembles several other serious conditions, including gastroenteritis, kidney stones, urinary tract infection, Crohns disease, pelvic inflammatory disease, and ovarian cysts.

Name five complications of cirrhosis.

As blood in the portal system backs up from the congested liver, the repercussions are felt throughout the body.

Splenomegaly. The spleen enlarges into a condition called splenomegaly because it can't get rid of its by-products from red blood cell breakdown.

Jaundice. Bilirubin (a by-product of the recycling of dead red blood cells) is produced in the spleen, and it is supposed to be broken down in the liver. When this is impossible because of cirrhosis, water-soluble components of bilirubin, which are strongly pigmented, accumulate in the bloodstream and turn the sclera of the eyes and the skin a yellowish color.

Ascites. When blood pressure in the portal system increases, plasma filtrates out of the venous capillaries into the peritoneal space, causing the abdominal distension known as ascites.

Systemic edema. Cirrhosis can cut blood flow leaving the liver, as well as blood flow going in. One of the critical proteins for maintaining fluid balance in the body, albumin, is significantly lowered in advanced cirrhosis. Without albumin, the body cannot maintain proper fluid levels. Edema accumulates, not just in the abdomen (ascites), but systemically in all interstitial spaces.

Internal varices. Pressure in abdominal veins grows as fluid backs up through the system. This can lead to internal venous distensions and varicosities. Pressure in the esophageal veins also grows; sometimes they'll bulge into esophageal varices, or varicose veins of the esophagus. These can hemorrhage during vomiting, leading to bloody vomit, shock, or even death.

Hormone disruption. The livers of men with cirrhosis no longer inactivate their normal low levels of estrogen; feminizing characteristics such as breast development, loss of chest hair, impotence, and atrophy of the testicles soon follow. For women, hormonal changes include the cessation of periods. Both men and women can expect decreased sex drives.

Encephalopathy. With advanced cirrhosis, the detoxifying agents in the liver are out of commission. No protection exists from the chemicals (ammonia, for instance) produced whenever food is metabolized. These toxins accumulate in the blood and eventually cause brain damage. Symptoms include somnolence, confusion, tremors, hallucinations, even coma.

Kidney failure. Advanced cirrhosis can affect blood flow to the kidneys, resulting in kidney failure. Hepatorenal syndrome is an emergency situation that requires a liver transplant in order for a person to survive.

Know why anemia is part of the profile for ulcerative colitis.

One of the most dependable complications of long-term ulcerative colitis is anemia, from the slow, constant blood loss.

List the recommendations for colon cancer screenings for people over 40 years old.

Basic screening for colon cancer begins with a digital rectal exam. Fecal occult blood tests, special examinations of stool samples that will indicate the presence of microscopic amounts of blood in the stool, are another early screening technique.

If stool samples are positive for abnormal levels of blood, the next step is either a barium enema, which reveals through x-rays any particular masses in the colon, or a sigmoidoscopy: an exploration of the colon via a small tube with a camera attached. This scope looks for polyps that may be malignant. The sigmoidoscopy is limited to the sigmoid colon; a full colonoscopy can be performed if tumors are suspected higher up in the structure.

If a test reveals the presence of suspicious polyps, tissue samples must be obtained to be examined for cancerous cells.

Identify the difference between diverticulosis and diverticulitis.

Diverticulosis is the presence of small sacs, or diverticula, in the colon. These sacs fill with fecal matter and bacteria, and the potential for infection is high. About 20% of the people diagnosed with diverticulosis will go on to develop diverticulitis, or inflammation of the diverticulae.

Name two complications gallstones can cause.

The most obvious complication of gallstones is an obstruction of the cystic or common bile duct, which can lead to jaundice. If the clog is distal to where the pancreas adds its secretions to the common bile duct, the pancreas can also sustain damage from a backup of its highly corrosive digestive juices; this is acute pancreatitis. The pooling of stagnant bile can also lead to infection of the gallbladder, or cholecystitis.

Name three possible causes of gastroenteritis.

Viruses. The most common cause of GI inflammation is an infection with rotavirus or Norwalk virus. Any of the hepatitis viruses can also cause it, as can the enterovirus.

Bacteria. Common bacterial pathogens include salmonella, shigella, and staphylococcus. "Travelers' diarrhea" is almost always from the E. Coli bacterium.

Other causes of gastroenteritis include parasites (e.g., Giardia), fungal infections (e.g., candida), toxins (e.g., poisonous mushrooms), dietary problems (e.g., food allergies), medications (e.g., antibiotics or magnesium-containing laxatives or antacids), or other conditions such as appendicitis, ulcerative colitis, or diverticulitis.

Name which variety of hepatitis is the most communicable.

Hepatitis A is the variety of hepatitis that is most communicable. This virus is transmitted through food or water contaminated with fecal matter. Hepatitis A is the reason for the signs about hand washing in restaurant bathrooms.

Name three ways in which bacteria can gain entry to the peritoneal space.

The bacteria that cause peritonitis can gain access to the peritoneal space through a variety of sources:

Rupture or perforation of an organ. This is a complication of appendicitis, perforated ulcers, and diverticulitis.

Abdominal abscesses. These can release bacteria for systemic infection.

Mechanical perforation. Perforation of the abdomen can introduce bacteria from the outside.

Spontaneous peritonitis. This is an occasional complication of advanced cirrhosis.

Peritoneal dialysis. This is a particular method of kidney dialysis for people with advanced kidney failure. It uses the peritoneal membrane as a filter to clean the blood.

Chapter Objectives: Urinary System Conditions

Name four structures that comprise the urinary system.

The urinary or excretory system is a relatively small system in the body, comprised of the kidneys, the ureters, the bladder, and the urethra.

Name three problems that could be present if red blood cells are found in the urine.

Any damage to the nephrons of the kidneys could result in red blood cells in the urine. Some examples include glomerulonephritis, kidney stones, pyelonephritis, and renal failure.

Name the difference between interstitial cystitis and urinary tract infection.

Interstitial cystitis is a condition in which the walls of the bladder become permeated with scar tissue, and the bladder can become smaller and less elastic.

Urinary tract infections usually begin as urethritis. If the bacteria are able to travel up the system, they may set up an infection in the bladder.

Name four possible causes for kidney stones.

In the case of calcium oxalate stones, the cause is almost always super-saturation of the urine.

A disorder of the parathyroid glands can cause a particular class of kidney stones.

An excess of Vitamin D can increase the amount of calcium absorbed from the diet, and this excess calcium can contribute to the formation of kidney stones.

A genetic predisposition for kidney stones may be present.

Certain foods can change the internal environment (these foods will be different for different people).

Difficulty with the processing of uric acid can lead to both gout and kidney stones.

A mechanical blockage of the urinary tract can cause kidney stones.

Chronic pyelonephritis contributes to the formation of kidney stones.

Some diuretics, which serve to concentrate the urine, cause stones to form.

Name the organism most often responsible for the development of pyelonephritis.

Most kidney infections are a complication of an E. coli infection in the urinary tract that travels up the ureters to set up an infection in the kidneys themselves.

Name one common cause for acute renal failure, and one common cause for chronic renal failure.

Acute kidney (renal) failure. This short-term problem is associated with severe ischemia from a lack of blood flow (which could happen for any number of reasons), a reaction to toxins, a tube blocked by a kidney stone or a tumor, direct damage to the kidney, or severe hemorrhaging.

Other causes of acute renal failure include acute tubular necrosis, or an infection of E. coli bacteria from undercooked meats, which produce enough toxins to interfere with kidney function.

Chronic kidney failure. This condition is directly linked to chronic high blood pressure. Other causes for chronic renal failure include glomerulonephritis, polycystic kidney disease, diabetes, and physical obstruction of the kidneys by a stone or tumor.

Chapter Review Questions: Urinary System Conditions

1. Describe how high blood pressure can lead to kidney dysfunction.

   Filtration, the movement of substances through a membrane by exterior mechanical pressure (in this case the blood pressure), is the mechanism by which most substances are exchanged between the circulatory system and the urinary system. Clearly, blood pressure and kidney health must be carefully intertwined. If blood pressure is consistently high, then the delicate tissue of the kidneys will be damaged and become less efficient.

2. Describe how kidney dysfunction can lead to high blood pressure.

   If the kidneys are not functioning adequately, the body accumulates excess fluid, which forces blood pressure up.

3. Why do people get kidney stones more often in hot environments than in other places?

   Kidney stones usually form in the absence of adequate fluids. Thus, they are very common in tropical environments where people tend to lose more liquid through sweat than they replace by drinking.

4. Why are women more likely to suffer from urinary tract infections than men?

   UTIs are almost always a women's disorder because the female urethra is so short, and it is located close to the anus, which allows bacteria that are harmless in the digestive tract to cause havoc if they gain access to the urinary tract.

5. How can renal failure lead to disconnected symptoms such as itching or mental incapacitation?

   The accumulation of toxins in the blood caused by renal failure can lead to several disconnected symptoms, including lethargy, fatigue, headaches, itchiness, loss of sensation in the hands and feet, discolored (yellowish or brownish) skin, tremors, seizures, easy bruising and bleeding, and muscle cramps. Changes in mental and emotional states can occur as the accumulation of toxins in the blood affect the brain.

6. Describe the relationship between long-term stress and urinary tract infections.

   A sympathetic nervous system component may contribute to the development of UTIs; anecdotal evidence links stress and bladder infections. Living in a sympathetic state may cause reduced blood flow to the bladder, possibly making it more susceptible to infection. However, clinical evidence to date shows that while stress may aggravate symptoms of UTIs, it has not been proven to cause them.

7. A client describes an accident in which she was sliding into home base and collided with the catcher. She complains of extreme pain on one side of her mid-back. Her muscles are not particularly tender, and she shows no signs of infection. What condition is likely to be present?

   This client needs to see a doctor. Although no signs of infection are visible, she may be suffering from pyelonephritis. Another possibility, however, is that she has bruised a kidney.

Chapter Objectives: Reproductive System Conditions

Know where in the reproductive system fertilization usually occurs.

The uterine tubes gently caress the ovaries, coaxing the eggs toward them. Once inside the fallopian or uterine tubes, the eggs make the 5-day journey to the uterus itself. If an egg is going to be fertilized, it will generally happen inside the fallopian tube.

Name the two most common types of breast cancer.

Although several different types of breast cancer are identified, the two most common are lobular and ductal carcinoma.

List four treatment options for breast cancer.

Surgery. Lumpectomies, partial mastectomies, total mastectomies, and modified mastectomies are surgical options for removing tumors and nearby lymph nodes.

Radiation. Radiation is aimed at tumors to slow or stop growth, or to shrink tumors in order to make them easier to remove surgically.

Chemotherapy. Chemotherapy is the treatment of cancer with highly toxic drugs to slow or stop the growth of tumors.

Hormone therapy. Some breast cancer tumors are sensitive to estrogen; they need access to this hormone in order to grow.

Know the connection between endometriosis and anemia.

The collection of blood in endometrial deposits routes blood away from where it is useful, causing anemia.

Name four risk factors for the development of ovarian cancer.

Familial history. Perhaps the greatest risk factor for ovarian cancer is having it in the family. Women who have a first-degree relative (mother, sister, daughter) with ovarian cancer have up to a 50% chance of developing the cancer themselves. Having a second-degree relative (grandmother, aunt, half-sister) with ovarian cancer also increases the chance of developing the disease. Families with a history of breast cancer also have statistically higher rates of ovarian cancer than the general population.

Reproductive history. Any woman who has never had a child or not taken birth control pills, or who has experienced multiple miscarriages is at increased risk for developing ovarian cancer. In addition, women who have taken fertility drugs without conceiving and bearing a child may also be at increased risk, although the statistics for these women are a bit inconsistent.

Health history. Women who have a history of breast cancer themselves have approximately twice the chance of developing ovarian cancer as the rest of the population.

Estrogen replacement therapy. Women who employ ERT against osteoporosis have a higher chance of developing ovarian cancer than others.

Other. Other risks involve exposure to radiation or asbestos; the use of talcum powder on the genitals; a high-fat diet; and age—the chance of developing ovarian cancer increases considerably between the ages of 40 and 60.

Know why ovarian cancer is so dangerous.

Ovarian cancer is a dangerous disease because early symptoms are practically nonexistent, or so subtle that they are easily passed over. When the cancer is finally identified, it has often metastasized beyond the point of control.

Name two types of ovarian cysts.

Follicular cysts. Occasionally, the follicle holding an egg never ruptures and releases it. In this case, a blister forms and the fluid isn't immediately reabsorbed into the body. Follicular cysts rarely grow bigger than 2 to 3 inches across, and they generally resolve within a few months.

Corpus luteum cysts. After a follicle releases an egg, it is referred to as the corpus luteum. Blisters can form over these structures, which changes the balance of hormones being secreted from the ovaries.

Polycystic ovaries. Also called Stein-Leventhal syndrome, this condition involves enlarged ovaries with multiple small cysts.

Know the most dangerous complication of pelvic inflammatory disease.

If an infection backs up from the vagina to the uterus to the uterine tubes, it can spread across to the ovaries, but it can just as easily start growing in the open pelvic cavity; this is peritonitis, and it can be a life-threatening situation.

Name three serious conditions associated with pregnancy.

In the vast range of things that could go wrong in a pregnancy, three conditions that massage therapists especially need to watch for are prenatal diabetes, pregnancy-induced hypertension, and ectopic pregnancy.

Know why one of the major signs for prostate cancer is difficulty with urination.

The prostate is a donut-shaped gland that lies inferior to the bladder and encircles the male urethra. If it becomes enlarged, thick, and hard, it interferes with the movement of urine through the urethra and out of the body.

Chapter Review Questions: Reproductive System Conditions

1. Describe how birth control pills work.

   Birth control pills work by introducing artificial hormones into the blood. These trick the pituitary into believing that the woman is pregnant, so she never ovulates.

2. Is the risk factor profile a very useful guideline for breast cancer? Why or why not?

   One of the most frustrating things about breast cancer is that no dependable profile exists of a woman who is likely to develop it. Statistically, women who began their menstrual periods early in life, who had children later in life or not at all, and who are obese are at a somewhat greater risk. However, the majority of women with some or all of these features may never develop breast cancer, and 25% of all women who develop breast cancer show none of these tendencies.

3. What are prostaglandins, and how are they involved in dysmenorrhea?

   Several different factors can contribute to primary dysmenorrhea. At the top of the list are prostaglandins: chemicals produced all over the body, but especially in the uterus. They cause smooth muscle contractions and also sensitize the body to pain.

4. Describe how stress can exacerbate menstrual pain.

   It is easy to see how physical or emotional stress fits into the picture of menstrual pain. Sympathetic reactions in the body exacerbate uterine ischemia, leading to pain, which reinforces spasm. The emotional state of dreading the pain and discomfort of menstrual periods can then become a self-fulfilling prophecy: the stress of anticipating an unpleasant event works to make that event even more unpleasant.

5. Under what circumstances may fibroid tumors cause symptoms?

   Usually fibroids create no symptoms at all. In very extreme cases, the fibroid may grow large enough to put pressure on the sensory nerves inside the uterus, or press on nearby structures such as the bladder, which can cause urinary frequency. If they press on the uterine tubes, they may interfere with pregnancies. They can also cause particularly heavy menstrual bleeding, and occasionally bleeding between menstrual periods.

6. How can endometriosis or pelvic inflammatory disease lead to sterility?

   In endometriosis, the development of the fibrous coverings for endometrial deposits can cause scarring and adhesions in or on the uterine tubes and ovaries.

   In PID, abscesses sometimes grow on the ovaries or uterine tubes. The body isolates these infections with fibrous connective tissue, and the growth of a scar often leads to a blockage of the tubes and subsequent sterility.

7. Ovarian cancer is the leading cause of death from gynecological diseases, yet it is a relatively rare condition. How can this be true?

   The prognosis for ovarian cancer is generally so poor because it is extremely difficult to make an early diagnosis. More than 50% of women diagnosed have already experienced some metastasis. The 5-year survival rate overall is 35 to 38%, but if the disease is identified early, that statistic rises to 85%.

8. Discuss the relationship between certain hormonal changes that occur in pregnancy and muscle spasm.

   One of the hormones secreted during pregnancy is relaxin. Its job is to loosen the ligaments in the pelvis to allow the baby to emerge. But relaxin starts working almost from day one, making all the ligaments in the body looser and more mobile. This can cause many problems, from unstable vertebrae to asymmetrical sacroiliac joints. Muscles then tighten up to stabilize the joints, causing spasm and pain.

9. Why may it be uncomfortable for a late-term pregnant woman to receive massage in a fully supine position?

Being fully reclined allows the fetus to rest directly on the big abdominal blood vessels, which will either limit blood flow to the legs, leading to cramping in the gastrocnemius, or limit blood flow up the vena cava, leading to dizziness and unconsciousness.

10. A client has been diagnosed with endometriosis, but has no particular symptoms at the time of her appointment. In order to help with her low back pain, her massage therapist works deeply on the psoas. Within a few hours the client has sharp shooting pains low in her abdomen and can't stand up straight. What may have happened?

Endometriosis sometimes displaces the pelvic contents, so the ovaries of a woman with endometriosis may not be in exactly the same place as they are in someone else. In this case, it is likely that the massage therapist inadvertently pressed or bruised an ovary.

Chapter Objectives: Miscellaneous Conditions

Name three criteria for a diagnosis of alcoholism.

An accepted definition for when alcohol use becomes abuse is when the patient must drink in order to feel "normal." Other criteria to determine the presence of alcoholism include:

Tolerance: an increasing tolerance to the effects of alcohol;

Withdrawal: the cessation of alcohol use creates withdrawal symptoms, including tremors, increased heart rate, sweating, insomnia, nausea and vomiting, anxiety, hallucinations, and seizures;

Can't stop: self-imposed efforts to limit or stop alcohol use are repeatedly unsuccessful;

Time loss: significant amounts of time are spent in alcohol use and recovery from hangovers;

Neglected responsibilities: responsibilities to family members, jobs, and personal health are neglected because of alcohol use;

Denial: denial that alcohol is seriously impeding in or damaging the user's life.

Name two external factors and two internal factors in the development of cancer.

External factors include carcinogens, which are chemical or environmental agents identified as cancer-causers. The hydrocarbons in cigarette smoke are carcinogens, as is UV radiation from the sun, especially for fair-skinned people. Viruses have long been known to cause cancer in some animals, but only recently has HIV been shown to actually cause, not just open the door for, Kaposi's Sarcoma.

Internal factors: Every cell in the body has a built-in capacity for self destruction. Some cells have a gene that prohibits this process. Therefore, cancer may be as much caused by cells that refuse to die as it is by new cells coming to life.

Some cancers result from or are connected to genetic features. This may mean a gene exists that is likely to cause cellular mutations sometime in the future, or a genetic susceptibility to factors that wouldn't be a threat to other people exists in some individuals.

Sometimes hormonal problems or immune system dysfunctions can also increase the risk for developing cancer.

Name five common signs that indicate the possibility of cancer, as presented by the American Cancer Society.

1. A change in bowel or bladder habits.

2. A sore that does not heal.

3. Unusual bleeding or drainage.

4. A thickening or lump in the breast or elsewhere.

5. Indigestion or swallowing difficulty.

6. A change in a wart or mole.

7. Persistent cough or hoarseness.

Name four suggestions for helping to prevent cancer, as presented by the National Research Council.

1. Eat more fruits, vegetables, and whole grain breads and cereals.

2. Reduce dietary fat.

3. Control weight.

4. Exercise regularly.

5. Use sunscreen.

6. Stop smoking and other tobacco use.

7. Limit alcohol consumption.

Name three types of cysts.

Baker's cysts are outpouchings of the synovial joint in the popliteal fossa. Ganglion cysts are pouches formed by tendonous sheaths. Ovarian cysts are usually harmless self-limiting growths on the ovaries at the site of egg release. Layers of connective tissue will also form around any foreign material that gets into the body. Unremoved shrapnel will be encysted, for example, and so will localized infections of tuberculosis. Massage therapists will most often encounter sebaceous cysts.

Know what conditions may be suspected if ongoing fatigue is not relieved by normal amounts of rest.

Fatigue that is not relieved with a reasonable amount of rest and recovery time may be a warning sign of chronic fatigue syndrome or anemia.

Name three contributing factors to insomnia.

Stress and anxiety. A precipitating event may begin the cycle of insomnia, but a pattern of sleeplessness can outlive the stress of the initial event. Eventually it can explode into a vicious circle in which a person lays awake, stressed about not being asleep, which increases stress, which decreases the ability to sleep, ad infinitum.

Depression. Clinical depression is both a cause and a symptom of chronic insomnia.

Counterproductive habits. These include changing time zones or sleep cycles frequently, napping, consuming caffeine close to bedtime, heavy smoking, or excessive alcohol consumption.

A poor sleeping environment. A room that is too cold or hot, has too much noise, too much light, or being forced to get adequate sleep during daylight hours may all contribute to insomnia.

Physical pain. If a person experiences pain when lying down, this can interfere with getting adequate sleep. In addition, not getting adequate sleep hinders the injury-repair process, prolonging the pain.

Mechanical pressure on the sympathetic trunk. If any cervical vertebrae are even slightly subluxated anteriorly, they can put pressure on the sympathetic trunk, the chain of ganglia that connect sympathetic neurons. This constant stimulus can literally lock someone into a fight-or-flight state that is not relieved until the mechanical pressure on the trunk is removed.

Other problems. These include sleep apnea, a breathing disorder; nocturia, the need to urinate frequently at night; and nocturnal myoclonus, a condition in which the legs involuntarily twitch during sleep, repeatedly waking the person.

Name three consequences of sleep deprivation.

The immune system is refreshed and rejuvenated during the deepest sleep cycles. Somatotrophin, the hormone that stimulates the action of fibroblasts for wound healing, is secreted primarily during deep sleep. In the absence of somatotrophin, people have a limited ability to heal from any kind of injury. Furthermore, lack of sleep depletes immune system activity. If the immune system isn't functioning well, the pathogens that live on the skin could turn into a life-threatening infection through any tiny hangnail or scrape.

In the short term, lack of sleep creates measurable changes in reflexes, memory capacity, reasoning skills, and the ability to do simple math problems. Lack of sleep is implicated in 200,000 automobile accidents every year, and costs the United States approximately $150 billion every year in costs from absenteeism.

In the long run, insomnia and other sleeping problems are part of the syndromes accompanying clinical depression, fibromyalgia, chronic fatigue syndrome, and chronic pain and injury patterns.

Name two major cautions for working with clients who are recovering from major surgery.

The two major cautions for massage following major surgery are immunosuppressant drugs and blood clots.

Define "abuse" as in "substance abuse."

The official definition of substance abuse makes no particular distinction between legal and illegal substances. Abuse is simply the use of a substance in ways or dosages that were never intended for that product. The substance is used to modify or control mood or state of mind in a way that is potentially harmful to the user or to other people.

Chapter Review Questions: Miscellaneous Conditions

1. Pick two body systems and describe the effects of alcohol on organs of those systems.

   The digestive system: Alcohol is highly irritating to the stomach lining, and high levels of consumption are responsible for a specific type of gastritis.

   People who have preexisting gastrointestinal problems are especially vulnerable to the worst effects of alcohol. It is implicated in the development of cancer in the upper gastrointestinal tract, especially in the esophagus, pharynx, larynx, and mouth. Alcoholism can cause ulcers, internal hemorrhaging, and pancreatitis. About 20% of long-term drinkers will develop cirrhosis.

The cardiovascular system: Alcohol use decreases the force of cardiac contractions and can lead to irregular heartbeats, or arrhythmia. Alcohol tends to agglutinate red blood cells, making them stick together. This leads to the possibility of thrombi, not only in the brain, but in the coronary arteries as well.

Moderate alcohol consumption can actually help prevent cardiovascular disease by increasing HDL levels (the "good" cholesterol) in the blood.

The nervous system: Memory loss frequently occurs for biochemical reasons as well as from agglutinated red blood cells becoming stuck in the cerebral capillaries, which causes brain cells to starve to death. Even some "social drinkers" sustain measurable brain damage from repeated agglutination. In the short term, alcohol slows reflexes, slurs speech, impairs judgment, and compromises motor control. In the long term, the same effects can happen on a permanent basis, in a condition known as organic brain syndrome. In advanced stages of cirrhosis, the blood is full of toxins that can cause brain damage, and several other brain disorders, which won't be discussed here, are associated with alcohol use.

The immune system: Prolonged alcohol use impedes resistance, especially to respiratory infections. Alcoholics are especially vulnerable to pneumonia.

The reproductive system: Alcoholism causes reduced sex drive, erectile dysfunction, menstrual irregularities, and infertility. Babies of alcoholic women are susceptible to fetal alcohol syndrome, the most common type of environmentally caused mental retardation in the United States. FAS affects 4,000 to 12,000 babies every year.

2. Briefly describe the staging process for cancer: what are the stages, and what do they mean?

Most types of cancer develop in predictable enough patterns to be "staged," or given a label to indicate how advanced the cancer is. Different systems exist for staging cancer, depending somewhat on what types of tissues are affected. Breast cancer, for instance, tends to progress very differently from colon cancer. The two widely recognized systems for staging cancer can be used independently or together to rate the degree of progression of the disease.

The TNM classification system rates tumors by: Tumor size (T); Nodal involvement (N); and extent of Metastasis (M).

The numerical staging system gives a number to indicate the degree of progression:

Stage 0 means some malignant cells may be present, but they are isolated and show no signs of spreading. Stage 0 cancer is sometimes called cancer *in situ*.

Stage I cancer involves a small tumor.

Stage II means the tumor may be larger or signs of metastasis to nearby lymph nodes are present.

Stage III indicates larger tumors and further signs of metastasis.

Stage IV generally means that the cancer has metastasized to distant parts of the body.

3. What are the possible risks of massaging a client who is living with cancer?

Massage that directly impacts blood and lymph flow may aid the process of metastasis.

4. What are the possible benefits of massaging a client who is living with cancer?

Massage may offer pain relief, parasympathetic balance during an especially stressful time, and immune system support to strengthen the activity of natural killer cells and other cancer-limiting mechanisms.

5. Describe the circular relationship between mental/emotional fatigue and physical fatigue.

   The two varieties of fatigue are usually inextricably blended together. Living in chronic stress (mental/emotional fatigue) can throw the neck muscles into an ongoing contraction (physical fatigue). This person always feels more tired than if those muscles were able to release their unnecessary tension. The feeling of always being tired is a self-fulfilling prophecy; feeling tired, the person moves less efficiently, which exacerbates that loss of energy.

6. Describe the relationship between inadequate sleep and limited capacity to heal from injury.

   Somatotrophin, the hormone that stimulates the action of fibroblasts for healing wounds, is secreted primarily during deep sleep. In the absence of somatotrophin, people have a limited ability to heal from any kind of injury.

7. What makes the difference between substance use and substance abuse?

   Substance use becomes abuse when the user continues to take the drug in order to seek out the pleasurable sensations it offers, or to avoid the negative effects of withdrawal, or both.

8. Describe the difference between physical addiction and psychological addiction.

   Psychological addiction is a dependency on pleasurable or satisfying sensations provided by a substance. Physical addiction is a dependency arising from the need to avoid withdrawal symptoms. Substance abuse is usually a combination of these two factors.

9. How have recent innovations in surgical techniques changed the way massage applies to postoperative patients?

   Today many surgeries are performed with lasers, balloons, and microscopic tools through tiny incisions in the skin. Procedures used to involve general anesthesia and hospital stays; now they are being performed on an outpatient basis, allowing patients to go home on the same day.

   The rapid development of new, less invasive surgical techniques is good news for massage therapists because the risks involved following major surgery (infection, blood clotting) are serious and frequently make doing massage impractical.

10. A client has a small (5 cm) undiagnosed lump on her upper back. It is dense but not painful, and it moves slightly on palpation. What is it most likely to be, and what should a responsible massage therapist do about it?

    A couple of conditions are possible in this situation. The lump is likely a sebaceous cyst, or a small lipoma. Neither one of these is particularly dangerous, but it is absolutely outside the scope of practice for massage therapists to diagnose the lump. A responsible practitioner will avoid the area and recommend that the client have it diagnosed by a physician.

Quick Reference Charts

Appendix 5

Read this first!

This appendix provides a reference for massage students and practitioners who need fast answers to simple questions. It is *not* intended as a substitute for reading the complete article for each condition, and will not provide enough information to make a well-informed decision without that background. Some conditions, however, are not detailed in text. These have been marked with an *.

Several things are important to remember while using these quick reference charts:

- The label "indicated" does *not* mean that a condition will always be improved by massage. It means that massage will not make the situation worse, and the support and comfort massage gives can certainly be beneficial to the client, if not to the particular condition.
- The term "massage" refers to circulatory-based massage that has a direct effect on blood and lymph flow. If a condition is labeled "contraindicated," it's usually because the influence of massage on circulation would have a negative impact on the client. This does not necessarily rule out touch altogether, however, and many conditions that contraindicate vigorous circulatory massage are perfectly appropriate for less mechanically based bodywork modalities.
- When massage is considered appropriate or indicated, it is a systemic recommendation. When massage is contraindicated, guidelines for whether those cautions are local or systemic have been provided.
- The specific kind of impact that massage may have on various conditions is discussed in the complete articles rather than here in the abbreviated version.

The most important thing to remember is that it is impossible to make a foolproof judgment about whether massage is a good choice strictly from a book. Every client is different; every practitioner has a different kind of approach. These recommendations are just that: *recommendations* that may help to shape well-informed decisions about the appropriateness of massage.

Condition Name	What Is It/ What Are They?	How Is It Recognized/ How Are They Recognized?	Is Massage Indicated or Contraindicated?
Abortion, Spontaneous and Elective (page 325)	Spontaneous and elective abortions are pregnancies that are ended, unintentionally or intentionally, before the fetus is born naturally.	Generalized or pelvic pain and bleeding may be present, but often no outward signals indicate a woman is recovering from a spontaneous or elective abortion.	Massage is locally contraindicated (no deep abdominal work) for women recovering from a recent spontaneous or elective abortion, until her bleeding has stopped, and she is free of any signs of infection.
Acne (page 19)	Acne is a bacterial infection of sebaceous glands usually found on the face, neck, and upper back. It is closely associated with adolescence, or liver dysfunction that results in excess testosterone in the system.	It looks like raised, inflamed pustules on the skin, sometimes with white or black tips.	Massage is locally contraindicated for acne because of the risk of spreading infection, causing pain, and exacerbating the symptoms with the application of an oily lubricant.
Acromegaly*	Acromegaly is an endocrine disorder in which too much pituitary growth hormone is available to tissues in individuals post-puberty.	Acromegaly is recognized by abnormal growth rates in certain areas, specifically the skull, hands, and feet.	Acromegaly is frequently caused by pituitary tumors. If the client has been cleared for massage by his or her doctor, conservative massage may be appropriate, as long as the bones and circulatory system are basically healthy.
Alcoholism (page 356)	Alcoholism is the dependence on alcohol use to feel "normal" and the lack of ability to limit or stop consumption.	Symptoms of alcoholism include increased tolerance to the effects of alcohol, solitary drinking, memory loss (blackouts), and the neglect of responsibilities and personal health.	Massage can be appropriate for persons recovering from alcohol use in rehabilitative settings, under medical supervision. Massage is always appropriate for alcoholics who no longer consume alcohol, providing they have no other contraindicating conditions. Massage is contraindicated for persons under the influence of alcohol at the time of their appointment.
Alzheimer's Disease*	Alzheimer's disease is a progressive degenerative disease of the brain leading to deterioration and dementia.	Many signs and symptoms indicate Alzheimer's disease. Some of the most common include memory loss, anxiety, delusions, depression, personality changes, restlessness, sleeplessness, social withdrawal, and intellectual decline.	Massage will not reverse the process of Alzheimer's disease, but it's unlikely to do any harm, as long as the client is comfortable. Therefore, with medical clearance, and within the comfort levels of the client, massage may be indicated for Alzheimer's disease.
Amyotrophic Lateral Sclerosis (page 133)	Amyotrophic lateral sclerosis (ALS) is a progressive disease that begins in the central nervous system. It involves the degeneration of motor neurons and the subsequent atrophy of voluntary muscle.	Symptoms of ALS include weakness, fatigue, and muscle spasms. It appears most frequently in men between 40 and 70 years of age.	Massage is indicated for ALS, with caution and under a doctor's supervision.

Condition Name	What Is It/ What Are They?	How Is It Recognized/ How Are They Recognized?	Is Massage Indicated or Contraindicated?
Anemia (page 178)	Anemia is a symptom rather than a disease in itself. It indicates a shortage of red blood cells or hemoglobin or both.	Symptoms of anemia include pallor, shortness of breath, fatigue, and poor resistance to cold. Other symptoms may accompany specific varieties of anemia.	Massage is indicated for idiopathic and nutritional deficiency anemias (except advanced pernicious anemia). Hemolytic, most aplastic, and secondary anemias contraindicate massage.
Aneurysm (page 190)	An aneurysm is a delicate dilation or outpouching in an artery, usually part of the aorta or at the base of the brain.	Symptoms of aneurysms are hard to pin down. Thoracic aneurysms may cause chronic hoarseness; abdominal aneurysms may cause local discomfort, reduced urine output, or severe backache. Cerebral aneurysms may be silent, or may cause extreme headache when they are at very high risk for rupture.	Massage is systemically contraindicated for diagnosed aneurysms, and is strongly cautioned for clients who fit the profile for aneurysms, but have not been diagnosed.
Ankylosing Spondylitis (page 69)	Ankylosing spondylitis (AS) is a progressive arthritis of the spine.	It generally begins as stiffness and pain around the sacrum, with occasional referred pain down the back of the buttocks and into the legs. It has acute and subacute episodes. People with advanced AS are locked in a flexed position.	Massage is indicated in the subacute stages of AS only, and then only under a doctor's supervision. During acute episodes, massage is at least locally contraindicated in areas of pain and inflammation.
Appendicitis (page 280)	Appendicitis is inflammation of the vermiform appendix, often due to infection, but sometimes related to physical obstruction, as well as pathogens.	The symptoms of appendicitis are widely variable, but include general abdominal pain that gradually settles in the lower right quadrant. Fever, nausea, vomiting, food aversion, and diarrhea may also be present.	Massage is systemically contraindicated for acute appendicitis. Postoperative massage may be appropriate.
Asthma (page 259)	Asthma is the result of spasmodic constriction of bronchial smooth muscle tubes in combination with excess mucus production and mucosal edema.	Asthma attacks are sporadic and involve coughing, wheezing, and difficulty with breathing, especially exhaling.	Massage is indicated for asthma as long as the individual is not in the throes of an attack. Between episodes, massage can be useful to reduce stress and deal with some of the muscular problems that accompany difficulty with breathing.
Atherosclerosis (page 193)	Atherosclerosis is a condition in which the arteries become partially or completely occluded due to atherosclerotic plaques.	Atherosclerosis has no symptoms until it is very advanced. However, it is connected to several other types of circulatory problems, including hypertension, arrhythmia, coronary artery disease, cerebrovascular disease, and peripheral vascular disease.	Circulatory massage is systemically contraindicated for advanced atherosclerosis.

Condition Name	What Is It/ What Are They?	How Is It Recognized/ How Are They Recognized?	Is Massage Indicated or Contraindicated?
Baker's Cysts (page 92)	Baker's cysts are fluid-filled extensions of the synovial membrane at the knee. They protrude into the popliteal fossa.	Baker's cysts are usually painless sacs that are palpable deep to the superficial fascia in the popliteal fossa.	Massage is locally contraindicated in the popliteal fossa anyway, and especially if the client has a Baker's cyst. In addition, if any signs of circulatory disruption (coldness, clamminess, edema) are distal to the cyst, that whole area is a contraindication, and the client needs to be cleared of the possibility of thrombosis.
Bell's Palsy (page 151)	Bell's palsy is a flaccid paralysis of one side of the face caused by inflammation or damage to cranial nerve VII.	Symptoms of Bell's palsy include drooping of the muscles on the affected side, difficulty with drinking and eating, and difficulty in closing the eye on one side. There may also be some pain, headaches, hypersensitivity to sound, and drooling.	Massage is indicated for Bell's palsy, in the absence of contraindicated underlying causes.
Boils (page 4)	Boils are local staphylococcus infections similar to acne, but they are not related to adolescence or liver dysfunction.	Boils look like acne, too, except that the lesions are bigger and they usually occur singly rather than being spread over a large area. They are also more painful than typical acne lesions.	Boils at least locally contraindicate massage, and care should be taken to make sure the infection is not systemic (screen the client for other symptoms such as swelling, fever, or discomfort other than at the site of the lesion). The bacteria that cause boils are extremely virulent and communicable. The sheets of a client with boils should be treated with extra care.
Breast Cancer (page 332)	Breast cancer is the growth of malignant tumor cells in breast tissue; these cells can invade skin and nearby muscles. If they invade lymph nodes, they can metastasize to the rest of the body.	The first sign of breast cancer is a small painless lump or thickening in the breast tissue or near the axilla. The lump may be too small to palpate, but may show on a mammogram. Later, the skin may change texture, the nipple may change shape, and the nipple may release discharge.	This is a topic of some controversy. It is impossible to make a blanket statement; advantages and disadvantages of massage for the breast cancer patient must be weighed on a case-by-case basis.
Bronchitis*	Bronchitis is an inflammation of the trachea, bronchi, and bronchioles, generally from a respiratory tract infection.	Symptoms of bronchitis include fever, fatigue, difficulty in breathing, chest burning, coughing, wheezing, and rales.	Massage is contraindicated for acute bronchitis, as it is for all acute infections. Clients recovering from a bronchitis infection may receive massage safely.
Bunions (page 94)	A bunion is a protrusion at the metatarsal-phalangeal joint of the great toe that occurs when the toe is laterally deviated.	Bunions are recognizable by the large bump on the medial aspect of the foot. If they are inflamed, they will be red, hot, and possibly edematous.	Vigorous massage is locally contraindicated at the point of a bunion regardless, and especially when or if it is inflamed. Massage elsewhere on the foot or body is very much indicated within pain tolerance to help with compensation patterns that occur when it is difficult to walk.

Condition Name	What Is It/ What Are They?	How Is It Recognized/ How Are They Recognized?	Is Massage Indicated or Contraindicated?
Burns (page 34)	Burns are caused by damage to the skin that causes the cells to die. They can be caused by fire, overexposure to the sun, dry heat, wet heat, electricity, radiation, extreme cold, and toxic chemicals.	First-degree burns involve mild inflammation. Second-degree burns include blistering and damage at the deeper levels of the epidermis. Third-degree burns penetrate the dermis itself and will often show white or black charred edges. In the postacute stage, serious burns will often develop shrunken, contracted scar tissue over the area of affected skin.	Massage is locally contraindicated for all burns (except, perhaps, mild sunburns) in the acute stage. In the subacute and postacute stages, massage may be performed around the damaged area within pain tolerance of the client.
Bursitis (page 95)	A *bursa* is a fluid-filled sack that acts as a protective cushion at points of recurring pressure, eases the movement of tendons and ligaments moving over bones, and cushions points of contact between bones. Bursitis is the inflammation of a bursa.	Acute bursitis is painful and will be aggravated by both passive and active motion. Muscles surrounding the affected joint will often severely limit range of motion. It may be hot or edematous.	Massage is locally contraindicated in the acute phase of noninfectious bursitis. Massage elsewhere on the body during an acute phase, and directly on the muscles of the affected joint (within pain limits) in a subacute phase, is perfectly appropriate.
Cancer (page 358)	Cancer is the growth of malignant cells into tumors that invade tissues and spread throughout the body.	Cancer in early stages is often difficult to detect. Early signs depend on what part of the body is affected.	The decision of whether to include massage as part of a treatment plan with cancer is a complicated one. Many benefits are possible, along with some risks. Circulatory massage that is not vigorous may be appropriate for persons dealing with cancer, but it should be performed with medical approval.
Candidiasis*	This is a fungal infection of any of a number of systems. The usual cause is an organism called Candida albicans, although several other fungi can cause similar symptoms. Candidiasis infections can affect the skin, gastrointestinal tract, urinary and reproductive systems, and the lungs. In an extreme form, it can develop into *acute systemic candidiasis*, which has several life-threatening complications. Acute systemic candidiasis is a medical emergency.	Symptoms of candidiasis depend on which systems are affected. Some possibilities include fever, malaise, hypotension, and skin rashes. Acute systemic candidiasis may also involve tachycardia, altered mental state, and enlarged spleen and liver.	Massage is locally contraindicated in the presence of acute skin rashes of any kind. Acute systemic candidiasis systematically contraindicates massage. For other candidiasis infections, massage may be appropriate with medical clearance.

Condition Name	What Is It/ What Are They?	How Is It Recognized/ How Are They Recognized?	Is Massage Indicated or Contraindicated?
Carpal Tunnel Syndrome (page 111)	Carpal Tunnel Syndrome (CTS) is irritation of the median nerve as it passes under the transverse carpal ligament into the wrist. It has several different causes.	CTS will cause pain, tingling, numbness, and weakness in the part of the hand supplied by the median nerve.	Massage is indicated with extreme caution for CTS. Work on or around the wrist must stop immediately if any symptoms are elicited, but some types of CTS will respond well to massage. It is necessary to get a medical doctor's diagnosis in order to know which type of CTS is present.
Cerebral Palsy*	Cerebral palsy (CP) is a general term for a group of signs and symptoms of central nervous system damage that occurs prenatally or in early infancy.	Symptoms of CP depend on what part of the brain is affected. They can include variable amounts of motor dysfunction and/or mental retardation.	Massage is indicated for CP as long as sensation is present.
Chondromalacia/ Patellofemoral Syndrome (page 71)	Chondromalacia is a pathological softening of the patellar cartilage. Patellofemoral syndrome (PFS) is an overuse syndrome that can lead to this sort of damage.	Chondromalacia causes pain at the knee, stiffness after immobility, and discomfort in walking down stairs.	Massage is indicated for chondromalacia and PFS, assuming the knee is not acutely inflamed. Massage may or may not be useful to correct these problems, but it will certainly do no harm.
Chorea (page 134)	Chorea is involuntary twitching, usually due to essential tremor, Huntington's disease, or Parkinson's disease.	Chorea is identified through uncontrolled gross motor movements.	Massage is indicated for most kinds of chorea, as long as medical clearance has been obtained.
Chronic Fatigue Syndrome (page 229)	Chronic fatigue syndrome (CFS) is a collection of signs and symptoms that indicate an ongoing immune response. The original stimulus of the response may be an identifiable pathogen, or it may simply be a dysfunction of the immune system.	The central symptom to CFS is debilitating fatigue. It may be accompanied by swollen nodes, slight fever, muscular and joint aches, headaches, excessive pain after mild exercise, and non-restorative sleep.	Massage is indicated for CFS except during fever, and can be a very helpful part of a treatment plan.
Cirrhosis (page 291)	With cirrhosis normal liver cells are replaced with scar tissue.	The symptoms of cirrhosis can be subtle until the disease is very far advanced. Early symptoms include loss of appetite, nausea, vomiting, and weight loss. Later symptoms include jaundice, ascites, and vomiting blood.	Massage is contraindicated for people with advanced cirrhosis.

Condition Name	What Is It/ What Are They?	How Is It Recognized/ How Are They Recognized?	Is Massage Indicated or Contraindicated?
Colon Cancer (page 282)	Colon cancer is the development of malignant tumors in the colon or rectum. Growths can block the bowel and/or metastasize to other organs, particularly the liver.	Colon cancer has different symptoms, depending on what part of the colon is affected. The most dangerous symptoms are extreme changes in bowel habits— diarrhea or constipation—that last more than 10 days. Other symptoms include blood in the stool, iron-deficiency anemia, and weight loss.	Circulatory massage is contraindicated for active cases of colon cancer, as it is for most cases of cancer, although decisions must be made on a case-by-case basis.
Common Cold (page 249)	The common cold (or upper respiratory tract infection— URTI) is a viral infection from any of about 200 different types of viruses.	The symptoms of colds are nasal discharge, sore throat, mild fever, dry coughing, and headache.	Massage is indicated for colds in the subacute stage only.
Contractures (page 49)	Contractures are permanently shortened muscles or muscle groups that are surrounded by thick, contracted fascia.	Contractures usually happen in flexion rather than extension. The muscles lose bulk and the tissue is hard and unyielding.	Massage is indicated for contracture in which sensation is present, although it may do little to reverse the process if it's gone too far. Massage can be a good preventative measure for contractures.
COPD/ Emphysema (page 262)	Emphysema is a condition in which the alveoli of the lungs become fibrous and inelastic. They merge with each other, decreasing surface area, and limiting oxygen-carbon dioxide exchange. It is one of a group of diseases called *chronic obstructive pulmonary disease*, or COPD.	Symptoms of emphysema include shortness of breath with mild or no exertion, rales, cyanosis, and susceptibility to secondary respiratory infection.	Massage is indicated for emphysema under medical supervision.
Crohn's Disease*	Crohn's disease is an idiopathic inflammatory condition, usually of the small intestine and sometimes of the large intestine. It is slowly progressive, involving isolated lengths of intestine, with normal areas remaining in between damaged tissue.	Signs and symptoms of Crohn's disease depend on the affected part of the intestines. They include diarrhea, abdominal pain, and weight loss. Crohn's disease is badly aggravated by any intestinal bacterial infection.	Crohn's disease at least locally contraindicates massage. Massage to areas outside the abdomen may be appropriate, under a doctor's supervision.
Cysts (page 362)	Cysts are layers of connective tissue surrounding and isolating something that shouldn't be in the body, e.g., a piece of shrapnel or a localized infection.	Palpable cysts are generally small, painless, distinct masses that move slightly under the skin.	Massage is locally contraindicated for cysts.
Decubitus Ulcers (page 36)	Decubitis ulcers, or bedsores, are ulcers caused by impaired circulation to the skin. Lack of blood supply leads to irreplaceable tissue death.	Unlike other sores, ulcers don't crust over; they remain open wounds that are highly vulnerable to infection.	Once the tissue has been damaged, massage is *strictly* locally contraindicated until the sores have completely healed over.

Condition Name	What Is It/ What Are They?	How Is It Recognized/ How Are They Recognized?	Is Massage Indicated or Contraindicated?
Dermatitis/ Eczema (page 21)	Dermatitis is an umbrella term for inflammation of the skin. Eczema is a type of *atopic* dermatitis, a non-contagious skin rash usually brought about by an allergic reaction. Contact dermatitis is a related but slightly different type of hypersensitivity reaction.	Dermatitis presents itself in various ways, depending on what type of skin reactions are elicited. Exposure to poison oak or poison ivy results in large inflamed wheals; metal allergies tend to be less inflamed and more isolated in area. Eczema usually appears as one of two varieties: very dry and flaky skin (seborrheic eczema) or blistered, weepy skin (dyshidrotic eczema).	The appropriateness of massage depends completely on the source of the problem and the condition of the skin. If the skin is very inflamed or has blisters or other lesions, massage is at least locally contraindicated until the acute stage has passed. If signs indicate a rash could spread (e.g., with poison oak), massage is systemically contraindicated while the irritation is present. Dry, flaky eczema indicates massage. If the skin is not itchy and the affected area is highly isolated, as with a metal allergy to a watch band or earrings, massage is only locally contraindicated.
Diabetes Mellitus (page 210)	Diabetes is a group of metabolic disorders characterized by glucose intolerance or deficiency and disturbances in carbohydrate, fat, and protein metabolism.	Early symptoms of diabetes include frequent urination, thirstiness, and increased appetite along with weight loss, nausea, and vomiting.	Massage is indicated for people with diabetes as long as their tissue is healthy and they receive medical clearance.
Dislocations (page 72)	Dislocations are traumatic injuries to joints in which the articulating bones are forcefully separated.	Acute (new) dislocations are extremely painful. The bones may be visibly separated and a total loss of function occurs at the joint.	Massage is indicated in the sub-acute stage for dislocations, as long as work is conducted within pain tolerance. As the area heals, massage may be useful for managing scar tissue accumulation and muscle spasm around the affected joint.
Diverticulosis/ Diverticulitis (page 285)	Diverticulosis is the development of small pouches that protrude from the colon. Diverticulitis is the inflammation of these pouches when they become infected.	Diverticulosis is usually symptomless. When inflammation is present, lower left-side abdominal pain, cramping, bloating, constipation, or diarrhea will occur.	Deep abdominal massage is locally cautioned if the client knows diverticula are present. Massage is systemically contraindicated in the presence of active infection.
Dupuytren's Contracture (page 97)	Dupuytren's contracture is an idiopathic shrinking and thickening of the fascia on the palm of the hand.	It usually affects the ring and little fingers, pulling them into permanent flexion.	Massage is indicated for Dupuytren's contracture as long as sensation is present, although it may do little to reverse the process if it's gone too far.
Dysmenorrhea (page 326)	Dysmenorrhea is the technical term for menstrual pain that is severe enough to interfere with and limit the activities of women of childbearing age.	The symptoms of dysmenorrhea are dull aching or sharp severe lower abdominal pain, preceding and/or during the early stages of menstruation. Nausea and vomiting may accompany very severe cases.	Massage is appropriate for dysmenorrhea that is not linked to underlying pathology, although the abdomen is locally contraindicated for deep work during days of heavy menstrual flow.

Condition Name	What Is It/ What Are They?	How Is It Recognized/ How Are They Recognized?	Is Massage Indicated or Contraindicated?
Edema (page 224)	Edema is the retention of interstitial fluid either because of electrolyte or protein imbalances or because of mechanical obstruction in the circulatory or lymphatic systems.	Edematous tissue is puffy or boggy. It may be hot, if associated with local infection, or quite cool, if it is cut off from local circulation.	Massage is contraindicated for most edemas, particularly pitting edema, where the tissue does not immediately spring back from a touch. Indicated edemas include those due to subacute soft tissue injury or temporary immobilization caused by some factor that does *not* contraindicate massage.
Embolism or Thrombus (page 182)	Thrombi are stationary clots; emboli are clots that travel through the circulatory system. Emboli are usually composed of blood, but may also be fragments of plaque, fat globules, air bubbles, tumors, or bone chips.	Venous emboli land in the lungs, causing pulmonary embolism. Symptoms of PE include shortness of breath, chest pain, and coughing up sputum that is streaked with blood. Arterial emboli can lodge in coronary arteries (heart attack), the brain (transient ischemic attack or stroke), kidneys, legs, or some other organ.	Massage is systemically contraindicated in the presence of diagnosed thrombi or emboli, as it is for any disorder involving potential blood clots.
Encephalitis (page 143)	Encephalitis is inflammation of the brain usually brought about by a viral infection.	Signs and symptoms of encephalitis include fever, headache, confusion, and personality and memory changes. Encephalitis is diagnosed through examination of cerebrospinal fluid and analysis of CT or MRI scans.	Massage is systemically contraindicated for acute encephalitis, but if a client has had it in her history with no signs of present infection, massage is perfectly acceptable.
Endometriosis (page 328)	Endometriosis is the growth of endometrial cells in the peritoneal cavity (and possibly elsewhere). The cells swell and subside with the menstrual cycle.	Endometriosis often has no symptoms. When it does, they are generally infertility and abdominal pain during menstruation.	Massage is a local contraindication for diagnosed cases of endometriosis.
Epilepsy*	Epilepsy is a seizure disorder, caused by neurological damage, although it may be impossible to delineate exactly what the damage is.	Epilepsy is diagnosed through CT and MRI scans. Seizures may take different forms for different people; they range from barely noticeable to life-threatening.	Massage is contraindicated during seizures, but is indicated at all other times for clients with epilepsy.
Erysipelas (page 6)	Erysipelas is a streptococcus infection that kills skin cells, leading to painful inflammation of the skin. It usually occurs on the face or lower leg.	A distinct margin between the reddened, affected area and the surrounding unaffected areas marks this condition. When it occurs on the face, it often creates a red "butterfly" shape over the cheeks and bridge of the nose. Fever and signs of systemic infection can accompany it.	This is a bacterial infection that can invade both the lymph and circulatory systems. Massage is systemically contraindicated until the infection has completely passed.
Fatigue (page 364)	Fatigue is a state of less than optimal performance because the body has had inadequate rest and recovery time.	A person suffering from mental or physical fatigue feels tired, move inefficiently, and may be more prone to injury.	In the absence of other contraindicated conditions, massage is systemically indicated for fatigue.

Condition Name	What Is It/ What Are They?	How Is It Recognized/ How Are They Recognized?	Is Massage Indicated or Contraindicated?
Fever (page 232)	Fever is an increased core temperature brought about by immune system reactions, usually to invasion by some pathogens.	Fever is identifiable by thermometer.	Massage is systemically contraindicated for fever, which indicates that the body is fighting infection. This condition can be recognized at a glance (or touch). Massage therapists are not, by the way, usually required to keep thermometers in their offices.
Fibroid Tumors (page 330)	Fibroid tumors are benign growths in the muscle or connective tissue of the uterus.	Most fibroid tumors are asymptomatic. Some, however, cause increased menstrual bleeding or may put mechanical pressure on other structures in the pelvis.	Deep abdominal massage is locally contraindicated for large, diagnosed fibroid tumors. However, most fibroids are quite small and virtually symptomless. In these cases, massage is appropriate.
Fibromyalgia (page 50)	Fibromyalgia is a condition that involves chronic muscle pain, trigger points, tender points, and nonrestorative sleep.	Fibromyalgia is diagnosed when other diseases have been ruled out, and seven to ten active trigger points are identified.	Massage is indicated for fibromyalgia. Care must be taken not to overtreat, however, because patients are extremely sensitive to pain and may have accumulations of waste products in the tissues that are difficult to flush out adequately.
Fractures (page 60)	A fracture is any kind of broken or cracked bone.	Most fractures are painful and involve loss of function at the nearest joints, but some may be difficult to diagnose without an x-ray.	Massage is locally contraindicated for acute fractures, but work done on the rest of the body can yield reflexive benefits. Massage is indicated for people in later stages of recovery from fractures.
Fungal Infections (page 7)	Fungal infections of human skin, also called *mycoses*, are caused by fungi called *dermatophytes*. When there is a fungal infection caused by dermatophytes, the characteristic lesions are called *tinea*. Thus, within this heading several different types of tinea are listed.	Most tinea lesions begin as one reddened circular itchy patch. Scratching the lesions will spread them to other parts of the body. As they get larger they tend to clear in the middle and keep a red ring around the edges. Athlete's foot, another type of mycosis, will involve moist blisters and cracking between the toes. If it affects the nails they will become yellow, thickened, and pitted.	Massage is at least locally contraindicated for fungal infections in all phases. If the affected areas are very limited—for instance, only the feet are involved or only one or two small, covered lesions appear on the body—massage may be administered to the rest of the body. If there is a large area involved, and especially if the infection is acute (i.e., not yet responding to treatment), then massage is systemically contraindicated.
Gallstones (page 294)	Gallstones are crystallized formations of cholesterol or bile pigments in the gall bladder. They can be as small as grains of sand or as large as a golf ball.	Most gallstones do not cause symptoms. When they do, long-term or short-term pain occurs in the upper right side of the abdomen, which may refer to the back and right scapula. Gallstones stuck in ducts may cause jaundice or pancreatitis.	Massage is appropriate for symptom-free gallstones although draining strokes over the liver are contraindicated.

Condition Name	What Is It/ What Are They?	How Is It Recognized/ How Are They Recognized?	Is Massage Indicated or Contraindicated?
Ganglion Cysts (page 98)	Ganglion cysts are small fluid-filled connective tissue sacks that are attached to tendons, tendinous sheaths, ligaments, or periosteum.	Ganglion cysts are small bumps that usually appear on the wrist or ankle. They are not usually painful, unless they are in a place to be injured by normal wear and tear.	Massage is locally contraindicated for ganglion cysts. It cannot make them better, and may irritate them through excess fluid flow.
Gastroenteritis (page 276)	Gastroenteritis is a form of gastrointestinal inflammation, which may be caused by a viral or bacterial infection, a parasite, fungus, toxic exposure, or other factors.	Symptoms of gastroenteritis include nausea, vomiting, and diarrhea.	Massage is at least locally contraindicated for anyone with acute gastrointestinal inflammation, and systemically contraindicated for people with acute intestinal infections.
Glomerulo- nephritis (page 309)	Glomerulonephritis is a condition in which the glomeruli (small structures that are part of nephrons) become inflamed and cease to function efficiently.	Early symptoms of glomerulonephritis include dark or rust-colored urine, foamy urine, or blood in the urine. Later symptoms indicate chronic renal failure: systemic edema, fatigue, headaches, decreased urine output, discoloration of the skin, and general malaise.	Massage is systemically contraindicated for glomerulonephritis. This inflammatory condition impairs the body's ability to manage fluid exchanges.
Gout (page 74)	Gout is an inflammatory arthritis caused by deposits of sodium urate (uric acid) in and around joints, especially in the feet.	Acute gout causes joints to become red, hot, swollen, shiny, and extremely painful. It usually has a sudden onset.	Massage is systemically contraindicated for gout in the acute stage, and locally contraindicated for gouty joints at all times.
Guillain Barré Syndrome*	Guillain Barré Syndrome is a disease of the nervous system brought about by autoimmune dysfunction, certain types of infections or vaccinations, Hodgkin's lymphoma, surgery, or exposure to some drugs.	This disease begins with reduced sensation in fingers and toes, which progresses up toward the central nervous system. Both sensation and motor innervation may be affected. In extreme cases, patients may need a ventilator to assist in breathing. Guillain Barré syndrome is usually a temporary situation, and most patients experience a full or nearly full recovery within weeks or months.	Sensation may be limited during the onset phase of this disease, and any sensory impairment contraindicates vigorous massage. If sensation is intact and medical clearance is obtained, massage may be a useful part of the recovery strategy for Guillain Barré syndrome.
Headaches (page 153)	Headaches are pain caused by any number of sources. Muscular tension is the most common source of pain; congestive headaches are less common; and headaches due to serious underlying pathology are the rarest of all.	Tension headaches may be bilateral and generally painful. Vascular headaches are often unilateral and have a distinctive "throbbing" pain from blood flow into the head. Headaches brought about by central nervous system disease are extreme, severe, and prolonged. They can have a sudden or gradual onset.	Massage is systemically contraindicated for headache due to infection or CNS disturbance. Massage is indicated for vascular headaches in the subacute stage. Massage is indicated for tension headaches.
Heart Attack (page 206)	A heart attack, or myocardial infarction (MI), is damage to the myocardium caused by a clot or plaque fragment getting lodged somewhere in a coronary artery, or atherosclerosis so complete that it deprives the cardiac muscle of oxygen.	Symptoms of heart attacks include angina, shortness of breath, a feeling of great pressure on the chest, and pain around the left shoulder and arm, jaw, and back.	Massage is contraindicated for patients recovering from heart attacks. After complete recovery, heart attack patients may be good candidates for massage but not without medical clearance.

Condition Name	What Is It/ What Are They?	How Is It Recognized/ How Are They Recognized?	Is Massage Indicated or Contraindicated?
Hematoma (page 186)	A hematoma is a deep bruise (leakage of blood) between muscle sheaths.	Superficial hematomas are simple bruises. Deep bleeds may not be visible, but they will be painful, and if extensive bleeding is present, the affected tissue will have a characteristic "gel-like" feel.	Massage is locally contraindicated for acute hematomas because of the possibility of blood clots and pain. In the subacute stage (at least two days later), when the surrounding blood vessels have been sealed shut and the body is in the process of breaking down and reabsorbing the debris, gentle massage within pain tolerance around the perimeter of the area and hydrotherapy can be helpful. Watch for signs of thrombophlebitis or deep vein thrombosis, and if there is any doubt, consult a doctor.
Hemophilia (page 184)	Hemophilia is a genetic disorder in which certain clotting factors in the blood are either inactive or missing altogether.	Hemophilia can cause superficial bleeding that persists for longer than normal, or internal bleeding into joint cavities or between muscle sheaths with little or no provocation.	Massage is systematically contraindicated for most cases of hemophilia unless the case is very mild and the client gets medical clearance.
Hepatitis (page 296)	Hepatitis is inflammation of the liver, usually due to viral infection.	All types of hepatitis produce the same symptoms, with variable severity. Symptoms, when any exist, include fatigue, jaundice, abdominal pain, nausea, and diarrhea. Sometimes no symptoms are present.	Massage is systemically contraindicated for acute hepatitis. For clients with chronic hepatitis, the appropriateness of massage will depend on their general health.
Hernia (page 99)	A hernia is a hole or rip in the abdominal wall or the inguinal ring through which the small intestines may protrude. A hiatal hernia forms where the diaphragm opens to allow the esophagus to pass; when this hole becomes wider, the stomach protrudes upwardly.	Abdominal hernias usually show some bulging and mild-to-severe pain, depending on whether or not a portion of the small intestine is trapped. Hiatal hernias are usually distinguished by the presence of chronic heartburn.	Massage is locally contraindicated for unreduced hernias, and systemically contraindicated for unreduced hernias that show signs of infection. For recent surgeries, postoperative protocols should be observed. For old hernia surgeries, massage is indicated.
Herniated Disc (page 114)	A herniated disc is a situation in which the nucleus pulposis or the surrounding annulus fibrosis of an intervertebral disc protrudes in such a way that it puts pressure on nerve roots or on the spinal cord itself.	The symptoms of nerve root pressure include referred pain along the dermatome, specific muscle weakness, paresthesia, and numbness.	Massage is indicated in the subacute stage of herniated discs.

Condition Name	What Is It/ What Are They?	How Is It Recognized/ How Are They Recognized?	Is Massage Indicated or Contraindicated?
Herpes Simplex (page 10)	Herpes simplex is a viral infection resulting in cold sores or fever blisters on the face or in the mouth (type I) or around the genitals, thighs, or buttocks (type II).	Herpes outbreaks are often preceded by two to three days of tingling, itching, or pain. Blisters then appear, which gradually crust and disappear, usually within two weeks.	Massage is locally contraindicated for any kind of herpes in the acute stage, and systemically contraindicated if the client is showing any systemic signs of infection. The sheets of clients with herpes must be isolated and sterilized. For clients with histories of herpes but no active symptoms, massage is indicated.
Herpes Zoster (page 144)	Herpes Zoster, or shingles, is a viral infection of sensory neurons from the same virus that causes chicken pox.	Shingles creates extremely painful blisters along the dermatomes, usually around the ribs, but occasionally of the trigeminal nerve. It is almost always unilateral.	Massage is systemically contraindicated during the acute stage of shingles, because this is such a painful condition. After the blisters have healed and the pain has subsided, massage is appropriate.
HIV/AIDS (page 233)	Acquired Immune Deficiency Syndrome (AIDS) is a disease caused by the Human Immunodeficiency Virus (HIV), which attacks and disables the immune system, leaving a person vulnerable to a host of diseases that are not a threat to uninfected people.	Most people with HIV will experience a week or two of flu-like symptoms within a few weeks of being infected. Then an interval passes with no symptoms. When the virus has successfully inactivated the immune system, infections will occur by opportunistic conditions such as cytomegalovirus or pneumocystis carinii. At this point, the HIV infection becomes AIDS.	Massage is indicated for all stages of HIV infection as long as the practitioner is healthy and doesn't pose any risk to the client, and the client is able to keep up with the changes that massage brings about in the body.
Hives (page 24)	Hives are an inflammatory skin reaction to an allergen or emotional stressor.	They can be small red spots or large wheals that are warm to the touch and itchy. They generally subside within a few hours.	Massage is systemically contraindicated in the acute stage and locally contraindicated in the subacute stage of hives. By bringing even more circulation to the skin, massage would only make a bad situation worse.
Hodgkin's Disease (page 225)	Hodgkin's disease is a slow-growing lymphoma that typically begins in the lymph nodes of the neck, axilla, or inguinal areas, but may spread to attack internal organs.	Painless swelling of lymph nodes is the cardinal sign of this disease, along with the possibility of fatigue, low-grade fever, night sweats, itchiness, and loss of appetite.	Rigorous circulatory massage is generally not recommended for a person who is fighting cancer, although this may be a case-by-case decision. For someone who has been cancer-free for 5 years or more, massage is appropriate. Noncirculatory types of massage may be appropriate for Hodgkin's patients, with medical clearance.
Hyperesthesia (page 156)	Hyperesthesia is extreme sensitivity in the skin, often because of stress or irritated nerves.	Hyperesthesiac clients are extremely sensitive and have very low pain thresholds.	This depends entirely on the root cause of the problem.

Condition Name	What Is It/ What Are They?	How Is It Recognized/ How Are They Recognized?	Is Massage Indicated or Contraindicated?
Hypertension (page 199)	Hypertension is the technical term for high blood pressure.	High blood pressure has no dependable symptoms. The only way to identify it is by taking several blood pressure measurements over time.	For borderline or mild high blood pressure, massage may be useful as a tool to control stress and increase general health, but other pathologies related to kidney or cardiovascular disease must be ruled out. High blood pressure that requires medication usually contraindicates circulatory massage, but under some circumstances, massage may be appropriate with a doctor's approval.
Hyperthyroidism*	Hyperthyroidism is a reaction to the secretion of too much thyroid hormone, which regulates metabolism. The most common type of hyperthyroidism is an autoimmune condition called Graves' disease. Other varieties of hyperthyroidism cause the growth of goiters.	Signs and symptoms of hyperthyroidism include nervousness, increased sweating, heat intolerance, and palpitations.	Massage may be appropriate for hyperthyroidism, depending on the underlying causes. Always work under a doctors supervision.
Hypothyroidism*	Hypothyroidism is a condition in which inadequate levels of thyroid hormone are circulating, or the body has built up a resistance to the hormone so that it no longer stimulates normal responses.	Signs and symptoms of hypothyroidism include weakness, fatigue, and lethargy; intolerance to cold; decreased memory; and possible constipation, muscle cramps, and weight gain.	Hypothyroidism can be caused by several different factors, including autoimmune reactions and radiation therapy. If the underlying cause of the problem does not contraindicate, massage may be appropriate for hypothyroidism, under the supervision of a doctor.
Ichthyosis (page 39)	Ichthyosis is pathologically dry skin—much more severe than average dry skin.	Ichthyosis creates distinctive diamond-shaped "scales" on the skin, usually on the lower legs.	Massage is definitely indicated for this condition. It probably won't be a permanent solution to this congenital problem, but it can certainly make it better in the short run. Take care to avoid areas where cracking exposes the blood to the possibility of infection.
Impetigo (page 12)	Impetigo is a bacterial (staphylococcus or streptococcus) infection of the skin.	There is a rash with fluid-filled blisters and honey-colored crusts. It usually begins somewhere on the face, but can appear anywhere on the body.	Until the lesions have completely healed, massage is systematically contraindicated for this highly contagious condition.

Condition Name	What Is It/ What Are They?	How Is It Recognized/ How Are They Recognized?	Is Massage Indicated or Contraindicated?
Inflammation (page 237)	Inflammation is a protective device in response to injury or infection. It involves localized swelling and chemical reactions to isolate the area and to resolve the damage through immune response.	The signs of inflammation are redness, pain, swelling, heat, and loss of function.	Massage is contraindicated for acute inflammation, but may be appropriate for subacute situations, depending on the causative factors.
Influenza (page 251)	Influenza ("flu") is a viral infection of the respiratory tract.	The symptoms of flu include high fever, and muscle and joint achiness that may last for up to 3 days, followed by a runny nose, coughing, sneezing, and general malaise.	Massage is indicated for the flu in the subacute stage only.
Insomnia (page 365)	Insomnia is the inability to attain adequate amounts of sleep.	Signs of insomnia include general fatigue, reduced mental capacity, and slow healing processes.	Massage is systemically indicated for insomnia.
Interstitial Cystitis (page 317)	Interstitial cystitis is a chronic inflammation of the bladder, involving scar tissue, stiffening, decreased capacity, bleeding, and sometimes ulcers in the bladder walls.	Symptoms of interstitial cystitis are similar to those of urinary tract infections: burning, frequency, urgency of urination; decreased capacity of the bladder may become a problem, along with pain, pressure, and tenderness.	Massage is only locally contraindicated for interstitial cystitis, as long as no signs of generalized infection (i.e., fever, chills, malaise) are present.
Irritable Bowel Syndrome (page 288)	Irritable bowel syndrome (IBS) is a collection of signs and symptoms related to a functional problem of the digestive system. It is aggravated by stress and diet.	The symptoms of IBS include alternating bouts of constipation and diarrhea, bloating or abdominal distension, and moderate to severe abdominal cramps that are relieved with defecation.	Massage is indicated for IBS with caution against aggravating an already hypersensitive GI tract.
Jaundice (page 299)	Jaundice is a symptom of liver dysfunction, involving the presence of excess bilirubin in the blood, which is then dissolved in subcutaneous fat, mucous membranes, and the sclera of the eyes.	Jaundice gives the skin, eyes, and mucous membranes a yellowish cast.	Massage is contraindicated for jaundice, which is usually a sign of significant congestion and dysfunction in the liver or gall bladder.
Kidney Stones (page 310)	A kidney stone is a deposit of crystalline substances inside the kidney or the ureters.	Small stones may show no symptoms at all, but larger stones can cause extreme pain that may be accompanied by nausea and vomiting. Pain may refer from the back into the groin and hips.	Massage is contraindicated for someone experiencing renal colic (a kidney stone attack) although it is appropriate for people with a history of stones, but no current symptoms.

Condition Name	What Is It/ What Are They?	How Is It Recognized/ How Are They Recognized?	Is Massage Indicated or Contraindicated?
Lice and Mites (page 13)	Lice and mites are tiny arthropods that drink blood. They are highly contagious and spread through close contact with skin or infested sheets or clothing.	The mites that cause scabies are too small to see, but they leave itchy trails where they burrow under the skin. They prefer warm, moist places such as the axillae or between fingers. Head lice are easy to see, but they can hide. A more dependable sign is their eggs: nits are small, white, rice-shaped flecks that cling strongly to hair shafts. Pubic lice look like tiny white crabs. All three of these parasites create a lot of itching.	Massage is contraindicated for all three infestations, until the infestation has been completely eradicated. If a massage therapist is exposed to any of these parasites, every client he or she subsequently works on will also be exposed even before the therapist shows any symptoms. Parasitic infestations are something every massage therapist fears. Therapists are so very vulnerable to whatever is crawling around on clients' skin. But here, as for all things fearful, the best defense is information.
Liver, Enlarged (page 300)	Enlarged liver, or hepatomegaly, is a condition in which the liver becomes distended and may displace other internal organs.	Hepatomegaly may have no symptoms, but it can sometimes cause abdominal discomfort or ascites: fluid accumulation in the abdomen.	Massage is contraindicated for persons whose livers are distended because of internal dysfunction.
Lung Cancer (page 266)	Lung cancer is the development in the lungs of malignant tumors that quickly spread to the lymph system and other organs in the body.	The early symptoms of lung cancer are a chronic cough, blood-stained sputum, and recurrent bronchitis or pneumonia.	Massage is systemically contraindicated for lung cancer.
Lupus (page 241)	Lupus is an autoimmune disease in which antibodies attack various types of connective tissue throughout the body. Three varieties have been identified, of which *systemic lupus erythematosis* is the most serious.	Eleven specific criteria are used to identify lupus. They include, among other things, arthritis in two or more joints, pleurisy, pericarditis, and kidney and nervous system dysfunction.	Massage is systemically contraindicated for acute flares of lupus. It *may* be indicated in the subacute stage, depending on the health of the tissues.
Lyme Disease*	Lyme disease is an infection of several body systems, brought about by exposure to the spirochete *Borrelia burgdorferi*. It is transmitted by deer ticks.	Lyme disease has three stages. Stage 1 appears as a skin rash and flu-like symptoms. Stage 2 involves one or more systems; the nervous and circulatory systems are most frequently involved. Stage 3 is chronic Lyme disease, and can involve arthritis and chronic neurological syndromes.	Massage is systematically contraindicated in the acute stages of this and any other types of systemic infections.

Condition Name	What Is It/ What Are They?	How Is It Recognized/ How Are They Recognized?	Is Massage Indicated or Contraindicated?
Lymphangitis (page 227)	Lymphangitis is an infection of lymph capillaries. If it proceeds to the nodes, it is called *lymphadenitis*. If it travels past the lymphatic system, it is called blood poisoning (*septicemia*), and it can be life threatening.	Lymphangitis includes all the signs of local infection: pain, heat, redness, swelling. It also often shows red streaks from the site of infection running toward the nearest lymph nodes.	Massage is systemically contraindicated for lymphangitis until the infection has been completely eradicated.
Marfan's Syndrome*	Marfan's syndrome is a genetic disorder that can affect the musculoskeletal system, the circulatory system, and the eyes.	Symptoms of Marfan's syndrome include abnormally long, thin fingers; systemic ligament laxity; and tall stature. Cardiovascular symptoms include mitral valve prolapse and the regurgitation of blood through the mitral valve. Symptoms in the eye include subluxation of the lens and myopia.	If cardiovascular problems are addressed, a patient with Marfan's syndrome has a virtually normal life expectancy. Therefore, with medical clearance, massage is appropriate for most Marfan's syndrome patients with normal heart function.
Meningitis (page 146)	Meningitis is an infection of the meninges, specifically the pia mater and the arachnoid layers.	Symptoms of acute meningitis include very high fever, rash, photophobia, headache, and stiff neck. Symptoms are not always consistent, however; they may appear in different combinations for different people.	Meningitis is strictly contraindicated in the acute phase. People who have recovered from meningitis are perfectly fine to receive massage.
Moles (page 25)	Moles are small isolated areas where the pigment cells in the epidermis have produced excess melanin.	Moles are usually black or brown (not mixed). They tend to be raised from the skin.	Massage will not help or hurt moles, but massage therapists may be able to see changes in a mole of which the client may be unaware.
Multiple Sclerosis (page 135)	Multiple sclerosis (MS) is an idiopathic disease that involves the destruction of myelin sheaths around both motor and sensory neurons in the CNS.	MS has many symptoms, depending on the nature of the damage. These can include fatigue, eye pain, spasticity, tremors, and a progressive loss of vision, sensation, and motor control.	Massage is indicated in subacute stages of MS, when the client is in remission, rather than during acute periods, when function is diminishing.
Myasthenia Gravis*	Myasthenia gravis (MG) is an autoimmune disorder in which the acetylcholine receptors at neuromuscular junctions of skeletal muscles are damaged. This limits the strength of nerve transmissions and causes the muscles to become weak.	MG causes muscle weakness, often of muscles that control the eyes and mouth, but the limbs can also be involved. This weakness progresses for several years and then reaches a plateau and stabilizes. Muscles that control breathing and coughing may become weak enough to cause respiratory crises. Skin sensation is normal but pain may be present if muscles of the neck and the head become weak and go into chronic spasm.	Massage may be indicated for MG patients with a doctor's supervision. Medication for this condition often compromises the immune system, so take care to avoid exposing the client to infectious agents.

Condition Name	What Is It/ What Are They?	How Is It Recognized/ How Are They Recognized?	Is Massage Indicated or Contraindicated?
Myositis Ossificans (page 54)	This is the growth of a bony deposit in soft tissues. It usually follows trauma that involves significant leakage of blood between fascial sheaths.	An x-ray is the best way to see this problem, but it is palpable as a dense mass where, anatomically, no such thing should be.	Massage is always locally contraindicated for myositis ossificans, but work around the edges of the area—within pain tolerance—may stimulate the reabsorption of the bone tissue without doing further damage.
Neuritis (page 157)	Neuritis means inflammation of a nerve. It is usually a symptom or complication of some other problem.	Hyperesthesia is the primary symptom of this condition. Numbness, weakness, and paresthesia may also be present.	Massage is at least locally contraindicated for any acute neuritis. Whether massage is systemically contraindicated will depend on the underlying pathology.
Open Wounds and Sores (page 38)	These include any injury to the skin that has not healed and that is vulnerable to infection if exposed to bacteria or other microorganisms. Skin injuries are vulnerable as long as there is a visible crust or scab.	A crust or scab appears at the site of the injury.	Massage is locally contraindicated for any unhealed skin injury with which bleeding has occurred. When the underlying epidermis has been completely replaced, the scab will fall off and the wound will no longer be at risk for infection. Massage may be systemically contraindicated if the skin injury is connected to a contraindicated underlying condition such as diabetes.
Osgood-Schlatter Disease*	Also called "growing pains," this condition is associated with adolescent growth spurts in which the bones, specifically the tibia, grow faster than the muscles and tendons.	Osgood-Schlatter disease usually hurts at the tibial condyle. It is exacerbated by exercise and resisted extension of the lower leg.	This inflammatory condition must be left alone during acute episodes. When the area is not painful and inflamed, and when stress fractures or other bone problems have been ruled out, massage can be appropriate to ease pain and improve local circulation.
Osteoarthritis (page 77)	This is joint inflammation brought about by wear and tear causing cumulative damage to articular cartilage.	Affected joints are stiff, painful, and occasionally palpably inflamed. Osteoarthritis most often affects knees, hips, and distal joints of the fingers.	Massage is locally contraindicated in the acute stage and indicated in the subacute stage, when it can contribute to muscular relaxation and mobility of the affected joint.
Osteogenesis Imperfecti*	This large group of inherited conditions involves abnormally fragile bones, which may break with minimal trauma.	Signs and symptoms of osteogenesis imperfecti include deformity of long bones, unusually lax ligaments, and a bluish tint to the sclerae of the eye.	Depending on the severity of the condition, vigorous massage may be contraindicated for osteogenesis imperfecti. Therapists need to work with primary care physicians to make case-by-case decisions concerning clients with this condition.

Condition Name	What Is It/ What Are They?	How Is It Recognized/ How Are They Recognized?	Is Massage Indicated or Contraindicated?
Osteoporosis (page 62)	This is loss of bone mass and density brought about by endocrine disorders and poor metabolism of calcium.	Osteoporosis in the early stages is identifiable only by x-ray and bone-density tests. In later stages, compression or spontaneous fractures of the vertebrae, wrists, or hips often result. Kyphosis brought about by compression fractures of the vertebrae is a frequent indicator of osteoporosis.	Very gentle massage is indicated for persons with osteoporosis. Massage will not affect the progression of the disease once it is present, but may significantly reduce associated pain. Massage for acute fractures, however, is contraindicated.
Ovarian Cancer (page 338)	Ovarian cancer is the development of malignant tumors on the ovaries; they rapidly metastasize to other structures in the abdominal cavity.	Symptoms of ovarian cancer are generally extremely subtle until the disease has progressed to life-threatening levels. Early symptoms include a feeling of heaviness in the pelvis, vague abdominal discomfort, occasional vaginal bleeding, and weight gain or loss.	As with all cancers, the appropriateness of massage depends on whether a client wishes to include it in a treatment program. Massage for ovarian cancer patients must be done under medical supervision.
Ovarian Cysts (page 341)	Ovarian cysts are benign, fluid-filled growths on the ovaries.	Ovarian cysts may exhibit no symptoms, or they may cause a change in the menstrual cycle. Also possible are constant pain in the pelvis, pain with intercourse, or symptoms similar to early pregnancy: nausea, vomiting, and breast tenderness.	Massage is locally contraindicated for diagnosed ovarian cysts.
Paget's Disease (page 65)	This is a bone disorder in which healthy bone is rapidly reabsorbed and replaced with fibrous connective tissue.	Bone pain is the primary symptom. X-rays are used for a definitive diagnosis.	Due to the lack of knowledge about the actual causes of Paget's disease, massage is systemically contraindicated in all but the mildest cases, and those should be massaged under a doctor's supervision.
Parkinson's Disease (page 139)	Parkinson's disease is a degenerative disease of the substantia nigra cells in the brain. These cells produce the neurotransmitter dopamine, which helps the basal ganglia to maintain balance, posture, and coordination.	Early symptoms of Parkinson's include general stiffness and fatigue; resting tremor of the hand, foot, or head; stiffness; and poor balance. Later symptoms include a shuffling gait, a "mask-like" appearance to the face, and a monotone voice.	Massage is indicated for Parkinson's disease, under a doctor's supervision. Care must be taken for the physical safety of these clients, who cannot move freely or smoothly.
Pelvic Inflammatory Disease (page 346)	Pelvic inflammatory disease, or PID, is a bacterial infection of female reproductive organs. It starts at the cervix and can move up to infect the uterus, fallopian (uterine) tubes, ovaries, and entire pelvic cavity.	Symptoms of acute PID include abdominal pain, fever, chills, headache, lassitude, nausea, and vomiting. Chronic PID may produce no symptoms, or may involve chronic pain, pain on urination, and pain with intercourse.	Massage is systemically contraindicated for any active pelvic infection.

Condition Name	What Is It/ What Are They?	How Is It Recognized/ How Are They Recognized?	Is Massage Indicated or Contraindicated?
Peripheral Neuropathy (page 142)	Peripheral neuropathy is damage to peripheral nerves, usually of the hands and feet, as a result of some other underlying condition such as alcoholism, diabetes, or lupus.	Sensory damage, motor damage, or both may be present. Symptoms include burning or tingling pain beginning distally and slowly moving proximally; loss of movement or control of movement; hyperesthesia; and eventual numbness.	Massage is at least locally contraindicated for peripheral neuropathy, because it may irritate a hyperesthesiac condition. Many underlying causes of peripheral neuropathy may contraindicate massage systemically.
Peritonitis (page 301)	Peritonitis is inflammation, usually due to bacterial infection, of the peritoneal lining of the abdomen.	Acute peritonitis shows the signs of systemic infection: fever and chills, along with abdominal pain, distension, nausea, and vomiting.	Massage is contraindicated for acute peritonitis, which is a medical emergency.
Pes Planus (page 101)	This is the medical term for flat feet.	The feet lack arches. Pronation of the ankle will probably also be present.	Massage is very much indicated. In some cases, the health of intrinsic foot muscles and ligaments can be improved to the point where alignment in the foot is also improved. In other cases, where the ligaments are lax through genetic problems, massage may not correct the situation, but neither will it make it worse.
Plantar Fasciitis (page 102)	Plantar fasciitis is the pain and inflammation caused by injury to the plantar fascia of the foot.	Plantar fasciitis is acutely painful after prolonged immobility. Then the pain recedes, but comes back with extended use. It feels sharp and bruise-like just at the anterior calcaneus or deep in the arch.	Massage is indicated for plantar fasciitis. It can help release tension in deep calf muscles that put strain on the plantar fascia; it can also help to affect the development of scar tissue at the site of the tear.
Pneumonia (page 252)	Pneumonia is an infection in the lungs brought about by bacteria, viruses, or other pathogens.	The symptoms of pneumonia include coughing, occasional fever, pain on breathing, and shortness of breath.	Massage is indicated for pneumonia in the subacute stage, under medical supervision.
Polio (page 148)	Polio is a viral infection, first of the intestines, and then (for about 1% of exposed people) the anterior horn cells of the spinal cord.	The destruction on CNS motor neurons leads to degeneration, atrophy and finally paralysis of skeletal muscles.	Massage is fine for postacute polio survivors. Massage can be indicated for post polio syndrome, but only under a doctor's supervision.
Post Polio Syndrome (page 150)	Post polio syndrome is a group of signs and symptoms common to polio survivors, particularly those who experienced significant loss of function in the acute stage of the disease.	Symptoms of PPS include a sudden onset of fatigue, achiness, and weakness. There may also be breathing and sleeping difficulties.	Massage under medical supervision is indicated for people with PPS.
Postoperative Situations (page 367)	Postoperative situations are conditions in which a client is recovering from any kind of surgery.	Surgeries may be major and invasive, or they may be conducted through tiny holes in the abdomen or through long tubes inserted into blood vessels to get to a destination far away.	Massage can be appropriate for persons recovering from surgery, depending on the reason for the surgery, and the danger of possible complications.

Condition Name	What Is It/ What Are They?	How Is It Recognized/ How Are They Recognized?	Is Massage Indicated or Contraindicated?
Postural Deviations (page 67)	Postural deviations are overdeveloped thoracic or lumbar curves (kyphosis and lordosis) or an S-curve or a C-curve in the spine (scoliosis).	Extreme curvatures are visible to the naked eye, although x-rays are used to pinpoint the exact places where the problems begin and end.	Massage is indicated for all postural deviations as long as other underlying pathologies have been ruled out. Massage may or may not be able to reverse any damage, but it can certainly provide relief for muscular stress.
Pregnancy (page 347)	Pregnancy is the state of carrying a fetus.	The symptoms of advanced pregnancy are obvious, but symptoms that specifically pertain to massage include swelling, loose ligaments, muscle spasms, clumsiness, and fatigue.	Massage is indicated for all stages of uncomplicated pregnancy, with specific cautions relating to each trimester.
Premenstrual Syndrome*	Premenstrual syndrome (PMS) is a group of signs and symptoms that precede a woman's menstrual period. They may be severe enough to interfere with normal activities.	Signs and symptoms of PMS include depressed mood, mood swings irritability, headaches, tender breasts, systemic edema, and fatigue.	Massage is systematically indicated for PMS.
Prostate Cancer (page 344)	Prostate cancer is the growth of malignant cells in the prostate gland. The tumors may then metastasize, usually to nearby bones.	Symptoms of prostate cancer include problems with urination: weak stream, frequency, urgency, nocturia, and other problems arising from constriction of the urethra.	Massage may be appropriate in the presence of slow-growing prostate cancer, when medical clearance has been obtained.
Psoriasis (page 26)	Psoriasis is a noncontagious, nonspreading chronic skin disease with occasional acute episodes.	Psoriasis occurs in pink or reddish patches, sometimes with a silvery scale on top. It occurs most frequently on elbows and knees, but it can also be found on the trunk or scalp.	Massage is locally contraindicated in the acute stage of psoriasis, because the extra stimulation and circulation massage provides can make a bad situation worse. But in subacute stages, as long as the skin is intact, massage is a good idea.
Pyelonephritis (page 313)	Pyelonephritis is an infection of the kidney and/or renal pelvis.	Symptoms of pyelonephritis include cystitis, back pain, fever, chills, nausea, and vomiting.	Massage is systemically contraindicated for a person with a kidney infection, until the infection has been eradicated.
Raynaud's Syndrome (page 202)	Raynaud's syndrome is defined by episodes of vasospasm of the arterioles, usually in fingers and toes, but occasionally in the nose, ears, lips, and tongue.	Affected areas will often go through marked color changes of white, or ashy gray for dark-skinned people, to blue to red. Attacks can last for less than a minute or several hours. Numbness and/or tingling may accompany attacks and recovery.	Massage is indicated for Raynaud's syndrome that is not associated with underlying pathology. Otherwise, follow the guidelines for the precipitating condition.

Condition Name	What Is It/ What Are They?	How Is It Recognized/ How Are They Recognized?	Is Massage Indicated or Contraindicated?
Reflex Sympathetic Dystrophy*	Reflex sympathetic dystrophy (RSD) may also be called *causalgia syndrome*. This situation causes pain following soft tissue or bone injury not to follow a normal course. Instead, it continues after the healing process is complete, for no known reason.	Signs and symptoms of RSD include all varieties of pain—burning, aching, deep, and superficial—along with discolored and edematous skin. Joints are likely to be stiff, and hypersensitivity to cold and heat are often present.	If underlying pathologies have been ruled out, massage may be appropriate for RSD as long as it doesn't exacerbate symptoms.
Renal Failure (page 314)	Renal failure is a situation in which the kidneys are incapable of functioning at normal levels. It may be an acute or a chronic problem, but it can be life-threatening.	Symptoms of acute and chronic renal failure differ in severity and type of onset, but they have in common reduced urine output, systemic edema, and changes in mental state brought about by the accumulation of toxins in the blood.	Massage is systemically contraindicated for both acute and chronic renal failure.
Rheumatoid Arthritis (page 80)	Rheumatoid arthritis (RA) is an autoimmune disease in which synovial membranes, particularly of the joints in the hands and feet, are attacked by immune system agents. Other structures, such as muscles, tendons, and blood vessels, may also be affected.	In the acute phase, affected joints are red, swollen, hot, and painful. They often become gnarled and distorted. It tends to affect the body symmetrically, and it is not determined by age.	Massage is systemically contraindicated during acute episodes of RA. Massage is indicated in the subacute stages when it may be used to reestablish mobility and to reduce the stresses that can trigger another flare.
Scar Tissue (page 38)	It is the growth of new tissue, skin or fascia, after injury.	Scar tissue on the skin often lacks pigmentation and hair follicles.	Massage is locally contraindicated during the acute stage of any injury in which the skin has been damaged. In the subacute stage, massage may improve the quality of the healing process.
Sciatica (page 118)	Sciatica is inflammation of the sciatic nerve. The source of irritation may be inside or outside the spinal canal.	Symptoms of sciatic nerve irritation include shooting pain along the dermatome, numbness, or reduced sensation and paresthesia.	Massage is indicated for sciatica brought about by muscular or ligamentous forces, but for problems that begin in the spinal cord, the guidelines in the *herniated disc* or *spondylosis* sections must be followed.
Scleroderma*	Scleroderma is a chronic condition without a known cause. It involves general fibrosis and vascular abnormalities. It can be a mild, lifelong condition, or may be severe enough to cause death within a few months.	The many possible signs and symptoms of scleroderma include Raynaud's phenomenon, skin ulcers, scaling, and itching, as well as joint stiffness, neuropathy, and fascial pain.	Scleroderma can be appropriate for massage, under a doctor's supervision, if the skin is healthy and sensation is normal.

Condition Name	What Is It/ What Are They?	How Is It Recognized/ How Are They Recognized?	Is Massage Indicated or Contraindicated?
Seizure Disorders (page 166)	Seizure disorders are usually caused by neurological damage, although it may be impossible to delineate exactly what that damage is. Epilepsy is one type of seizure disorder.	Seizure disorders are diagnosed through CT scans and MRIs. Seizures may take very different forms for different people; they range from barely noticeable to life threatening.	Massage is contraindicated during seizures, but is indicated at all other times.
Septic Arthritis (page 83)	Septic arthritis is joint inflammation caused by infection inside the joint capsule.	This conditions shows the cardinal signs of inflammation: pain, heat, redness, and swelling. It is often accompanied by fever.	Massage is systemically contraindicated for septic arthritis until the infection is completely gone from the joint. At that time, massage may be useful to help restore function.
Shin Splints (page 55)	Shin splints are lower leg problems involving some combination of an injury to the anterior or posterior tibialis and possible hairline fractures of the tibia. They are usually brought about by overuse or misalignment in the ankle.	Pain along the tibia may be superficial or deep, mild or severe. It is often made worse by resisted dorsiflexion for anterior tibialis or resisted plantarflexion for posterior tibialis.	Massage is indicated for mild shin splints, but is advised only with caution for periostitis or stress fractures and is contraindicated entirely for anterior compartment syndrome.
Sinusitis (page 255)	Sinusitis is inflammation of the paranasal sinuses from infection, obstruction, or allergies.	Symptoms include headaches, localized tenderness over the affected area, runny or congested nose, facial or tooth pain, fatigue, and, if it's related to an infection, thick opaque mucus, fever, and chills.	Massage is contraindicated for acute infections, but for chronic or noninfectious situations, it can be appropriate.
Skin Cancer (page 28)	Skin cancer is cancer in the stratum basale of the epidermis (basal cell carcinoma or BCC); cancer of the keratinocytes in the epidermis (squamous cell carcinoma or SCC); or cancer of the melanocytes (pigment cells) of the epidermis (malignant melanoma).	For BCC and SCC, look for the cardinal sign: sores that never heal. These are the clearest indication of BCC or SCC. For malignant melanoma, look for a mole that exhibits the ABCDEs of melanoma.	For BCC, which does not tend to metastasize, massage is locally contraindicated, as long as the lesion has been diagnosed by a dermatologist. For SCC or malignant melanoma, circulatory massage, which moves material (including malignant cancer cells) into the lymphatic system, is systemically contraindicated until the client has been cleared by a doctor.

Condition Name	What Is It/ What Are They?	How Is It Recognized/ How Are They Recognized?	Is Massage Indicated or Contraindicated?
Spasms, Cramps (page 57)	Spasms and cramps are involuntary contractions of skeletal muscle. Spasms are considered to be low-grade, long-lasting contractions, while cramps are short-lived, very acute contractions.	Cramps are extremely painful with visible shortening of muscle fibers. Long-term spasms are achy and cause inefficient movement, but may not have acute symptoms.	Massage is locally contraindicated for acutely cramping muscle bellies, though origin/insertion work can trick the proprioceptors into letting go. Subacute cramps respond well to massage, which can reduce residual pain and clean up chemical wastes. Underlying cramp-causing pathologies must be ruled out before massage is applied. Massage is indicated for long-term spasm because it can break through the ischemia-spasm-pain cycle to reintroduce circulation to the area, as well as reduce muscle tone and flush out toxins.
Spinal Cord Injury (page 158)	Spinal cord injury is a situation in which some or all of the fibers in the spinal cord have been damaged, usually by trauma but occasionally from other problems such as tumors or bony growths in the spinal canal.	Spinal cord injury will cause the loss of some muscle function, as well as sensory deprivation. The affected muscles, in the absence of nerve conduction, atrophy quickly.	Mechanical types of massage are appropriate only if sensation is present and no underlying pathologies will be exacerbated by the work. Areas without sensation are contraindications for massage that intends to manipulate and influence the quality of muscle tissue.
Spondylolisthesis*	Spondylolisthesis is a condition in which the vertebral body of one of the lumbar vertebrae is anterior of the rest of the spine.	Spondylolisthesis causes irritation at the joints between the affected vertebrae, resulting in symptoms of spondylitis, or arthritis of the spine.	Massage can be indicated for spondylolisthesis; follow the same guidelines for spondylosis.
Spondylosis (page 84)	Spondylosis is osteoarthritis of the spine.	It is identifiable by x-ray, which shows a characteristic thickening of the affected vertebral bodies, facets, and ligamentum flava. Symptoms will be present if pressure is exerted on nerve roots. These will include pain, numbness, paresthesia, and specific muscle weakness.	Massage is indicated for spondylosis, with caution. Muscle splinting, which protects the joints against movement that may be dangerous, is often a feature of this condition; massage therapists should not interfere with this mechanism.
Sprains (page 87)	Sprains are injured ligaments.	In the acute stage, symptoms include pain, redness, heat, swelling, and loss of joint function. In the subacute stage, these symptoms will be abated, although perhaps not entirely absent. At all stages pain will be present on passive stretching of the affected ligament.	Massage is indicated for subacute sprains. It can influence the healthy development of scar tissue and reduce swelling and damage due to edematous ischemia. Care must be taken to rule out bone fractures.

Condition Name	What Is It/ What Are They?	How Is It Recognized/ How Are They Recognized?	Is Massage Indicated or Contraindicated?
Strains (page 59)	Strains are injured muscles.	Pain, stiffness, and occasionally palpable heat and swelling will be present. Pain is exacerbated by stretching or resisted exercise of the injured muscle.	Massage is indicated for muscle strains, to influence the production of useful scar tissue, reduce adhesions and edema, and reestablish range of motion.
Stroke (page 161)	A stroke is damage to brain tissue caused by either a clot lodged to block blood flow to brain tissue or an internal hemorrhage.	The symptoms of stroke are paralysis and/or numbness on one side, blurry or diminished vision, asymmetrically dilated pupils, dizziness, difficulty in speaking or understanding simple sentences, sudden extreme headache, and possibly loss of consciousness.	Massage may be indicated during recovery from a stroke, but only with medical clearance, since this problem is usually associated with cardiovascular disease.
Substance Abuse (page 368)	Substance abuse is the use of a material (not necessarily a drug) in methods or dosages for which it was never intended; this use results in damage to the user and other people whom the user contacts.	Symptoms of substance abuse depend entirely on what substances are being consumed.	Massage is indicated, with medical supervision, for people who are recovering from substance abuse, under medical supervision. Massage for people with a history of substance abuse but no lasting health problems is also indicated. Massage is contraindicated for people who are intoxicated at the time of their appointment.
Temporomandibular Joint Disorders (page 89)	TMJ disorders arise when constant strain, stress, and malocclusion of the jaw lead to arthritis, inflammation, and dislocation of the temporomandibular joint.	Symptoms of TMJ disorder include head, neck, and shoulder pain, ear pain, mouth pain, clicking or locking in the jaw, and loss of range of motion in the jaw.	Massage can be useful for TMJ problems, especially before arthritic irritation begins. However, this condition must be diagnosed by a physician.
Tendinitis (page 103)	Tendinitis is inflammation of a tendon, usually due to injury at the tenoperiosteal or musculotendinous junction.	Pain and stiffness will be present, as well as, in acute stages, palpable heat and swelling. Pain is exacerbated by resisted exercise of the injured muscle-tendon unit.	Massage is locally contraindicated for acute tendinitis. Massage is indicated for tendinitis in the subacute stage, to influence the production of useful scar tissue, reduce adhesions and edema, and reestablish range of motion.
Tenosynovitis (page 104)	Tenosynovitis is the inflammation of a tendon and/or surrounding synovial sheath. It can happen wherever tendons pass through these sheaths, but is especially common in the forearm, particularly in the extensor muscles.	Pain, heat, and stiffness will be present in the acute stage. In the subacute stage, only stiffness and pain may be present. The tendon may feel or sound creaky (crepitis) as it moves through the sheath. It is difficult to bend fingers with tenosynovitis, but even harder to straighten them.	Massage is locally contraindicated for tenosynovitis in the acute stage, and very much indicated in the subacute stage.

Condition Name	What Is It/ What Are They?	How Is It Recognized/ How Are They Recognized?	Is Massage Indicated or Contraindicated?
Thoracic Outlet Syndrome (page 120)	Thoracic outlet syndrome (TOS) is a collection of signs and symptoms brought about by occlusion of nerve and blood supply to the arm.	Depending on what structures are compressed, TOS will show shooting pains, weakness, numbness, and paresthesia along with a feeling of fullness and possible discoloration of the affected arm from impaired circulation.	This depends on the source of the problem. If it is related to muscle tightness, massage is indicated. TOS due to muscle degeneration or some other disorder such as spondylosis or herniated disc will not respond well to massage.
Thrombophlebitis or Deep Vein Thrombosis (page 187)	Thrombophlebitis and deep vein thrombosis (DVT) are inflammations of veins due to blood clots.	Symptoms for thrombophlebitis may or may not include pain, heat, redness, swelling, and local itchiness, and a hard cord-like feeling at the affected vein. Symptoms for DVT are often more extreme: possibly pitting edema distal to the site, often with discoloration, and intermittent or continuous pain that is exacerbated by activity or standing still for a long period of time.	Massage is strictly systemically contraindicated for thrombophlebitis or deep vein thrombosis.
Torticollis (page 106)	Torticollis is a unilateral spasm of neck muscles. The spasm may be related to a variety of causes.	Flexion and rotation of the head are the main symptoms. Torticollis may also refer pain into the neck, shoulders, and back.	This depends on the cause of the problem. One variety, called simple wryneck, resulting from trigger points, cervical misalignment, ligament sprain, or trauma may be appropriate for massage if no acute inflammation is present. Spasmodic torticollis patients may benefit from pain relief offered by massage, but work should be done under supervision. If symptoms don't improve or if any signs of systemic infection occur, a more thorough diagnosis should be sought.
Trigeminal Neuralgia (page 164)	Trigeminal neuralgia (TN) is pain along the trigeminal nerve, usually in the lower face and jaw.	The pain of trigeminal neuralgia is very sharp and severe. Patients report stabbing, electrical, or burning sensations. There may also be a muscular tic.	Massage is locally contraindicated when a client is having an acute episode of TN. Otherwise, massage is appropriate. Work on the face and head of a client who has TN with their specific guidance.
Tuberculosis (page 257)	Tuberculosis is a bacterial infection that usually begins in the lungs, but may spread to bones, kidneys, lymph nodes, or elsewhere in the body. It is a highly contagious airborne disease.	Infection with the tuberculosis bacterium may produce no symptoms. If the infection turns into the actual disease, symptoms may include coughing, bloody sputum, fatigue, weight loss, and night sweats.	Massage is contraindicated for active tuberculosis disease, unless the client has been on consistent medication for several weeks and has medical clearance. Massage for clients with tuberculosis infection but no disease is fine, but these people should be under medical supervision as well.

Condition Name	What Is It/ What Are They?	How Is It Recognized/ How Are They Recognized?	Is Massage Indicated or Contraindicated?
Ulcerative Colitis (page 290)	Ulcerative colitis is a condition in which the inner layer of the colon becomes inflamed and develops ulcers.	Symptoms of acute ulcerative colitis include abdominal cramping, pain, chronic diarrhea, blood and pus in stools, weight loss, and mild fever.	Massage is locally contraindicated for acute ulcerative colitis, and systemically contraindicated in the presence of fever. In subacute situations, gentle (not deep) abdominal massage may be helpful, but only within the tolerance of the client.
Ulcers (page 278)	Ulcers are sores that, for various reasons, don't experience a normal healing process, but instead, remain open and vulnerable to infection.	The symptoms of gastric and peptic ulcers include general burning or gnawing abdominal pain between meals that is relieved by taking antacids or eating.	Massage is locally contraindicated for someone with ulcers; specific work on the abdomen may exacerbate symptoms.
Urinary Tract Infection (page 318)	A urinary tract infection (UTI) is an infection of the urinary tract, usually by bacteria that live normally and harmlessly in the digestive tract.	Symptoms of UTIs include pain and burning sensations during urination, frequency, urgency, and cloudy or blood-tinged urine. In the acute stage, fever and general malaise may also present.	Circulatory massage is systemically contraindicated during acute UTIs, as it is for all acute infections. Massage may be appropriate in the subacute stage, although deep work on the abdomen is still locally contraindicated until all signs of infection are gone.
Varicose Veins (page 204)	Varicose veins are distended veins, usually in the legs, caused by valvular incompetence and a backup of blood returning to the heart.	Varicose veins are ropey, slightly bluish, elevated veins that twist and turn out of their usual course. They happen most frequently on the medial side of the calf, although they are also found on the posterior aspects of the calf and thigh.	Massage is locally contraindicated for extreme varicose veins and anywhere distal to them. Mild varicose veins contraindicate deep, specific work, but are otherwise safe for massage.
Warts (page 17)	Warts are neoplasms that arise from the keratinocytes in the epidermis; they are caused by extremely slow-acting viruses.	Typical warts (verruca vulgaris) look like hard, cauliflower-shaped growths. They usually occur on the hands. They can affect anyone, but teenagers are especially prone to them.	Massage is locally contraindicated for warts. The virus is contained in the blood and shedding skin cells, and it is possible to get warts from another person.
Whiplash (page 108)	Whiplash is an umbrella term referring to a series of injuries that may occur with cervical acceleration/deceleration. These injuries include sprained ligaments, strained muscles, misaligned or fractured vertebrae, herniated or ruptured discs, TMJ problems, and central nervous system damage.	Symptoms of whiplash will vary according to the nature of the injuries. Pain at the neck and referring into the shoulders and arms along with headaches are the primary indicators.	Massage is contraindicated for acute stages of whiplash, and very much indicated for the subacute stage, when in conjunction with chiropractic or manipulation, it can contribute to a thorough resolution of the problem.

Glossary of Terms

abrasion: A scrape involving injury to the epithelial layer of the skin or mucous membranes.

absence seizure: A type of seizure characterized by brief lapses in consciousness with rapid recovery.

acute: A stage of injury or infection; short term, severe.

adenoma: A benign neoplasm, usually occurring in epithelial tissue.

adhesion: The adhering or uniting of two surfaces. Layers of connective tissue may adhere, which limits movement and increases the risk of injury.

Adson's test: A test for thoracic outlet syndrome, during which the patient is seated with his head extended and rotated toward the affected side. With deep inspiration, a diminution or total loss of radial pulse is noticeable on that side.

adventitia: The outermost connective tissue layer that covers organs and vessels.

aerobic metabolism: Metabolism that occurs in the presence of adequate oxygen, which reduces the overall production of toxic waste products.

allergen: A substance that produces an allergic reaction.

alveolus, alveoli: A small cavity or socket. Specifically, the terminal epithelial structures in the lungs where gaseous exchange takes place.

amino acid: An organic acid in which one of the hydrogen atoms on a carbon atom has been replaced by NH_2. A building block of proteins.

amphiarthrosis: A form of joint in which the two bones are joined by fibrocartilage.

anaerobic metabolism: Metabolism that takes place without adequate supplies of oxygen, which may result in the excessive build up of toxic waste products.

anaphylactic shock: An immediate, transient allergic reaction characterized by systemic contraction of smooth muscle and dilation of capillaries.

angina: A severe, often constricting pain. Usually refers to *angina pectoris*.

angioneurotic edema: A situation in which hives appear on the face and neck, and swelling occurs to the point that breathing becomes difficult.

angioplasty: Recanalization of a blood vessel, usually by means of balloon dilation or the placement of a stent.

antibody: An immunoglobulin molecule produced by B cells and designed to react with a specific antigen.

anticoagulant: An agent that prevents or inhibits coagulation of the blood.

antigen: Any substance that, as a result of coming into contact with appropriate cells, elicits an immune response.

apoptosis: Programmed cell death.

arachnoid: A delicate membrane of spider-web–like filaments that lies between the dura mater and the pia mater.

arrhythmia: Electrical irregularity of the heart rhythm.

arteriogram: Radiographic demonstration of an artery after the injection of a contrast medium.

arteriole: A minute artery continuous with a capillary network.

arteriosclerosis: Hardening of the arteries; *atherosclerosis* is one type of arteriosclerosis.

ascites: The accumulation of serous fluid in the peritoneal cavity.

atopic: Relating to an allergic reaction.

atrium, atria: A chamber or cavity, connected to other cavities. Specifically, the superior chambers of the heart.

atrophy: A wasting of tissues from a number of causes, including diminished cellular proliferation, ischemia, malnutrition, and death.

autoimmune: Arising from and directed against the individual's tissues.

avulsion: A tearing away or forcible separation.

axon: The process of a nerve cell that conducts impulses away from the cell body.

barrel chest: An occasional symptom of emphysema, characterized by increased anteroposterior chest diameter due to trapping of air associated with airway damage.

basal ganglia: Large masses of gray matter at the base of the cerebral hemispheres.

basal layer: Also called the *stratum basale*; the deepest layer of the epidermis.

basophil: A phagocytic leukocyte.

461

benign: Denoting the mild character of an illness, or non-malignant character of a neoplasm.

benign prostate hypertrophy (BPH): A nodular hyperplasia of the prostate; the gland thickens in a way that may obstruct the urethra.

beta-blocker: A type of drug that limits sympathetic reactions, specifically as they relate to the cardiovascular system.

bile: Yellowish-brown or green fluid produced in the liver, stored in the gall bladder, and released into the duodenum to aid in the digestion of fats.

bilirubin: A red bile pigment formed from the hemoglobin of dead erythrocytes.

bone scan: A diagnostic test to look for bone cancer or infections, evaluate unexplained pain, or diagnose fractures.

bradykinesia: A decrease in the spontaneity of movement.

bruxism: Jaw clenching that results in rubbing and grinding of teeth, especially during sleep.

bulla, bullae: A bubble-like structure, specifically the air-filled blisters on the lung formed by fused alveoli in emphysema.

calcitonin: A hormone that increases the deposition of calcium and phosphate in bone.

callus: A thickening of the keratin layer of the epidermis as a result of repeated friction or intermittent pressure.

carbuncle: A group of localized infections of hair follicles, with the formation of connecting sinuses. A group of boils.

cellular immunity: Also called *cell mediated immunity*. Immune responses initiated by T cells and mediated by T cells, macrophages, or both.

cervical rib: An abnormally wide transverse process of a cervical vertebra, or a supernumerary rib that articulates with a cervical vertebra, but does not articulate with the sternum. C_7 is the vertebra usually affected.

chemonucleolysis: Injection of chymopapain into the nucleus pulposis of a herniated disc.

chemotherapy: The treatment of disease by chemical means, i.e., drugs. In modern use, this has come to mean the use of extremely cytotoxic drugs to treat cancer.

chondroitin sulfate: One of the substances present in the extracellular matrix of connective tissue.

chronic: Referring to a health-related state; low intensity, lasting a long time.

chyme: Semifluid mass of partly digested food in the stomach or small intestine.

clonic spasm: Alternating involuntary contraction and relaxation of a muscle.

colic: An abnormal contraction of smooth muscle, particularly in the digestive tract.

collagen: A major protein forming the white fibers of connective tissue.

colostomy: The establishment of an artificial opening from the skin to the colon.

consolidation: Solidification into a firm, dense mass, specifically with cellular exudate in the lungs during pneumonia.

constriction: A narrowed portion of a tubular structure.

contact inhibition: The tendency of basal cells involved in healing to stop reproducing when they encounter cells from the other side of the wound.

corticosteroid injection: An injection of a specific steroid into an injured area for its anti-inflammatory and/or connective tissue dissolving properties.

cortisol: A glucocorticoid secreted by the adrenal cortex, also known as hydrocortisone. Cortisol is the active form of this hormone. It acts upon carbohydrate metabolism and influences the growth and nutrition of connective tissue.

cortisone: A biologically inactive precursor to cortisol. A synthetically produced version of cortisone may be injected into specific areas to act as an anti-inflammatory or to help dissolve connective tissue.

coxsackie virus: A group of viruses first isolated in Coxsackie, New York. They may be responsible for several human diseases, including meningitis and juvenile diabetes.

crepitus: A crackling sound resembling the noise heard when hair is rubbed between the fingers. This is sometimes heard during joint movement.

crisis: A sudden change, usually for the better, in the course of an acute disease.

crust: A hard outer covering; a scab.

cyanosis: A bluish or purplish coloration of the skin and mucous membranes due to deficient oxygenation of the blood.

cytokine: Hormone-like proteins secreted by many different cells, involved in cell-to-cell communication.

cytomegalovirus: A group of viruses in the Herpesviridae family, which infect humans and animals.

cytotoxic drug: A drug that is detrimental or destructive to certain cells.

degeneration: A retrogressive pathologic change in tissues; may cause their functions to be impaired or destroyed.

dementia: The loss, usually progressive, of cognitive and intellectual functions, without impairment of perception or consciousness.

dendrite: The process of a nerve cell that carries impulses toward the cell body.

dermatome: The area of skin supplied by cutaneous branches from a single spinal nerve.

dermatophyte: A fungus that causes superficial infections of the skin, hair, and nails.

diarthrosis: Also called *synovial joint*; a joint in which articulating surfaces are covered by articular cartilage and held together by a capsular ligament, which is lined with a synovial membrane. Some degree of freedom of movement is possible with diarthrotic joints.

diastole: Normal post-systolic dilation of the heart cavities, during which they fill with blood.

dilation: The enlargement of a hollow structure or opening.

diplegia: Paralysis of corresponding parts on both sides of the body.

diuretic: A chemical agent that increases urine output.

DMSO (dimethyl sulfoxide): A penetrating solvent that enhances absorption of therapeutic agents from the skin.

dopamine: A neurotransmitter present in the basal ganglia.

dura mater: A tough, fibrous membrane forming the outer covering of the central nervous system.

dyshidrosis: A skin eruption involving blisters and itching that usually appears on the volar surface of the hands or feet.

dysphagia: Difficulty in swallowing.

dyspnea: Shortness of breath.

eclampsia: The occurrence of one or more convulsions not attributable to other cerebral conditions. In this case, related to pregnancy-induced hypertension.

edema: An accumulation of an excessive amount of watery fluid in cells, tissues, or serous membranes.

elastin: A yellow, elastic fibrous protein that contributes to the connective tissue of elastic structures.

electrolyte: Any compound that, in solution, conducts electricity and is decomposed by it.

endo-: A prefix indicating *within, inner, absorbing,* or *containing.*

endometrium: The inner layers of the uterine wall.

endomysium: The connective tissue sheath surrounding individual muscle fibers.

endosteum: A layer of cells lining the inner surface of bone in the central medullary cavity of long bones.

enzyme: A protein that acts as a catalyst to induce chemical changes in other substances, while remaining unchanged itself.

ephelis, epheli: Freckles.

epi-: Prefix indicating *upon, following,* or *subsequent to.*

epidermis: The superficial epithelial portion of the skin.

epimysium: The connective tissue membrane surrounding a skeletal muscle.

epinephrine: The chief hormone of the adrenal medulla; a potent stimulant of the sympathetic response.

epithelium: A purely cellular avascular layer covering all free surfaces including skin, mucous, and serous glands.

Epstein Barr virus: A herpesvirus that causes infectious mononucleosis and is implicated in Burkitt's lymphoma.

ERT (estrogen replacement therapy): A treatment for the prevention or slowing of osteoporosis by replacing some of the hormones that are lost or diminished with the onset of menopause.

erythrocyte: A mature red blood cell.

erythropoietin: A hormone secreted by the kidneys and possibly other tissues that stimulates the formation of red blood cells.

essential: Of unknown etiology, specifically in reference to hypertension.

estrogen: A group of hormones secreted by the ovaries, placenta, and possibly other tissues. Estrogens influence secondary sexual characteristics and the menstrual cycle.

external scar tissue: Scar tissue that develops outside of the injured structure, often binding that structure to other nearby structures in adhesions.

fascicle, fasciculi: A band or bundle of fibers, specifically muscle fibers.

fasciculation: Involuntary contractions or twitchings of fasciculi.

festinating gait: Gait in which the trunk is flexed, legs are flexed at the knees and hips, but stiff, while the steps are short and progressively more rapid.

fibrin: An elastic filamentous protein that aids in coagulation of the blood.

filtration: The process of passing a liquid or gas through a filter.

fimbria, fimbriae: Any fringe-like structure. Ovarian fimbriae extend over the ovaries.

fixation: The condition of being firmly attached or set. In regards to the spine, being excessively limited in movement between individual vertebrae.

flaccid paralysis: Paralysis with a loss of muscle tone, although sensation is present.

furuncle: A localized bacterial infection in a hair shaft; a boil.

gamma globulin: A preparation of proteins of human plasma containing the antibodies of healthy adults.

gastrostomy: Establishment of a new opening into the stomach.

glomerulus: A tuft of capillary loops at the beginning of each nephric tubule in the kidney.

glucagon: A hormone secreted by the liver which elevates blood sugar concentration.

glycogen: A substance found primarily in the liver and muscles that is easily converted into glucose.

grand mal seizure: Also called *generalized tonic clonic seizure.* Characterized by a sudden onset of tonic contraction of the muscles, giving way to clonic convulsive movements.

granulocyte: A mature granular leukocyte.

greater omentum: A fold of peritoneum holding fat cells that hangs like an apron in front of the intestines.

hallux valgus: A deviation of the great toe toward the lateral side of the foot.

hematuria: Any condition in which the urine contains blood or red blood cells.

hemiplegia: Paralysis of one side of the body.

hemo-: A prefix denoting anything to do with blood.

hemoglobin: Red protein of erythrocytes which binds to oxygen.

hemolytic: Destructive to blood cells.

hemorrhage: An escape of blood through ruptured or unruptured vessels.

histamine: A secretion of some cells that is a powerful stimulant of gastric secretion, a constrictor of bronchial smooth muscle, and a vasodilator.

hobnailed liver: Characteristically knobby, bumpy appearance of a liver with advanced cirrhosis.

Homan's sign: A pain at the back of the knee or calf when the ankle is slowly dorsiflexed with the knee bent. This test indicates incipient or established thrombosis in the veins of the leg.

homeostasis: A state of equilibrium in the body with respect to various functions and the chemical compositions of fluids and tissues.

humoral immunity: Immunity associated with circulating antibodies, as opposed to cellular immunity.

hyper-: A prefix denoting *excessive, above normal.*

hyperacusis: Abnormal acuteness of hearing due to irritability of sensory neural nerves.

hyperglycemia: An abnormally high concentration of glucose in the circulating blood.

hyperkinesia: Excessive muscular activity.

hyperreflexia: A condition in which the deep tendon reflexes are exaggerated.

hypersensitivity: An exaggerated response to the stimulus of a foreign agent.

hypertonic: Having a greater degree of tension.

hypertrophic scar: An elevated scar resembling a keloid but which does not spread into surrounding tissues.

hyperuricemia: Enhanced blood concentrations of uric acid.

hypo-: A prefix denoting *deficient, below normal.*

hypoglycemia: An abnormally low concentration of glucose in circulating blood.

hypokinesia: Diminished or slowed movement.

hypotonic: Having a lesser degree of tension.

hypoxia: Below normal levels of oxygen.

idiopathic: Denoting a disease of unknown cause.

incision: A cut or surgical wound.

infarction: Sudden insufficiency of arterial or venous blood supply due to emboli, thrombi, vascular torsion, or necrosis.

interferon: A class of proteins with antiviral properties.

Interleukin 1: A cytokine that enhances the proliferation of T helper cells and the growth and differentiation of B cells.

internal scar tissue: Scar tissue that accumulates within the injured structure, *e.g.,* tendon, muscle, or ligament.

interstitial: Relating to spaces within a tissue or organ, but excluding such spaces as body cavities or potential space.

intrinsic factor: A mucoprotein in the stomach necessary for the absorption of vitamin B_{12}.

ischemia: Local anemia due to a mechanical obstruction of the blood supply.

keloid scar: A nodular mass of scar tissue that may occur after surgery, a burn or cutaneous diseases.

keratin: A substance present in cuticular structures, *e.g.,* hair, nails, and horns.

keratinocyte: A cell of the epidermis that produces keratin.

ketoacidosis: Acidosis caused by the enhanced production of ketonic acids.

Kupffer cells: Specialized phagocytes found in the liver.

kyphosis: A deformity of the spine, characterized by extensive flexion.

laceration: A torn or jagged wound.

leiomyoma: A benign neoplasm derived from smooth muscle tissue.

lentigo: A brown macule or spot, resembling a freckle.

lesion: A wound or injury; a pathogenic change in tissues.

leukocyte: A type of blood cell formed in several different types of tissues, involved in immune reactions; a white blood cell.

Lhermitte's sign: Sudden electric-like shocks extending down the spine on flexion of the neck.

ligamentum flava: A pair of yellow elastic fibrous structures that bind the laminae of adjoining vertebrae.

lordosis: A deformity of the spine, characterized by excessive extension of the low back, which causes an abnormal convexity of the sacral and thoracic spine.

lumen: The space in the interior of a tubular structure.

lymphadenitis: Inflammation of a lymph node or nodes.

lymphangion: A lymphatic vessel.

lymphocyte: A white blood cell formed in lymphatic tissues.

lymphokines: A group of hormone-like substances, released by lymphocytes, that mediate immune responses.

macrophage: A type of phagocytic white blood cell.

malaise: A feeling of general discomfort or uneasiness.

malar rash: A rash of the cheeks or cheekbones.

malignant: Having the property of locally invasive and destructive growth and metastasis.

malocclusion: Any deviation from a physiologically acceptable contact of opposing teeth.

mast cell: A white blood cell found in connective tissue that contains heparin and histamine.

matrix: The intercellular substance of a tissue.

melanin: Dark brown to black pigment formed in the skin and some other tissues.

melanocyte: A pigment-producing cell located in the basal layer of the epidermis.

mesentery: A double layer of peritoneum attached to the abdominal wall and enclosing a portion of the abdominal viscera.

microbe: Any very minute organism.

mononeuropathy: Disorder involving a single nerve.

myalgic encephalomyelitis: Inflammation of the brain and spinal cord, characterized by muscle pain.

mycoplasma: A specialized type of bacteria that do not possess a true cell wall, but are bound by a three-layered membrane.

mycosis: Any disease caused by a fungus.

myelin: A membrane composed of fat and protein molecules that surrounds nerve fibers.

myofibril: One of the fine longitudinal fibers occurring in skeletal or cardiac muscle fiber.

necrosis: Pathologic death of one or more cells, or a portion of a tissue or organ.

neoplasm: An abnormal tissue that grows by cellular proliferation, more rapidly than normal, and continues to grow after the stimuli that initiated the new growth cease.

nephrolithiasis: Presence of renal calculi.

nephron: A long convoluted tubular structure; the functional unit of the kidney.

neurilemma: A cell that enfolds one or more axons of the peripheral nervous system.

neuron: The functional unit of the nervous system, consisting of the nerve cell body, the dendrites, and the axon.

neutrophil: A type of mature white blood cell formed in the bone marrow.

nevus, nevi: A malformation of the skin, colored by hyperpigmentation or increased vascularity.

NICO (neuralgia inducing cavitational osteonecrosis): A recently recognized problem in which tissue death occurs at the site of extracted teeth, which causes pain in the face. NICO is one form of *osteomyelitis*.

nit: The ovum of a head, body, or crab louse.

nociceptor: A peripheral nerve organ or mechanism for the reception and transmission of painful or injurious stimuli.

nocturia: Urinating at night.

norepinephrine: A hormone produced in the adrenal medulla, secreted in response to hypotension and physical stress.

noxious: Injurious, harmful.

NSAID: Nonsteroidal anti-inflammatory drug, *e.g.*, aspirin, ibuprofen.

numb-likeness: A condition characterized by reduced sensation, but not total numbness.

orthotics: The science concerned with the making and fitting of orthopaedic appliances. Also used to refer to orthopaedic appliances that are made to adjust the alignment and weight-bearing stress in the feet.

osteoblast: A bone-forming cell.

osteoclast: A cell functioning in the absorption and removal of osseus tissue.

osteomalacia: A disease characterized by the gradual softening and bending of the bones, with varying severity of pain.

osteophyte: A bony outgrowth or protuberance.

oxygen free radical: An atom or atom group carrying an unpaired electron and no charge. They may promote heart disease, cancer, Alzheimer's disease, and other progressive disorders.

palliative: Denoting the alleviation of symptoms without curing the underlying disease.

palpable: Perceptible to touch.

palpitation: Forcible or irregular pulsation of the heart perceptible to the patient, usually with an increase in frequency or force, with or without an irregularity in rhythm.

paraplegia: Paralysis of both lower extremities, and generally, the lower trunk.

paresis: Partial or incomplete paralysis.

paresthesia: An abnormal sensation, such as burning, prickling, tickling, or tingling.

pathogen: Any virus, microorganism, or substance that causes a disease.

perforation: Abnormal opening in a hollow organ.

peri-: Prefix denoting *around, about,* or *near.*

perimysium: The fibrous sheath enveloping each of the primary bundles of skeletal muscle fibers.

periosteum: The thick fibrous membrane covering every surface of a bone except the articular cartilage.

petit mal: A type of primary generalized seizure characterized by the sudden arrest of activity for a few seconds to minutes.

photosensitivity: Abnormal sensitivity to light, especially of the eyes.

pia mater: A delicate fibrous membrane firmly adherent to the brain and spinal cord.

plasmapheresis: Removal of whole blood from the body, separation of its cellular elements, and reinfusion of them suspended in saline or another plasma substitute.

plaque: A small differentiated area on a surface; atheromatous plaques form well-defined yellow areas or swellings on the intimal surface of an artery.

pleurisy: Inflammation of the pleurae.

plexus: A network or interjoining of nerves, blood vessels, or lymphatic vessels.

polydipsia: Excessive thirst that is relatively prolonged.

polyneuropathy: A disease process involving a number of peripheral nerves.

polyphagia: Excessive eating.

polyuria: Excessive excretion of urine.

preeclampsia: Development of hypertension with proteinuria or edema, or both, due to pregnancy.

proliferants: Injected substances designed to stimulate the growth of new collagen fibers, which, with appropriate stretching and exercise, will lay down in alignment with the original fibers.

prophylaxis: Prevention of a disease or of a process that can lead to a disease.

proprioceptor: Sensory end organs that relay information about position and muscle tension.

prostaglandin: Several substances present in many tissues with effects such as vasodilation, vasoconstriction, and stimulation of smooth muscle tissue.

prostatitis: Inflammation of the prostate.

protease inhibitor: A group of AIDS drugs that work to interrupt the maturing phase of the virus.

pseudogout: Acute episodes of synovitis caused by calcium pyrophosphate crystals as opposed to urate crystals, as in true gout.

PTH (parathyroid hormone): A hormone secreted by the parathyroid glands that raises serum calcium levels by causing bone resorption.

pustule: A small circumscribed elevation of the skin containing purulent material.

pyelogram: A radiograph of the kidneys and ureters, following the injection of a contrast medium.

pyrogen: A fever-inducing agent that causes a rise in temperature.

quadriplegia: Paralysis of all four limbs.

rales: Term for an abnormal sound heard on listening of breath sounds.

reduction: The restoration, by surgical or manipulative procedures, of a part to its normal anatomical relation.

Reed-Sternberg cells: Large transformed lymphocytes, indicative of Hodgkin's disease.

Reiter's syndrome: A combination of symptoms, including urethritis, cutaneous lesions, arthritis, and diarrhea. One or more of these symptoms may recur at intervals, but the arthritis may be persistent.

renal calculus: A stone or pebble formed in the kidney collection system.

renal colic: Severe pain caused by the impaction or passage of a calculus in the ureter or renal pelvis.

renin: An enzyme produced by the kidneys that is involved in vasoconstriction and hypertension.

reticulocyte: An immature red blood cell.

retinopathy: Noninflammatory degenerative disease of the retina.

retrovirus: A virus in the family of Retroviridae. They possess RNA that serves as a template for the synthesis of DNA in the host cell.

ringworm: A fungus infection of the keratin component of hair, skin, or nails; tinea.

rodent ulcer: A slowly enlarging ulcerated basal cell carcinoma, usually on the face.

sarcomere: The segment of a myofibril between Z lines; the functioning contractile unit of striated muscle.

Schwann cells: Cells forming a continuous envelope around each fiber of peripheral nerves.

scoliosis: Abnormal lateral curve of the vertebral column.

sebaceous gland: Gland in the dermis that usually opens into hair follicles and secretes an oily semi-fluid; sebum.

seborrhea: Overactivity of the sebaceous glands, resulting in an excessive amount of sebum.

seborrheic keratosis: Superficial benign skin lesions of proliferating epithelial cells.

sebum: The secretion produced by sebaceous glands.

septicemia: Systemic disease caused by the spread of microorganisms and their toxins in circulating blood.

Sjögren's syndrome: An autoimmune disorder with a collection of signs and symptoms, including conjunctivitis, dryness of mucous membranes, and bilateral enlargement of the parotid glands.

sodium urate: Uric acid.

spastic paralysis: Central nervous system damage resulting in permanent muscle contraction; combines aspects of hypertonia, hypokinesis, and hyperreflexia.

spasticity: A state of increased muscle tone with exaggerated muscle tendon reflexes.

specific immunity: The immune state in which an altered reactivity is directed solely against the antigens that stimulated it.

specific muscle weakness: Degeneration and weakening of muscles as they are specifically supplied by individual damaged motor neurons; as opposed to *general muscle weakness*, which is related to atrophy in whole areas, and may not be determined by specific individual nerve damage.

sphygmomanometer: An instrument used to indirectly measure arterial blood pressure.

spirochete: A type of bacteria shaped like undulating spiral-shaped rods.

sporadic: Occurring irregularly, haphazardly.

sputum: Expectorated matter, especially mucous or mucopurulent matter expectorated in diseases of the air passages.

squamous: Relating to or covered with scales.

staging: The classification of distinct phases or periods in the course of a disease.

staphylococcus: A type of bacteria formed of spherical cells that divide to make irregular clusters.

Starling's equilibrium: Also called Starling's hypothesis; the principle that the amount of fluid squeezed out of circulatory capillaries should be almost equal to the amount being drawn into lymphatic capillaries.

stenosis: A stricture of any canal.

stent: A device to hold tissue in place or provide support.

streptococcus: A type of bacteria formed of spherical cells that occur in pairs or in long or short chains.

subacute: Between acute and chronic, denoting a mild duration or severity.

subcutaneous: Beneath the skin.

subluxation: An incomplete dislocation; though a relationship is altered, contact between joint surfaces remains.

substantia nigra: A large mass composed of pigmented cells located in the brainstem. The site of dopamine synthesis.

superficial fascia: A loose fibrous envelope of connective tissue under the skin containing fat, blood vessels, and nerves.

synarthrosis: A fibrous joint, sometimes said to be immovable.

synovectomy: The excision of part or all of the synovial membrane of a joint.

synovial joint: A diarthrosis, or freely moveable joint.

systole: The contraction of the heart, specifically of the ventricles.

tachycardia: Rapid heart beat, usually applied to rates over 100 beats per minute.

testosterone: A naturally occurring androgen, found in testes and other tissues.

tetraplegia: Quadriplegia.

thrombocyte: Platelet.

tinea: A fungus infection of the keratin component of hairs, skin, or nails.

tonic/clonic seizure: The sudden onset of tonic contraction of muscles, giving way to clonic convulsive movements; grand mal seizure.

tonic spasm: Continuous involuntary spasm of skeletal muscle.

toxic megacolon: Acute nonobstructive dilation of the colon.

transcriptase: An enzyme that converts RNA to DNA in the AIDS virus.

transcutaneous: Denoting the passage of substances through unbroken skin.

trigger point: A small area in which muscle fibers have suffered injury and not gone through a normal healing process. Pressure on a trigger point elicits moderate to severe pain in specific referring patterns.

trophic ulcer: Ulcer resulting from cutaneous sensory denervation.

tumor: Any swelling, usually denoting a neoplasm.

tunica intima: The innermost coat of a blood or lymphatic vessel.

tunica media: The middle, usually muscular coat of a blood vessel or lymphatic vessel.

unilateral: Confined to one side only.

uremia: An excess of urea and other nitrogenous waste in the blood.

ureterolithiasis: A kidney stone lodged in the ureter.

varix, varices: A dilated vein.

vasculitis: Inflammation of a blood or lymphatic vessel.

ventricle: A normal cavity, specifically in the brain or heart.

venule: A venous branch continuous with a capillary.

verruca vulgaris: A wart composed of a thickened keratitic layer of the epidermis.

vesicle: A small circumscribed fluid-filled elevation of the skin, a blister.

virulent: Extremely toxic, denoting a markedly pathogenic microorganism.

Wolff's law: A law stating that every change in the form and or function of a bone is followed by changes in internal and external architecture of the bone.

Wright's test: A thoracic outlet syndrome test in which the hand is placed over the head and the head is turned toward the affected side. If this exacerbates symptoms or reduces the strength of the pulse of the affected side, impingement to the axillary artery and lower brachial plexus nerves is suspected.

yuppie flu: Vernacular for a set of signs and symptoms that may be diagnosed as chronic fatigue syndrome.

zygapophyseal joint: Relating to a zygapophysis or articular process of a vertebra.

Illustration Credits

COLOR PLATES

Color Plate 1. Reprinted with permission from Rassner G. Atlas of Dermatology. 3rd ed. Philadelphia: Lea & Febiger, 1994:228.

Color Plate 2. Reprinted with permission from Rassner G. Atlas of Dermatology. 3rd ed. Philadelphia: Lea & Febiger, 1994:228.

Color Plate 3. Reprinted with permission from Rassner G. Atlas of Dermatology. 3rd ed. Philadelphia: Lea & Febiger, 1994:51.

Color Plate 4. Reprinted with permission from Willis MC. Medical Terminology: The Language of Health Care. 1st ed. Baltimore: Williams & Wilkins, 1996:100. Courtesy of Laurence J. and Richard D. Underwood, Mission Viejo, CA.

Color Plate 5. Reprinted with permission from Rassner G. Atlas of Dermatology. 3rd ed. Philadelphia: Lea & Febiger, 1994:65.

Color Plate 6. Reprinted with permission from Rassner G. Atlas of Dermatology. 3rd ed. Philadelphia: Lea & Febiger, 1994:42.

Color Plate 7. Reprinted with permission from Rassner G. Atlas of Dermatology. 3rd ed. Philadelphia: Lea & Febiger, 1994:49.

Color Plate 8. Reprinted with permission from Rassner G. Atlas of Dermatology. 3rd ed. Philadelphia: Lea & Febiger, 1994:46.

Color Plate 9. Reprinted with permission from Rassner G. Atlas of Dermatology. 3rd ed. Philadelphia: Lea & Febiger, 1994:47.

Color Plate 10. Reprinted with permission from Rassner G. Atlas of Dermatology. 3rd ed. Philadelphia: Lea & Febiger, 1994:241.

Color Plate 11. Reprinted with permission from Rassner G. Atlas of Dermatology. 3rd ed. Philadelphia: Lea & Febiger, 1994:101.

Color Plate 12. Reprinted with permission from Rassner G. Atlas of Dermatology. 3rd ed. Philadelphia: Lea & Febiger, 1994:95.

Color Plate 13. Reprinted with permission from Willis MC. Medical Terminology: The Language of Health Care. 1st ed. Baltimore: Williams & Wilkins, 1996:A5. Courtesy of American Academy of Dermatology, Schamburg, IL.

Color Plate 14. Reprinted with permission from Rassner G. Atlas of Dermatology. 3rd ed. Philadelphia: Lea & Febiger, 1994:196.

Color Plate 15. Reprinted with permission from Rassner G. Atlas of Dermatology. 3rd ed. Philadelphia: Lea & Febiger, 1994:29.

Color Plate 16. Reprinted with permission from Rassner G. Atlas of Dermatology. 3rd ed. Philadelphia: Lea & Febiger, 1994:173.

Color Plate 17. Reprinted with permission from Rassner G. Atlas of Dermatology. 3rd ed. Philadelphia: Lea & Febiger, 1994:169.

Color Plate 18. Reprinted with permission from Rassner G. Atlas of Dermatology. 3rd ed. Philadelphia: Lea & Febiger, 1994:170.

Color Plate 19. Reprinted with permission from Rassner G. Atlas of Dermatology. 3rd ed. Philadelphia: Lea & Febiger, 1994:171.

Color Plate 20. Reprinted with permission from Rassner G. Atlas of Dermatology. 3rd ed. Philadelphia: Lea & Febiger, 1994:176.

Color Plate 21. Reprinted with permission from Rassner G. Atlas of Dermatology. 3rd ed. Philadelphia: Lea & Febiger, 1994:319.

Color Plate 22. Reprinted with permission from Rassner G. Atlas of Dermatology. 3rd ed. Philadelphia: Lea & Febiger, 1994:207.

Color Plate 23. Reprinted with permission from Judd RL, Ponsell PP. Mosby's First Responder. 2nd ed. St. Louis: Mosby-Year Book, Inc., 1988.

Color Plate 24. Reprinted with permission from Rassner G. Atlas of Dermatology. 3rd ed. Philadelphia: Lea & Febiger, 1994:82.

Color Plate 25. Reprinted with permission from Judd RL, Ponsell PP. Mosby's First Responder. 2nd ed. St. Louis: Mosby-Year Book, Inc., 1988.

Color Plate 26. Reprinted with permission from Willis MC. Medical Terminology: The Language of Health Care. 1st ed. Baltimore: Williams & Wilkins, 1996:A5.

Color Plate 27. Reprinted with permission from Rassner G. Atlas of Dermatology. 3rd ed. Philadelphia: Lea & Febiger, 1994:25.

Color Plate 28. Reprinted with permission from Rassner G. Atlas of Dermatology. 3rd ed. Philadelphia: Lea & Febiger, 1994:44.

Color Plate 29. Reprinted with permission from Rassner G. Atlas of Dermatology. 3rd ed. Philadelphia: Lea & Febiger, 1994:271.

Color Plate 30. Reprinted with permission from Rassner G. Atlas of Dermatology. 3rd ed. Philadelphia: Lea & Febiger, 1994:302.

Color Plate 31. Reprinted with permission from Wallace DJ, Hahn BH. Dubois' Lupus Erythematosus. 5th ed. Baltimore: Williams & Wilkins, 1997:Plate 3.

CHAPTER 1

Figure 1.1. Reprinted with permission from Willis MC. Medical Terminology: The Language of Health Care. 1st ed. Baltimore: Williams & Wilkins, 1996:90.

Figure 1.2. Reprinted with permission from Rassner G. Atlas of Dermatology. 3rd ed. Philadelphia: Lea & Febiger, 1994:228.

Figure 1.3. Reprinted with permission from Rassner G. Atlas of Dermatology. 3rd ed. Philadelphia: Lea & Febiger, 1994:228.

Figure 1.4. Reprinted with permission from Rassner G. Atlas of Dermatology. 3rd ed. Philadelphia: Lea & Febiger, 1994:51.

Figure 1.5. Reprinted with permission from Willis MC. Medical Terminology: The Language of Health Care. 1st ed. Baltimore: Williams & Wilkins, 1996:100. Courtesy of Laurence J. and Richard D. Underwood, Mission Viejo, CA.

Figure 1.6. Reprinted with permission from Rassner G. Atlas of Dermatology. 3rd ed. Philadelphia: Lea & Febiger, 1994:65.

Figure 1.7. Reprinted with permission from Rassner G. Atlas of Dermatology. 3rd ed. Philadelphia: Lea & Febiger, 1994:42.

Figure 1.8. Reprinted with permission from Rassner G. Atlas of Dermatology. 3rd ed. Philadelphia: Lea & Febiger, 1994:49.

Figure 1.9. Reprinted with permission from Zitelli BJ, Davis HW. Atlas of Pediatric Physical Diagnosis. 3rd ed. St. Louis: Mosby-Year Book, Inc., 1997.

Figure 1.10. Reprinted with permission from Willis MC. Medical Terminology: The Language of Health Care. 1st ed. Baltimore: Williams & Wilkins, 1996:100.

Figure 1.11. Reprinted with permission from Willis MC. Medical Terminology: The Language of Health Care. 1st ed. Baltimore: Williams & Wilkins, 1996:100.

Figure 1.12. Reprinted with permission from Rassner G. Atlas of Dermatology. 3rd ed. Philadelphia: Lea & Febiger, 1994:46.

Figure 1.13. Reprinted with permission from Rassner G. Atlas of Dermatology. 3rd ed. Philadelphia: Lea & Febiger, 1994:47.

Figure 1.14. Reprinted with permission from Rassner G. Atlas of Dermatology. 3rd ed. Philadelphia: Lea & Febiger, 1994:241.

Figure 1.15. Reprinted with permission from Rassner G. Atlas of Dermatology. 3rd ed. Philadelphia: Lea & Febiger, 1994:101.

Figure 1.16. Reprinted with permission from Rassner G. Atlas of Dermatology. 3rd ed. Philadelphia: Lea & Febiger, 1994:95.

Figure 1.17. Reprinted with permission from Willis MC. Medical Terminology: The Language of Health Care. 1st ed. Baltimore: Williams & Wilkins, 1996:A5. Courtesy of American Academy of Dermatology, Schamburg, IL.

Figure 1.18. Reprinted with permission from Rassner G. Atlas of Dermatology. 3rd ed. Philadelphia: Lea & Febiger, 1994:196.

Figure 1.19. Reprinted with permission from Rassner G. Atlas of Dermatology. 3rd ed. Philadelphia: Lea & Febiger, 1994:29.

Figure 1.20. Reprinted with permission from Rassner G. Atlas of Dermatology. 3rd ed. Philadelphia: Lea & Febiger, 1994:173.

Figure 1.21. Reprinted with permission from Rassner G. Atlas of Dermatology. 3rd ed. Philadelphia: Lea & Febiger, 1994:169.

Figure 1.22. Reprinted with permission from Rassner G. Atlas of Dermatology. 3rd ed. Philadelphia: Lea & Febiger, 1994:170.

Figure 1.23. Reprinted with permission from Rassner G. Atlas of Dermatology. 3rd ed. Philadelphia: Lea & Febiger, 1994:171.

Figure 1.24. Reprinted with permission from Rassner G. Atlas of Dermatology. 3rd ed. Philadelphia: Lea & Febiger, 1994:176.

Figure 1.25. Reprinted with permission from Rassner G. Atlas of Dermatology. 3rd ed. Philadelphia: Lea & Febiger, 1994:319.

Figure 1.26. Reprinted with permission from Rassner G. Atlas of Dermatology. 3rd ed. Philadelphia: Lea & Febiger, 1994:207.

Figure 1.27. Reprinted with permission from Judd RL, Ponsell PP. Mosby's First Responder. 2nd ed. St. Louis: Mosby-Year Book, Inc., 1988.

Figure 1.28. Reprinted with permission from Rassner G. Atlas of Dermatology. 3rd ed. Philadelphia: Lea & Febiger, 1994:82.

Figure 1.29. Reprinted with permission from Judd RL, Ponsell PP. Mosby's First Responder. 2nd ed. St. Louis: Mosby-Year Book, Inc., 1988.

Figure 1.30. Reprinted with permission from Willis MC. Medical Terminology: The Language of Health Care. 1st ed. Baltimore: Williams & Wilkins, 1996:A5.

Figure 1.31. Reprinted with permission from Rassner G. Atlas of Dermatology. 3rd ed. Philadelphia: Lea & Febiger, 1994:25.

CHAPTER 2

Figure 2.1. Reprinted with permission from Travell JG, Simons DG. Myofascial Pain and Dysfunction: The Trigger Point Manual: Volume 1: The Upper Extremities. 1st ed. Baltimore: Williams & Wilkins, 1983:33.

Figure 2.3. Reprinted with permission from Wilkins EW Jr. MGH Textbook of Emergency Medicine. 1st ed. Baltimore: Williams & Wilkins, 1978:575.

Figure 2.4. Reprinted with permission from Travell JG, Simons DG. Trigger Point Pain Patterns: Wall Charts. 1st ed. Baltimore: Williams & Wilkins, 1996.

Figure 2.5. Reprinted with permission from Travell JG, Simons DG. Myofascial Pain and Dysfunction: The Trigger Point Manual: Volume 1: The Upper Extremities. 1st ed. Baltimore: Williams & Wilkins, 1983:60.

Figure 2.6. Reprinted with permission from Clemente CD. Anatomy: A Regional Atlas of the Human Body. 4th ed. Baltimore: Williams & Wilkins, 1997:Plate 349.

Figure 2.9. Reprinted with permission from Willis MC. Medical Terminology: The Language of Health Care. 1st ed. Baltimore: Williams & Wilkins, 1996:132.

Figure 2.10. Reprinted with permission from Edeiken J. Roentgen Diagnosis of Diseases of Bone, Volume 2. 3rd ed. Baltimore: Williams & Wilkins, 1981:841. Courtesy of Herbert M. Stauffer, Temple University Hospital, Philadelphia, PA.

Figure 2.11. Reprinted with permission from Edeiken J. Roentgen Diagnosis of Diseases of Bone, Volume 2. 3rd ed. Baltimore: Williams & Wilkins, 1981:975.

Figure 2.12. Reprinted with permission from Willis MC. Medical Terminology: The Language of Health Care. 1st ed. Baltimore: Williams & Wilkins, 1996: 135.

Figure 2.13. Reprinted with permission from Macnab I, McCulloch J. Neck Ache and Shoulder Pain. 1st ed. Baltimore: Williams & Wilkins, 1994:201.

Figure 2.14. Reprinted with permission from Baker CL. The Hughston Clinic Sports Medicine Book. 1st ed. Baltimore: Williams & Wilkins, 1995: 534.

Figure 2.15. Reprinted with permission from Baker CL. The Hughston Clinic Sports Medicine Book. 1st ed. Baltimore: Williams & Wilkins, 1995:365.

Figure 2.16. Reprinted with permission from Barker LR, Burton JR, Zieve PD. Principles of Ambulatory Medicine. 4th ed. Baltimore: Williams & Wilkins, 1995:935.

Figure 2.18. Reprinted with permission from Harris JH Jr, Harris, WH, Novelline RA. The Radiology of Emergency Medicine. 3rd ed. Baltimore: Williams & Wilkins, 1993:440, 467.

Figure 2.19. Reprinted with permission from Macnab I, McCulloch J. Neck Ache and Shoulder Pain. 1st ed. Baltimore: Williams & Wilkins, 1994:45.

Figure 2.20. Reprinted with permission from Macnab I, McCulloch J. Neck Ache and Shoulder Pain. 1st ed. Baltimore: Williams & Wilkins, 1994:45.

Figure 2.21. Reprinted with permission from Travell JG, Simons DG. Myofascial Pain and Dysfunction: The Trigger Point Manual: Volume 1: The Upper Extremities. 1st ed. Baltimore: Williams & Wilkins, 1983:175.

Figure 2.22. Reprinted with permission from Barker LR, Burton JR, Zieve PD. Principles of Ambulatory Medicine. 4th ed. Baltimore: Williams & Wilkins, 1995:946.

Figure 2.23. Reprinted with permission from Barker LR, Burton JR, Zieve PD. Principles of Ambulatory Medicine. 4th ed. Baltimore: Williams & Wilkins, 1995:946.

Figure 2.25. Reprinted with permission from Salter RD. Textbook of Disorders and Injuries of the Musculoskeletal System. 2nd ed. Baltimore: Williams & Wilkins, 1983:Figure 6.125.

Figure 2.26. Reprinted with permission from Basmajian JV. Primary Anatomy. 8th ed. Baltimore: Williams & Wilkins, 1982:Figure 6.46.

Figure 2.27. Reprinted with permission from Moore KL, Agur AMR. Essential Clinical Anatomy. 1st ed. Baltimore: Williams & Wilkins, 1995:326.

Figure 2.28. Reprinted with permission from Zitelli BJ, Davis HW. Atlas of Pediatric Physical Diagnosis. 3rd ed. St. Louis: Mosby-Year Book, Inc., 1997.

Figure 2.29. Reprinted with permission from Benninghoff/Goerttler, Lehrbuch der Anatomie des Menschen, edited by H. Ferer and J. Staubesand, Urban & Schwarzenberg. As seen in Clemente CD. Anatomy: A Regional Atlas of the Human Body. 3rd ed. Munchen, Germany: Urban & Schwarzenberg, 1987:Figure 506.

Figure 2.30. Reprinted with permission from Baker CL. The Hughston Clinic Sports Medicine Book. 1st ed. Baltimore: Williams & Wilkins, 1995:604.

Figure 2.31. Reprinted with permission from Clemente CD. Anatomy: A Regional Atlas of the Human Body. 4th ed. Baltimore: Williams & Wilkins, 1997:Plate 63.

Figure 2.32. Reprinted with permission from Moore, KL. Clinically Oriented Anatomy. 3rd ed. Baltimore: Williams & Wilkins, 1992:791.

Figure 2.33. Reprinted with permission from Foreman SM, Croft AC. Whiplash Injuries: The Cervical Acceleration/Deceleration Syndrome. 2nd ed. Baltimore: Williams & Wilkins, 1995:295.

Figure 2.34. Reprinted with permission from Clemente CD. Anatomy: A Regional Atlas of the Human Body. 4th ed. Baltimore: Williams & Wilkins, 1997:Plate 68.

Figure 2.35. Reprinted with permission from Macnab I, McCulloch J. Neck Ache and Shoulder Pain. 1st ed. Baltimore: Williams & Wilkins, 1994:459.

Figure 2.36. Reprinted with permission from Moore, KL. Clinically Oriented Anatomy. 3rd ed. Baltimore: Williams & Wilkins, 1992:327.

Figure 2.37. Reprinted with permission from Willis MC. Medical Terminology: The Language of Health Care. 1st ed. Baltimore: Williams & Wilkins, 1996: 133.

Figure 2.38. Reprinted with permission from Agur AMR. Grant's Atlas of Anatomy. 9th ed. Williams & Wilkins, 1991. As seen in Moore, KL. Clinically Oriented Anatomy. 3rd ed. Baltimore: Williams & Wilkins, 1992:418.

Figure 2.39. Reprinted with permission from Travell JG, Simons DG. Myofascial Pain and Dysfunction: The Trigger Point Manual: Volume 1: The Upper Extremities. 1st ed. Baltimore: Williams & Wilkins, 1983:604.

CHAPTER 3

Figure 3.3. Reprinted with permission from Okazaki H, Scheithauer BW. Atlas of neuropathology. 1st ed. London: Gower Medical Publishing, 1988. Copyright by Mayo Clinic, Rochester, Minnesota. By permission of the Mayo Foundation.

Figure 3.4. Reprinted with permission from Barclay L. Clinical Geriatric Neurology. 1st ed. Baltimore: Williams & Wilkins, 1993:156.

Figure 3.5. Reprinted with permission from Rassner G. Atlas of Dermatology. 3rd ed. Philadelphia: Lea & Febiger, 1994:44.

Figure 3.6. Reprinted with permission from Sobotta. Atlas der Anatomie des Menschen, edited by H. Ferner and J. Staubesand, Urban & Schwarzenberg. As seen in Clemente CD. Anatomy: A Regional Atlas of the Human Body. 3rd ed. Munchen, Germany: Urban & Schwarzenberg, 1987: Figures 404 and 406.

Figure 3.7. Reprinted with permission from Clemente CD. Anatomy: A Regional Atlas of the Human Body. 4th ed. Baltimore: Williams & Wilkins, 1997:Plate 463.

Figure 3.8. Reprinted with permission from Moore KL, Agur AMR. Essential Clinical Anatomy. 1st ed. Baltimore: Williams & Wilkins, 1995:353.

Figure 3.9. Reprinted with permission from Davis RL, Robertson, DM. Textbook of Neuropathology. 3rd ed. Baltimore: Williams & Wilkins, 1997:758.

Figure 3.10. Reprinted with permission from Benninghoff/Goerttler, Lehrbuch der Anatomie des Menschen, edited by H. Ferer and J. Staubesand, Urban & Schwarzenberg. As seen in Clemente CD. Anatomy: A Regional Atlas of the Human Body. 3rd ed. Munchen, Germany: Urban & Schwarzenberg, 1987:Figure 611.

CHAPTER 4

Figure 4.1. Reprinted with permission from Willis MC. Medical Terminology: The Language of Health Care. 1st ed. Baltimore: Williams & Wilkins, 1996:A16. White blood cells. Wintrobe's Clinical hematology. 9th ed. Philadelphia: Lea & Febiger, 1993.

Figure 4.2. Reprinted with permission from Willis MC. Medical Terminology: The Language of Health Care. 1st ed. Baltimore: Williams & Wilkins, 1996:162.

Figure 4.3. Reprinted with permission from Hart CA, Broadhead RL. Color Atlas of Pediatric Infectious Diseases. 1st ed. London: Mosby-Wolfe, 1992.

Figure 4.4. Reprinted with permission from Willis MC. Medical Terminology: The Language of Health Care. 1st ed. Baltimore: Williams & Wilkins, 1996:164.

Figure 4.6. Reprinted with permission from Willis MC. Medical Terminology: The Language of Health Care. 1st ed. Baltimore: Williams & Wilkins, 1996:165.

Figure 4.7. Reprinted with permission from Willis MC. Medical Terminology: The Language of Health Care. 1st ed. Baltimore: Williams & Wilkins, 1996:171.

Figure 4.8. Reprinted with permission from Rassner G. Atlas of Dermatology. 3rd ed. Philadelphia: Lea & Febiger, 1994:271.

Figure 4.9. Reprinted with permission from Willis MC. Medical Terminology: The Language of Health Care. 1st ed. Baltimore: Williams & Wilkins, 1996:173. From Sheldon H. Boyd's Introduction to the Study of Disease. 11th ed. Philadelphia: Lea & Febiger, 1992:90.

Figure 4.10. Reprinted with permission from Willis MC. Medical Terminology: The Language of Health Care. 1st ed. Baltimore: Williams & Wilkins, 1996:172.

Figure 4.11. Reprinted with permission from Rassner G. Atlas of Dermatology. 3rd ed. Philadelphia: Lea & Febiger, 1994:302.

CHAPTER 5

Figure 5.2. Reprinted with permission from Skarin AT. Atlas of Diagonstic Oncology. 2nd ed. London: Times Mirror International Publishers, 1996.

Figure 5.3. Reprinted with permission from Mindel A. AIDS: A Pocket Book of Diagnosis and Management. 1st ed. Baltimore: Urban & Schwarzenberg, 1990:116.

Figure 5.5. Reprinted with permission from Wallace DJ, Hahn BH. Dubois' Lupus Erythematosus. 5th ed. Baltimore: Williams & Wilkins, 1997:Plate 3.

CHAPTER 6

Figure 6.1. Reprinted with permission from Willis MC. Medical Terminology: The Language of Health Care. 1st ed. Baltimore: Williams & Wilkins, 1996:A18.

Figure 6.2. Reprinted with permission from Willis MC. Medical Terminology: The Language of Health Care. 1st ed. Baltimore: Williams & Wilkins, 1996:A18.

Figure 6.3. Reprinted with permission from Fletcher CDM, McKee PH. An Atlas of Gross Pathology. 1st ed. London: Gower Medical Publishing, 1987.

Figure 6.4. Reprinted with permission from Willis MC. Medical Terminology: The Language of Health Care. 1st ed. Baltimore: Williams & Wilkins, 1996:233.

Figure 6.6. Roche Lexikon Medizin, 3. Auflage, Urban & Schwarzenberg. Munich, Germany.

CHAPTER 7

Figure 7.2. Reprinted with permission from Fletcher CDM, McKee PH. An Atlas of Gross Pathology. 1st ed. London: Gower Medical Publishing, 1987.

Figure 7.4. Reprinted with permission from Willis MC. Medical Terminology: The Language of Health Care. 1st ed. Baltimore: Williams & Wilkins, 1996:374.

Figure 7.5. Reprinted with permission from Willis MC. Medical Terminology: The Language of Health Care. 1st ed. Baltimore:

Williams & Wilkins, 1996:371. From West J Med 1981;134:415.

Figure 7.6. Reprinted with permission from Willis MC. Medical Terminology: The Language of Health Care. 1st ed. Baltimore: Williams & Wilkins, 1996:377.

Figure 7.7. Reprinted with permission from Moore KL, Agur AMR. Essential Clinical Anatomy. 1st ed. Baltimore: Williams & Wilkins, 1995:97.

CHAPTER 8

Figure 8.1. Reprinted with permission from Willis MC. Medical Terminology: The Language of Health Care. 1st ed. Baltimore: Williams & Wilkins, 1996:407.

Figure 8.2. Reprinted with permission from Massry SG, Glassock R. Textbook of Nephrology, Volume 2. 1st ed. Baltimore: Williams & Wilkins, 1983:6.281.

CHAPTER 9

Figure 9.2. Reprinted with permission from Beckmann CRB. Obstetrics and Gynecology for Medical Students. 1st ed. Baltimore: Williams & Wilkins, 1992:306.

Figure 9.3. Reprinted with permission from Beckmann CRB. Obstetrics and Gynecology for Medical Students. 1st ed. Baltimore: Williams & Wilkins, 1992:398.

Figure 9.4. Reprinted with permission from Mitchell GW. The Female Breast and Its Disorders. 1st ed. Baltimore: Williams & Wilkins, 1990:140.

Figure 9.6. Reprinted with permission from Moore KL, Agur AMR. Essential Clinical Anatomy. 1st ed. Baltimore: Williams & Wilkins, 1995:163.

APPENDIX 1

Unfigure 1. Reprinted with permission from Travell JG, Simons DG. Myofascial Pain and Dysfunction: The Trigger Point Manual: Volume 1: The Upper Extremities. 1st ed. Baltimore: Williams & Wilkins, 1983:48.

Unfigure 2. Reprinted with permission from Travell JG, Simons DG. Myofascial Pain and Dysfunction: The Trigger Point Manual: Volume 1: The Upper Extremities. 1st ed. Baltimore: Williams & Wilkins, 1983:47.

Index

Page numbers in *italics* denote figures; those followed by a t denote tables.